AF848360

EXERCISE MANAGEMENT FOR REFERRED MEDICAL CONDITIONS

Exercise referral describes the process of consultation, planning and instructing physical activity programmes and applying appropriate behaviour change strategies for clients presenting a range of low- to medium-risk medical conditions. *Exercise Management for Referred Medical Conditions* is the first book to integrate exercise prescription with the development of healthy behaviours and the promotion of physical activity and well-being and provides students with an evidence-based, applied guide to becoming effective exercise referral practitioners.

The book draws upon the latest research and recommends best practices for creating referral pathways, providing exercise programmes and engaging clients in healthy lifestyles. Covering the pathology, medical management, role of exercise and recommendations for programming in each case, it discusses a range of conditions, including:

- Obesity and type I and II diabetes
- Hypertension and dyslipidaemia
- Asthma
- Low back pain, osteoarthritis and joint replacement, rheumatoid arthritis and osteoporosis
- Depression, anxiety and stress disorders

Consistently organised and laden with pedagogical features, including learning objectives, key terms, case studies, future developments and chapter summaries, no other book offers such a clear, holistic model for exercise referral. This is a vital resource for any student undertaking vocational courses in exercise referral and an important reference for exercise scientists, physical therapists, fitness professionals or local policy-makers interested in the use of physical activity in healthcare.

Andrew Scott is Senior Lecturer and Course Leader for the MSc Clinical Exercise Science programme in the School of Sport, Health and Exercise Science at the University of Portsmouth. He is a researcher, lecturer and practitioner in exercise and physical activity for people with long-term conditions to support their health and quality of life. His main interest is applying research to support education in clinical exercise for implementation in routine health-care practice.

David Broom is Professor of Physical Activity, Exercise and Health with over 20 years of experience working in health promotion and academia. Notable achievements include being an appointed member of the expert working group that updated the UK Chief Medical Officers Adult Physical Activity Guidelines published in 2019 and chair of BASES Division of Physical Activity for Health. He has recently submitted evidence to the Houses of Commons and House of Lords select committees regarding national plans for sport and recreation and the impact of major sporting and cultural events.

EXERCISE MANAGEMENT FOR REFERRED MEDICAL CONDITIONS

Edited by Andrew Scott and David Broom

Routledge
Taylor & Francis Group
LONDON AND NEW YORK

Cover image: Wavebreakmedia / Getty Images

First published 2022
by Routledge
4 Park Square, Milton Park, Abingdon, Oxon OX14 4RN

and by Routledge
605 Third Avenue, New York, NY 10158

Routledge is an imprint of the Taylor & Francis Group, an informa business

© 2022 selection and editorial matter, Andrew Scott and David Broom; individual chapters, the contributors

The right of Andrew Scott and David Broom to be identified as the authors of the editorial material, and of the authors for their individual chapters, has been asserted in accordance with sections 77 and 78 of the Copyright, Designs and Patents Act 1988.

All rights reserved. No part of this book may be reprinted or reproduced or utilised in any form or by any electronic, mechanical, or other means, now known or hereafter invented, including photocopying and recording, or in any information storage or retrieval system, without permission in writing from the publishers.

Trademark notice: Product or corporate names may be trademarks or registered trademarks, and are used only for identification and explanation without intent to infringe.

British Library Cataloguing-in-Publication Data
A catalogue record for this book is available from the British Library

Library of Congress Cataloging-in-Publication Data
A catalog record for this book has been requested

ISBN: 978-1-138-10399-3 (hbk)
ISBN: 978-1-138-10400-6 (pbk)
ISBN: 978-1-315-10239-9 (ebk)

DOI: 10.4324/9781315102399

Typeset in Bembo
by Apex CoVantage, LLC

CONTENTS

FIGURES

TABLES

BOXES

CONTRIBUTORS

Alberto Alves, PhD
University Institute of Maia, Maia, Portugal

Oluwaseun Anyiam, PhD
Derby Hospital, Derby, UK

Richard Bracken, PhD
Swansea University, UK

David Broom, PhD
Coventry University, UK

Benjamin J R Buckley, PhD
Liverpool John Moores University, UK

John P Buckley, PhD
University of Keele, Staffordshire, UK

Kate Button, PhD
Cardiff Metropolitan University, UK

Diane Crone, PhD
University of Gloucestershire, UK

Gill Crowther, PhD
Canterbury Christ Church University, UK

John Dickinson, PhD
School of Sport and Exercise Sciences, University of Kent, UK

Michael Eynon, PhD
St Mary's University, Twickenham, UK

Jason Feavers
Cancer Research UK, UK

Mary Finn, PhD
Adelaide and Meath Children's Hospital, Tallaght, Dublin, Ireland

James Fisher, PhD
Solent University, Southampton, UK

Zoë Franklin, PhD
Manchester Metropolitan University, UK

Bonnie Furzer, PhD
University of Western Australia, Australia

Paul Gorczynski, PhD
University of Portsmouth, UK

Paul Hendrick, PhD
University of Nottingham, UK

Joseph Henson, PhD
University of Leicester, UK

Louisa Herring, PhD
University Hospitals of Leicester NHS Trust

Charlotte Hilton, PhD
Director of Hilton Health Consultancy, UK

Lynne Johnston, PhD
South Tyneside and Sunderland NHS Foundation Trust, UK

Karen Knapp, PhD
University of Exeter, UK

Hopin Lee, PhD
Oxford University, UK

Steven Mann
Places for People and UKactive, UK

George Metsios, PhD
University of Thessaly, Greece

Hayley Mills, PhD
Canterbury Christ Church University, UK

Joseph M. Moore, PhD
University of Portsmouth, UK

Othmar Moser, PhD
University of Bayreuth and University of Graz, Austria

Becky Murphy, PhD
Liverpool John Moores University, UK

Emily Newton
Sheffield Hallam University, UK

Matthew Pearce
West Berkshire Council, UK

Nicola Pease, MB BCh, FRCP
Velindre NHS Trust, UK

Linda Pescatello, PhD
University of Connecticut, USA

Andy Pringle, PhD
University of Derby, UK

Suraj Rajput
Medway Community Healthcare, UK

Fernando Ribeiro, PhD
University of Aveiro, Aveiro, Portugal

Simon Rosenbaum, PhD
University of New South Wales, Australia

Zoe H Rutherford, PhD
The University of Queensland, Brisbane, Australia

Andrew Scott, PhD
University of Portsmouth, UK

Liba Sheeran, PhD
Cardiff Metropolitan University, UK

Antonis Stavropoulos-Kalinoglou, PhD
Leeds Beckett University, Leeds, UK

Victoria Stiles, PhD
University of Exeter, UK

Michelle G Swainson, PhD
Lancaster University, UK

Dave Thompson
Fairfield General Hospital, Bury, UK

Dane Vishnubala, PhD
University of Leeds, UK

Paula M Watson, PhD
Liverpool John Moores University, UK

Kemi Wright, PhD
University of New South Wales, Australia

Jeannie Wyatt-Williams
National Exercise Referral Scheme Manager for Wales, Welsh Local Government Association, UK

Jane Yardley, PhD
University of Alberta, Canada

Stephen Zwolinsky, PhD
West Yorkshire & Harrogate Cancer Alliance, UK

GLOSSARY

Activator protein one (AP-1) Transcription pathway involved in the development of rheumatoid arthritis.

Antipsychotics A class of psychotropic medication primarily used to manage psychosis, principally schizophrenia, and a range of other psychotic disorders.

Anxiety The body's natural response to stress; a feeling of fear or apprehension about what is to come.

Artificial pancreas A system consisting of a continuous glucose-sensing device and an insulin pump than can sense the interstitial glucose value and adjust the insulin pump rate to euglycaemic values based on glucose measurement.

Basal insulin Synthetic insulin usually taken once a day by injection.

Biological therapies/biologics Novel therapies under the family of DMARDs. They target specific molecules involved in the process of inflammation and tend to work rapidly.

Bolus insulin Synthetic insulin usually taken with food at mealtimes either with a pump or as an injection.

Bone mineral density (BMD) A surrogate measure of bone strength that quantifies the amount of mineralised tissue (bone mass) per unit area of bone (g/cm2) assessed by dual energy X-ray absorptiometry (DXA).

Brain-derived neurotrophic factor (BDNF) A nerve growth factor found in the brain and the periphery.

Cognitive behavioural therapy (CBT) Classification of psychotherapeutic approaches informed by cognitive and behavioural therapy in which individuals work alongside a therapist to explore their cognitive (thinking) and behavioural (actions) patterns, which may be contributing to their mental disorder or are preventing/impacting recovery.

COM-B model A model of behaviour change based on competency, opportunity and motivation.

Continuous glucose monitoring (CGM) A glucose-management strategy in which people with type 1 diabetes are tethered to an insulin pump, and insulin is automatically delivered in a more discreet, continuous fashion than injection; intermittently scanned glucose-monitoring (isCGM) systems or real-time (rtCGM) continuous-glucose monitoring devices for which a sensor is placed in the interstitium of the arm or abdomen and which display resultant glucose values via a reader or mobile phone application.

Continuous subcutaneous insulin infusion (CSII) A glucose-management strategy in which people with type 1 diabetes are tethered to an insulin pump, and insulin is automatically delivered in a more discreet, continuous fashion than injection.

Co-production The involvement of public service users in any of the design, management, delivery and/or evaluation of public services.

Counter-regulatory hormones Fight-or-flight hormones such as adrenaline, noradrenaline, cortisol and glucagon, which serve to increase hepatic glycogenolysis and release glucose into the circulation.

C-reactive protein (CRP) Acute-phase reactant that is commonly assessed in inflammatory conditions.

Depression A low mood that lasts for weeks or months and affects daily life.

Disease activity score 28 (DAS28) A common assessment of disease activity composed of the number of swollen and painful joints, a visual analogue scale for the perceived severity of the disease and an ESP or CRP value.

Disease-modifying anti-rheumatic drugs (DMARDs) A group of drugs including conventional DMARDs and biological therapies. They act by altering the underlying disease rather than treating symptoms. While they are not painkillers, they reduce pain, swelling and stiffness and decelerate disease progression.

Downstream Interventions that focus on providing equitable access to care and services to those who need them (i.e. will target sub-populations).

DSM-5 *Diagnostic and Statistical Manual of Mental Disorders*, Fifth Edition

Effectiveness The extent to which an intervention achieves its intended effect in the usual real-world setting.

Efficacy The extent to which an intervention has the ability to bring about its intended effect under ideal circumstances.

Electroconvulsive therapy (ECT) A medical treatment whereby across a course of treatment, electrical currents are passed through the brain while the individual is under a general anaesthetic with the aim of inducing a seizure and stimulating regions of the brain.

Erythrocyte sedimentation rate (ESR) The rate at which erythrocytes (red blood cells) sediment within one hour. It is a measure of non-specific inflammation.

Euglycaemia Blood glucose concentrations between 4 and 10 mmol/L (> 70 to < 180 mg/dL).

Evaluation The systematic investigation of the merit, worth or significance of an object (Scriven, in Centres for Disease Control, 1999).

Exercise A subset of physical activity that is planned, structured and repetitive and has as a final or an intermediate objective the improvement or maintenance of physical fitness.

Exercise referral Interventions that seek to increase PA and involve:

- An assessment involving a primary care or allied health professional to determine that someone is sedentary or inactive
- A referral by a primary care or allied health professional to a PA specialist or service
- A personal assessment involving a PA specialist or service to determine what programme of PA to recommend for the patient's specific needs
- An opportunity to participate in a PA programme

Feeding and eating disorders A group of related conditions including anorexia, bulimia and binge eating.

Fragility fracture Also known as a low-trauma fracture or osteoporotic fracture, this typically occurs at the hip, wrist or spine (key fracture sites) as a result of falling from a standing height or lower.

Glycaemic index (GI) The blood glucose response to ingestion of a carbohydrate foodstuff. Carbohydrate-containing foods that quickly enter the circulation and swiftly raise blood glucose are termed high GI, whereas foods that contain low amounts of carbohydrates or slowly digested carbohydrates that enter the circulation gradually are called low GI.

Hard-to-reach groups Refers to people who are difficult to access and/or engage due to specific factors such as accommodation, age, ethnicity, gender, income, language, location and religion.

HbA1c The amount of glycosylated haemoglobin in the circulation, represented as a percentage value, or in mmol per mol. This value is a clinical marker of glycaemic control.

Health assessment questionnaire (HAQ) A commonly used questionnaire assessing the functional ability of the patients. It involves questions on everyday activities such as sitting and standing, opening doors and lifting cups and the ability of the person to perform them with or without any difficulty or aids.

Human leukocyte antigen (HLA) A gene complex located in chromosome 6, encoding MCH proteins.

Hyperglycaemia High blood glucose (> 10 mmol/L (180 mg/dL)).

Hypoglycaemia Low blood glucose (< 3.9 mmol/L (70 mg/dL)).

ICD International Classification of Disease.

Interleukins (IL) A groups of cytokines that were initially observed to be expressed by white blood cells, thus obtained the *-leukin* suffix. They are now recognised as modulating inflammation in various ways.

Intervention An effort or policy that attempts to improve mental and physical health on a population level.

Major histocompatibility complex (MCH) This plays a major part in acquired immunity. It is composed of a number of cell surface proteins responsible for the recognition of peptide fragments from pathogens with the aim of presenting them to the appropriate T-cells.

Mechanosensitivity The receptiveness of bone cells to respond to mechanical stimuli.

Mechanostat theory Similar to the role of a thermostat in temperature control, the mechanostat is a prevailing paradigm originally proposed by Frost in 1964 that describes the mechanism(s) that continually monitor the mechanical loading of bone (mechanical usage of bone from normal daily activities) relative to a minimum effective strain (set-point) in order to detect and direct mechanical signals into an appropriate bone mass response (e.g. increasing bone mass to regain homeostasis with prevailing mechanical usage of bone).

Mechanotransduction External mechanical stimuli are converted into a bone-remodelling response as a result of chemicals being released by bone cells.

Mental disorders Encompass a wide variety of signs, symptoms, experiences and disorders which are diagnosed by a medical professional and significantly interfere with an individual's cognitive, emotional or social abilities.

Mental health A state of well-being in which the individual realises his or her own abilities, can cope with the normal stresses of life, can work productively and is able to make a contribution to his or her community.

Mental health crisis When a person requires urgent help due to feeling extremely anxious and having panic attacks or flashbacks, feeling suicidal or self-harming.

Mental health disorders Disorders that affect a person's mood, thinking and behaviour, including depression, anxiety disorders, schizophrenia, eating disorders and addictive behaviours.

Mental illness A disorder that affect a person's mood, thinking and behaviour, including depression, anxiety disorders, schizophrenia, eating disorders and addictive behaviours.

Moderate-impact activity Moderate-impact weight-bearing activity in which both feet leave the floor for a brief period of time and yield impact forces > 2 BW upon landing is the target intensity to promote bone health in those living with osteoporosis who are not at risk from falling and do not have vertebral fractures. Example activities include running, rope-jumping, low jumps, Highland-type dancing, dynamic side steps and hops. Certain group exercise classes (e.g. Zumba) that include a mixture of these activities together with racquet sports, track athletics, team sports/ball games and martial arts that include foot stamping are all accepted ways to experience moderate-impact activities.

Moving Medicine An interactive, evidence-based, web-based tool to support brief advice in PA across a range of diseases and conditions. The intervention includes a series of modules linked to a range of conditions on which PA can have an impact. It offers health-care professionals a number of strategies, time-bound consultations, promotional materials and resources to assist patients through the process of being more physically active.

Multiple-dose insulin injections (MDII) A glucose-management strategy in which people with type 1 diabetes take a number of daily insulin injections consisting of long- and short-acting insulins.

National Institute for Health and Care Excellence (NICE) Their role is to improve outcomes for people using the NHS and other public health and social care services.

National Institute for Health Research (NIHR).

Non-steroidal anti-inflammatory drugs (NSAIDs) Drugs aimed at reducing inflammation and, as a result, pain, swelling and general discomfort. They do not stop disease progression, however.

Nuclear factor kappa beta (NF-κB) A group of transcription factors induced by a variety of cytokines. It controls a wide range of genes involved in various immune and inflammatory processes.

One repetition max (1RM) The maximum amount of weight someone can lift in one repetition.

Osteoblasts Effector cells responsible for the synthesis and mineralisation of new bone (bone formation) within the cavity created by bone resorption.

Osteoclasts Effector cells responsible for the resorption of old, damaged or excess bone.

Osteopenia Low bone mass defined as a BMD between 1.0 and 2.5 SD below the mean of sex-matched young adults (WHO, 2004).

Osteoporosis A progressive skeletal disease characterised by low bone mass, deterioration of the bone's microarchitecture and an increased susceptibility to fragility (low-trauma) fracture. A diagnosis of osteoporosis is made in individuals who have a BMD of more than 2.5 SD below the mean value for sex- and ethnicity-matched young adults (WHO, 2004).

Participatory research An approach in which those being researched are involved in decisions in the research process.

Physical activity Any bodily movement produced by skeletal muscles that results in increased energy expenditure.

Positive cardiometabolic health An intervention framework for people experiencing psychosis and schizophrenia.

Post-traumatic stress disorder (PTSD) Trauma- and stressor-related mental health disorders can develop following exposure to a potentially life-threatening or traumatic event and are highly prevalent among those exposed to occupational trauma, including emergency service workers (e.g. police, fire, ambulance) and veterans.

Pre-activity readiness questionnaire (PAR-Q) A simple screening tool that can and should be used by anyone who is planning to start an exercise program to assess potential risk.

Premier League Men's Health Programme A national intervention of men's health improvement delivered through 16 English Premier League football clubs.

Progressive resistance training (PRT) A strength-training protocol in which weight equivalent to 80% of 1RM is lifted 12 reps/set × three sets and, as muscle strength increases over time, to create a new progressive overloading stimulus, a heavier weight representing a new intensity at 80% 1RM is lifted for fewer reps (e.g. 8 or 10).

Quality-adjusted life years (QALY) One quality-adjusted life year (QALY) is equal to one year of life in perfect health. QALYs are calculated by estimating the years of life remaining for a patient following a particular treatment or intervention and weighting each year with a quality-of-life score (on a 0 to 1 scale).

Rheumatoid arthritis (RA) A chronic autoimmune inflammatory condition that affects the joints but has several systemic manifestations as well.

Rheumatoid cachexia Altered body composition characterised by reduced muscle mass at the presence of stable or even slightly increased body weight. This indicates an increase in fat mass to compensate for muscle mass losses.

Stakeholder A person with an interest in or concern for something, especially a business.

Strain A measure of a material's change in shape (deformation) in response to an applied load, which is calculated by the amount of deformation divided by the initial (reference) length of the material.

Substance use disorders (SUDs) Mental health disorder that occurs in cases when substance use becomes habitual, resulting in a cluster of cognitive, behavioural and physiological symptoms, with the diagnosis of SUD based on evidence of impaired control, social impairment, risky use and pharmacological criteria.

Tumour necrosis factor alpha (TNFα) A cell-signalling protein, released as an acute phase reactant that modulates acute inflammation.

Type 1 diabetes A condition defined by an absolute or relative lack of insulin due to autoimmune destruction of the insulin-secreting β-cells within the pancreas.

Underserved groups Groups identified as not having their health and physical needs met by mainstream health and physical activity services.

Upstream Interventions and strategies that focus on improving fundamental social and economic structures (i.e. will target everyone).

Weight-bearing activity The weight of the body (load) is supported typically through the feet and legs during movement (activity), which creates additional load and levels of 'impact' that can vary, depending on the type and speed of movement performed.

World Health Organisation (WHO) A specialised agency of the United Nations responsible for international public health.

1

INTRODUCTION

Andrew Scott, Paul Gorczynski and David Broom

Chapter Aims

The aims of this chapter are to:

- Provide an introduction to the book
- Provide the rationale of physical activity for public health guidance
- Introduce the concept of exercise referral schemes
- Introduce the role of the exercise referral practitioner and its international counterparts
- Provide guidance on the layout of the chapters and how to use them
- Provide an online resources section for further training

Introduction

The aim of this chapter is to introduce the reader to the field of exercise referral, with the aim of supporting the development of the reader into an exercise referral practitioner and for the book to be used as an occupation-long resource. The book is written largely from the UK context but can be applied to any setting where the health and fitness sectors might work within a similar space. The book has been written in a style to provide contemporary information on exercise for health conditions where evidence suggests that exercise might prove beneficial for supporting the management of these conditions and contributing to enhanced quality of life. There is, therefore, a practitioner focus to the chapters, rather than solely reporting data from laboratory studies, and, importantly, there are four chapters that are focused on the soft skills of engaging sedentary individuals in becoming more physically active using evidence-based research and the professional experiences of the authors.

Physical Activity for Public Health

Physical activity is essential for the promotion of good health, including improving both physical and mental health; physical activity has also been shown to improve social health, or the way we stay connected with others (Kokkinos, 2012; Lee et al., 2012; McKinney et al., 2016;

DOI: 10.4324/9781315102399-1

Warburton et al., 2006). Many rigorous studies from all around the world, examining diverse populations, have consistently shown that regularly engaging in physical activity is, quite simply, good for us. Yet despite this consistent evidence of physical activity benefits and the pleas of public health researchers and practitioners, many people remain inactive and do not achieve weekly recommended amounts of physical activity (NHS Digital, 2020). There are a lot of complex individual and environmental determinants as to why people do not engage in regular physical activity. The better our understanding of individuals and their social contexts, the more likely that behaviour change interventions, like exercise referral schemes (ERS), can be employed to successfully help people become active and ultimately improve their health.

Physical Activity Guidelines

For adults between the ages of 19 and 64 years, the United Kingdom Physical Activity Guidelines UK Chief Medical Officers recommend that to achieve good health, individuals should aim to be active on a daily basis (Department of Health and Social Care, 2019). Specifically, over the course of one week, individuals should accumulate 150 minutes of moderate-intensity physical activity. Activities of moderate intensity have an energy cost of three to six metabolic equivalents (METs), which often produces a noticeable increase in heart rate, respiration rate and perspiration. Examples of moderate-intensity physical activity includes brisk walking, gardening and housework (Ainsworth et al., 2011). Alternatively, individuals may also reach recommended levels of aerobic activity by accumulating 75 minutes of vigorous-intensity activity. Vigorous-intensity activities have an energy cost of greater than six METs and require large amounts of effort, which causes rapid breathing and a substantial increase in heart rate. Examples of vigorous-intensity activities include running, fast cycling, aerobics, fast swimming and heavy shovelling (World Health Organization [WHO], 2010). In addition to aerobic activity, individuals should perform strength-training exercises at least two days per week. Strength training should be done using one's own body weight or some form of resistance and involve all major muscle groups. Some examples of strength training include exercise with weights, calisthenics and simply carrying or moving heavy objects like boxes or groceries. Lastly, the physical activity guidelines suggest individuals minimise time spent being sedentary. This includes time spent sitting and watching television, reading or using the computer. It is recommended that individuals break up sedentary time by taking regular activity breaks or, when possible, substitute sedentary activities with more active options, such as undertaking active travel such as walking or cycling instead of driving.

Exercise Referral Schemes

Given that many individuals in the UK are not aware of current physical activity guidelines and don't meet recommended levels of moderate- to vigorous-intensity physical activity (MVPA), ERS were implemented by the National Institute for Health and Care Excellence (NICE) to help individuals, especially those who were inactive and had existing health conditions or other factors that increased their risk of ill health, to become active (NICE, 2014). An exercise referral scheme consists of the following components:

- An assessment by a primary care or allied health-care professional to determine that an individual is sedentary or inactive and not meeting the physical activity guidelines

- A referral by a primary care or allied health-care professional to see a physical activity specialist or service
- An assessment by a physical activity specialist or service to determine the best physical activity programme to meet the needs of the individual
- The opportunity to participate in a physical activity programme

Physical activity may be differentiated from exercise, and often an ERS may be referred to as a physical activity referral scheme (PARS) to reflect the emphasis on encouraging not only supervised/structured exercise in a leisure-centre setting but also self-directed everyday activities which may be better integrated into an individual's daily routines (e.g. active modes of transport). A common understanding of physical activity is that it refers to any movement of the body that results in energy expenditure above that of resting level (Caspersen et al., 1985). For the purpose of this chapter, it is acknowledged that exercise refers to a component of PA that is more structured and purposefully undertaken (e.g. gym attendance, jogging or attending an exercise class), though the reader is directed to Winter and Fowler (2009) for wider discussion on the definition of exercise.

The NICE guidelines state that physical activity programmes should be designed on established behaviour change models and theories and be evidenced based (NICE, 2014). These ERS follow a developed framework and usually take place in public leisure centres (Department of Health (DOH), 2001; Williams et al., 2007). They are reportedly cost effective for individuals with multiple disease risk factors, including obesity (NICE, 2014). The aim of exercise referral schemes is to improve health through physical activity (NICE, 2014). Typically, a programme of physical activity is provided for 10 to 12 weeks and may be subsidised or free of charge; however, this varies nationwide. The programme involves an initial assessment and programme development followed by monitoring and supervision throughout (Williams et al., 2007). A systematic review by Pavey et al. (2012) examined uptake and adherence to ERS, reporting a wide range for both uptake (28–100%) and adherence (12–93%). When looking at adherence to completing the referral period across study types, the pooled mean was 43% (observational studies) versus 49% (randomised controlled trials [RCT]) (Pavey et al., 2012).

Following NICE guidance that ERS were not as effective as they could be, recent research has been performed to characterise and evaluate ERS more thoroughly (NICE, 2014). In a survey of 30 ERS in England, with a combined total of 85,259 exercise referral scheme participants, schemes were typically 12 weeks in length, offering participants two exercise sessions in a fitness gym or studio per week using a combination of exercises, with adherence typically being measured through attendance (Rowley et al., 2021). There were often variations in programme delivery, non-exercise components and programme management methods. In a study of four ERS services in Scotland, the exercise referral practitioners prescribed exercise to improve activities of daily living and promote independence and autonomy of participants, rather than explicitly targeting the referral condition (Shore et al., 2021a). This is not surprising since the aims of ERS are to enhance physical activity behaviours of participants from low active to at least moderately active, which is associated with the largest improvement in health and well-being if maintained according to public health guidelines. However, whilst over-medicalising the exercise approach may not be as conducive to behaviour change as we would think, having an understanding of the reasons for the referral can help inform targeted exercise prescriptions that might bring about improved biofeedback to support PA behaviour change and perhaps enhance public health on a larger scale.

Systematic review evidence suggests that longer-length schemes of more than 20 weeks improve adherence to the prescribed physical activity, resulting in improved health outcomes compared to 8- to 12-week schemes for people with cardiovascular, mental health and musculoskeletal disorders (Rowley et al., 2018). The review also found that schemes tend not to tailor services to suit the participants' health conditions, which does not fit with consumers' needs or support self-determined physical activity choices, potentially reducing adherence and improvement in quality of life. A review of studies reporting the uptake, attendance, prescribed exercises and adherence to ERS found that the reporting of these key performance indicators was insufficient (Shore et al., 2019). This information is important to indicate the populations that may benefit from engaging in an ERS but who do not, the populations that engage in particular types of ERS activities and those who do not and which ERS components are associated with enhanced adherence. Such data might be used locally within a scheme but also as part of the national ERS database. A study of uptake, attendance and session count in an ERS in Scotland reported that in this scheme, there were no sociodemographic differences between attenders and non-attenders, yet there was a 68% exit rate at five sessions or fewer (Shore et al., 2021b). This is significant since health benefits can only be attained by adhering to the exercise prescription. This is not to say that the participants had not begun to self-manage their PA away from the leisure-based ERS. In an analysis of a national ERS database, the majority of people referred were already in the moderately active category yet managed to increase their PA further by engaging in more vigorous-intensity PA as part of the ERS (Rowley et al., 2020). This suggests that people already in an action phase of PA behaviour change are making use of services and are reporting increased PA behaviour anyway but are still within the moderately active category. The indication in this study suggests an increased focus on supporting PA contemplators and preparers for PA to engage in ERS should be encouraged.

The Role of the Exercise Referral Practitioner

We refer to an ERS within the context of the structured exercise component of services that typically requires fitness professionals or exercise physiologists to be trained to work with clinical populations: e.g. as a Chartered Institute for the Management of Sport and Physical Activity (CIMSPA)–registered exercise referral practitioner or equivalent elsewhere in the world. The professional must be trained to develop and manage an ERS, perform consultations, apply and interpret initial and follow-up assessments, prescribe personalised exercise, apply personalised behaviour change techniques and goal setting and deliver exercise training activities for the particular population they are working with. In the context of this book, the long-term conditions considered are low to moderate risk, where exercise is recommended to manage or even ameliorate the client's referred condition(s) to prevent future significant disease or disability. Generally, people considered eligible for entry to an ERS are classified as physically inactive (i.e. not meeting physical activity guidelines) and presenting one or more of the long-term conditions in Table 1.1.

For this reason, the pathophysiology of these conditions, fitness assessment methods, exercise prescription adaptations and exercise leadership guidance are provided in this book to help guide current and future professionals in working with people with long-term conditions in the exercise referral setting.

TABLE 1.1 The health conditions included in ERS

Cardiovascular conditions	**Metabolic conditions**
Hypertension	*Obesity*
Hypercholesterolaemia	*Type 1 diabetes*
Respiratory conditions	*Type 2 diabetes*
Asthma	
Musculoskeletal conditions	**Mental health**
Osteopenia	*Stress*
Simple mechanical low back pain	*Anxiety*
Osteoarthritis	*Depression*
Rheumatoid arthritis	*Substance/alcohol misuse*
Joint replacement	

Graduate Exercise Referral Practitioners

It is possible for graduates to progress in the broad field of exercise referral with sufficient education and experience to be British Association of Sport and Exercise Sciences (BASES)–certified exercise practitioners or, with higher-level training, to become an accredited clinical exercise physiologist through the American College of Sports Medicine (ACSM), the Biokinetics Association of South Africa (BASA), Clinical Exercise Physiology UK (CEP-UK), the Canadian Society of Exercise Physiology (CSEP) or the Exercise and Sports Science Australia (ESSA), depending on where you reside and wish to practice. Further details of career progression as a clinical exercise physiologist are available in the resources section at the end of this chapter, and an example of developing a career as an exercise referral practitioner or a clinical exercise physiologist is illustrated in Box 1.1.

BOX 1.1 STUDENT GRADUATING FROM UNIVERSITY WITH AN EXERCISE REFERRAL AWARD

Jonathan graduated from New University with a 2.1 class BSc in Sport and Exercise and was hopeful that prospective employers would recognise his hard work to achieve this. He wanted to be a specialist exercise instructor.

Jonathan developed his interest in promoting physical activity for health through his varied taught modules in exercise science but particularly developed his personal and technical skills by studying a series of vocational awards alongside his degree, including gym instructor, personal trainer and exercise referral certifications. He was able to make use of these qualifications to gain paid experience in a local sport and leisure facility. With sufficient experience, he was able to gain experience in the centre's exercise referral scheme and utilise this experience in his degree's professional development module.

Immediately following graduation, he began working professionally as an exercise referral specialist at the fitness centre where he gained his work experience during his studies, based on the good impression he had made and his qualifications. He was soon enrolled on specialist exercise instructor courses, such as cardiac rehabilitation, since the service was becoming more popular with higher-risk clients. Within one year, he was a full-time employee and managing the scheme's referral pathway for high-risk medical conditions.

His employer is now paying for him to study an accredited MSc in clinical exercise physiology so that he can improve his research skills in order to fully evaluate their service provision and develop knowledge, skills and experience in working with people with higher risk health conditions as a clinical exercise physiologist.

Using This Book

The book should be read in its entirety to provide information about ERS and being an ER practitioner. The chapters have been compiled in such a way that they can be read as standalone chapters. This chapter and Chapters 2 and 3 provide the experiences of the chapter authors in developing an ERS (Chapter 2) and leading a national ERS (Chapter 3). Chapter 4 details best-practice methods for working with a referred person and applying relevant person-centred health-fitness assessments. Chapters 5 through 9 detail the often-neglected approach of engaging people to change their health-physical activity behaviour, particularly in the ERS setting. These include personalising the experience for the person through to supporting the maintenance of newly found physical activity behaviours following completion of a scheme. Finally, Chapters 10 through 20 cover condition-specific considerations to support you in your understanding of these conditions in the exercise setting. Each chapter relating to heath conditions (Chapters 10–20) contains the following sub-sections:

- Introduction to the condition
- Medication and medical management
- Effect of condition/treatment on the exercise response
- Effects of exercise training
- Exercise prescription principles
- Chapter summary and key points
- Study tasks

Pedagogic aids are provided to support your learning. Figures, tables and boxes are used to illustrate and consolidate information provided in the text. Case studies are provided in each chapter to illustrate the application of the principles communicated in the chapter to an exercise-referral example, and study tasks are presented to encourage you to think independently about each chapter. The references that are used provide additional relevant information, which you are also encouraged to read. Lastly, in each of the condition-specific chapters, we present a table illustrating the effect of common medications on the exercise response and a one-page at-a-glance guide to encapsulate each chapter for ease of reference in your practice.

We hope you enjoy reading the book and applying the information in your practice.

Resources

The following are professional training routes that you can undertake to work towards becoming an exercise specialist for people with health conditions:

- CIMSPA Exercise Referral Practitioner: https://www.cimspa.co.uk/membership/sport-and-physical-activity-practitioner/exercise-referral-practitioner-%E2%80%93-membership-entry-requirements

- BASES Certified Exercise Practitioner: www.bases.org.uk/sspage-professional_development-accreditation_and_endorsement-certified_exercise_practitioner__cep_.html
- Registered Clinical Exercise Physiologist with CEP-UK: www.clinicalexercisephysiology.org.uk/
- Accredited Exercise Physiologist with ESSA: www.essa.org.au/Public/Consumer_Information/What_is_an_Accredited_Exercise_Physiologist_.aspx
- Certified Clinical Exercise Physiologist:
- With ACSM: www.acsm.org/get-stay-certified/get-certified/cep
- With CSEP: https://csep.ca/csep-certification/csep-professional-standards-program-cep/
- Biokineticist with BASA: https://biokineticssa.org.za/biokineticist-info/#qualifications

References

Ainsworth, B., Haskell, W.L., Herrmann, S.D., Meckes, N., Bassett, D.R. Jr., Tudor-Locke, C., Greer, J.L., Vezina, J., Whitt-Glover, M.C., & Leon, A.S. (2011). 2011 Compendium of physical activities: A second update of codes and MET values. *Medicine and Science in Sports and Exercise*, 43(8), 1575–1581.

Caspersen, C.J. Powell, K.E., & Christenson, G.M. (1985). Physical activity, exercise, and physical fitness: Definitions and distinctions for health-related research. *Public Health Reports*, 100(2), 126–131.

Department of Health (DOH) (2001). *Exercise referral systems: A national quality assurance framework*. London: TSO.

Department of Health and Social Care (2019). *Physical activity guidelines: UK chief medical officers report*. London: TSO.

Kokkinos, P. (2012). Physical activity, health benefits, and mortality risk. *ISRN Cardiology*, 718789.

Lee, I-M., Shiroma, E.J., Lobelo, F., Puska, P., Blair, S.N., & Katzmarzyk, P.T. (2012). Effect of physical inactivity on major non-communicable diseases worldwide: An analysis of burden of disease and life expectancy. *The Lancet*, 380(9838), 219–229.

McKinney, J., Lithwick, D.J., Morrison, B.N., Nazzari, H., Isserow, S., Heilbron, B., & Krahn, A.D. (2016). The health benefits of physical activity and cardiorespiratory fitness. *British Columbia Medical Journal*, 58(3), 131–137.

National Institute for Health and Care Excellence (2014). *Physical activity: Exercise referral schemes*. London: TSO. Available at: www.nice.org.uk/guidance/ph54

NHS Digital (2020). *Statistics on obesity, physical activity and diet, England – 2020*. Available at: www.gov.uk/government/statistics/statistics-on-obesity-physical-activity-and-diet-england-2020-ns

Pavey, T.G., Taylor, A., Hillsdon, M., Fox, K., Campbell, J., Foster, C., Moxham, T., Mutrie, N., Searle, J., & Taylor, R. (2012). Levels and predictors of exercise referral scheme uptake and adherence: A systematic review. *Journal of Epidemiology and Community Health*, 66, 737–744.

Rowley, N., Mann, S., Steele, J., Horton, E., & Jimenez, A. (2018). The effects of exercise referral schemes in the United Kingdom in those with cardiovascular, mental health, and musculoskeletal disorders: A preliminary systematic review. *BMC Public Health*, 18(1), 949. doi: 10.1186/s12889-018-5868-9.

Rowley, N., Steele, J., Mann, S., Jimenez, A., & Horton, E. (2021). Delivery approaches within exercise referral schemes: A survey of current practice in England. *Journal of Physical Activity and Health*, 18(4), 357–373. doi: 10.1123/jpah.2020-0388.

Rowley, N., Steele, J., Wade, M., Copeland, R.J., Mann, S., Liguori, G., Horton, E., & Jimenez, A. (2020). Are exercise referral schemes associated with an increase in physical activity? Observational findings using individual patient data meta-analysis from the national referral database. *Journal of Physical Activity and Health*, 17(6), 621–631. doi: 10.1123/jpah.2019-0435.

Shore, C.B., Hubbard, G., Gorely, T., Hunter, A.M., & Galloway, S.D. (2021a). The match between what is prescribed and reasons for prescribing in exercise referral schemes: A mixed method study. *BMC Public Health*, 21(1), 1003. doi: 10.1186/s12889-021-11094-z.

Shore, C.B., Hubbard, G., Gorely, T., Hunter, A.M., & Galloway, S.D.R. (2021b). Associated sociodemographic and facility patterning of uptake, attendance, and session count within a Scottish exercise referral scheme. *Journal of Physical Activity and Health*, 18(5), 557–562. doi: 10.1123/jpah.2020-0539.

Shore, C.B., Hubbard, G., Gorely, T., Polson, R., Hunter, A., & Galloway, S.D. (2019). Insufficient reporting of factors associated with exercise referral scheme uptake, attendance, and adherence: A systematic review of reviews. *Journal of Physical Activity and Health*, 16(8), 667–676. doi: 10.1123/jpah.2018-0341.

Warburton, D., Nicol, C.W., & Bredin, S.S. (2006). Health benefits of physical activity: The evidence. *Canadian Medical Association Journal*, 174(6), 801–809.

Williams, N., Hendry, M., France, B., Lewis, R., & Wilkinson, C. (2007). Effectiveness of exercise-referral schemes to promote physical activity in adults: Systematic review. *British Journal of General Practice*, 57(545), 978–986.

Winter, E., & Fowler, N. (2009). Exercise defined and quantified according to the Systeme International d'Unites. *Journal of Sports Sciences*, 27, 447–460.

World Health Organization [WHO] (2010). *Global recommendations on physical activity for health*. Geneva: WHO Press.

2

CO-PRODUCTION IN EXERCISE REFERRAL SCHEMES

Benjamin J R Buckley, Paula M Watson, Becky Murphy, Matthew Pearce and Diane Crone

Chapter aims

The aims of this chapter are to:

- Highlight emerging challenges for exercise referral schemes
- Make a case for using co-production approaches
- State the importance of stakeholder perspectives in exercise referral settings
- Use case studies to provide pragmatic examples of how a real-world participatory approach was undertaken to co-produce an evidence-based exercise referral scheme

Introduction

The emerging challenge for exercise referral schemes

Exercise referral schemes (ERS) and physical activity referral schemes (PARS), sometimes referred to as exercise on prescription schemes, were first developed in the early 1990s. They involve the referral of a patient from primary care – for example, a general practitioner (physician), practice nurse etc. – following or during a period of poor health to a programme of exercise (Gidlow et al., 2005). They have been identified as a suitable means to promote exercise to improve health, in its broadest sense, for patient well-being as both treatment and preventative options in healthcare (Crone & James, 2016; Gidlow, Crone, & Huws-Thomas, 2016). These programmes continue to be thought of as the most prevalent type of physical activity intervention programme in the UK (Crone & James, 2016).

As the evidence underpinning the use of exercise as an adjunct to treatment in a range of medical conditions has developed, so, too, has the evidence underpinning the effectiveness of the exercise referral for health enhancement. However, despite the rise in prevalence of referral schemes and the range of evidence of their effectiveness for certain patient groups, there is still controversy over their worth for long-term behaviour change. (For a review, see Gidlow et al., 2016.)

DOI: 10.4324/9781315102399-2

Initially, ERS were set up as a relationship between a GP practice and the local leisure provider (Crone, Johnston, & Grant, 2004). However, as their prominence grew, the links and referral pathways between health referrers and physical activity providers became more sophisticated and integrated into existing patient referral pathways in healthcare. As that formal relationship developed, the various roles of the multiple stakeholders in those pathways were found to be an important influence on uptake, adherence and outcomes (Crone & James, 2016; James et al., 2008; James et al., 2009; Queen, Parker, & Crone, 2016).

Over the past 20 years since the development of the first exercise referral schemes, there has been substantial funding for their development and delivery across the UK, despite the controversy over their efficacy and effectiveness. It has become increasingly important for stakeholders to work together to deliver such schemes and co-produce them due to the various complex processes involved. Furthermore, as these programmes became formalised into health-care systems, the complex processes, including pathway development, referral mechanism, patient journey and evaluation framework, became increasingly more prominent. Similar to other contemporary public health challenges, researchers have been acknowledging for some time the inadequacy of some of the linear, more traditional approaches to evidence generation and recommending more complex evaluation frameworks that combine both process and outcome evaluation (Gidlow et al., 2008; Moore et al., 2015; Rutter et al., 2017). Alternative methods of evidence generation, such as co-production, that engage multiple stakeholder groups, are a 'contemporary' way forward for the next generation of exercise referral schemes in UK healthcare.

Making the case for co-production

What is it?

The importance of trans-disciplinary partnerships has long been recognised in public health (Roussos & Fawcett, 2000). There has been recent renewed interest in and advocacy for the adoption of co-production as a means of co-creating value across the public sector (Clarke et al., 2017). The concept was first coined in 1970 when social policy recognised the benefits of including end-users in the delivery of their own public services (Realpe & Wallace, 2016). Co-production therefore emphasises the importance of collaboration between service providers and service users. Since conceptualisation, various terminology has evolved, yet a recent definition appears to be popular within the medical and public health literature: 'the involvement of public service users in any of the design, management, delivery and/or evaluation of public services' (Osborne, Radnor, & Strokosch, 2016). In a health-care context, such participatory co-production methods should draw on stakeholder knowledge in addition to the available scientific evidence in both the design and, crucially, the delivery of services (Hunter & Ritchie, 2007; Batalden et al., 2016). Participatory research has been described as moving away from a 'them and us' mentality and involves actively engaging local stakeholders from all levels (end-users, practitioners and policy-makers), also termed a 'bottom-up' approach, alongside academics in the co-production of interventions (Bergold & Thomas, 2010). The key difference between participatory research and more traditional methodologies lies in the location of power (Cornwall & Jewkes, 1995). Adopting a co-production approach means stakeholder knowledge and scientific evidence are equally valued.

Why is it important? Efficacy, effectiveness and the translation of evidence to practice

A primary problem for the public health sector is a lack of successful implementation of research knowledge into community settings where it can have the most impact (Nutbeam, 1996; Brownson et al., 2006). Furthermore, it has been loosely accepted that when successful, the process of translation of evidence to clinical practice takes an estimated 17 years on average (Westfall, Mold, & Fagnan, 2007; Green et al., 2009). Though a crude estimate (Morris, Wooding, & Grant, 2011), it highlights a clear gap in the transition from research evidence to evidence-based practice. One emerging area of scrutiny is the inappropriate use of efficacy trials used to directly inform real-world practice. Efficacy, demonstrated in phase I–III trials, denotes 'the extent to which a drug has the ability to bring about its intended effect under ideal circumstances' (Hill, 2012, p. 2). In contrast, effectiveness demonstrated in phase IV trials denotes 'the extent to which a drug achieves its intended effect in the usual clinical setting' (Hill, 2012, p. 3). Replace *drug* with your intervention of choice (e.g. physical activity), and it becomes clear that effectiveness is what matters to commissioners and patients (Beedie et al., 2016).

Whilst efficacy studies (e.g. randomised controlled trials) represent the gold standard in the academic domain, these highly controlled environments lack ecological validity and provide little information about the challenges faced by policy-holders and practitioners when implementing interventions in real-world settings (Watson et al., 2013). Consequently, when lab-based interventions are implemented in practice, the true magnitude of effect (effectiveness) may be diminished. If sport and exercise medicine is to produce evidence that is of value to improving physical activity levels in clinical populations, alternative research methodologies are urgently needed (Beedie et al., 2016).

Participatory co-production research may be a tool to help bridge the gap between scientific evidence and clinical practice. Multi-stakeholder involvement provides important insights into the feasible implementation of interventions in the real world, in turn leading to interventions that are context sensitive, effective and sustainable within local infrastructures (Harden et al., 2016). A participatory research approach can facilitate knowledge translation and production, often described as action-orientated collaborative research. Knowledge translation is designed to fill the gap between what is known regarding evidence-based practice and actual implementation (Dent et al., 2016; Grimshaw et al., 2012). It is this balance of available evidence and pragmatic stakeholder knowledge that should be a target for public health initiatives adopting co-production.

Challenges and considerations

Co-production is a promising method for primary and secondary prevention services, yet it should not be viewed as a panacea. Associated challenges and limitations need to be carefully considered prior to its use. A collaborative approach, as previously discussed, involves multiple levels of engagement including researchers, policy-makers, managers, practitioners and service-users, all of whom should have an equal influence in the research process, regardless of their individual roles. Yet in practice, it is acknowledged this is easier said than done and therefore requires careful negotiation of group politics to enable productive discussions that result in meaningful actions (Rycroft-Malone et al., 2016). The involvement of such a diverse, multidisciplinary stakeholder group in the design, delivery and/or evaluation phase(s) is inevitably going to be a time-consuming process. It is therefore essential that commissioners have a realistic awareness of appropriate time frames from the beginning of the development phase. Finally, there may be times when a conceptual gap emerges between stakeholder-desired outcomes and researcher-desired outcomes. An important step is at the beginning of a co-production approach. Here, the goal should be to facilitate a consensus on an appropriate agenda and well-aligned outcome objectives among stakeholders. In the instance of disagreement, however, discussion of tensions and differences between stakeholders should be encouraged, and the involvement of the wider community should be viewed as a resource, not a threat (Hunter & Ritchie, 2007).

In order to support a collaborative environment, some level of leadership is required to bring multiple stakeholders and researchers together, at least in the first instance. Rycroft-Malone et al. (2016) highlighted several transferable qualities that facilitators of a collaborative and co-production process may find helpful. These included the ability to be generalistic, be tolerant of 'messiness', have diverse communication skills, be able to manage conflict and be adaptable whilst maintaining research rigor. The authors also noted that stakeholders need to be aware that expectations and constraints are often set by funders and thus have a direct impact on potential outcomes. The following four (simplified) steps highlight the skeleton of a co-production approach: 1) Identify and understand the problems (needs analysis), 2) co-produce ideas for change, 3) co-deliver the intervention or service and 4) co-evaluate the intervention or service (Needham & Carr, 2009).

The importance of stakeholder perspectives in exercise referral settings

There is a dearth of evidence that has examined the process of an exercise referral programme from the perspectives of all key stakeholders involved. Information obtained from key stakeholders with regard to their attitude towards the exercise referral service and the opinions of programme processes at an operation level may have implications for their involvement and subsequent improvement of the referral process. In addition, obtaining stakeholder opinions and working practices of the services to which they refer can be a valuable means of improving a service.

Qualitative methods have been used to understand a participant's overall experience of an ERS and, more specifically, factors that influence decisions to adopt and maintain exercise. The methods utilised have included focus groups (Wormald & Ingle, 2004; Crone, Smith, & Gough, 2005), interviews (Hardcastle & Taylor, 2001 and a combination of both (Crone et al., 2005; Stathi et al., 2003), with participants who are at different stages of the exercise referral process. A small number of studies have interviewed the same sample of participants as they have progressed through the exercise referral scheme (Crone et al., 2005; Hardcastle & Taylor, 2001).

Health professionals are the primary gatekeepers for clients entering the exercise referral process and, hence, play a pivotal role in current programme delivery. Advice from a health professional is an important factor in a participant's decision to adopt exercise (Graham, 2006). In this sense, an examination of the reasons why and the mechanisms of how health professionals refer participants to an ERS is essential to successful programme implementation

(Taylor, 2003). Information obtained, in terms of operation and programme processes, at the primary care level may have implications for health professional involvement and subsequent improvement of the referral process. Health professionals, attitudes, opinions and working practices with regard to their engagement in physical activity promotion and preventive activity have been examined in both UK (McKenna & Vernon, 2004; Moore, Moore, & Murphy, 2011, 2012) and non-UK populations (Anis et al., 2004). There is some evidence to suggest that UK health professionals have a positive attitude towards disease prevention (McAvoy et al., 1999), but they also have reservations about their own personal involvement in such practices (Graham, Dugdill, & Cable, 2005).

A range of barriers inhibit health professionals' willingness to provide lifestyle advice to patients. These include lack of time (McKenna & Vernon, 2004), lack of confidence in the efficacy of health promotion in general practice, a perceived limited ability to modify patients' lifestyles (McKenna & Vernon, 2004), lack of confidence in counselling skills, a perceived lack of patient motivation towards health behaviour change (McAvoy et al., 1999; Moore et al., 2011), insufficient education with regards to exercise at medical school (Kennedy & Meeuwisse, 2003) and concerns that patients will suffer a myocardial infarction or cardiac arrest during the advised programme of activity (Morey & Sullivan, 2003).

Exercise professionals undertake a multifaceted role in exercise referral scheme operation (Department of Health (DoH), 2001). The integral role of the exercise professionals to the operation of ERS mean that the skills and abilities that they exhibit and their relationships with other stakeholders may be vital to programme success (Graham, 2006). Despite this, limited literature has explored exercise professionals' perspectives on the exercise referral process or their perspectives on communication/operational processes associated with such schemes.

The success of an ERS depends on the characteristics of the key personnel involved and maintenance of communication between key organisations and professionals (Riddoch, Puig-Ribera, & Cooper, 1998). The National Quality Assurance Framework for exercise referral systems (Department of Health (DoH), 2001) suggests that an adequate level of communication (amongst the various professionals involved) is a precursor to programme success. Further, Mills et al. (2012) found success to be a multidimensional concept in the context of exercise referral. Traditional markers of success (such as attendance/adherence, weight loss and blood pressure) are commonly reported according to those commissioning, developing and evaluating referral schemes (McNair et al., 2005). However, in practice, ERS impact has been documented as a more holistic concept incorporating psychological and social components (Mills et al., 2012). Broadening the focus beyond physical outcomes to psychosocial factors associated with behaviour change has provided a better understanding of success (Abildso et al., 2010).

Stakeholder perspectives make an important contribution to health policy development and also health service intervention design (Henderson et al., 2017). Stakeholders of an ERS can vary, depending upon the delivery model adopted. Broadly speaking, key stakeholders involved in the practical implementation process include end users (i.e. participants/patients), health professionals (i.e. general practitioner or practice nurse) and exercise professionals (DoH, 2001). An additional key stakeholder is the professional or organisation responsible for commissioning the scheme and/or public health specialists with responsibility for the delivery of physical activity strategy.

Perspectives from a public health commissioner

Public sector commissioners are facing unprecedented challenges to improve health outcomes against a backdrop of an ageing population, complex illnesses and real-term reductions in health-care expenditure. Despite the strong economic argument for prevention, it is estimated that only 4% of the total health-care budget is spent on prevention, compared to 70% expended on treating long-term conditions (Butterfield, Henderson, & Scott, 2009). The need for high-quality, cost-effective services has never been greater. Despite the mixed evidence concerning the effectiveness of exercise on referral schemes, they remain a popular intervention amongst public sector commissioners (Pavey et al., 2011). This popularity likely derives from evidence that shows that schemes improve health outcomes for individuals with the early onset of disease or established chronic conditions (NICE, 2014). Whilst targeting individuals with existing medical needs can often be perceived as being 'downstream', the pressing need to save money across healthcare means that exercise on referral programmes have the potential to yield short-term financial benefits (PHE, 2016).

This pressure to demonstrate return on investment has led to greater scrutiny of investment in public services. Whilst the old saying that 'prevention is better than cure' continues to sound intuitively sensible, commissioners are increasingly having to make the case for prevention and identify where savings will be realised across local systems. The barriers for greater investment in public health have been well documented (Hemenway, 2010; Brownson, Chriqui, & Stamatakis, 2009). These include greater evidence of return on investment, the belief that overall prevention may cost more than treatment, the gestation period required for public health interventions to generate savings and the 'identifiable victim effect', whereby the public may prefer relieving the suffering of an individual to funding an intervention which does not address current ill health (Richardson, 2012).

Overcoming these challenges within a politically charged arena is not straightforward, but it has been suggested that there should be greater fairness in the assessment and resource allocation across populations which look at cost effectiveness rather than cost savings (Pinto et al., 2012). Quality-adjusted life years (QALY) are the common currency used to evaluate new and innovative health-care treatments; however, these are rarely used by commissioners in isolation to make investment decisions (Klein & Maybin, 2012). Commissioning intentions are often determined using multiple criteria such as local and nationally determined priorities, health needs, acceptability to patients and evidence of effectiveness.

As ERS continue to develop, they will need to collect more robust data to assess the overall impact on their local populations and strengthen the case for investment. In England, a major policy drive is the development of accountable care systems, for which collaborations are being formed consisting of health-care providers, local authorities and the voluntary sector. This shift toward greater integration and pooling of resources will provide new opportunities for areas to link datasets and assess the outcomes of individuals and populations across multiple organisations. Although this will enable areas to measure changes in health outcomes (e.g. weight, blood pressure, physical activity levels, mental well-being) and health service utilisation (e.g. reduction in A&E visits, unplanned admissions, reductions in demand for social care), it will also enable systems to look at broader social, economic and environment benefits, otherwise known as 'social value' (Health and Social Care Act, 2012). For example, ERS could measure the impact of increased physical activity on social capital or employment.

As the public sector embarks on unprecedented changes to services and the development of new 'local systems', commissioners will look for greater involvement of individuals and communities in the design, delivery and evaluation of services. Despite co-production being relatively new within commissioning circles, it is an attractive concept as it can mobilise individual and community assets that can then become effective agents of change (Boyle & Harris, 2009). Most importantly, it brings together the expertise of professionals with the lived experience of individuals, which can lead to services which are outcome focused and, in the long term, more sustainable. For ERS, this may potentially mean diversifying the physical activity offer away from the gym and delivering a range of opportunities across different settings, communities, and disease pathways. For example, dance for older adults, which reduces loneliness and maintains independence, and generic exercise programmes for individuals with multi-morbidity. In many areas, this is already happening, with the growing popularity of social prescribing leading to a greater recognition of utilising non-medical interventions to improve health and well-being (Bickerdike et al., 2017).

Despite the benefits associated with embedding co-production in public services, it is not without its challenges. For example, commissioners are often required to balance commissioning decisions against the needs and demands of individuals and communities alongside the existing supply of services or assets. By giving service users a voice in commissioning, there is a risk that what individuals 'demand' may be different from what they may 'need' or are able to benefit from. Commissioning that leans too heavily towards the individual's viewpoint could lead to the commissioning of services that, while demanded, may provide little in the way of health benefit to patients (Stevens & Gillam, 1998). In addition, the choices that individuals demand can sometimes conflict with what is known about the effectiveness of an intervention. For example, if individuals demand investment in ERS, it could be argued that due to the limited evidence of its effectiveness, commissioners would contest whether this is a good use of public funds. This raises important questions facing local health systems about understanding what we mean by value and the balance between commissioning for populations and commissioning for individuals (National Voices, 2015; Klein & Maybin, 2012).

Co-production in exercise referral: Case study examples

The following case studies provide pragmatic examples of how a real-world participatory approach was undertaken to co-produce evidence-based ERS. The case studies are the initial phases of a project that aimed to co-develop (phase 1), pilot (phase 2) and evaluate (phase 3) an evidence-based ERS for clinical populations. This approach is underpinned by the Medical Research Council (MRC) guidelines for complex interventions (Craig et al., 2008; Skivington et al., 2021). Case study 1 aims to provide an example of a co-production approach involving multiple stakeholders (Buckley et al., 2018). Case study 2 aims to provide insight into the practitioner training and development process during the pilot phase (Buckley et al., 2019).

Case study 1 Co-production of an evidence-based exercise referral scheme

Recommendations from the National Institute for Health and Care Excellence (NICE, 2014) state that ERS should only be commissioned if they incorporate behaviour change theory and collect long-term evaluation data. A lack of effectiveness evidence may be somewhat attributable to the use of highly controlled research to inform practice, which provides limited information regarding challenges faced at the coal face by policy-makers and practitioners working in the real world (Watson, 2017). To improve the implementation and effectiveness of long-term PA behaviour change interventions, there is a demand for ecologically valid, multi-stakeholder-developed interventions (Gates et al., 2016; Harden et al., 2016) that reflect the pragmatic needs of end users in programme design (Farrance, Tsofliou, & Clark, 2016). Therefore, the aim of this study was to co-produce an evidence-based PARS for clinical populations that was feasible to implement in practice (Buckley et al., 2018).

Design: A development group was formed, consisting of public health commissioners (n = 4), a fitness centre area manager (n = 1), a general practitioner (GP; n = 1), exercise referral practitioners (n = 2), a health trainer (n = 1), a health trainer coordinator (n = 1), patients (n = 5), plus academic experts in exercise referral (n = 1), exercise psychology (n = 1) and exercise physiology (n = 1). Multi-level stakeholders were recruited based on a professional and/or personal involvement with the original exercise referral scheme in operation. The role of academic group members was to provide theoretical knowledge and scientific evidence, whilst local stakeholders (commissioners, managers, practitioners and patients) contributed local knowledge and experiences to inform the pragmatic feasibility of the intervention.

Figure 2.1 provides an overview of the co-production protocol used for this study. Five development group meetings were organised to facilitate the iterative co-production of the intervention. Objectives were predetermined for each meeting, although content and timescales were dynamic and responsive to stakeholder input. Each meeting was facilitated by a member of the research team who was skilled in facilitating group discussion and was deemed relatively independent as exercise referral was not their specialty. Anecdotally, a skilled facilitator is vital to help reduce bias in conclusions and to ensure every level of stakeholder will contribute.

During each development meeting, small-group activities (four to five participants per subgroup) were used to facilitate collaboration and ensure all stakeholders were given a voice. Each subgroup was presented with open questions to discuss and asked to record their views on a white board or flip chart. Following subgroup discussions, a whole group discussion collated any issues raised in relation to each meeting's objectives. Efforts were made to facilitate co-production by providing a clear rationale for decisions and tasks and structuring activities to allow the development group to come up with their own solutions. Through the development process, intervention components were iteratively mapped to the Template for Intervention Development and Replication (TIDieR) checklist (Hoffmann et al., 2014). To check that stakeholders' views had been accurately interpreted in the proposed intervention model following the development meetings, an online survey was sent via email to stakeholders (paper format to patients).

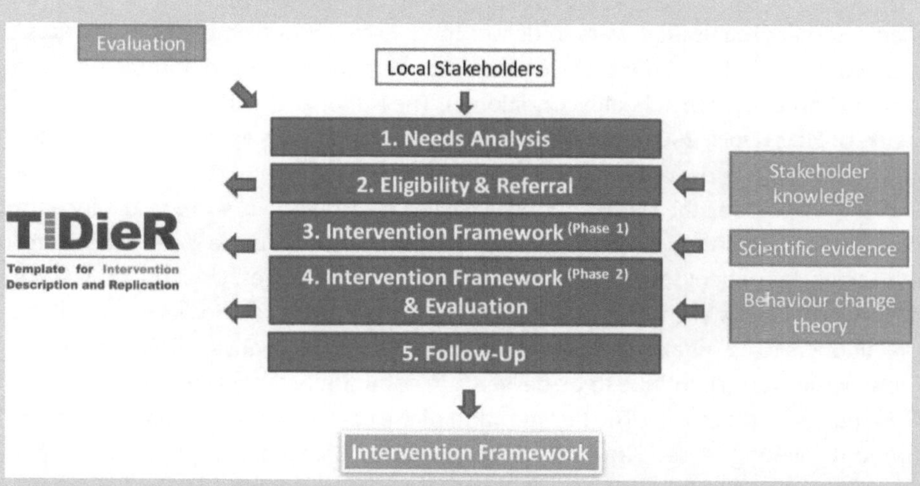

FIGURE 2.1 Co-production protocol for phase 1 of 'Making a Move in Exercise Referral' project. Numbers 1 to 5 represent the development meetings in chronological order

This provided an opportunity to confirm their individual agreement and provide any final comments.

Findings: Several factors emerged that must be considered when translating evidence to practice in an exercise referral setting.

A cultural shift from exercise to physical activity: Following development meeting 1, there was a consensus amongst stakeholders that the focus of the ERS should be on individual PA behaviour change. In contrast, traditional ERS typically have a 12-week 'exercise prescription' model. For exercise referral to develop a more holistic PA approach aligned with DoH PA guidance (DoH, 2004), a cultural shift is needed. A small yet potentially instigating step is a re-branding of exercise referral to PA referral.

Patient safety and accountability: Having established the importance of a PA behaviour change focus, consideration was given to how such support could be provided within existing resources. External organisations such as a health trainer service were discussed regarding viability to provide PA behaviour change support. The health trainer service is a UK initiative that employs lay health workers to provide individualised behaviour change support for a broad spectrum of health issues. Such health behaviours include PA, nutrition, smoking cessation and alcohol consumption. It was initially proposed that health trainers could act as the primary referral route and provide behaviour change support to patients. Other titles with very similar roles include health and lifestyle coaches.

> [Health trainers] *are very skilled, they're very good at working with people and supporting them, so that makes a big difference, having the right type of people.*
>
> *(Exercise Referral Practitioner)*

If an external organisation were to deliver the scheme, however, the question arose as to who would be accountable for ensuring the patient's PA programme was safe and appropriate for their health condition(s). The National Quality Assurance Framework for ERSs (DoH, 2001) and the British Heart Foundation's exercise referral toolkit contain detailed information regarding exercise prescription and clinical populations and PA support for the general public. Yet the document lacks clear guidance for broader PA support for clinical populations. Consequently, advice is needed regarding liability for patient safety within PA-focused referral schemes. Until such guidance is developed, the stakeholder group concluded it was necessary for level 3 qualified practitioners to assess all patients and provide appropriate PA advice. This meant that the scheme would continue to be delivered in community fitness centres.

Resources and capacity: The first iteration of the co-developed framework (development meeting 3; see Figure 2.1) was evidence based and represented stakeholder needs. Yet group discussion found that the proposed bi-weekly support was 'time and resource intensive' (GP and Public Health Commissioner); further, it was considered as 'not always necessary or even potentially intrusive' (Patient). Such discussions highlighted a lack of congruence between the perceived 'ideal' (i.e. what would be delivered to produce optimal results) and the 'real' (i.e. what could feasibly be delivered within current resources). It took further discussion and co-production to arrive at an intervention model that was still evidence based yet, importantly, feasible to implement in the real world (see Figure 2.2).

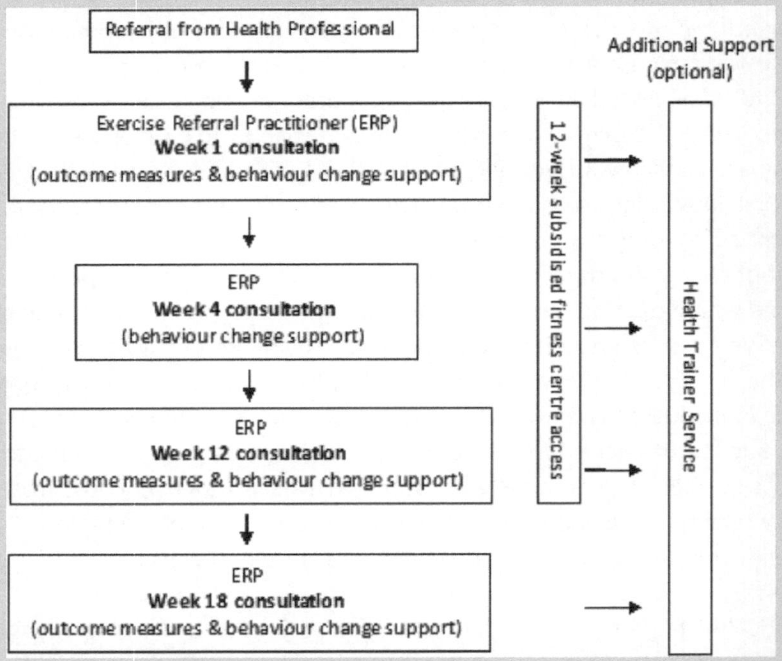

FIGURE 2.2 Co-developed PA referral scheme, including regular behaviour change consultations with ERPs

TABLE 2.1 Summary of pragmatic facilitators and challenges of a participatory research process

Facilitators	*Challenges*
• Using the first meeting as a 'needs analysis' allowed the stakeholders to share their perceptions of the existing scheme and expectations of the process.	• Multidisciplinary group discussion meant that occasionally, different stakeholders had contrasting views on topics that were not always resolved. In these instances, follow-up meetings with individuals, email and telephone contact allowed for finer details to be decided upon.
• Open questions and use of subgroups facilitated input and discussion from stakeholders, ensuring that their knowledge and experience informed the intervention.	• Irregular stakeholder attendance meant content had to be repeated for participants who missed previous meetings.
• Multidisciplinary debate and problem solving allowed for various areas of expertise and experience to inform the intervention. Stakeholders included researchers, public health commissioners, a GP, health trainers, fitness centre managers, exercise referral practitioners and service users/patients.	• Understanding translational research methodology: Stakeholders may have initially seen research and practice as separate entities rather than a collaboration of the two to try and achieve effectiveness.
• Reflective practice contributed to the iterative intervention development and facilitated knowledge translation. For example, researcher discussions following stakeholder development meetings involved summarising key topics and forming actions going forward.	

Source: Buckley et al., 2018

Table 2.1 provides a summary of the facilitators and challenges whilst undertaking the co-production approach described here (Buckley et al., 2018). It is hoped that this information will assist any researchers/stakeholders/practitioners planning to undergo such a process.

Implications for practice: Incorporating a multidisciplinary group of local stakeholders and academics in the co-production of an intervention from its conception may facilitate the creation of interventions that are both evidence based and feasible to implement in real-world clinical practice. If UK exercise referral is to evolve from the typical 12-week 'exercise prescription' model to a more holistic 'physical activity behaviour change' focus, consideration must be given to patient safety and accountability, provision of behaviour change support and feasibility within available resources.

Case study 2 Working towards co-ownership with exercise practitioners (a trainer's perspective)

The co-production process outlined in case study 1 resulted in an intervention outline of an evidence-based PA referral scheme (see Figure 2.1). The scheme was aimed at supporting PA behaviour change through a series of one-to-one consultations at 1, 4, 12 and 18 weeks, with exercise referral practitioners (ERPs), alongside 12 weeks of subsidised access to the fitness centre. The follow-up consultation took place at 18 weeks, as this was deemed by patients in the co-production group to be an appropriate length of time (when compared with the more typical 24-week follow-up, which was deemed too long to wait). Similarly, patients and practitioners felt the first progress consultation should be early in the scheme (four weeks), in an effort to prevent the common dropout seen at five to eight weeks in the city's existing ERS (The Murray Consultancy, 2013). Behaviour change consultations were to be underpinned by self-determination theory (SDT) (Ryan & Deci, 2000), with the aim of enhancing patients' autonomous motivation for PA (i.e. the volitional desire to engage in PA, as opposed to engaging because of other pressures), since it is well established that autonomous motivation is associated with a greater likelihood of long-term PA participation (Teixeira et al., 2012). This service model differed from the existing ERS being delivered in the city, in which the only formal one-to-one contact was at week 1 (followed by 12 weeks of subsidised access to the fitness centre). Thus, ERPs would be required to integrate an additional three consultations for each patient, whilst also moving away from an approach focused on 'advising patients what exercise to do' and towards 'supporting patients to fit PA into their lifestyles'.

In the section that follows, Dr Paula Watson (HCPC-registered sport and exercise psychologist) reflects on the process of training ERPs to foster autonomous motivation for PA and considers the role of co-production in this process. Results from this pilot phase of the project are reported in Buckley et al. (2019).

Philosophical considerations and approach: In developing training for ERPs to deliver the PA behaviour change intervention, we were mindful of several factors: 1) only one of the six ERPs to be trained had been involved in the co-production phase, and this ERP was also the team leader; 2) SDT-based delivery can be challenging for non-experts to learn, and previous research attempting to train ERPs to deliver autonomy-supportive behaviour change consultations had seen limited success (Duda et al., 2014); and 3) none of the ERPs had received any behaviour change training previously, and their traditional training had focused on 'prescribing exercise for patients'. Given these factors, a didactic model of training was unlikely to achieve any meaningful outcomes. We therefore continued to draw on co-production principles throughout the training process; that is, we aimed to deliver training activities in such a manner that ERPs felt (co-)ownership of the intervention and autonomously motivated to make the changes required.

As well as being the focus of the behaviour change intervention, SDT provided a useful framework for the training process itself. A key component of SDT is the premise that there are three basic psychological needs essential for human well-being and optimal functioning (Ryan & Deci, 2000). These are autonomy (the need to feel behaviour is self-determined), competence (the need to feel capable of achieving the desired outcomes) and relatedness (the need to feel connected with others). Satisfaction of these basic psychological needs fosters autonomous motivation, which in turn promotes sustained and authentic engagement in tasks (rather than paying 'lip service' or taking shortcuts to reach the desired outcomes). Therefore, by designing training activities in a way that supported ERP needs for autonomy, competence and relatedness (see Table 2.2), we aimed to foster volitional and sustained engagement, which in turn would promote a sense of 'co-ownership' of the intervention.

TABLE 2.2 Training strategies used to support ERP autonomy, competence and relatedness, as a means of working towards co-ownership

Basic psychological need	*Example strategies*
Autonomy	Providing a clear and relevant rationale for the project (i.e. coming from the ERP perspective)
	Involving ERPs in decision making about training and programme delivery (and taking their lead in pragmatic issues)
	Listening to ERP needs – encouraging open, honest feedback and (most importantly) responding to feedback
	Reducing power imbalances by acknowledging the two-way learning process
Competence	Acknowledging ERP expertise and their crucial contribution to the project
	Providing structured one-to-one support and feedback
	Tailoring support to the different starting points of ERPs
Relatedness	Personalised, informal communication to build rapport with ERPs (e.g. emails, informal chats during visits)
	Demonstrating compassion, empathy, care
	Promoting shared ownership (e.g. using terms such as 'we'/'our' project)

Note: Although strategies are organised into categories, it is likely strategies contributed to satisfying more than one psychological need.

Methods: Training consisted of an initial three-hour workshop, following by regular one-to-ones and group meetings as and when required. We also observed ERPs conducting baseline consultations prior to the start of training (needs analysis) and during delivery of the intervention at a later stage (progress tracking and personalised feedback). As training lead, I engaged in reflective practice (Gibbs, 1988) throughout the process, using a reflective log to record what was working well, what challenges were arising and to what extent the sense of co-ownership was being achieved.

Reflections on the process: To what extent did we achieve 'co-ownership'? Although ERPs were open to participation in the project and keen to improve delivery, the reflective process exposed several gaps between the intervention we were attempting to deliver and how the ERPs were experiencing the process. When training others, we must be mindful that the message practitioners hear may be different from the message we intend to convey. For example, the following extract from my reflective log demonstrates how personal context can influence the way messages are interpreted.

> *I realised as I was chatting to one of the ERPs . . . whilst I was talking about psychosocial needs, they were hearing it as 'physical needs' . . . so in their minds they are already tailoring programmes to client's needs.*

These crossed wires led to confusion amongst some of the ERPs (who perceived themselves to already be delivering 'needs-supportive' consultations). Yet I was blind to the underlying cause of this confusion until I took the time to sit back and reflect on my interactions with the ERP. This demonstrates the importance of reflective learning in moving forward collaboratively (Ghaye et al., 2008) since this realisation allowed us to clarify the issue and re-align practitioner and trainer goals.

Whilst at times I felt we were achieving the desired 'shared ownership' of the project, there were other occasions when ERPs expressed feelings of 'you want us to do it this way', suggesting a lack of internalisation of the project objectives. Whilst evidence is held in high esteem for academics, it remains a basic human condition that experience holds 'the highest authority' (Rogers, 1961). That is, if we have tried and tested it ourselves, the effect is far more powerful than someone telling us that it has been tried and tested with a large sample of strangers. It is therefore important to understand the personal and professional beliefs of the individuals we are training since these values will influence their responses to the concepts being introduced. For example, despite fitness instructor training stating that programmes are to be negotiated and agreed on with clients, one ERP struggled to internalise the notion that the patient could have a say in directing their own exercise programme:

> *He* [ERP] *felt he had to set the client's gym programme because he knew what were the right exercises for his condition.*

Strengths of co-production: By creating an open, equal environment in which ERPs felt their views were valued (and would be acted upon), we were able to identify and overcome delivery challenges rather than ploughing on with protocols that were not working. For example, part of the intervention involved ERPs tracking participant progress by using the International Physical Activity Questionnaire (IPAQ, Craig et al., 2003). After several weeks of following this protocol, the ERP team leader contacted us to note the questionnaire was proving challenging to administer in the time they had and presented an idea for how this might be delivered more efficiently (by incorporating the validated questions into a more user-friendly format). We consequently made this change, thus providing evidence to ERPs that we were serious about listening to them (thus increasing the likelihood of future two-way dialogues). This example highlights the importance of being able to tolerate 'messiness' when engaging in co-production (as outlined by Rycroft-Malone et al., 2016) since flexibility is essential in establishing a delivery protocol that meets both trainer and practitioner needs.

Conclusion: The aim of this project was to foster shared ownership of a PA behaviour change intervention through adopting an SDT-based approach to ERP training and support. Whilst the reflective process revealed challenges in working towards co-ownership, these were crucial training issues that needed to be brought to our awareness (and it was ultimately the co-production approach that allowed this to happen). Perhaps the best way to illustrate the beneficial effects of co-production is to imagine how this case study scenario would have played out had we taken a didactic approach to training. We would have delivered training and left ERPs to deliver (on the assumption they had digested what we had taught them); they would have struggled to implement what we asked, and the training would have been considered ineffective (without any understanding of why). In contrast, the co-production approach opened up possibilities to work iteratively and collaboratively with ERPs, ensuring teething problems were overcome and allowing the intervention to be developed to the extent it could be expected to have a worthwhile effect (Craig et al., 2008; Skivington et al., 2021).

The future of UK exercise referral: Design, delivery and evaluation

The National Quality Assurance Framework (DoH, 2001) states that ERS should go beyond 'advice giving, recommending exercise, or offering patients vouchers to attend exercise facilities' (p. vii). Yet anecdotal evidence suggests that ERS are typically gym based and 'exercise prescription' focused. This, among other considerations, likely explains the ambiguous effectiveness evidence for UK exercise referral. As previously discussed, NICE guidance has recommended that UK ERS should only be commissioned if 1) data is available for evaluation, and 2) they are underpinned by behaviour change components (NICE, 2014). According to the MRC guidance for complex interventions, 'before undertaking a substantial evaluation you should first develop the intervention to the point where it can reasonably be expected to have a worthwhile effect' (Craig et al., 2008; Skivington et al., 2021). It is believed that this has not been the case for UK exercise referral, and as a result, systematic review evidence has made conclusions based on evaluations of interventions that are not evidence based or underpinned by behaviour change theory.

The case study examples included within this chapter are the initial stages of a project that aimed to co-develop (phase 1), pilot (phase 2) and evaluate (phase 3) an evidence-based PARS for clinical populations. Case study 1 provides a practical example of a co-production phase, and case study 2 provides a practical example of a pilot phase of an approach underpinned by MRC guidance for complex interventions (Craig et al., 2008; Skivington et al., 2021). In brief summary, the co-production approach allowed for intervention teething problems to be overcome and the intervention itself and staff training to be iteratively developed, and, consequently, staff were continually supported through the behaviour change training process. In contrast, adopting a more didactic research design might have resulted in failure of the staff to successfully adopt and implement the new behaviour change techniques. In addition, the research team would have attempted to implement an intervention that was too time and resource intensive. Ultimately, this would have increased the risk of a premature evaluation concluding the intervention to be ineffective and wasting valuable public health resources.

Co-production approaches are strongly advocated, not just for ERS but for complex health interventions more generally. This is particularly the case for interventions that involve multiple stakeholders from various levels, often the case in public health. It is therefore vital that co-production work is piloted prior to conducting an evaluation. Further, ongoing collaboration with local stakeholders during evaluation and implementation phases is necessary if interventions are to evolve with the constantly changing public health climate. The phased approach is cyclic in nature: In an ideal scenario, following implementation phases, collaboration would continue back to co-production work when necessary; this would enable an intervention to remain adaptable and more likely to be an efficient use of public health resources (Craig et al., 2008; Skivington et al., 2021).

A co-production approach can result in a feasible solution to pragmatic challenges. For example, exercise professionals undertake a multifaceted role in ERS operation (DoH, 2001). The integral role of the exercise professionals in the operation of exercise referral schemes means that the skills and abilities that they exhibit and their relationships with other stakeholders may be vital to programme success (Graham, 2006). Despite this, limited literature has explored exercise professionals' perspectives of the exercise referral process or their perspectives on communication/operational processes associated with such schemes. Gaining such viewpoints from stakeholders at all levels can facilitate the creation of interventions that are more context sensitive and have increased chances of implementation success (Henderson et al., 2017).

However, as previously identified in this chapter, public health commissioners need to be mindful that demand from individuals may differ from what they actually need or will be able to benefit from in practice. For example, demand and choices can create a conflict if there is no parity between them. Thus, raising important questions and challenges for those involved in the decision making of commissioning services and in managing the co-production process is an important process to consider. This viewpoint is rarely presented or considered in academic literature, but it raises critical considerations and highlights the importance of transparency, agreed-upon objectives and expectations from the start of a multidisciplinary co-production approach. Careful planning, inclusion of a well-represented development group and skilled facilitation is required to balance 'commissioning for populations and individuals'.

Key points

- The translation of scientific evidence to real-world practice is a well-known challenge for public health researchers and stakeholders. The effectiveness of UK exercise referral schemes is ambiguous, yet this has been deemed an unfair assessment of its potential to impact public health.
- Co-production is a potential tool to facilitate the development of evidence-based interventions that draw on local needs and are feasible to implement within existing resources. Allowing researchers, commissioners, exercise professionals and users to contribute to design, development and delivery of the intervention can improve context sensitivity and, therefore, chances of implementation success.
- Public health commissioners need to be mindful that demand from individuals in a co-production approach may differ from what they actually need or will benefit from in practice.
- Pragmatic evaluation researchers need to carefully consider both the feasibility and appropriate use of highly controlled research trials. In addition, researchers and stakeholders need to be cautious of prematurely evaluating an intervention that may not yet be delivered as intended.
- Following the MRC guidance for complex interventions can help us evaluate interventions that are likely to have a worthwhile effect on public health. By focusing on intervention co-production and pilot testing as a priori to conducting evaluations should improve chances of implementation success and, thus, real-world effectiveness.

Short questions

1. What is co-production?
2. Why is co-production important in public health?
3. What are the four simple steps in a co-production approach?
4. What is the estimated health-care budget spent on prevention and treatment as a percentage?
5. What barriers inhibit health professionals' willingness to provide lifestyle advice to patients?
6. What are QALY?
7. Recommendations from the National Institute for Health and Care Excellence (NICE, 2014) state that ERS should only be commissioned if they include what?

References

Abildso C, Zizzi S, Gilleland D, Thomas J, and Bonner, D. (2010) A mixed methods evaluation of a 12-week insurance-sponsored weight management program incorporating cognitive-behavioral counseling. *Journal of Mixed Methods Research* 4(4): 278–294.

Anis NA, Lee RE, Ellerbeck EF, et al. (2004) Direct observation of physician counseling on dietary habits and exercise: Patient, physician, and office correlates. *Preventive Medicine* 38(2): 198–202. DOI: 10.1016/j.ypmed.2003.09.046.

Batalden M, Batalden P, Margolis P, et al. (2016) Coproduction of healthcare service. *BMJ Quality & Safety* 25(7): 509–517. DOI: 10.1136/bmjqs-2015-004315.

Beedie C, Mann S, Jimenez A, et al. (2016) Death by effectiveness: Exercise as medicine caught in the efficacy trap! *British Journal of Sports Medicine* 50(6): 323. DOI: 10.1136/bjsports-2014-094389.

Bergold J, and Thomas S. (2010) *Partizipative Forschung*. Berlin: Springer.

Bickerdike L, Booth A, Wilson PM, et al. (2017) Social prescribing: Less rhetoric and more reality. A systematic review of the evidence. *BMJ Open* 7(4): e013384. DOI: 10.1136/bmjopen-2016-013384.

Boyle D, and Harris, M. (2009) *The challenge of the co-production: How equal partnerships between professionals and the public are crucial to improving public services*. London: New Economics Foundation.

Brownson RC, Chriqui JF, and Stamatakis KA. (2009) Understanding evidence-based public health policy. *American Journal of Public Health* 99(9): 1576–1583. DOI: 10.2105/ajph.2008.156224.

Brownson RC, Kreuter MW, Arrington BA, et al. (2006) Translating scientific discoveries into public health action: How can schools of public health move us forward? *Public Health Reports (Washington, D.C.: 1974)* 121(1): 97–103. DOI: 10.1177/003335490612100118.

Buckley BJR, Thijssen DH, Murphy RC, et al. (2018) Making a move in exercise referral: Co-development of a physical activity referral scheme. *Journal of Public Health* 40(4): e586–e593. DOI: 10.1093/pubmed/fdy072.

Buckley BJR, Thijssen DH, Murphy RC, et al. (2019) Preliminary effects and acceptability of a co-produced physical activity referral intervention. *Health Education Journal* 78(8): 869–884. DOI: 10.1177/0017896919853322.

Butterfield R, Henderson J, and Scott R. (2009) *Public health and prevention expenditure in England. Report No. 4*. Penn State University, PA: The College of Information Sciences and Technology.

Clarke D, Jones F, Harris R, et al. (2017) What outcomes are associated with developing and implementing co-produced interventions in acute healthcare settings? A rapid evidence synthesis. *BMJ Open* 7(7): e014650. DOI: 10.1136/bmjopen-2016-014650.

Cornwall A, and Jewkes R. (1995) What is participatory research? *Social Science & Medicine* 41(12). DOI: 10.1016/0277-9536(95)00127-S.

Craig CL, Marshall AL, Sjöström M, et al. (2003) International physical activity questionnaire: 12-country reliability and validity. *Medicine and Science in Sports and Exercise* 35(8): 1381–1395. DOI: 10.1249/01.MSS.0000078924.61453.FB.

Craig P, Dieppe P, Macintyre S, et al. (2008) Developing and evaluating complex interventions: The new Medical Research Council guidance. *BMJ* 337. DOI: 10.1136/bmj.a1655.

Crone D, and James D. (2016) Evidence-based practice in physical activity promotion. In *Clinical Exercise Science* (edited by A. Scott and C. Gidlow). Abingdon: Routledge.

Crone D, Johnston L, and Grant T. (2004) Maintaining quality in exercise referral schemes: A case study of professional practice. *Primary Health Care Research and Development* 5(2): 96–103. DOI: 10.1191/1463423604pc189oa.

Crone D, Smith A, and Gough B. (2005) 'I feel totally at one, totally alive and totally happy': A psycho-social explanation of the physical activity and mental health relationship. *Health Education Research* 20(5): 600–611.

Dent E, Hoon E, Kitson A, et al. (2016) Translating a health service intervention into a rural setting: Lessons learned. *BMC Health Services Research* 16(1): 62. DOI: 10.1186/s12913-016-1302-0.

Department of Health (DoH) (2001) *Exercise referral systems: A national quality assurance framework*. London: Department of Health.

Department of Health (2004) *At least five a week: Evidence on the impact of physical activity and its relationship to health*. A report from the Chief Medical Officer. London: Department of Health.

Duda JL, Williams GC, Ntoumanis N, et al. (2014) Effects of a standard provision versus an autonomy supportive exercise referral programme on physical activity, quality of life and well-being indicators: A cluster randomised controlled trial. *The International Journal of Behavioral Nutrition and Physical Activity* 11: 10. DOI: 10.1186/1479-5868-11-10.

Farrance C, Tsofliou F, and Clark C. (2016) Adherence to community based group exercise interventions for older people: A mixed-methods systematic review. *Preventive Medicine* 87: 155–166. DOI: 10.1016/j.ypmed.2016.02.037.

Gates AB, Kerry R, Moffatt F, et al. (2016) Movement for movement: Exercise as everybody's business? *British Journal of Sports Medicine* 0(0). DOI: 10.1136/bjsports-2016-096857.

Ghaye T, Wikman A, Kisare M, et al. (2008) Participatory and appreciative action and reflection (PAAR) – Democratizing reflective practices. *Reflective Practice* 9(4). DOI: 10.1080/14623940802475827.

Gibbs G. (1988) *Learning by doing: A guide to teaching and learning methods.* Oxford, UK: Oxford Brookes University, Further Education Unit.

Gidlow C, Crone D, and Huws-Thomas M. (2016) Physical activity promotion in primary health care and the community. *Clinical Exercise Science* 1: 263–284.

Gidlow C, Johnston LH, Crone D, et al. (2005) Attendance of exercise referral schemes in the UK: A systematic review. *Health Education Journal* 64(2): 168–186. DOI: 10.1177/001789690506400208.

Gidlow C, Johnston LH, Crone D, et al. (2008) State of the art reviews: Methods of evaluation: Issues and implications for physical activity referral schemes. *American Journal of Lifestyle Medicine* 2(1): 46–50. DOI: 10.1177/1559827607308733.

Graham RC. (2006) *Stakeholder perspectives of an exercise referral scheme.* Dissertation Thesis.

Graham RC, Dugdill L, and Cable NT. (2005) Health professionals' perspectives in exercise referral: Implications for the referral process. *Ergonomics* 48(11–14): 1411–1422. DOI: 10.1080/00140130500101064.

Green LW, Ottoson JM, García C, et al. (2009) Diffusion theory and knowledge dissemination, utilization, and integration in public health. *Annual Review of Public Health* 30(1): 151–174. DOI: 10.1146/annurev.publhealth.031308.100049.

Grimshaw JM, Eccles MP, Lavis JN, et al. (2012) Knowledge translation of research findings. *Implementation Science* 7(1): 1–17. DOI: 10.1186/1748-5908-7-50.

Hardcastle S, and Taylor AH. (2001) Looking for more than weight loss and fitness gain: Psychosocial dimensions among older women in a primary-care exercise-referral program. *Journal of Aging and Physical Activity* 9(3): 313–328. DOI: 10.1123/japa.9.3.313.

Harden SM, Johnson S, Almeida FA, et al. (2016) Improving physical activity program adoption using integrated research-practice partnerships: An effectiveness-implementation trial. *Translational Behavioral Medicine* 7(1): 28–38. DOI: 10.1007/s13142-015-0380-6.

Health and Social Care Act (2012) Chapter 3. Available at: www.legislation.gov.uk/ukpga/2012/3/pdfs/ukpga_20120003_en.pdf (Accessed 11 November 2017).

Hemenway D. (2010) Why we don't spend enough on public health. *The New England Journal of Medicine* 362(18): 1657–1658. DOI: 10.1056/nejmp1001784.

Henderson H, Evans AB, Allen-Collinson J, et al. (2017) The 'wild and woolly' world of exercise referral schemes: Contested interpretations of an exercise as medicine programme. *Qualitative Research in Sport, Exercise and Health.* DOI: 10.1080/2159676X.2017.1352018.

Hill TP. (2012) Conducting phase IV clinical studies: A moral imperative? *Ecancermedicalscience* 6. Available at: www.ncbi.nlm.nih.gov/pmc/articles/PMC3493021/.

Hoffmann TC, Glasziou PP, Boutron I, et al. (2014) Better reporting of interventions: Template for intervention description and replication (TIDieR) checklist and guide. *BMJ* 348(March 7). DOI: 10.1136/bmj.g1687.

Hunter S, and Ritchie P. (2007) *Co-production and personalisation in social care: Changing relationships in the provision of social care.* London: Jessica Kingsley Publishers.

James D, Mills H, Crone D, et al. (2009) Factors associated with physical activity referral completion and health outcomes. *Journal of Sports Sciences* 27(10): 1007–1017. DOI: 10.1080/02640410903214248.

James DVB, Johnston LH, Crone D, et al. (2008) Factors associated with physical activity referral uptake and participation. *Journal of Sports Sciences* 26(2): 217–224. DOI: 10.1080/02640410701468863.

Kennedy MF, and Meeuwisse WH. (2003) Exercise counselling by family physicians in Canada. *Preventive Medicine* 37(3): 226–232. DOI: 10.1016/s0091-7435(03)00118-x.

Klein R and Maybin J. (2012) Thinking about rationing. *Kings Fund.* Available at: www.kingsfund.org.uk/sites/default/files/field/field_publication_file/Thinking-about-rationing-the-kings-fund-may-2012.pdf (Accessed 11 November 2017).

McAvoy BR, Kaner EF, Lock CA, et al. (1999) Our healthier nation: Are general practitioners willing and able to deliver? A survey of attitudes to and involvement in health promotion and lifestyle counselling. *The British Journal of General Practice: The Journal of the Royal College of General Practitioners* 49(440): 187–190.

McKenna J and Vernon M. (2004) How general practitioners promote 'lifestyle' physical activity. *Patient Education and Counseling* 54(1): 101–106. DOI: 10.1016/s0738-3991(03)00192-7.

McNair F, Graham RC, Dudgill L, et al. (2005) Determining the indicators of success in exercise referral schemes. *Journal of Sports Science* 23: 220–222.

Mills H, Crone D, James DV, et al. (2012) Exploring the perceptions of success in an exercise referral scheme. *Evaluation Review* 36(6): 407–429. DOI: 10.1177/0193841X12474452.

Moore GF, Audrey S, Barker M, et al. (2014) Process evaluation in complex public health intervention studies: The need for guidance. *Journal of Epidemiology and Community Health* 68(2). DOI: 10.1136/jech-2013-202869.

Moore GF, Audrey S, Barker M, et al. (2015) Process evaluation of complex interventions: Medical Research Council guidance. *BMJ* 350(6) (March 19): h1258. DOI: 10.1136/bmj.h1258.

Moore GF, Moore L, and Murphy S. (2011) Facilitating adherence to physical activity: Exercise professionals' experiences of the National Exercise Referral Scheme in Wales. A qualitative study. *BMC Public Health* 11: 935.

Moore GF, Moore L, and Murphy S. (2012) Integration of motivational interviewing into practice in the national exercise referral scheme in Wales: A mixed methods study. *Behavioural and Cognitive Psychotherapy* 40(3): 313–330. DOI: 10.1017/S1352465811000531.

Morey MC, and Sullivan RJ. (2003) Medical assessment for health advocacy and practical strategies for exercise initiation. *American Journal of Preventive Medicine* 25(3): 204–208. DOI: 10.1016/s0749-3797(03)00180-6.

Morris Z, Wooding S, and Grant J. (2011) The answer is 17 years, what is the question: Understanding time lags in translational research. *Journal of the Royal Society of Medicine* 104(12): 510–520. DOI: 10.1258/jrsm.2011.110180.

The Murray Consultancy Ltd (2013) *Lifestyles' exercise for health evaluation: Liverpool*. National Institute for Health and Care Excellence (NICE) Physical activity: Exercise referral schemes [PH54].

National Institute for Health and Care Excellence (2014) *Physical activity: Exercise referral schemes*. London: TSO. Available at: www.nice.org.uk/guidance/ph54

National Voices (2015) *How should we think about value in health and care?* Discussion Paper. September 2015. Available at: www.health.org.uk/publication/how-should-we-think-about-value-health-and-care (Accessed 2 November 2017).

Needham C, and Carr S. (2009) *SCIE Research briefing 31: Co-production: An emerging evidence base for adult social care transformation*. London: Social Care Institute for Excellence.

Nutbeam D. (1996) Achieving "best practice" in health promotion: Improving the fit between research and practice. *Health Education Research* 11(3): 317–326.

Osborne S, Radnor Z, and Strokosch K. (2016) Co-production and the co-creation of value in public services: A suitable case for treatment? *Public Management Review* 18(5): 639–653.

Pavey T, Taylor A, Fox K, et al. (2011) Effect of exercise referral schemes in primary care on physical activity and improving health outcomes: Systematic review and meta-analysis. *BMJ* 343. DOI: 10.1136/bmj.d6462.

PHE (2016) Local health and care planning: Menu of preventative interventions. *Public Health England*. Available at: www.gov.uk/government/uploads/system/uploads/attachment_data/file/565944/Local_health_and_care_planning_menu_of_preventative_interventions.pdf (Accessed 11 November 2017)

Pinto D, Robertson MC, Hansen P, and Abbott JH. (2012) Cost-effectiveness of nonpharmacologic, nonsurgical interventions for hip and/or knee Osteoarthritis: Systematic review. *Value in Health* 15(1): 1–12.

Queen M, Parker A, and Crone D. (2016) Gender perceptions and their impact when referring obese patients for exercise. *Qualitative Research in Sport, Exercise and Health* 8(3): 287–300.

Realpe A, and Wallace LM. (2016) What is co-production? *The Health Foundation* 1–19.

Richardson AK. (2012) Investing in public health: Barriers and possible solutions. *Journal of Public Health* 34(3), 1: 322–327.

Riddoch C, Puig-Ribera A, and Cooper A. (1998) *Effectiveness of physical activity promotion schemes in primary care: A review.* London: Health Education Authority.

Rogers C. (1961) On becoming a person. In *The Carl Rogers reader* (edited by H. Kirschenbaum and V.L. Henderson, 1990), 17–29. London: Constable.

Roussos ST, and Fawcett SB. (2000) A review of collaborative partnerships as a strategy for improving community health. *Annual Review of Public Health* 21: 369–402.

Rutter H, Savona N, Glonti K, et al. (2017) The need for a complex systems model of evidence for public health. *Lancet* 17(3). DOI: 10.1016/S0140-6736.

Ryan RM and Deci EL. (2000) Self-determination theory and the facilitation of intrinsic motivation, social development, and well-being. *The American Psychologist* 55(1): 68–78.

Rycroft-Malone J, Burton CR, Bucknall T, et al. (2016) Collaboration and co-production of knowledge in healthcare: Opportunities and challenges. *International Journal of Health Policy and Management* 5(4): 221–223. DOI: 10.15171/ijhpm.2016.08.

Skivington K, Matthews L, Simpson SA, Craig P, Baird J, Blazeby JM, et al. (2021) A new framework for developing and evaluating complex interventions: Update of Medical Research Council guidance. *British Medical Journal* 374: n2061.

Stathi A, McKenna J, and Fox KR. (2003) The experiences of older people participating in exercise referral schemes. *Journal of the Royal Society for the Promotion of Health* 124(1): 18–23.

Stevens A and Gillam S. (1998) Needs assessment: From theory to practice. *BMJ: British Medical Journal* 316(7142): 1448–1452.

Taylor A. (2003) The role of primary care in promoting physical activity. In *Perspectives on exercise and health* (edited by J. McKenna and C. Riddoch), 153–180. Hampshire: Palgrave Macmillan.

Teixeira PJ, Carraça EV, Markland D, et al. (2012) Exercise, physical activity, and self-determination theory: A systematic review. *International Journal of Behavioural Nutrition and Physical Activity* 9: 78. DOI: 10.1186/1479-5868-9-78.

Watson P. (2017) Stuck in the "exercise" trap: Current issues and future directions for UK exercise referral schemes. *European Journal of Public Health* 27(3): ckx187.057.

Watson P, Dugdill L, Murphy R, et al. (2013) Moving forward in childhood obesity treatment: A call for translational research. *Health Education Journal* 72(2): 230–239.

Westfall J, Mold J, and Fagnan L. (2007) Practice-based research – 'Blue Highways' on the NIH roadmap. *JAMA* 297: 403–406. DOI: 10.1001/jama.297.4.403.

Wormald H, and Ingle L. (2004) GP exercise referral schemes: Improving the patient's experience. *Health Education Journal* 63: 362–373.

3

THE EXERCISE REFERRAL PROCESS

Jeannie Wyatt-Williams

Contents

Chapter aims

The aims of this chapter are:

- Describe the exercise referral process
- Explain the differences between referral and recommendation

Introduction

The purpose of this chapter is to describe the process of a referral to exercise. The question of delineating between 'referral' and 'recommendation' is an important one in a medico-legal context. Where physical activity is simply 'recommended', the health professional gives advice about exercising directly to the patient and, in some cases, may recommend a specific exercise programme. In this case, the health professional is responsible for any advice given. He or she may be liable for damages if that advice is given negligently, and the patient

DOI: 10.4324/9781315102399-3

experiences an injury as a result of the recommendations given if contraindicated or not appropriate.

However, if a medical professional refers a patient to a programme of physical activity that follows a formal process, the health professional is liable to assess the patient, ensuring they meet the exercise referral scheme (ERS) inclusion criteria, and the exercise professional is responsible for designing and delivering a safe and effective programme of exercise to meet that patient's individual needs. Referral is therefore not the same as a 'recommendation' to exercise.

A formal agreement needs to exist between the referrer and the referral programme or an individual exercise specialist prior to the start-up of any programme. It is the reason many health professionals are reluctant to recommend exercise in the absence of a formal process, and, in many instances, they are very cautious about referring to ERS. Consequently, it is important to know the benefits of physical activity as a suitable rationale for setting up ERS and to encourage health professionals to engage in referral to your scheme.

A useful document illustrating these benefits is a summary of the research to date in the UK Chief Medical Officers' Physical Activity Guidelines (2019). The document concludes that despite the widely reported benefits of physical activity, most adults and many children across the UK are insufficiently active and therefore not meeting the guidelines. In summary, the guidelines:

- Present a UK-wide consensus on the amount and type of physical activity that is needed to benefit health across the life course
- Have been updated using the best available evidence and reflect what we know now about the relationship between physical activity and health
- Apply across the population, irrespective of gender, age, or socioeconomic status

We know there are clear health inequalities in relation to physical inactivity, and therefore, interventions to promote physical activity must consider ways to emphasise and educate the public about the impact of physical inactivity or sedentary lifestyles, ensuring that these are identified as a major casual factor in chronic disease and are as important as smoking cigarettes and an unhealthy diet. In summary, and related specifically to ERS-related issues, the guidelines highlight:

- Inactive and unfit people have almost double the risk of dying from coronary heart disease (CHD) compared with their more active and fitter counterparts.
- Active people have a 33% to 50% lower risk of developing type 2 diabetes than inactive people, while the risk of premature death is much lower in active and fit persons with type 2 diabetes than in those who are inactive and unfit.
- Weight-bearing physical activity increases bone mineral density in adolescents, maintains it in young adults and slows its decline as we age.
- People who lead an active lifestyle over a number of years have a reduced risk of suffering symptoms of clinical depression, while physical activity also ameliorates the effects of mild, moderate or severe clinical depression.
- The most active individuals have a 40% to 50% lower risk of developing colon cancer. There is also some evidence of reduced risk of breast cancer among postmenopausal women and possibly a reduction in the risk of lung cancer.

Whilst the evidence of the benefits of physical activity on health is firmly established, evidence on effective interventions to encourage people to be more active is not so well developed. With regards to ERS, in 2006, the National Institute for Clinical Excellence (NICE) published 'A Rapid Review of the Effectiveness of Exercise Referral Schemes'. The document included a number of studies and concluded that there was evidence from two studies to suggest that exercise referral can have positive effects on physical activity in the short term (6–12 weeks), but evidence from four trials suggested that it may be ineffective in the longer term (over 12 weeks) or very longer term (over one year).

The document concluded that 'further research, using a controlled research design, is required to determine the impact that exercise referral schemes may have on reducing health inequalities and their effectiveness in increasing physical activity levels in adult populations'. This addressed the need not only to develop good quality schemes that meet best practices but also to collate sufficient data to prove effectiveness.

In response, the Welsh government sought to address this lack of evidence by conducting a randomised controlled trial (RCT) to determine the effectiveness of ERS as an intervention to increase physical activity and improve health. In doing so, the Welsh government brought together health, leisure and research partners to discuss the opportunities and barriers to setting up a funded National Exercise Referral Scheme (NERS) with standardised protocols and to evaluate it using a RCT which was launched in 2007.

With the evaluation of the National Exercise Referral Scheme in Wales concluding that, at that time, the NERS was 89% likely to be cost effective at just over £12,000 per QALY and, for those who adhere to the full programme, is likely to be marginally cost saving (-£367 per QALY) *(Murphy et al., 2010).*

NICE has suggested that interventions delivering a cost per QALY of under £20,000–£30,000 are likely to be an acceptable use of NHS resources. Primary care referral to the NERS falls well within this range or is potentially cost saving, particularly where participants pay a nominal fee per exercise class. This and subsequent studies have ensured that funding of the NERS has continued in Wales, and it operates across all 22 local authority areas (Tudor Edwards et al., 2013).

A National Institute for Health Research (NIHR)–funded systematic review of exercise referral found that ERS increased physical activity in people who had no or little physical activity to begin with compared with usual care or advice. But these schemes do not appear to be cost effective for all people, as identified in 'NHIR: Exercise Referral Schemes Increase Physical Activity for Some' (14 October 2015).

Prior to publication, the findings of this review informed the 2014 update to the NICE public health guideline on ERS. The updated guideline recommends ERS only for people who have existing health conditions or other health risk factors and undertake excessive sedentary behaviour and/or are inactive.

The referral process

The Medical Protection Society Statement (2000), whilst outdated, highlights some key issues that exercise referral practitioners should be aware of:

> The MPS endorses the provision of supervised exercise sessions for patients and appreciates that general practitioners have an important role in facilitating the use of exercise programmes.

> In order to encourage GPs to become involved in referring patients for exercise it is important that guidelines are simple, and GPs do not feel that they are being asked to take on responsibilities for which they are ill-equipped. It would be helpful for there to be either national or local guidelines which set out specific conditions for which referral for a structured exercise programme is appropriate.
>
> The introduction of the exercise professional that will be registered with a national body and have an indemnity in respect of his or her work is welcomed. We see no difficulty in GPs providing the exercise professional with details of the patient's past medical history with the consent of the patient and it will then be for the exercise professional to assess the suitability of the patient for a planned programme of exercise, the content of which would be his or her responsibility.
>
> It would be expected that the exercise professional would feed back to the GP any problems that are encountered and the progress that is made through the programme.
>
> With this framework we would see the GP's involvement as forming part of their responsibilities as a general practitioner and provided they were paying the appropriate subscription then they could look to the Society for advice and an indemnity in respect of their practice.

These considerations were taken into account when developing the Welsh NERS and are still relevant and need to be adhered to in the present day in relation to developing a quality-assured referral process and delivery options. When unpacking the statement, a number of key terms and points emerge:

- Supervised exercise sessions – highlights the need for supervision
- Referring patients – specifies 'referral' as opposed to a 'recommendation'
- National or local guidelines are simple – suggests the need for clear yet concise guidelines
- The exercise professional should be registered with a professional body and hold indemnity cover – should help reassure both health professionals and patients
- Past medical history and feedback to GP – supports the need for continuity of care between the health and exercise professions

The decision to refer is a matter for the health professional, but where the health professional does not have relevant qualifications to prescribe an exercise programme, it may be more appropriate to refer the patient to an exercise professional. However, the health professional is responsible for ensuring the patient is being referred to an exercise professional who has the relevant exercise referral instructor qualification, has appropriate personal indemnity insurance and is registered on a professional register.

There are some essential components to consider and agree on with all stakeholders in relation to developing a referral process. A needs assessment should be conducted to identify the target population for the referral programme and the entry criteria.

- Agree on what the aims of the programme should be
- Agree what outcome measures will be undertaken to evidence these aims
- Agree at what intervals and how the outcomes will be shared with referral partners and/or funding providers
- Agree on the referral form content and design

- Establish the method(s) for sending the referral form to named contact in compliance with GDPR
- Establish a set of roles and responsibilities for all parties

It is useful to design a service development scope document and a logic model to aid discussions with all parties and to visually check all steps are in place to ensure the programme offers a person-centred approach. This should be capable of supporting someone through a physical activity programme, encouraging positive healthier choices using motivational interviewing and behavioural change techniques, enabling them to improve their health and well-being outcomes and giving them the knowledge and confidence to continue their physical activity programme independently, effectively forming a 'Bridge from Health into Mainstream Leisure Activities'.

See Figure 3.1 for a sample template for a service development scope document highlighting the components you should consider when developing your bid for funding and engaging with collaborative partners.

Alongside this scoping document, it is useful to develop a logic model or process chart to further aid discussions with commissioners, referral partners and multidisciplinary teams you may wish to engage with. A logic model is a graphic which represents the theory of how an intervention produces its outcomes. It represents, in a simplified way, a hypothesis or 'theory of change' about how an intervention works. A logic model should allow everyone to:

- Visually check all steps are in place to achieve successful outcomes and a good return on investment
- See details on every step in the referral process
- Identify the person responsible for completing each task

If just one link is incomplete, then the process fails. For further guidance on developing logic models, you can look up the Public Health England Guidance Introduction to Logic Models (7 August 2018). Figure 3.2 is the logic flow chart developed by Graham Moore, developing a mix of methods framework for process evaluations of complex interventions in the case of the NERS policy trial in Wales. This is part of an unpublished doctoral dissertation (Cardiff University).

Template of a Service Development Scope Document
Scope
Objective
Duration of programme
Location of sessions
Delivery team
Team lead
Proposed start date
Quality standards
Referral documents and data collection
Frequency of reporting and identify who will receive the report

FIGURE 3.1 Sample template of a service development scope document

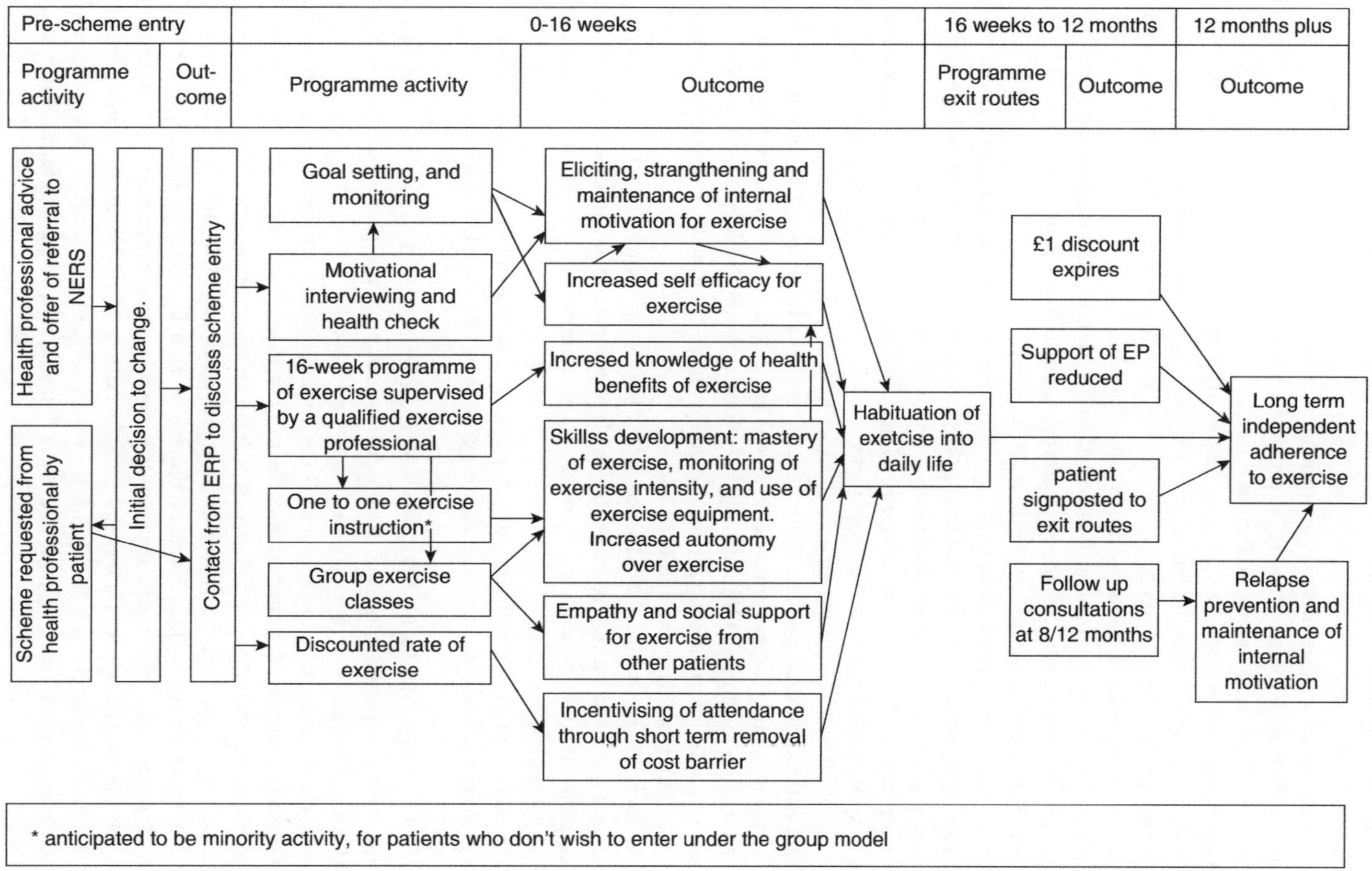

FIGURE 3.2 Developing a mix of methods framework for process evaluations of complex interventions

From the logic model, we can identify all processes that are essential to ensure compliance with the approved pathway and provide evidence to support ongoing funding:

- The patient has an assessment with a primary care or allied health professional to determine if they meet the programme criteria and are inactive: that is, they are not meeting current UK physical activity guidelines (2019).
- A formal referral is made by a primary care or allied health professional to an individual physical activity specialist or the exercise referral programme coordinator.
- On receipt, the referral form should be checked for completeness, and it should be established that the referral meets the programme criteria.
- An invite is sent to the patient to attend a consultation to fully explain the programme and discuss their current health, establish their current lifestyle and activity level and set their short-, medium- and long-term goals.
- Once the patient's physical activity capabilities have been assessed utilising evidence-based fitness or function tests and their goals have been discussed, a planned programme of activities to meet their specific needs is jointly discussed and agreed on.
- A start date is scheduled, and advice is offered for those unfamiliar with leisure centres (e.g. type of clothing to wear, show them around the facility explaining where everything is and how to use changing room lockers etc.).
- Gain patient's written permission for all collected data to be stored in a secure database that meets with UK government GDPR guidance. It is also useful to review the Information Commissioner's Office Guidance, which is the UK's independent authority set up to uphold information rights in the public interest, promoting openness by public bodies and data privacy for individuals.
- The exercise professional should schedule the follow-up review consultations to ensure the programme continues to meet the needs of the patient and complete all the same pre-programme assessments at the end of the programme to evidence success and feedback to referrer.
- The exercise professional should also offer advice to the patient on appropriate exit route sessions to maintain activity to further improve their health and well-being.

Figure 3.3 highlights the Welsh NERS process chart from referral to first consultation and identifies who is responsible for each action. It is essential that this process is reviewed regularly to ensure it remains compliant with national guidance.

A flow chart's purpose is to highlight all the considerations and identify the appropriate action, ensuring that everyone understands their roles and responsibilities. The NERS process chart references an operational handbook, which is a culmination of over 30 years' experience of ERS delivery. It was specifically written as an induction manual for new NERS instructors but is also used as an aid to ensure there is compliance with all protocols and procedures. This handbook is currently subject to copyright. It is the role of the programme's coordinator to check that the referrals received meet the criteria and to inform the health professional and client if they are ineligible. It is the coordinator who assigns the referral to the appropriately qualified exercise professional to meet the patient's needs. The exercise referral practitioner's role is to:

- Assess, monitor and manage risk to clients arising from exercise participation throughout the referral period

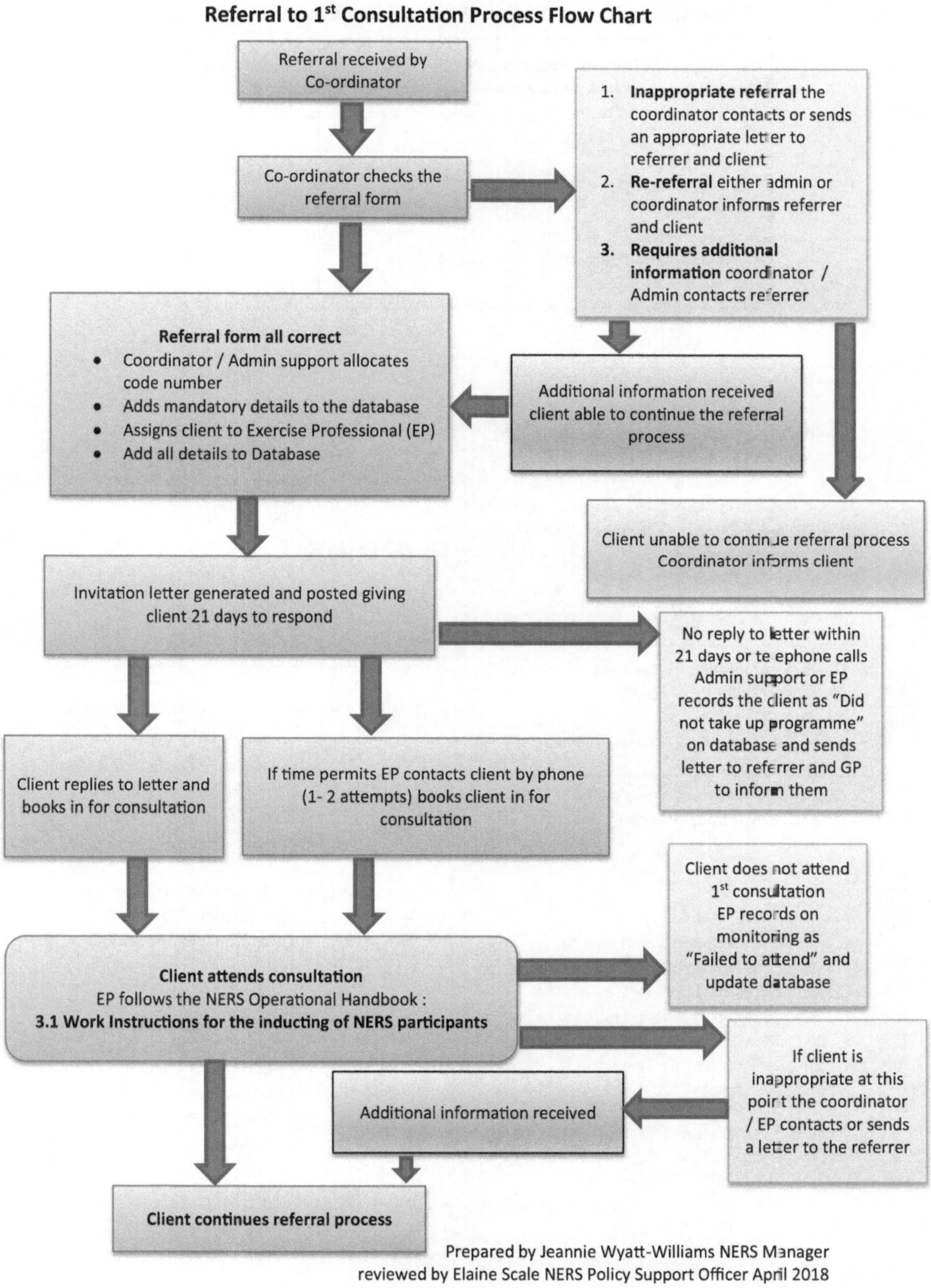

FIGURE 3.3 Welsh NERS process chart from referral to first consultation (April 2018)

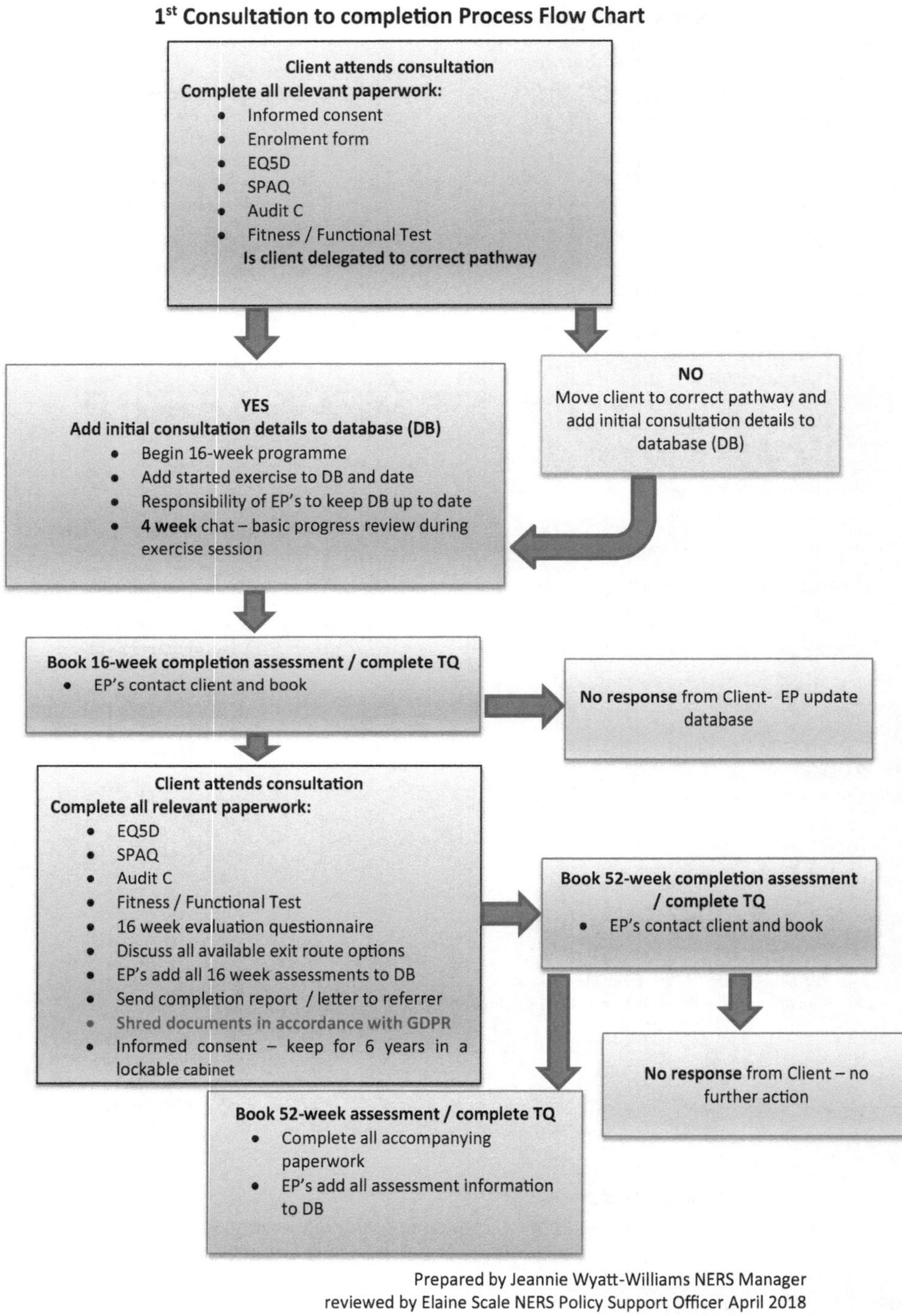

FIGURE 3.3 (Continued)

- Analyse information relating to individual clients about safe and effective programme design
- Identify, agree on and review short-, medium- and long-term goals to ensure the effectiveness of exercise programmes
- Promote a range of physical activity opportunities in accordance with the needs and health status of the client
- Tailor progressive exercise appropriate to the client's medical condition, using results from the physical/exercise assessments, medical information, national guidelines and client goals and objectives
- Develop and apply strategies to motivate clients to adhere to an exercise programme during the referral period
- Keep up to date with health and fitness industry developments and exercise guidelines for medical conditions
- Make the appropriate decisions relating to clients; where required, refer the client to a more appropriate professional

Occupational competence

It is important that the exercise referral professionals are aware of the boundaries of their role and qualification and are able to make the appropriate decisions and, when required, refer the person to a more appropriate professional (e.g. a specialist exercise instructor for a specific medical condition or a health professional). To ensure successful programmes, the exercise professional is responsible for:

- Completing a fitness and/or function test, ensuring that they use the correct protocol so the tests can be replicated at the end of the programme
- Delivering the exercise referral programme that meets the individual's needs
- Reviewing the individual's activity programmes regularly to ensure they are progressively improving their fitness and functional abilities and build rapport and trust with the individual
- Completing fitness inductions to promote confidence so individuals can safely get on with their programme independently in between supervised sessions
- Completing and recording all appropriate outcome measures to ensure all members of the MDT are aware of the results and any actions that may need addressing
- Reviewing progress and completing all pre/post assessments with the client

If the condition of the client changes during the scheme and they are no longer eligible, the exercise professional should inform the coordinator so appropriate action can be taken. The overall objective of consultations and data collection is to motivate and support people to take up the offer of the programme and contribute to evidencing improved physical activity levels and thereby improvements in the health and well-being of the people referred. At the first consultation the exercise professional carries out specific baseline measures and a health status and medication check, which help indicate the most effective outcome measures to complete as a baseline, and these results identify the type of activity most appropriate for the person. Time and careful consideration during this first consultation will help build the necessary rapport with the person and gain their trust, which will aid positive outcomes for both the person and the programme. The following provides an example of measures and tests that should form part of an effective consultation:

- Health check tool (e.g. Irwin and Morgan), including a review of current medication to look at any that may affect their ability to engage in or tolerance for physical activity
- Height
- Weight
- Waist circumference
- Blood pressure
- Resting heart rate
- Scottish Physical Activity Questionnaire: Seven-day recall physical activity questionnaire
- EQ-5D-5L Quality of Life questionnaire
- An appropriate fitness/function test such as a six-minute walk test, shuttle walk, timed up and go, sit-to-stand

These measures, tools and methods will enable you to create meaningful reports evidencing your participants improved health and well-being and help support bids for continued funding.

Exercise referral policies

It is important to have knowledge of any policies that support ERS to help convince the health professionals who express concern about their personal and professional liability if they send or refer a patient to the gym and they have a sudden medical event. In April 2001, the Department of Health published 'Exercise Referral Systems: National Quality Assurance Framework (NQAF), which provides guidelines for exercise referral systems, with the aim of improving standards among ERS and helping the development of new schemes. The framework focuses primarily on the most common model of exercise referral system, in which the GP or practice nurse refers patients to facilities such as local authority leisure centres or private gyms for supervised exercise programmes. The guidance also covers issues including patient selection, evaluation and long-term follow-up.

The Exercise Referral Toolkit (2010) was developed and written by the British Heart Foundation National Centre for Physical Activity and Health to support professionals to design, deliver, commission and evaluate ERS. The toolkit is now hosted by the National Centre Sports and Exercise Medicine (NCSEM). It is a practical guide for all professionals involved in the delivery, coordination, commissioning and evaluation of exercise referral schemes. This resource has been developed in consultation and collaboration with a range of professionals involved with ERS and key national stakeholders. It draws on current government policy for the design and delivery of quality-assured exercise referral schemes; it is not a replacement for national policy and should be used in conjunction with the NQAF. It uses the evidence base and local scheme practice to support schemes in meeting the guidelines set out within the NQAF and to raise standards within schemes.

This document states that ERS should consist of all the following components:

- An assessment involving a primary care or allied health professional to determine that someone is sedentary or inactive: that is, they are not meeting current UK physical activity guidelines (see Start active, stay active)

- A referral by a primary care or allied health professional to a physical activity specialist or service
- A personal assessment involving a physical activity specialist or service to determine what programme of physical activity to recommend for their specific needs
- An opportunity to participate in a physical activity programme

Some schemes also review participants' progress at completion of the scheme. This opportunity to gather outcome data and evidence programmes success is useful in obtaining continued funding. It also provides a recommendation for exercise referral for people who are sedentary or inactive but otherwise healthy.

Recommendation 1

Policy-makers and commissioners should not fund ERS for people who are sedentary or inactive but otherwise apparently healthy.

Primary care practitioners should not refer people who are sedentary or inactive, but otherwise apparently healthy, to ERS.

Referral to an appropriate exercise service is recommended for people who are sedentary or inactive and have a health condition or other health risk factors.

Recommendation 2

Policy-makers and commissioners should only fund ERS for people who are sedentary or inactive and have existing health conditions or other risk factors that put them at increased risk of ill health. ERS are encouraged to incorporates the core techniques outlined in 'Behaviour change: individual approaches' (NICE public health guidance 49).

These include:

- Recognising when people may or may not be more open to change
- Agreeing on goals and developing action plans to help change behaviour
- Advising on and arranging social support
- Tailoring behaviour-change techniques and interventions to individual need
- Monitoring progress and providing feedback
- Developing coping plans to prevent relapse
- Collecting data in line with the 'essential criteria' outlined in the standard evaluation framework for physical activity interventions

Specifically:

- Programme details
- Evaluation details
- Demographics of individual participants
- Baseline data
- Follow-up data (impact evaluation), process evaluation
- Make the data collected available for analysis, monitoring and research to inform future practice

Primary care practitioners should only refer people who are sedentary or inactive and have existing health conditions or other factors that put them at increased risk of ill health to an ERS if they meet these criteria. It is worth pointing out that NICE have also updated their guidance for the role of structured exercise programmes in the management of, and rehabilitation following, a health condition.

It is important to stress that there are phase 4 rehabilitation programmes that are structured, tailored with supervised activities and 'must only be delivered by a specialist physical activity and exercise instructor trained in exercise for relevant chronic condition(s)'. As an exercise referral practitioner, should you receive an inappropriate referral that your qualification does not allow you to accept, you need to either:

- Return the referral form, explaining your inclusion/exclusion criteria to better inform future referrals.
- Forward the referral to the relevant department, if you are working as part of a multidisciplinary team. You must inform the referrer where you have forwarded the referral form so they know for the future and explain your inclusion/exclusion criteria to better inform future referrals to yourself.
- Find a local, appropriately qualified specialist exercise instructor who would be willing to accept the referral. You must inform the referrer where you have forwarded the referral form so they know for the future and explain your inclusion/exclusion criteria to better inform future referrals to yourself.

As the exercise referral practitioner, you should familiarise yourself with:

- NICE Guidance in Relation to Physical Activity: Exercise Referral Schemes (Public Health Guideline [PH54], September 2014)
- Physical Activity Guidelines: Guidance from the Chief Medical Officers in the UK on the Amount and Type of Physical Activity People Should Be Doing to Improve Their Health (Department of Health and Social Care, 7 September 2019)
- Behaviour Change: Individual Approaches (NICE Public Health Guidance 49, 2 January 2014)

Exercise referral in healthcare

Health-care professionals have a crucial role to play in promoting physical activity with patients and ensuring they are offered the safest and most appropriate physical activity pathway to meet their health-care needs and personal preferences. The NICE Guidance 'Physical Activity: Exercise Referral Schemes' (Public Health Guideline [PH54], September 2014) has highlighted specific conditions that must be met before health-care providers will refer into physical activity programmes, and, despite this guidance only being targeted at primary care practitioners, this same quality assurance is required by secondary care providers if and when you or your exercise referral staff are appropriately trained to provide exercise for higher-risk target populations, as highlighted in Recommendation 2 earlier.

Programmes must also incorporate the core techniques outlined in 'Behaviour Change: Individual Approaches' (NICE Public Health Guidance 49). The key concern for many health-care professionals is the time it takes to complete a referral form to transfer the necessary medical information from a health-care practitioner to an appropriately qualified exercise referral practitioner. It is essential to make your referral form as accessible and easy to complete as possible and to set up a secure transfer procedure compliant with the UK government's GDPR Guidance and Information Commissioner's office to assure participant data protection and minimise the risk of poor uptake of your service.

The multidisciplinary team

A multidisciplinary team (MDT) is a group of different professionals who specialise in specific disciplines to support a patient in managing their health and well-being. Within primary care, you may have a general practitioner, a practice and/or specialist nurse, a health advisor and, in some areas, you may have physiotherapists or exercise specialists. Each person on the multidisciplinary team is responsible for the provision of services or treatments in which they specialise. Most multidisciplinary teams will have a key worker assigned to the patient, serving as that person's primary contact point to the rest of the team. The patient is then able to follow an all-inclusive specific care plan that all professionals have collaborated to develop. Ultimately, their aim is to provide the patient with the specific services they require to maintain an independent life.

As an exercise professional, you should offer your expertise to these multidisciplinary teams to gain their trust by working closely with and informing them of your qualifications, details of your sessions and any case studies or evidential outcome measures you may have to encourage referrals into your programme. There are advantages and disadvantages to consider when looking at the structure and services that a multidisciplinary team is able to provide as follows:

Advantages:

- **It gives a patient access to an entire team of experts.**
  - When a multidisciplinary team is formed, it allows a patient to receive collaborative support from a wide range of experts.
  - Each person contributes from their own perspective, which can then enhance the treatments which are offered by others.
  - This process works to ensure that every patient is given access to the best possible treatment options that are currently available.
- **It improves service coordination.**
  - Although there are greater time commitments involved for members of an MDT, there are greater efficiencies offered to the patient.
  - When the services are coordinated, there is a framework of uniformity provided to each person that improves treatment delivery.
- **It speeds up the referral process.**
  - MDT are often composed of experts in their specific fields of practice. That means a patient who must receive a referral for a specific treatment will already have access to the people who need to make that happen.
  - The MDT can work together to get processes approved, delays minimised and treatments started to give that person the best possible chance to restore or maintain their health status.

- **It creates new avenues for service implementation.**
  - One of the best reasons to have an MDT is that it provides the patient with access to resources from multiple departments and organisations, making the service patient centred and offering a more comprehensive intervention with better patient outcomes.
- **It allows patients to create goals for themselves.**
  - An MDT team offers patients a chance to set specific daily, weekly, monthly and yearly goals for themselves. This allows the team to engage with the goals, holding themselves and the patient accountable for the desired outcome.
  - It also gives the MDT a chance to encourage family participation with the goals, which can improve care coordination and even reduce inpatient stays in some situations.
  - Although there may be personality conflicts to manage, most patients see more progress with an MDT than without one.

Disadvantages:

- **Time pressure involved in providing service and communicating with MDT.**
  - When working with a MDT, there are two key elements to consider for each person instead of one. Not only are they responsible for finishing their own work with the patient; they must also spend time communicating with the rest of the patient's team.
  - They must respond to any modifications that happen to the treatment plan, sometimes even those that do not apply to them. Even though it is a collaborative process, there are non-collaborative elements which take place.
- **Different team members come from unique backgrounds.**
  - An MDT succeeds when there is similarity in member backgrounds and educational experiences. The reality of the modern team is that you get a wide mix of people, some just starting their careers while others may be approaching retirement.
  - Different jobs happen on different schedules as well, which creates challenges when trying to provide services.
  - Then there is the issue of a behavioural psychologist not necessarily knowing what a social worker or exercise professional's roles is within the MDT, and vice-versa.
- **It requires frequent collaboration to be effective.**
  - MDTS must meet frequently to provide collaboration and communication to keep everyone on the same page. Although some time can be saved by having each person offer information at specific times, then review notes of the entire meeting later, a large MDT meeting might last two to three hours for the patient involved. For most people, that is a lot of time that they are forced to take out of their day.
- **It is dependent on available resources.**
  - MDTs are forced to rely on whatever resources, including manpower, are available to the patient at the time. That means it may not be possible for all the

recommendations of the team to be implemented at the same time. In that kind of circumstance, the treatments which take the top priority would be implemented first, forcing other members of the team to attend meetings even though they are not playing an active role in the outcomes being achieved.

- **Incomplete decisions happen without complete information.**
    - MDTs work best when everyone present is working within a defined role on the patient's behalf. To create these roles, there must be complete information access, including evaluations, surveys and other unique data points. Without this information, the decisions that the team makes will be unable to maximise the potential benefits that the patient may need to receive.
- **If it was not documented, then it did not happen.**
    - Over the course of any given day, a member of an MDT might be working with more than a dozen patients, but if they fail to document any facts or information, then it effectively did not happen. Many governments provide oversight of MDT meetings, which means there can be civil or criminal investigations as an outcome of missed services.

With regard to the advantages and disadvantages of an MDT, it is clear they can provide more effective care. The quality of that care is dependent on the resources that are available from the community, each service provider, and the patient themselves. When everyone works together to achieve an outcome, then good things can happen.

Funding exercise referral services

Funding of exercise referral continues to be challenging, especially for an independent exercise professional; therefore, it is essential that you understand that commissioning is the process of assessing needs, planning and prioritising, purchasing and monitoring health services. To get the best health outcomes, it is essential that your offer is for a high-quality service that meets the local needs and priorities, and you have the means to verify that your service can be delivered efficiently and effectively. The use of a logic model indicating a clear and concise offer will help this process of approaching potential funders. In many cases, the commissioning will be carried out by clinical commissioning groups, public service boards or the local health board. There may also be joint commissioning arrangements and other single commissioning organisations, and in some circumstances, the commissioners and providers may exist within the same organisation, as in the case of a charitable trust. Commissioners will need to comply with their internal procurement processes and procedure to ensure they:

- Ensure best value for money
- Meet world-class commissioning competencies
- Allow commissioners to evaluate a range of market providers and ensures the 'best fit' for the service specification
- Review current contracts towards performance improvement
- Fulfil legal obligations under European Union procurement rules

Case study

In 2007, to specifically address the concerns of funding exercise referral schemes as highlighted in the National Institute for Clinical Excellence publication regarding ERS, 'A Rapid Review of the Effectiveness of Exercise Referral Schemes' (Williams et al., 2007), the Welsh government (WG) agreed to fund an RCT to determine the effectiveness of exercise referral as an intervention to increase physical activity and improve health. WG brought together health, leisure and research partners to discuss the opportunities and barriers to setting up a funded National Exercise Referral Scheme (NERS), with standardised protocols and to include an RCT. Several local authorities and corresponding health partners signed up to the programme, and in 2007, the WG established the NERS to address this lack of evidence by conducting an RCT to determine the effectiveness of exercise referral as an intervention to increase physical activity and improve health.

The scheme was fully evaluated to monitor the impact on long-term adherence to physical activity, improvements in health and potential cost savings to the health service. NERS was designed to build on the best practices from the UK and the current evidence base and to operate to national standards. Initial funding by Welsh government in 2007 was for three years and only available to areas that agreed to deliver the programme as part of a robust evaluation. Eleven local authority areas signed up, and the results were published in 2010. The aim of the NERS programme was to reduce the inequalities in ill health by providing access to tailored and supervised physical activity and behavioural change intervention for those aged 16+ across Wales who were inactive and at risk of or currently experiencing a long-term or chronic health condition.

The full results can be obtained at https://gov.wales/evaluation-national-exercise-referral-scheme-wales-0.

These results and continued improvement in retention and outcome measures have secured ongoing funding; this approach has strengthened the collaborative approach to exercise referral delivery in Wales.

Currently, the programme annually receives in excess of 30,000 referrals from suitably qualified NHS health professionals.

Retention currently stands at 56.85%, which is steadily growing year on year and a huge increase from the 44% retention reported in the evaluation report that evidenced that the NERS programme was cost effective.

NERS management is by WLGA because its primary purposes are to promote better local government and its reputation and to support authorities in the development of the policies and priorities which will improve public service and democracy. It represents the 22 local authorities is Wales that deliver the NERS programme.

The WLGA promotes equality and fairness for all with a priority theme for 2018–2019 to health and social care services and integration and investment in preventative services, based on an improvement evidence base with appropriate investment, to encourage a focus on preventative and well-being services to help reduce demand on health and social care services.

The NERS quality standards are maintained by regularly reviewing all protocols used in the programme to ensure they continue to meet the latest national guidance.

The NERS programme continues to be supported by the Welsh government (WG) working in partnership with the Welsh Local Government Association (WLGA), local authorities (LA), Public Health Wales (PHW), local health boards (LHBs) and primary and secondary care health professionals.

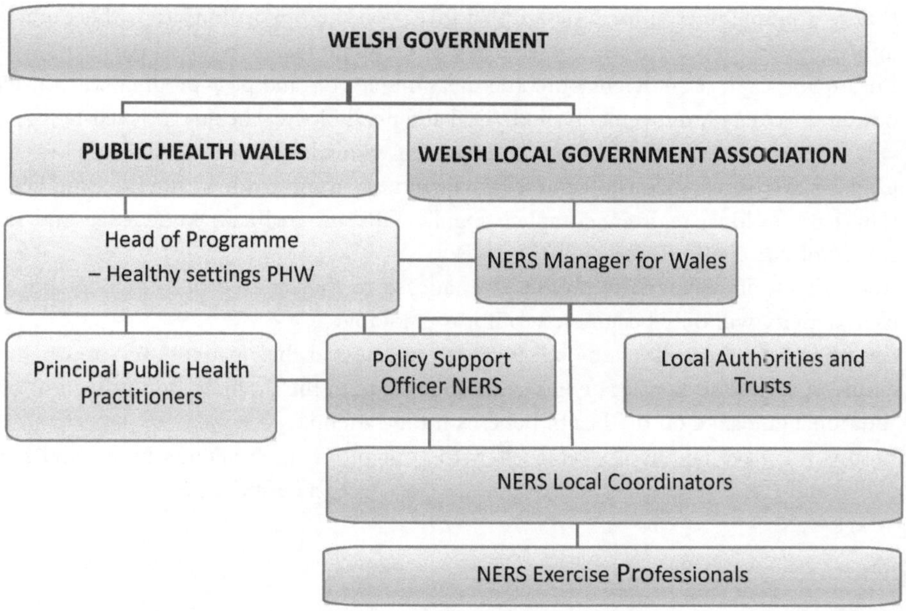

FIGURE 3.4 NERS organisational chart

The WLGA's primary purposes are carefully incorporated in NERS delivery across the local authorities of Wales.

Here is the link to the NERS website for more information and case studies: www.wlga.wales/national-exercise-referral-scheme-ners.

Chapter summary

This chapter and example are not written as a 'blueprint' for how ERS must be designed, implemented and evaluated, but they offer some best-practice principles for all those involved in the delivery, management and commissioning of ERS.

It is for you as individuals to consider whether the implementation of these principles will improve the design, delivery and effectiveness of your programme, given the capacity and resources available to you and your ERS.

Make as many contacts as possible with your local health professionals and try wherever you are able to become part of their MDT; this may open doors for additional funding, but it will definitely provide you with some 'free' continuing professional development that will enhance your CV and professional practice.

Ensure you keep up to date with all relevant UK government and NICE guidance, which may require you to amend your referral programme to ensure you are compliant with all latest standards.

Key points

- Ensure you develop a clear and concise referral process.
- Engage with your local health partners and develop a working relationship to develop mutually agreed inclusion/exclusion criteria for your programme.

- Ensure a simple referral form design that gives you the opportunity to gather sufficient information to develop a safe and effective programme for the referred person.
- Ensure you capture sufficient outcome measures at pre- and post-programme consultations to evidence improvements in physical and psychological health and well-being; this will support you with funding bids or engaging with additional referral routes.
- Understand the parameters of your level 3 qualification and work within these guidelines.
- Join a professional register, complete regular CPD to maintain knowledge and keep abreast of current guidance.
- Always prescribe an activity programme tailored to the referred person's likes and dislikes; activity will only be adhered to if it is enjoyable.
- Ensure you report back to the referrer with updates on their patient's progress but also ensure you inform them of people who do not attend the programme so they can offer additional guidance on the health benefits if they attend.
- Ensure you have familiarised yourself with your programme venue's health and safety policy and risk assessments and that you have access to a defibrillator.

Study tasks

1. Define the difference between referral and recommendation to exercise.
2. Research a minimum of two exercise referral programmes to inform the development of a flow process for your intended exercise referral programme.
3. Request other exercise referral programmes' forms to inform the development of your own forms.
4. Identify your programme's inclusion and exclusion criteria using an evidenced-based risk stratification health check for guidance.
5. Prepare a draft for a patient information leaflet and a health professionals information leaflet; identify how and why they would differ.
6. Identify three conditions that would be excluded from your programme and explain why.
7. Research suitable outcome measures and select which of them you will use and when to evaluate your programme's success; describe how and when could you use this.
8. How would you approach a health professional to describe your programme?
9. What are the benefits of joining a professional register?
10. How would you report your outcome measures to a health professional?

References

Behaviour change: Individual approaches'. NICE Public Health Guidance 49. Published: January 2014. www.nice.org.uk/Guidance/PH49

Dept of Health Publication (2001): Exercise referral systems: A national quality assurance framework. https://webarchive.nationalarchives.gov.uk/+/www.dh.gov.uk/en/Publicationsandstatistics/Publications/PublicationsPolicyAndGuidance/DH_4009671

The Exercise Referral Toolkit (2010): This resource was written and produced by the British Heart Foundation National Centre for Physical Activity and Health. www.ncsem-em.org.uk/resources/exercise-referral-toolkit/

Information Commissioner's Office: GDPR guidance. https://ico.org.uk/

Irwin and Morgan Stratification Tool- V02-Iss 2 – October 19. www.cntw.nhs.uk/content/uploads/2017/12/HS-PGN-14-App9-Irwin-Morgan-RiskStratTool-V02-Iss-2-Oct-19.pdf#:~:text=Irwin%20and%20Morgan%20Risk%20Stratification%20Tool%20The%20Irwin,categories%20of%20risk%20are%20demonstrated%20below%3A%20Low%20Risk

Murphy, Simon, Larry Raisanen, Graham Moore & Lawrence Moore (2010): *The evaluation of the National Exercise Referral Scheme in Wales*. Published: 2010. Cardiff Institute of Society and Health, School of Social Sciences, Cardiff University, Cardiff, Wales,

NHIR: Exercise referral schemes increase physical activity for some. Published: 14 October 2015. Produced by the University of Southampton and Bazian on behalf of NIHR through the NIHR Dissemination Centre. https://evidence.nihr.ac.uk/alert/exercise-referral-schemes-increase-physical-activity-for-some/

NICE Guidance Physical activity: Exercise referral schemes. Public Health Guideline [PH54]. Published: 24 September 2014. www.nice.org.uk/guidance/ph54/resources/physical-activity-exercise-referral-schemes-pdf-1996418406085

Public Health England Guidance: Introduction to logic models. Published: 7 August 2018. www.gov.uk/government/publications/evaluation-in-health-and-well-being-overview/introduction-to-logic-models

Tudor, Edwards, Rhiannon Pat Linck, Natalia Hounsome, Larry Raisanen, Nefyn Williams, Laurence Moore & Simon Murphy (2013): Cost-effectiveness of a national exercise referral programme for primary care patients in Wales: Results of a randomised controlled trial. *BMC Public Health* 13, 1021.

UK Chief Medical Officers': Physical activity guidelines. Published: September 2019. www.gov.uk/government/collections/physical-activity-guidelines

UK Government: GDPR Guidance. www.gov.uk/government/publications/guide-to-the-general-data-protection-regulation

Williams, NH, M Hendry, B France, R Lewis & C Wilkinson (2007): Effectiveness of exercise-referral schemes to promote physical activity in adults: Systematic review. *British Journal of General Practice* 57(545), 979–986.

4

HEALTH-FITNESS CONSULTATION AND ASSESSMENT SKILLS

Michelle G Swainson, Zoe H Rutherford and John P Buckley

4.1 Chapter aims

The aims of this chapter are to:

- Provide information to understand key aspects and conduct within the initial consultation and assessment
- Develop understanding of screening procedures and risk stratification
- Indicate the value and importance of key communication skills during the phases of exercise referral
- Illustrate general assessment skills that would be required and know how to adapt them, depending on the referred person
- Indicate methods for monitoring and reviewing the progress and outcomes of people with long-term conditions

4.2 The initial consultation

Once a person is referred to an exercise referral scheme (ERS), the initial consultation and assessment is their first meeting with the exercise referral (ER) practitioner, which will ultimately inform the mutually agreed-upon approach, goals and personalised programme, which is typically 12 weeks. This chapter addresses the core components of the consultation which focus on establishing communication and building rapport, identifying the current stage of change, setting achievable goals via the implementation of motivational interviewing and establishing the referred person's baseline information to assist with programme design, monitoring and reviewing. Figure 4.1 provides a simple schematic to illustrate four phases of the initial consultation, each of which will be covered in more detail as we progress through this chapter.

Phase 1 is initiated even before the consultation begins. The referred person should be properly introduced to the ER practitioner who will inform the referred person of their name and title. The purpose of the consultation is to gather information from the referred

DOI: 10.4324/9781315102399-4

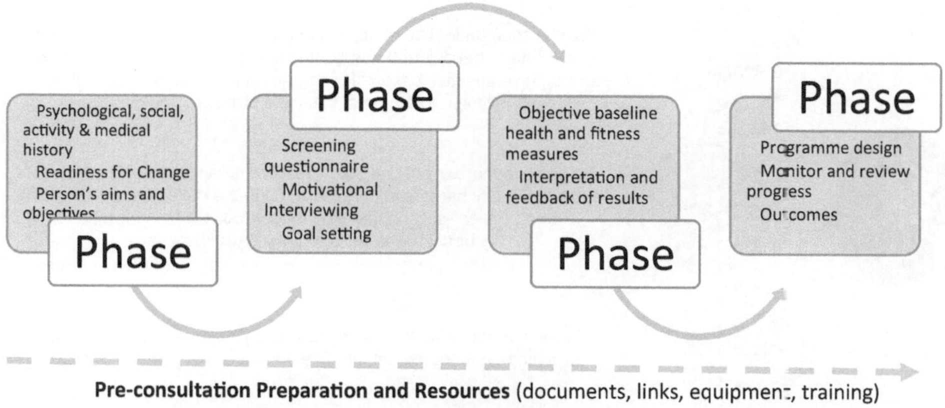

FIGURE 4.1 Schematic highlighting four phases of the phased diagram of the initial consultation

person, but it is advisable that the ER practitioner provide some information about themselves and the process in the first instance. This can support the notion of relatedness, which is a basic psychological need that requires satisfying when building a strong practitioner-referred person relationship (Williams et al., 2014). This rapport building will help the referred person understand the type of practitioner who will be supporting them over the course of the referral programme and help establish trust and show empathy. For the purpose of this chapter, we will follow the phases in order, but it is worth noting that an ER practitioner must be adaptable and prepared to alter their approach, depending on the referred person (section 4.3.2). Always remember the referred person is a key part of the process, so promote personal concordance and self-management rather than a paternalistic approach. For example, the practicalities of a consultation mean that in many cases, the referred person may make remarks that do not always follow this defined order, so effort is needed to demonstrate good listening skills, thus avoiding repetition. Allowing the discussion to flow freely as a conversational approach allows for better communication and rapport, but the ER practitioner must prompt for key information to ensure the required data are gathered to fulfil the consultation objectives.

Getting to know the referred person from Phase 1 onwards is paramount, and establishing a warm, positive interpersonal relationship early is key to personal engagement in the process, largely because this personalised time investment will confirm that you are considering their wants and needs. Before the official aspects of the consultation, it is important to gain an initial perception of how the referred person feels about attending the consultation and any apprehensions they may have (section 4.3.2). Phase 1 provides the ER practitioner with the opportunity to ask several questions that will help develop a clear picture of the referred person's subjective psychological, social, activity and medical history. We will briefly outline the type of information you should be trying to acquire during this phase and an example framework that can be used to document this pre-activity, health and lifestyle profile (Figure 4.1). Refer to the communication kills section for more detail about ways to encourage a referred person to provide information (section 4.3). In addition, Phases 1 and 2 also help establish the referred person's current stage of change, which relates to the Transtheoretical

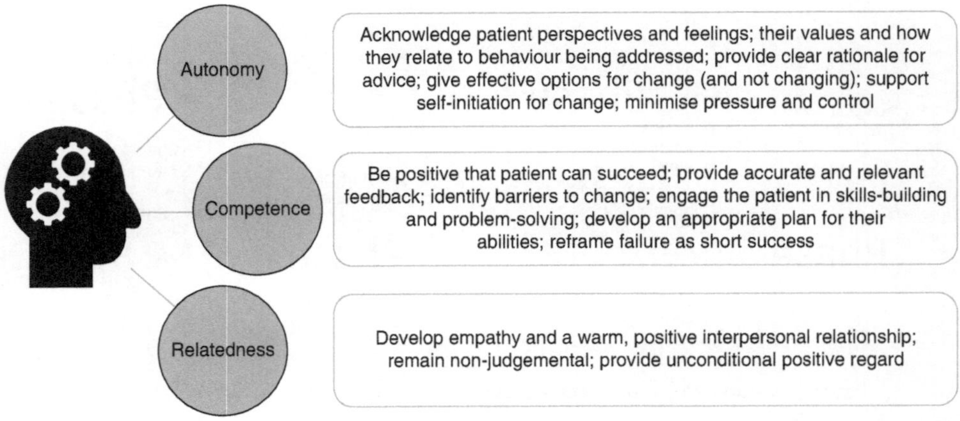

FIGURE 4.2 Self-determination theory with practical support points to facilitate an effective practitioner-patient person relationship

Source: Adapted from Williams et al., 2014

Model of Behaviour Change, which identifies the 'readiness' of a referred person to engage in the exercise referral process. In brief, most people will be in the preparation phase as they intend to take action, and the role of the ER practitioner and other relevant health-care professionals (HCP) is to encourage the referred person to progress into the action phase, in which they practice the desired behaviour, and then the maintenance phase for long-term benefits (Prochaska and Prochaska, 2014). In addition, ER practitioners should feel empowered to frame the consultation around the Self-Determination Theory (Figure 4.2). Refer to Chapter 6 for more information about behaviour change.

4.2.1 Personal, psychological, social and activity history

This includes gaining information that the referred person knows or perceives about themselves, including their name, date of birth, occupation, previous and current physical activity or exercise habits, smoking status, alcohol intake and diet. Much of this is subjective and based on self-reported recall (Figure 4.3), but the information is easily generated and helps ease the referred person into the process before the more 'probing' aspects of phase 2 (section 4.3.2) and the somewhat physically demanding aspects of phase 3 (section 4.5). Identifying any lifestyle habits that fall outside the remit of exercise referral is likely, so you should be familiar with professional services within your centre or area for referral e.g. smoking cessation.

The simple confirmation of name can be overlooked, but it is essential for a good working relationship to form. This gives the referred person the opportunity to inform the ER practitioner of their preferred or shortened name, and it is of utmost importance that their preference is respected. We cannot assume that all people will feel comfortable with the relaxed 'first-name terms' approach, and some may prefer to be called Mr or Mrs, especially if there is a notable age gap between themselves and the ER practitioner. Also, asking the referred person for their age can be somewhat sensitive, so confirming their date of birth is the best and most professional option. It is the ER practitioner's role to explain the reasons

Name	
ID number	
Consultation date	
DOB (age)	
Main reason for referral	
Occupation/social domestic responsibilities	Role: Desk-based [] Driving [] Stress level: High [] Moderate [] Low []
Daily activity *(if not using a validated PA questionnaire)*	Sedentary time: < 4 hours [] 4–7 hours [] > 7 hours [] Strength activities []; Flex/mobility []; Balance coord [] Aerobic – Light minutes/week _______ Aerobic – Mod/vig minutes/week _______
Activity/Exercise History	
Past 3 months	
Past 12 months	
Since Childhood	
Social Behaviour	
Alcohol	
Smoking	
Healthy diet awareness	
Medical	
High BP/cholesterol	Yes [] No [] Details:
Asthma/COPD	Yes [] No [] Details:
Obesity	Yes [] No [] Details:
Diabetes	Yes [] No [] Details:
Mental health	Yes [] No [] Details:
Family history of any above	Yes [] No [] Details:
Current Medications	Yes [] No [] Details:
Main reasons for them	Yes [] No [] Details:
Side effects/effects on exertion	Yes [] No [] Details:
Musculoskeletal	**Neck [] Shoulder [] Back [] Pelvis/Hips [] Elbow [] Wrist/Hands Knees [] Ankles [] Feet []** **Details:**
Clinical diagnoses	Yes [] No [] Details:
Treatments	Yes [] No [] Details:
Any other medical, physical, mental health problem?	Yes [] No [] Details:
Informed Consent	Yes [] No []
Patient signature	
Key elements related to goal setting	What are your initial thoughts/feelings (fears, anxieties or anticipated concerns) about following this exercise referral? What do you feel were the referring practitioner's reasons for making this referral? Are you comfortable with these reasons. or are there other reasons you'd like to consider? Do you have any questions before we go any further?

FIGURE 4.3 Example framework for information gathering during phase 1

this information is required; in this case, age is needed to calculate exercise prescription parameters, especially when heart rate is considered.

Given the rise in certain referred conditions amongst middle-aged adults, it should not be assumed that people will be 'older' and retired. Therefore, finding out about a referred person's occupation and social and caring responsibilities can provide an insight into their lifestyle, especially with the growing trend in sedentary workplaces and inactive commuting options. Asking about their average working week can provide information on time availability, which is often deemed a significant barrier to physical activity, as well as environment, education, socioeconomic status and attitudes that may impact on communication as well as their understanding of physical activity and accessibility to local provision (Borodulin et al., 2016). It also provides an insight into identifying options for reducing sedentary behaviour in addition to increasing their physical activity: for example, having active breaks, taking the stairs and organising walking meetings (Owen et al., 2010; Benatti and Reid-Larson, 2015). All this information can be noted on a form similar to Appendix A. Establishing their current physical activity behaviour is also very important at this stage to determine the referred person's starting point as well as finding out about their activity preferences. The referred person should complete a validated physical activity questionnaire (refer to section 4.5.2). See Appendix A for an information-gathering framework to assist with the consultation.

4.2.2 Medical history and screening

The ER practitioner should be aware of the medical condition that has led to the referred person entering into an ERS; however, it is good practice to ask the referred person why they think they have been referred in order to develop autonomy. It is important that the referred person document their medical history and any musculoskeletal issues that may impact their involvement as this will form part of the screening procedures. Prior to a person being referred into an ERS, they should have been suitably examined by their general practitioner (GP) or referring HCP and deemed safe to exercise. Early in the consultation, it is essential to check for any absolute contraindications to exercise (Table 4.1), and in the event of one or more of these being present, the referred person must be referred back to their referring HCP. It is most likely that the ER practitioner will receive information about their medical history, but the referred person must confirm their medications and any known associated side effects that may have important exercise considerations. This is covered in more detail within condition-specific chapters, but it is advisable that ER practitioners access the *British*

TABLE 4.1 Absolute contraindications to exercise

Unstable angina
Unstable or acute heart failure
Unstable diabetes
New or uncontrolled arrhythmias
Resting or uncontrolled tachycardia
Resting SBP > 180 mmHg or
Resting DBP > 100 mmHg
Symptomatic hypotension
Febrile illness
Valvular heart disease/aortic stenosis

National Formulary or utilise NHS-approved websites, including www.patient.info, to have a better understanding of medications.

There are both absolute and relative contraindications to exercise, and it is important to ensure the referred person's safety, but ER practitioners should also do everything possible to get people exercising. For example, a referred person may state that they have a contraindication, but this is a historical issue and would no longer affect their exercise safety. You need to develop interviewing skills to draw out current information by asking additional questions to determine whether a contraindication exists or not.

On confirmation that the referred person has no contraindications to exercise, they will enter a thorough screening programme prior to any specific discussions about their exercise referral programme. The purpose of the screening is to ensure the individual is safe to exercise, by means of both questionnaire and a number of resting measurements associated with cardiovascular risk. There is more detail provided on this within the General Assessment Skills section (section 4.5). On completion of the screening, further assessments provide additional baseline characteristics or 'outcome measures' that form part of phase 4, and these will be monitored over time, contributing to the review process (Section 4.6).

Traditionally in the exercise and fitness domain, the standard screening questionnaire used in practice is the Physical Activity Readiness Questionnaire (PAR-Q) (Figure 4.3), recommended in the Exercise Referral Toolkit (NCSEM, 2010). Although it is likely that an ER practitioner would follow up the standard PAR-Q with questions, there is no set guidance to be sure the correct questions have been asked for safe clearance to exercise in this group. In response to this, support exists to move towards the more recent development of the PAR-Q+ (Warburton et al., 2021, http://eparmedx.com/?page_id=79). Firstly, there is no specified age range, so it is suitable for everyone, and it allows for a more comprehensive account of the referred person's readiness to exercise, providing a structured approach to extracting further relevant information. This is the recommended tool to use in exercise referral. The very nature of receiving a person with a referred condition is that they are 'at higher risk' than the general healthy population. We should emphasise that it is the HCP who will initiate the referral, so we therefore assume the patient-doctor relationship has been effective in highlighting the risks of exercise. In the event of a referred person answering yes to one or more questions on the screening questionnaire, it is important that the ER practitioner has a record of the screening, understands the exercise risks posed by any issues on the questionnaire and can liaise directly with the HCP to avoid referring back unnecessarily. The e-PARMEDx form can supplement the PAR-Q+ if there are any positive responses; it is available at http://eparmedx.com/?page_id=79.

Risk stratification should not solely be considered a single risk score for categorising people into a classification of low, moderate or high risk. This approach is, however, commonly used in exercise referral via the Irwin and Morgan risk stratification tool (Figure 4.4).

In addition to this simplified traffic-light system, there are a number of other elements that need risk stratifying individually, including the risk of a disease developing or progressing and/or the risk of mortality, either acutely or prematurely in the future. In relation to exercise, the primary concern is to stratify based on the risk of experiencing an acute event due to exertion (i.e. during or after exercise) and the degree of supervision required to minimise this risk across different medical conditions. For example, to minimise a cardiac event, it is important to ensure a good warm-up and prolonged cool down as there is a greater likelihood of ischaemic angina on commencement and of arrhythmias during recovery (Fletcher

Low risk	
Overweight	No complications
High normal blood pressure	130–139/85–89 mmHg/not medication controlled
Deconditioned	Due to age or inactive lifestyle
Type 2 diabetes	Diet controlled
Older people aged > 65	No more than two cardiac risk factors and not a falls risk
Antenatal	No symptoms of pre-eclampsia/no history of miscarriage
Postnatal	Provided six-week check complete and no complications
Osteoarthritis	Mild where physical activity will provide symptomatic relief
Mild bone density changes	Bone mineral density (BMD) > 1 SD and < 2.5 SD below young-adult mean
Exercise-induced asthma	Without other symptoms
Smoker	One other cardiac risk factor and no known impairment of respiratory function
Stress/mild anxiety	Asymptomatic
Seropositive HIV	Asymptomatic
Medium risk	
Hypertension stage 1	140–159/90–99 mmHg or medication controlled
Type 2 diabetes	Medication controlled
Type 1 diabetes	With adequate instructions regarding modification of insulin dosage, depending on timing of exercise and warning signs
Physical disabilities	No other risk factors
Moderate osteoarthritis/rheumatoid arthritis	With intermittent mobility problems
Clinically diagnosed osteoporosis	BMD −2.5 SD at spine, hip or forearm or ≥ 4 on fracture index, with no history of previous low-trauma fracture
Surgery – pre and post	General or orthopaedic; *not cardiac*
Intermittent claudication	No symptoms of cardiac dysfunction
Stroke/transient ischaemic attack (TIA)	> 1 year ago; stable CV symptoms; ambulatory without assistance
Asthma	Mild – ventilatory limitation does not restrain submaximal exercise
Chronic obstructive pulmonary disease (COPD)	Without ventilatory limitation but would benefit from optimisation of respiratory system mechanics and correction of physical deconditioning
Neurological conditions	e.g. early-onset Parkinson's disease, multiple sclerosis
Early symptomatic HIV	Moderately diminished CD4 cells; intermittent or persistent signs and symptoms: e.g. fatigue, weight loss, fever, lymphadenopathy
Chronic fatigue syndrome	Significantly deconditioned due to long-standing symptoms

FIGURE 4.4 Irwin and Morgan risk stratification tool

Source: Adapted from *NCSEM, 2010*

Depression	Mild or moderate
Fibromyalgia	Associated impaired functional ability, poor physical fitness, social isolation, neuroendocrine and autonomic system regulation disorders
High risk	
Older people > 65 at risk of falls; frail older people with osteoporosis and history of fracture	REFER DIRECTLY TO THE FALLS SERVICE BMD ≥ 2.5 at spine, hip or forearm in the presence of one or more documented low-trauma or fragility fractures.
Unstable and uncontrolled cardiac disease	
Claudication with cardiac dysfunction	
Orthostatic hypotension	Fall in systolic blood pressure (SBP) > 20 mmHg or diastolic blood pressure (DBP) > 10 mm/Hg within three minutes of standing
Stroke/TIA	Recent (< 3 months ago)
Severe OA/RA	With associated immobility
Type 1 or type 2 diabetes –advanced	With accompanying autonomic neuropathy or advanced retinopathy
Moderate to severe asthma	Where ventilatory limitation restrains submaximal exercise
COPD	With true ventilatory limitation
AIDS	With accompanying neuromuscular complications, severe depletion of CD4 cells, malignancy or opportunistic infection
Psychiatric illness/cognitive impairment/ dementia	Abbreviated Mental Test (AMT) score < 8

Low-risk referrals	
Definition	People with minor, stable physical limitations or two or fewer cardiac risk factors (see following)
Exercise setting	Exercise referral schemes or other suitable community setting
Medium-risk populations	
Definition	People with significant physical limitations related to chronic disease or disability
Exercise setting	Exercise referral schemes or other suitable community setting
High-risk populations	
Definition	People with current severe disease or disability. Not suitable for exercise referral schemes
Exercise setting	Secondary or tertiary health-care settings only
Cardiac risk factors	
Family history	Cardiac event or cardiac surgery for female first-degree relatives (mother, father, brother, sister) aged < 45 years for male and < 55 years for female
Cigarette smoking	Current or given up in the past six months.
Hypertension	≥ 140 mmHg SBP/≥ 90 mmHg DBP

FIGURE 4.4 (Continued)

Hypercholesterolaemia	Total > 5.2 mml/L OR HDL < 0.09 mm/L OR LDL > 3.4 mmol/L
Sedentary lifestyle	Not meeting minimum recommendation ≥ 30 minutes of moderate intensity physical activity every day
Obesity	BMI ≥ 30 kg/m² or waist circumference > 100 cm
Impaired fasting glucose	≥ 6.1 mmol/L
Conditions indicating cardiac rehabilitation – phase IV	
Angina	Stable and controlled with no pain at rest
Cardiac surgery	If successful operation and has been discharged from phase III
Arrhythmia	Provided full cardiologist screening and approval
Valvular heart disease	Provided full cardiologist screening and approval
Congestive heart failure	Stable, on medical therapy without absolute contraindications (particularly obstruction to left ventricular outflow, decompensated CHF or threatening arrhythmias) and have an exercise capacity > 3 METs

FIGURE 4.4 (Continued)

et al., 2013). Most importantly, it is vital that the ER practitioner knows when not to exercise a referred person and when to refer back to the HCP.

4.3 Communication skills

To ensure a successful consultation, the ER practitioner and referred person must communicate effectively with one another and other relevant HCPs. However, the ER practitioner will have no direct control of the referred person's immediate communication skills, so the focus of this section is based on the ER practitioner's approach to verbal and non-verbal communication. It should be appreciated that this is not a 'phase' but an insight into key communication forms and skills that can relate to one or multiple phases of the consultation (Figure 4.5).

4.3.1 Non-verbal communication and considerations

There are several key considerations to be aware of to ensure the referred person feels comfortable before, during and after the consultation, which will consequently promote greater cooperation and engagement throughout the process. Primarily, environmental aspects, including the general room set-up and respecting personal space are highly important. Providing a non-clinical environment provides a more relaxed feel for the referred person. ER practitioners should consider motivational posters, testimonials, colourful and comfortable décor and furnishings with the purpose of functionality but also making it a welcoming space for people.

Positive body language from the ER practitioner is vital to help the referred person feel at ease in this potentially new environment. Positive body language is largely subjective and encompasses non-verbal attributes of an individual's personality, approachability, empathy and professionalism. The experienced ER practitioner should be able to gauge information about the referred person by observing their body language in the first instance, which should then

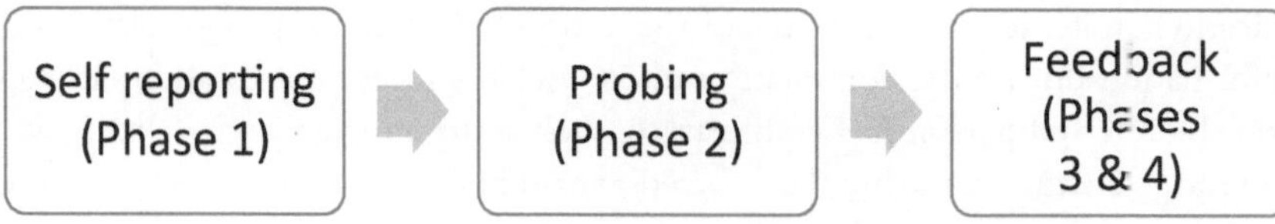

FIGURE 4.5 Stages of communication during the consultation

inform their initial approach in the consultation. For example, if a referred person is quiet, avoiding eye contact and fidgeting, this could be suggestive of apprehension. The ER practitioner must initially focus on helping them feel more comfortable and at ease – this is where investing time in 'getting to know the referred person' is fundamental to building rapport for a fruitful professional relationship (Figures 4.1 and 4.5).

Written communication plays a fundamental part of exercise referral, whether this is the completion of questionnaires within phases 1 and 2, documenting health and fitness measures in phase 3 or writing/reading progress reports in phase 4. Prior to the consultation, there will be written communication between the referring HCP and the ER practitioner, and this will continue when relaying progress reports expressing any concerns regarding their safety and suitability to the programme, which may result in referring back to the HCP. You can refer to an example letter that can be used to relay confidential information back to the HCP at agreed timescales (NCSEM, 2010; Section 5). Note that it is good practice to identify the psychosocial benefits first as these are likely to be the most prominent changes and potentially align more closely with the referred person's goals. There are a number of ethical considerations that must be attended to throughout the consultation but primarily respecting confidentiality, especially when communicating with colleagues involved in the exercise referral process.

The use of paper-based appointment cards allows the referred person to record their attendance and progress during each session, which can be checked by the ER practitioner, but primarily acts as a self-monitoring tool. There may, however, be mobile phone, tablet or computer apps that clients can now use to record this information. Following phase 3, the ER practitioner will collate information from phases 1 through 3 to formulate a paper-based exercise programme card, and this can act as the referred person's guide for supervised and non-supervised exercise. Written communication between the referred person and the ER practitioner should adhere to non-clinical terminology, use lay language and be concise for enhanced readability. As part of this relationship, the ER practitioner can signpost the referred person to additional resources to help them on their exercise referral journey. This may include various websites (e.g. the British Heart Foundation) or leaflets of local providers of physical activity opportunities that can be utilised outside the supervised sessions (e.g. yoga classes, swimming timetables, walking groups). This is one way to work towards continued physical activity and long-term behaviour change.

4.3.2 Verbal communication and motivational interviewing

Exercise referral is about changing people's physical activity behaviour to improve their current and future health, and so behaviour change should be the emphasis of the programme. In order change people's behaviour effectively, ER practitioners should adopt the most effective communication strategies to help facilitate this process. To build a strong relationship and gather information during the consultation interview, it is important to adopt an approach that makes the referred person feel comfortable, such as an informal-style 'chat', yet have a clearly outlined structure, ensuring the referred person knows what to expect from the consultation. Ensuring transparency throughout the process should allow the referred person to feel they are the driving force in the decision-making and therefore empowered to take ownership of their own commitment and progress (Teixeira et al., 2012). The way that you speak to someone is extremely important, as it is likely to be a deal breaker when you are trying to build rapport and trust with someone. Avoid familiarity too early, as calling someone 'love', 'darling' or 'mate' when you first meet them might cause offence and may imply that there is a lack of respect (refer to Section 4.2.1). The professional relationship is the single most important aspect of service delivery and should not be underestimated (Andersen and Speed, 2010), but it is a skill that will develop with experience, and ER practitioners are encouraged to observe and shadow other colleagues.

One of the most recognised forms of a client-centred consultation processes for exercise referral is motivational interviewing (Downey et al., 2021). Once trust and rapport has been established between the referred person and the ER practitioner in the initial part of the consultation, the deployment of a motivational interviewing–consistent conversation between the two is strongly advised. A general tip would be to use open questions at the start to gauge how the referred person feels about the consultation and upcoming programme, and through motivational interviewing, the ER practitioner should guide the discussion towards points that are relevant for designing the programme. Often, their own behavioural perspectives of being referred for exercise can be linked directly to current levels of intrinsic motivation, physical and social capabilities and opportunities to be active (Michie et al., 2009; Michie et al., 2011). Although the referred person has been referred for a particular condition with a focus on improving clinical outcomes, it should not be forgotten that the referred person plays the greatest role, and the programme should be based on what they want to achieve. For example, if they have been referred by their GP due to obesity, a key outcome will be weight loss; however, the referred person may want to focus more on improving their self-confidence and mood. Psychosocial benefits are widely reported within the 12-week referral period, and these are potentially the key to longer-term behaviour change and therefore warrant equal focus to physical benefits (Lederman et al., 2016).

4.4 General assessment skills

4.4.1 Pre-assessment considerations

What to do before the referred person arrives . . . be prepared!

Review your referred person

Before beginning a consultation, it is imperative that the ER practitioner knows who is attending. While phase 1 will require the review of these details (4.2.1), reviewing the referred person's notes beforehand in terms of their name, age, gender and the condition that they have been referred for will enable the ER practitioner to prepare for the consultation in a couple of ways:

1. Determine what equipment they will need to have ready and calibrated and ensure that it is working and appropriate (e.g. if they are referred for weight-loss purposes, it is important to ensure that the tape measure, callipers, scales and blood pressure cuff are the correct size).
2. Ensure that they are familiar with the referred person's condition to ensure that they consider any contraindications; it may prompt them to ask any additional questions that will help them better understand the referred person's needs, their PA history and any barriers to physical activity that may be associated with their condition.

These details might also help you moderate/tailor your language or approach when you first greet them. Picking out details from the referred person's notes (if you have them) will show that the ER practitioner is organised and has paid attention, something that will help them to build and maintain trust and is likely to develop 'buy-in' from the referred person. These points are also relevant to follow-up consultations – the ER practitioner should ensure they have familiarised themselves with who is attending and review their progress before they begin. One of the worst things that will undermine an ER practitioner's relationship with the referred person is to read their notes and ignore them for the first five minutes of the session. This does not give the impression that they care and suggests that they are not prepared.

Review the environment

Ensuring that the environment the consultation takes place in is private and appropriate for the activities that will take place is vital. If a referred person is uncomfortable for any reason (it's too hot or cold) or the consultation is being interrupted (e.g. people coming in and out, telephone ringing), then it is not going to make for a productive first impression, consultation or exercise session and may well influence whether they return for the following appointment.

1. Consider whether the consultation room is appropriate for the conversations that will be had and the measurements that will be taken.
    a. Is it sufficiently private to ensure that the referred person is comfortable sharing personal information and that this information will remain confidential?
    b. Ensure that the room is private and that there is a 'do not disturb' notice outside.
2. Consider whether the temperature and ventilation of the room are adequate for the activity being performed.
    a. Is the room too hot or cold or 'stuffy'?
    b. Is there air conditioning, and is it in good working order?
    c. Is there a water fountain in the room or close by?

Review the equipment

By knowing the attending referred person and at which point in their programme they are, the ER practitioner will be better prepared. Ensuring that the appropriate equipment is on hand for the measurements that are being taken is imperative. This doesn't just mean that the tool measures what it is supposed to measure (validity) but also that it is working correctly and that it has been calibrated for accuracy and reliability. It is also necessary to ensure that the tool being used is suitable for the person being measured (e.g. size).

Review training

Ensuring that staff have had enough training, with an excellent familiarity with all equipment and test procedures, is paramount. If an ER practitioner enters a consultation and assessment session looking like they don't know what they are doing or floundering with a new type of assessment technique or scale, then this may become a source of ill trust for a referred person. To avoid this, the key is to practice and become fluid so the delivery of the session appears second nature and, ultimately, puts a referred person at ease. It is essential that ER practitioners review their practice from time to time, keeping up to date with CPD opportunities and the latest literature. This will help inform and improve practice and ultimately improve the experience of the referred person and their likelihood of success.

Review your health and safety procedures

Adhering to health and safety policies and procedures is another vital aspect of delivering a successful exercise referral programme and should be reviewed before each session. This includes ensuring that the risk assessments conducted (see the section that follows) have been completed and actions taken. This will ensure the safety of the referred person, as well as the ER practitioner and other staff.

Risk assessment

Conducting a risk assessment of the activities that are being undertaken is of paramount importance to ensure that any hazards and risk of anything going wrong are minimised. This includes any measures, exercises and space that are being used. ER practitioners should be encouraged to work with colleagues at the venue for the exercise referral session to ensure risk assessments are in place.

Accessibility

It is likely that some of the people referred will have co-morbidities or physical disabilities that prevent them from taking part in traditional physical activities or exercise, and this may largely be related to a lack of access. It is important that the space being used for the consultation is accessible for people with impairments (again, this goes back to knowing who is being referred so that any necessary arrangements can be made) and that the physical activity and exercise space can be adapted to accommodate their needs. Indeed, this also refers to equipment. Ensure that there is wheelchair access and lifts available for those with limited mobility if sessions take place upstairs.

4.4.2 Questionnaires to support the consultation

A questionnaire is an instrument for collecting data on a given subject and involves asking the respondent to answer a set of oral or written questions. They are a quick and affordable way of collecting data in a standardised way. This means that you can measure any given variable in the same way across a number of people and across different time points. Depending on the condition that the person is being referred for, an ER practitioner may need to document (for GP reporting) or demonstrate the referred person's progress as part of their personal goals, and using a standardised questionnaire may be the best way to do this. Depending on the variable being measured, there may be numerous questionnaires available that seem to measure the same thing, but it can be confusing to decide which one is best. Whichever questionnaire is being used, the important factors to consider are:

- Does the questionnaire measure the variable or construct that it is required for?
- Is it written in a way that people will understand (both the language and the terminology used)?
- What is the time burden for the referred person (how long will it take for them to complete)?

The following are examples of variables and their associated questionnaires that may be useful across different conditions.

Physical activity

As stated in section 4.2.1, the measurement of physical activity and sedentary time using a validated questionnaire is not standard practice yet, but as with other direct measures, ensuring that the data collected is valid and reliable is essential. Furthermore, having a more comprehensive view of an individual's physical activity behaviour will help the ER practitioner support individuals to make habitual changes to their physical activity and sedentary behaviour. It will also allow them to demonstrate change over time that will help provide feedback to the referred person about their progress and the subsequent effects on their health – even if the scales or blood pressure monitor does not necessarily show change after 12 weeks.

There are a number of questionnaires that have been devised and validated for different populations (infants, children, adults, older adults, pregnant women etc.), different languages and different uses (e.g. population surveillance, test-retest, physical activity history, seven-day recall, diary), and a number of them have both a short and a long version, depending on what physical activity variable is of interest (frequency, intensity, duration, volume, mode, timing of bouts). An extremely useful resource available to help support this choice is the Diet, Anthropometry and Physical Activity (DAPA) Measurement Toolkit, which was produced by the University of Cambridge: www.measurement-toolkit.mrc.ac.uk/physical-activity/pa-splash. It is a free web-based resource to assist end users in being better equipped at using and interpreting existing data or reaching an appropriate decision on choosing methods that are fit for purpose.

One of the most widely used questionnaires is the International Physical Activity Questionnaire (IPAQ), devised by the World Health Organisation. There is both a long and a short version of this questionnaire. The short IPAQ form, 'last seven-day recall', is recommended for national monitoring and the long form for research requiring more detailed assessment

(Craig et al., 2003). The IPAQ can be found at the following link: https://sites.google.com/site/theipaq/questionnaire_links.

Quality of life

As previously discussed, the focus of any exercise referral consultation is to determine what is important to the client as much as it is to achieve the goals of improving the health risk factors that they have been referred for. To that end, one of the most important variables that we advise you to measure is health-related quality of life (QoL), as this is something that is 1) likely to be most important to the referred person and 2) likely to change over and above most physical measures over a 10- to 12-week period (Department of Health, 2002). Furthermore, guidance for the implementation and evaluation of exercise referral schemes specifically states the necessity of including QoL as an outcome measure (NICE, 2014). Use this weblink for the up-to-date recommended QoL scale and scoring chart: https://euroqol.org/ (Brooks, 1996; Hilton et al., 2015).

Fatigue

Being constantly tired or fatigued is one of the many symptoms that individuals who are referred to physical activity and exercise exhibit and may well be an important factor that an individual would like to see change over the programme. There is a dearth of evidence showing that people who attend exercise interventions for a number of chronic conditions see a significant reduction in fatigue after 12 weeks. There are several reasons for this, such as the increase in metabolism experienced as a result in an increase in muscle mass; increases in cardiovascular fitness and stamina mean that everyday tasks become easier. An obvious contributor to feeling less fatigued is the increase in sleep duration and sleep quality that many people exhibit following exercise (Dolezal et al., 2017; Kovacevic et al., 2017). The Chalder Fatigue Scale (CFQ 11) is a short questionnaire, phrased in simple English with a straightforward answering system that provides a brief tool to measure both physical and psychological fatigue (Jackson, 2015): www.goodmedicine.org.uk/files/assessment,%20chalder%20fatigue%20scale.pdf.

Sleep

Sleep is an exceptionally important factor that affects individuals' health, well-being and productivity and, paradoxically, is affected by an individual's health and physical activity status. Indeed, impaired sleep quality and quantity are associated with future morbidity and mortality (Kovacevic et al., 2017). The amount and quality of sleep is vital to ensuring that the body can repair and maintain homeostasis, as well as that learning is processed and filed in the long-term memory. One freely accessible measure of sleep quality is the Pittsburgh Sleep Quality Assessment (PSQI): http://uacc.arizona.edu/sites/default/files/psqi_sleep_questionnaire_1_pg.pdf.

Pain

If a person is referred to an ER practitioner for a musculoskeletal condition or with musculoskeletal co-morbidities, then it is highly likely that one of their goals will be to reduce their feeling of pain. Indeed, pain may be a perceived barrier to physical activity and exercise, so measuring this variable may help manage their exercise prescription as well as demonstrate progression and progress. In general, people will be more comfortable using a 0–10 pain scale and should note their pre-exercise/resting pain level (e.g. 3) as the intention is to select an appropriate exercise intensity to ensure they return to the resting level within two hours of finishing their exercise session. In the event they remain above their resting level, then the patient needs to inform the ER practitioner so changes can be made to the exercise prescription (e.g. longer rest times or lower-intensity exercises).

4.4.3 Resting baseline health measurements

In the first instance, a number of resting measurements, including resting heart rate, blood pressure, height and weight, will be measured as an extension of the standard screening questionnaire procedures (Section 4.2.2). These are measured to control for cardiovascular risk even if a person is not referred for a cardiovascular-related condition. They are valuable parameters to measure at baseline, midway through the programme and at the end to identify any changes/improvements.

Blood pressure

It is advisable to measure blood pressure (BP) even in people who have not been referred for hypertension (BP > 140/> 90 mmHg) because uncontrolled high BP is an absolute contraindication to exercise (Table 4.1). However, controlling the environmental conditions is important to ensure accuracy. Ideally, the referred person should have been seated for around ten minutes prior to the recording to have more assurance they are at ease. Being apprehensive generates a physiological response whereby the systolic BP may exceed 140 mmHg. To avoid referring the person back to the HCP due to elevated BP, allow the person more time to relax and take the measurement again. There are several other methodological considerations to ensure an accurate measure, including:

- People should be advised to refrain from caffeine, alcohol, smoking and high-intensity exercise prior to the consultation as these will temporarily increase BP. This guidance should be provided in the pre-consultation information sent via the referral scheme provider.
- Take the measurement in a quiet room to ensure the heart sounds can be clearly detected.
- Ensure legs are uncrossed with feet flat on the floor.
- The BP cuff must be the correct size for the person as if it is too small or too big, it will generate inaccurate measurements; push the sleeves out of the way so the cuff is fully wrapped around bare skin.
- Ideally, use manual BP monitoring. If the ER specialist is not competent in manual assessment, then a valid automatic monitor should be used (Wan et al., 2010). There is evidence to suggest that using automatic BP monitors reduces the 'white-coat' response associated with apprehension (Myers et al., 2011), and in general, any changes are relative to the person and the tool used, so avoid measuring pre- and post-exercise BP with different devices.

Heart rate

Resting heart rate (RHR) is classed as normal if it is between 60 and 80 beats per minute; however, a person would not be told they have tachycardia (high HR) unless it was > 100 beats per minute. It is most accurate within the exercise referral setting to have access to a HR chest strap and watch, although some automatic BP monitors do also record HR. If such equipment is not available, then manually taking the person's pulse from the radial or carotid artery provides a fallback plan (count beats for 15 seconds and multiply by four). Similar methodological considerations to BP apply here, especially around the avoidance of stimulants (food, drink, cigarettes).

As with BP, the RHR is likely to be elevated as a sympathetic response to apprehension, so provide enough time prior to taking the measurement or repeat the measurement after additional rest. A RHR < 60 beats per minute is referred to as bradycardia (slow HR), but it is not uncommon and is not always something to be concerned with. Neither is it always associated with 'fitter' hearts, so be aware that underlying cardiac conditions can contribute. As the ER specialist, if you are concerned by a slow or fast RHR in a person who would be categorised with low aerobic fitness, then you should consider contacting the HCP for confirmation/reassurance to continue. The GP may decide to send the person for some further cardiac screening, such as an ECG, to determine if there are any electrical abnormalities that are associated with their RHR. If this is the case, refer back and await further information.

Anthropometry

This umbrella term refers to the measurements of body size, shape and composition – including height, weight, body mass index (BMI) (weight/height^2) and waist circumference. BMI and waist circumference are considered in some risk stratification tools due to the association between obesity and cardiovascular risk, so they will be recorded even if the person has not been referred due to obesity. Height is measured using a free-standing stadiometer and recorded to the nearest 0.1 cm following a full inspiration, and weight is measured to the nearest 0.1 kg with shoes and heavy items removed (Lohman et al., 1991). Some people may be uncomfortable having these measurements taken, but it is the role of the ER specialist to inform them that weight (for instance) is required to predict fitness as well as for setting appropriate speeds, resistance and step heights for weight-bearing activities.

We are fully aware that BMI has its limitations at an individual level, although it remains useful for population-level epidemiological studies, but what else could you measure? Because of growing evidence linking high abdominal fat storage with disease risk, there is greater implementation of a simple waist circumference assessment. This should be measured to the nearest 0.1 cm at the same point each time to ensure accurate monitoring over time. There are two suggestions:

- *Preferred option* – the midway point between the bottom rib and top of the iliac crest (hip bone)
- *Alternative option* – the level of the umbilicus, although this tends to be favoured more for men than women

It is advised that there is limited use of the waist-to-hip ratio (WHR) (waist divided by hip circumference); despite its use in some practices, it is not consistently associated with disease outcomes and has scope to remain unchanged despite changes in body shape. For example, a female patient may have a waist circumference of 100 cm and hip circumference of 100 cm, calculating a WHR of 1.0. Following a 12-week programme, the patient may lose 10 cm from only the hips, which is fantastic, but their WHR increases to 1.11, so it is not always an effective monitoring or motivational tool. A simple and effective alternative that can be used in practice is the waist-to-height ratio (WHtR), with the general guidance being that a person's waist should be less than half their height (i.e. < 0.5) (Ashwell and Gibson, 2016).

The assessment of body composition is unlikely in exercise referral as access to gold-standard measurement tools such as DXA scanners is highly unlikely, so although several validated alternative methods exist, there are methodological issues. Using bioelectrical impedance analysis via specialised scales allows for quantification of fat, muscle and water. The skill level of the ER specialist does not influence the reliability or validity of the assessment, but people must be advised to be hydrated to avoid over-estimations of body fat content. However, there is a long-standing understanding that at least a 3% error is produced in comparison to gold-standard measurement. Some people may prefer to use skinfold callipers; however, this requires training and a considerable amount of time and practice to be deemed competent in valid and reliable assessment. It can also be argued that this method is invasive and not comfortable for the majority of referred people, and therefore, we do not advise its use in exercise referral.

4.4.4 Baseline fitness measurements

It is well documented that fitness is an independent predictor of disease outcome and mortality (Myers et al., 2002), and it is understood that people who engage in more physical activity/exercise are fitter than their less active counterparts. Choosing the most appropriate fitness test depends on available time, resources, expertise, space and the person's willingness to engage. The gold-standard assessment of aerobic fitness is usually not feasible in exercise referral settings, so alternatives are needed. We outline some validated options, but the exact protocols are well documented in other exercise testing resources.

Submaximal tests with no equipment

These typically involve walking, including the Rockport one-mile walk test and the six-minute walk test. For both tests, you ideally require a flat surface and an accurately marked-out course. The six-minute walk test is often used for older adults; the distance in metres covered within six minutes is measured, and the assessment has good test-retest reliability (Jones et al., 1998). Its focus is on functional capacity as opposed to providing a fitness prediction, but it does provide a good benchmark for monitoring people's progress, plus clinically meaningful distance changes have been reported (Bohannon and Crouch, 2017). The protocol guidelines are documented to ensure standardised testing (American Thoracic Society, 2002), and Figure 4.6 illustrates the set-up of a 60 m circuit with chairs provided for when rest is required.

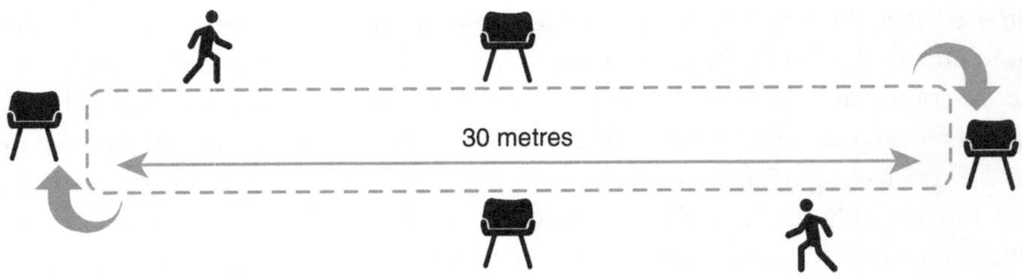

FIGURE 4.6 Six-minute walk test

For the Rockport one-mile test, HR is monitored at each quarter-mile point; the person need to walk continuously, as fast as they can, and the overall time to complete one mile is recorded. Fitness is calculated via the following equation:

$$\text{Predicted } VO_2\text{max} = 132.853 - (0.0769 \times \text{weight}) - (0.3877 \times \text{age}) + (6.3150 \times \text{sex}) - (3.2649 \times \text{time}) - (0.1565 \times \text{heart rate})$$

Weight (lbs); Sex (1 = male, 0 = female); Time (minutes)

It should be noted that not all facilities will have space for the 30 m distance or to accommodate the one mile. The Incremental Shuttle Walk Test (ISWT) typically used in UK cardiac and pulmonary rehabilitation has a similar set-up to the six-minute walk test but uses a shorter 10 m distance, with the aim being to walk as long as possible at the pace set by an audio signal (beeps quicken as progress continues through the levels), but there is an associated cost for the resources. Information can be found at this link: www.leicestershospitals.nhs.uk/aboutus/departments-services/pulmonary-rehabilitation/for-health-professionals/incremental-shuttle-walk/.

Submaximal tests with equipment

These tests include a variety of step-, cycle- and treadmill-based protocols, and it is important to select appropriately for the person and to acknowledge the validity and reliability of the tests. It is worth noting that cycle and treadmill ergometers may not be available in exercise referral facilities, so consider the suitability of step tests while acknowledging they can be quite difficult for those with balance issues and quite intense for those with low aerobic fitness.

Step tests include the Queens College step test (McArdle et al., 1972), Chester step test (Sykes and Roberts, 2004) and YMCA step test, to name a few, and these provide a quick and affordable option, but which is best? Some protocols, such as the Harvard step test, require a high step height, cadence and longer test duration that may be more suitable for those with higher aerobic fitness and not necessarily appropriate for people referred for exercise.

The Queens College step test protocol requires:

- Step up and down on a 41.3 cm–high platform at a rate of 22 steps per minute for women and 24 steps per minute for men.
- Participants are to step using a four-step cadence – 'up-up-down-down' – for three minutes.

- Stop immediately upon completion of the test and record recovery HR for one minute. This can be achieved by manual pulse monitoring if no HR monitor is available.
- Calculate predicted VO_2max using these equations (McArdle et al., 1972):
    - *Men:* VO_2max (ml/kg/min) = 111.33 − (0.42 × heart rate (bpm)
    - *Women:* VO_2max (ml/kg/min) = 65.81 − (0.1847 × heart rate (bpm)

If there is access to a cycle ergometer and a HR monitor, then the standard six-minute Astrand submaximal protocol is commonly used, whereby VO_2max predictions are based on the Astrand-Ryhming nomogram (Figure 4.7). The key requirements of this test are to encourage the person to maintain a cadence of 50 rpm and be able to record an accurate HR

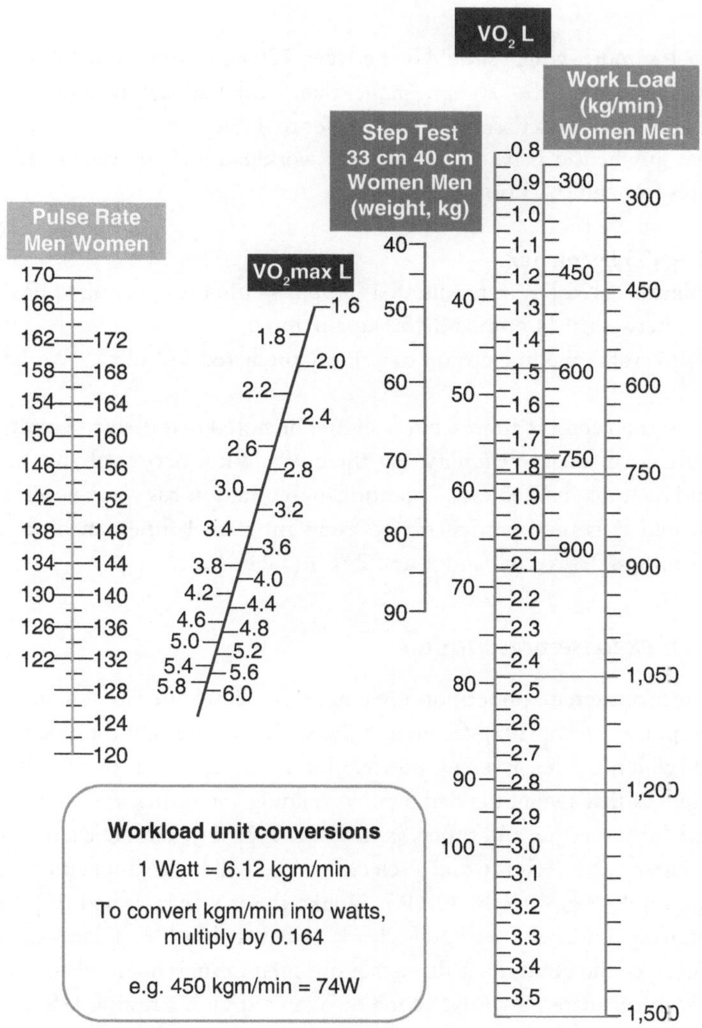

FIGURE 4.7 Astrand-Rhyming nomogram

Source: ACSM, 2018

TABLE 4.2 Guide to exercise workloads for the Astrand-Ryhming cycle test

	Untrained/Inactive	*Trained/Active*
Men	300–600 kg/m/min (50–100W)	600–900 kg/min (100–150W)
Women	300–450 kg/m/min (50–75W)	450–600 kg/min (75–100W)

TABLE 4.3 Functional tests included in the Senior Fitness Test

Strength	30-second sit-to-stand; number of arm curls in 1 minute
Flexibility	Back scratch; chair sit-and-reach test
Aerobic	6-minute walk test; 2-minute step test (if limited space)
Balance/Agility	8-feet timed up and go

at the end of each minute, which should be between 120 and 170 bpm (ACSM, 2018). If the HR is below or above the 120–170 bpm range, then workloads can be adjusted accordingly. In order to set appropriate exercise workloads, refer to Table 4.2.

The VO_2max prediction is based on the final workload and the calculated average HR between minutes five and six. Using Figure 4.7 as an example:

- Workload = 450 kg/m/min
- HR recording = 142 bpm (5 minutes), 146 bpm (6 minutes), average HR 144 bpm
- Draw a line between 144 bpm and 450 kg/m/min
- Read the VO_2 value the line crosses to identify predicted VO_2max = 2.6 L/min

We have focused on aerobic fitness, but it should be noted that there are multiple tests that relate to strength, balance and flexibility, but these would not necessarily be standard assessment and would be implemented on a condition-by-condition basis. However, one example battery of validated tests used particularly to assess functional fitness in older adults is the updated Senior Fitness Test (Rikli and Jones, 2013) (Table 4.3).

4.4.5 Basics of exercise prescription

In very simple terms, exercise prescription relates to the 'dose' of exercise required to initiate a favourable 'response', comprising frequency (how often), intensity (how hard), time (how long) and type (which mode). Exercise prescription is not the focus of this chapter, but the point to highlight is that recommended aerobic training intensities are often based on HR zones determined from resting and fitness assessment. Typically, aerobic exercise is prescribed based on heart rate reserve (HRR), and a selected range will be used specific to guidance for the referred condition (e.g. 40–60% HRR). Unlike the well-established ACSM guidelines, the exercise intensity guidelines are not as clearly stated within UK documentation, but the 'best' dose for each of the conditions/diseases is outlined in subsequent chapters.

For example, to calculate 60% HRR for a 65-year-old with a resting HR of 70 beats per minute, you must:

1. Calculate the maximum HR – estimated by [220 − age]: 220 − 65 = 155 bpm
2. Deduct the resting RHR: 155 − 70 = 85 (HRR)

3. Multiply HRR by 0.6: 85 × 0.6 = 51
4. Add the RHR back on: 51 + 70 = 121 beats per minute

The exercise prescription may be based on the subjective Borg's Ratings of Perceived Exertion 6–20 scale, which can sometimes be replaced by a 1–10 scale (e.g. when a person is taking beta-blocker medication). Exercise prescription for resistance training can be based on the ten-repetition maximum or using pain scales for musculoskeletal conditions.

4.5 Reviewing progress and outcomes

The standard exercise referral programme is relatively short, meaning that significant improvement in clinical and/or disease-related outcomes is not always achievable or clinically significant (Pavey et al., 2011). The dose-response relationship between exercise prescription and physiological improvements for key medical conditions will be covered in subsequent chapters. However, psychosocial outcomes must be measured and documented as per suggestions in Section 4.4. It should be noted that the first point of review is phase 4 of the consultation, when ER practitioners will provide feedback on a person's baseline results (Figure 4.1). This is an effective approach to ensure the person knows where they are starting from and also to better inform or refine the agreed-upon goals set via motivational interviewing prior to programme design. Although many exercise referral sessions take place in a group setting, people will be more likely to adhere to a programme and engage in physical activity thereafter if the programme is composed of specifically tailored advice, as opposed to a one-size-fits-all approach.

It is important for the person, as well as the ER practitioner, to review progress during and at the end of the exercise referral programme. The specific outcomes will vary from one person to the next, as outcomes will differ depending on the referred condition, but it is strongly encouraged that all conditions document changes in physical activity behaviour and psychosocial measures. Reviewing a person's progress will take place in one of two ways across the exercise referral programme.

1. During and after each session

   a. During each session, it is important that you observe the person, make notes on their movement quality and highlight any aspects of the exercises that they find difficult or can perform with ease – this information can help you determine the regression or progression of their next session. One key example is you may need to alter heart-rate training zones according to their responses and/or the presence of symptoms.
   b. At the end of each session, it is important that you provide the person with some feedback and also ask them to reflect on their session and provide you with feedback – this will help you to adapt the next session, and using a motivational interviewing–consistent conversation will ensure that you agree on these changes together and help the person feel that they have some control over the process, which will facilitate their feelings of autonomy.

2. In the interim and 12-week consultations

   a. Repeat each of the measures that took place during the initial consultation (Section 4.5) that will inform the reports that will be returned to the GP and other health-care professionals.

While interim data may not always be returned to the reporting HCP, these data will help you show the person that they are making progress and help reinforce the goal-setting process and psychological state. As previously mentioned, progress reports will highlight key psychosocial outcomes including mood and quality of life, as well as general and condition-specific physiological outcomes, including blood pressure, resting heart rate, anthropometry and fitness. The progress reviews will allow you to provide feedback to the person, but as mentioned in the communication skills section, you must always keep in mind the use of appropriate language, lay explanations and positive reinforcement to promote ongoing motivation for long-term behaviour change. You can provide the referring HCP with updates and an end-of-programme review letter that may encompass more technical terminology.

Overuse of normative data and comparing a person to a table with the use of categories from 'very poor' to 'excellent' is counterproductive. In many cases, especially over short interventions, the changes may not lead to much movement between categories or may lead to the demotivating realisation that they have moved from 'very poor' to 'poor'! It is worth highlighting that we should avoid comparing people to normative data and instead compare them to themselves to showcase relative improvements. In addition, the results and changes over 12 weeks may not seem much, but they may be clinically significant, and having an awareness of the clinically significant changes for select clinical outcomes is important.

The review process also provides an important opportunity to adapt the programme to encourage further improvements. This may involve increasing exercise intensity, including new exercises or greater encouragement to engage in additional physical activity outside the referred sessions. Exercise programme design is not the focus of this chapter, but we encourage you to engage with relevant material to ensure effective progression.

One final point to mention is that not all people who start the programme will choose to complete the 12 weeks, but it could be argued that this can be minimised if effective communication, motivational interviewing and personalised exercise programming take place. There are a whole variety of reasons why a person may drop out, and that is ultimately their choice, but it is highly advised that you conduct an exit interview to find out if their discontinuation could be avoided. This ultimately provides feedback to the ER practitioner and the referral team.

4.7 Case study: Behavioural considerations for exercise consultations

Case: Female, 47 years

Social history: Married, 3 children aged 10 to 16 years, works as care assistant in a nursing home

Current health status:

- Diagnosed reason for referral: hypertension and obesity
- Height 163 cm
- Body mass: 95 kg
- Body mass index 36 kg/m^2
- Resting heart rate 60 bpm
- Blood pressure: 145/95 mmHg

- Medication: Losartan 100 mg/day
  - This angiotensin receptor blocker (Losartan) has been prescribed to improve blood pressure because of its efficacy in African-Caribbean populations and also because the effects of using beta blockers or calcium channel blockers or diuretics could exacerbate her propensity of vaso-vagal fainting (see past medical history) (NICE, 2019).

Past medical history:

- No significant events, normal childbirths
- Transient post-natal depression with first child
- Lifelong propensity of occasional vaso-vagal fainting stimulated by external stressors (e.g. needles, pain, blood, visual gore, sickness)

Familial health and social history:

- African-Caribbean ethnicity
- Hypertension and strokes
- Mary was never 'sporty', avoided competitive games and has always perceived herself as a non-exerciser and has lived with the 'social tag' of being overweight ever since she started school.

4.7.1 Introduction to the case study

This case study of a client named Mary represents one of the most typical reasons for an exercise referral, which include risks of cardiovascular disease, diabetes and cancer associated with high body weight and high blood pressure (Wade et al., 2020; Steele et al., 2021; Rowley et al., 2021). This brief section on guidance towards supporting Mary simply aims to highlight how to value Mary's own behavioural perspectives on being referred for exercise, which is linked directly to her current levels of intrinsic motivation, physical and social capabilities and opportunities to be active (Michie et al., 2011; Michie et al., 2009). The following narrative aims to highlight, though very briefly, some of the contemporary approaches (cited earlier) for exercise professionals to help guide and increase physical activity. Specific training and experience in behaviour change and motivational interviewing are necessary for the ER practitioner.

4.7.2 Core behavioural and psychosocial considerations for supporting the client

Some key hallmarks of supporting Mary's behaviour change to becoming more regularly active include the practitioner's ability to be empathetic and collaborative; respecting that Mary will likely display ambivalence (moments of uncertainty) towards changing her behaviour; creating a communication environment that creates the opportunity for Mary to reveal comments of 'change talk', helping her achieve autonomy in her own action plan and working; and helping Mary plan for preventing and managing expected relapses in her behaviour (Fortune et al., 2019; Scott et al., 2019). When considering the implementation of these counselling processes, HCPs need to be aware that they may inadvertently become less empathetic towards clients as they pursue the desire to make use of their more advanced technical knowledge and skills (e.g. advancing clinical practice skills in the exercise referral process) (Miller and Rose, 2009).

A first step in working with Mary is to respect that the extrinsic biomedical goals for her have, in fact, been set by the referrer: in this case, the GP who recommended that she lose weight and reduce her blood pressure. The medical assumptions are that exercise can influence both weight loss and blood pressure, and weight loss in itself can also influence blood pressure (Perk et al., 2012). Mary followed up the GP's referral for exercise and made an appointment to meet with the exercise referral practitioner at her local leisure centre. From the simple application of the trans-theoretical model of behaviour change, it would appear Mary has moved from a stage of behavioural contemplation to preparation (Biddle and Mutrie, 2008). However, Mary's accepting the behavioural opportunity to take up the referral should not be mistaken for a sincere intrinsic motivation or the capability of wanting or being able to successfully become more regularly active (Michie et al., 2009; Michie et al., 2011).

At this point, it is important to respect the state of behavioural ambivalence likely to be in her mind. Even the act of commencing an exercise programme, which could occur on her first visit to the leisure centre, should not be inferred as Mary sincerely moving into an action phase of behaviour. Such categorisation of people into a simple behavioural stage (e.g. preparation, action, maintenance) can be fraught with challenges as Mary's attitudes towards changing her behaviour have not yet proven to be stable (controlled, autonomous, non-ambivalent) (Thompson et al., 2011). Coming to grips with simply participating in an exercise programme, including the activity environment (class, gym equipment programme, home programme, being with others during exercise, engaging with an exercise coach/professional) is in itself a preparation towards action which tested Mary's capabilities and motivations to fulfil the longer-term behaviour change of health-enhancing physical activity. In many cases, people take up an exercise referral or any lifestyle health improvement programme to please others, including their GP, or to allay concerns or fulfil the wishes of close relatives or friends (Waitzkin, 1984; Klitzman, 2006).

What therefore needs to be evaluated with Mary is how much she believes, values and is honestly willing to pursue a plan to improve her health through physical activity. If performed well, this will be revealed in 'change talk', which in this case will be Mary talking about the desire and need to change her behaviour. Mary was actually stating ways in which she considered the amount of time she could make available in and around her work and family obligations. ('On Wednesdays I have an early shift, finishing at 2:30, and where the children are at music and drama clubs until 5:30, so I was thinking this could be a time for my exercise. I would have to sacrifice my regular Wednesday meet-up with Gill for a coffee, and maybe she could come along to the gym too?')

In starting out with Mary's programme, it needs to be respected that the strong biomedical aims proposed by the GP may need to be addressed immediately. Mary's physical activity and nutrition needs are actually a part of a longer-term process. The time it will take to make behavioural adjustments that then result in biomedical changes is different for each person and, for Mary, completely controlled by her ability to psychologically and socially adjust her daily life (Ntoumanis et al., 2018). It is, in fact, the balance between the client and the exercise professional of who has control over the exercise programme which ultimately affects the long-term adherence required to achieve the desired health outcomes (weight loss and blood pressure) (Ntoumanis et al., 2018). In light of this evidence, it has been shown that when exercise professionals are faced with an overweight versus a normal-weight client, their beliefs and attitudes towards managing these two client categories differ significantly. If a client is overweight (compared to a typically defined normal-weight person), exercise instructors' attitudes unfortunately tend towards taking control of the client's behaviour and being over-prescriptive. This has been shown to actually impede the client's ability to become autonomous in managing their own health. The desire of the exercise professional to be too helpful can thus be counterproductive as this approach removes client ownership of the programme. For Mary, this is likely to simply reinforce that she has a health problem but worse, one which is the cause of her lifelong social stigma of being overweight. It is the social stigma created in her childhood, over which she had little control that will potentially resurface every time she meets with the ER practitioner, which may create a strong barrier to her successful participation. If the ER practitioner inadvertently takes too much control, it will prevent Mary from developing a personal sense of mastery. Personal senses of mastery are linked to the development of personal self-confidence and a related state of mental health required to meet the challenge of the desired behaviour (regular exercise), a new priority, amongst many other responsibilities, in Mary's daily/weekly life (Buckley et al., 1999).

4.7.3 Key aims of the short- and mid-term exercise programme goals: Banishing misconceptions and creating an appropriate supportive psychosocial environment

The key challenges and barriers (not necessarily in the order presented) to Mary's participation in a new programme of physical activity requires careful application of the supportive counselling techniques discussed earlier. The process of motivational interviewing does not have to occur in a single consultation session; it can be built up to gradually ease Mary into physical activity opportunities that demonstrate where she is most likely to have some social confidence to participate. For people like Mary at risk of cardiovascular disease, further reading is recommended on the more specific types and modes of behaviour change support for this population (Murray et al., 2012; Murray et al., 2013b). Within the process, the points of discussion listed next will likely include elements of both education to resolve misconceptions about weight and health and practically overcoming a number of psychosocial determinants (barriers) so as to create the best possible chance of the positive experiences eventually leading Mary to maintaining physical activity as a normal behaviour.

1. The points to follow all have hallmarks that can help to detract Mary's attention from the unfortunate lifelong body-image stigma that she has had. Physical activity has so many benefits to offer beyond the very oversimplified goal of losing weight, which is unrelentingly found across all media forms (including official government concerns) of promoting sport and exercise as a perceived 'simple' solution to an obesity epidemic. This unfortunately actually neglects to respect so many other benefits that physical activity offers beyond the single, perhaps over-sensationalised, issue of obesity.
2. Mary learning to appreciate that, whether or not the programme actually leads to fulfilling the GP's aims for losing weight and reducing blood pressure, the UK's chief medical officer's guidelines actually report that when inactive people take up and maintain regular

exercise, important health and social benefits can still be gained, including reducing some risk of cardiovascular disease, musculoskeletal dysfunction and breast and bowel cancer, and mental health and well-being can improve (CMOs-Guidelines, 2019).

3. In furthering point 2., any increase in physical activity above what Mary is currently doing, and wherever it occurs (at home, with the children, a social walk with friends) will be of physical and mental benefit. In Mary's work situation as a care assistant, the work is likely to be both emotionally and physically demanding, so asking her to increase her activity levels in and around work will likely have a negative connotation. She should, however, be encouraged to know that her work already contributes to her weekly levels of reduced sedentary time as recommended by the government (CMOs-Guidelines, 2019) and that she is far better off than so many other non-exercisers who have an office or desk job or sit all day at a supermarket till (Ekelund et al., 2019; Bull et al., 2020).
4. In relation to attending more formalised activities with the ER practitioner, whilst there will be an eventual goal of attaining 75 to 150 minutes per week of moderate to vigorous aerobic exercise (FITT), plus strength-building activities, it is far more important at this point to review, explore and experience (even through taster sessions) the type of social situations that will suit Mary best. Once a positive environment (or choice of different positive environments) has been achieved, that will help towards a sense of autonomous control by Mary, and then the exercise plan can start to be geared towards the individual recommended FITT targets.
5. Intertwined with all the previous points will no doubt be the point on the where and how Mary feels she will be able to fit any physical activity (including any formal exercise referral sessions) into her current normal weekly routine.
6. Linked to points 1 and 2 are the misconceptions around the types and amounts of fat loss, weight fears and risk of diabetes typically raised in many public and media domains. It will be important for Mary to understand that issues of fat and health risk are more closely linked to the visceral fat around her vital organs (liver, kidney, heart, bowel) and not what she sees and feels on her arms and legs. Regular exercise, independent of changes in BMI, weight and appearance of externally visible fat, will reduce visceral fat as well if not better than dieting (Verheggen et al., 2016). In relation to the risk of type 2 diabetes, unless Mary has a known family history of diabetes, only 15% of people who are obese actually go on to develop it (Malone and Hansen, 2019). If Mary has been concerned about this, then again, it will be encouraging to report that physical activity can be a part of reducing her risks. This point, however, needs to be reviewed with the GP to assess for diabetes risk, if this has not already been done, given Mary's age, blood pressure, ethnicity and family history of strokes.
7. The final point, which does bring the discussion back to the issue of weight loss first raised by the GP, will have certainly reminded Mary of her lifelong concerns (conscious or subconscious) about her body image. If, however, she is to lose weight, and she has set this as a goal, and in keeping with the UK CMO guidelines (CMOs Guidelines, 2019), this will require dietary changes alongside the physical activity programme. The most successful long-term weight loss programmes are those that involve both physical activity and dietary changes, rather than diet alone (Curioni and Lourenco, 2005). As a final encouraging note for Mary, if she gains some autonomous (intrinsic) control over her physical activity, she will be more likely to be successful in changing her eating and nutritional behaviours (Panao and Carraca, 2020).

4.8 Summary/Key points

- Establishing client history is key to an ER practitioner's preparation and ability to build positive rapport during a consultation and to devise a tailored programme that aligns with the wants and needs of the person.
- A thorough screening process and risk stratification should always be conducted to ensure the safety of the person engaging in exercise referral as well as inform the ER practitioner of a potential reason to refer back to the HCP.
- Building rapport and trust with a person requires a combination of effective non-verbal and verbal communication and a clear appreciation by the ER practitioner that people play a key contributing role in their own programme development.
- Assessment plays a valuable role in establishing baseline health and fitness outcomes, determining the most appropriate exercise prescription and being repeated at one or two points in the 12-week programme to provide a progress review. It is important that the ER practitioner does not focus on comparing a person's outcomes to normative tables and instead uses them as their own comparator to enhance motivation.
- Reviewing progress goes beyond the outcome of tests, and the key is to ask for feedback and provide feedback on a regular basis, not just at the end of the programme.

4.9 Study tasks

1. If the conversations during the consultation deviate from your predefined plan and process of gathering key information, how would you adapt your approach to ensure you still acquire a full history?
2. Using the case study of Mary, what is the communication approach used to develop a collaborative person-led discussion? Consider two or three open questions you might ask her to find out about barriers to and facilitators of physical activity.
3. What would you do if a person (referred for a non-cardiovascular condition) arrived for their consultation and mentioned in the medical history screening that they experience periods of heart palpitations that can last for varying periods of time and with no predictable pattern?
4. What is the primary purpose of completing risk stratification prior to commencing an exercise referral programme?
5. If a 57-year-old male person arrives for their consultation with medication-controlled type 2 diabetes (although fasting blood glucose 6.8 mmol/L), a body weight of 85 kg, BMI of 28.9 kg/m^2 and a waist circumference of 112 cm, into which risk category would they be placed?
6. Which risk stratification category would you place Mary from the case study in?
7. Identify three key considerations to ensure a person feels comfortable when they arrive for their consultation and provide an example for each.
8. How would you assess Mary's baseline physical activity levels, and how would you track whether they improve over the 12-week exercise referral programme?
9. The determination of baseline fitness is useful in exercise referral. If the person in question 4 completed the Rockport one-mile test in 17 minutes with an average HR of 139 bpm, calculate his predicted VO_2max.
10. When and how would you ask for and provide feedback to ensure your programme is being effectively reviewed?

References

ACSM (2018). *ACSM's Guidelines for Exercise Testing and Prescription* (10th Edition). Philadelphia: Wolters Kluwer.

American Thoracic Society (2002). ATS statement: Guidelines for the six-minute walk test. *American Journal of Respiratory and Critical Care Medicine*, 166(1), 111–117.

Andersen MB, Speed HD. (2010). Therapeutic relationships in applied sport psychology. In SJ Hanrahan, MB Andersen (Eds.), *Routledge Handbook of Applied Sport Psychology* (pp. 3–11). London: Routledge.

Ashwell M, Gibson S. (2016). Waist-to-height ratio as an indicator of 'early health risk': Simpler and more predictive than using a 'matrix' based on BMI and waist circumference. *British Medical Journal Open*, 6(3), e010159.

Benatti FB, Reid-Larson M. (2015). The effects of breaking up prolonged sitting time: A review of experimental studies. *Medicine and Science in Sport and Exercise*, 47(10), 2053–2061.

Biddle SJ, Mutrie N. (2008). *Psychology of physical activity* (2nd Edition). Oxford: Routledge.

Bohannon RW, Crouch R. (2017). Minimal clinically important difference for change in 6-minute walk test distance of adults with pathology: A systematic review. *Journal of Evaluation in Clinical Practice*, 23(2), 377–381.

Borodulin K, Sipilä N, Rahkonen O, Leino-Arjas P, Kestilä L, Jousilahti P, Prättälä R. (2016). Sociodemographic and behavioural variation to leisure-time physical activity. *Scandinavian Journal of Public Health*, 44(1), 62–69.

Brooks R. (1996). EuroQoL: The current state of play. *Health Policy*, 37(1), 53–72.

Bull FC, Al-Ansari SS, Biddle S, Borodulin K, Buman MP, Cardon G, Carty C, Chaput JP, Chastin S, Chou R, Dempsey PC, DiPietro L, Ekelund U, Firth J, Friedenreich CM, Garcia L, Gichu M, Jago R, Katzmarzyk PT, Lambert E, Leitzmann M, Milton K, Ortega FB, Ranasinghe C, Stamatakis E, Tiedemann A, Troiano RP, van der Ploeg HP, Wari V, Willumsen JF. (2020). World Health Organization 2020 guidelines on physical activity and sedentary behaviour. *Br J Sports Med*, 54, 1451–1462.

CMOs Guidelines. (2019). *UK Chief Medical Officers' Physical Activity Guidelines*. London: The Stationary Office.

Craig CL, Marshall AL, Sjöström M, et al. (2003). International physical activity questionnaire: 12-country reliability and validity. *Medicine and Science in Sports and Exercise,* 35(8), 1381–1395. DOI: 10.1249/01.MSS.0000078924.61453.FB.

Curioni CC, Lourenco PM. (2005). Long-term weight loss after diet and exercise: A systematic review. *Int J Obes (Lond)*, 29, 1168–1174.

Department of Health (2002). *Exercise Referral Systems: A National Quality Assurance Framework*. London: Department of Health.

Dolezal BA, Neufeld EV, Boland DM, Martin JL, Cooper CB. (2017). Interrelationship between sleep and exercise: A systematic review. *Advances in Preventive Medicine*, 2017, 1364387.

Downey J, Shearn K, Brown N, Wadey R, Breckon J. (2021). Behaviour change practices in exercise referral schemes: Developing realist programme theory of implementation. *BMC Health Service Research*, 21, 335.

Ekelund U, Tarp J, Steene-Johannessen J, Hansen BH, Jefferis B, Fagerland MW, Whincup P, Diaz KM, Hooker SP, Chernofsky A, Larson MG, Spartano N, Vasan RS, Dohrn IM, Hagströmer M, Edwardson C, Yates T, Shiroma E, Anderssen SA, Lee IM. (2019). Dose-response associations between accelerometry measured physical activity and sedentary time and all-cause mortality: Systematic review and harmonised meta-analysis. *British Medical Journal*, 366, l4570.

Fletcher G, Ades PA, Kligfield P, Arena R, Balady GJ, Bittner VA, Coke LA, Fleg JL, Forman DE, Gerber TC, Gulati M, Madan K, Rhodes J, Thompson PD, Williams MA. (2013). Exercise standards for testing and training: A scientific statement from the American Heart Association. *Circulation*, 128, 873–934.

Fortune J, Breckon J, Norris M, Eva G, Frater T. (2019). Motivational interviewing training for physiotherapy and occupational therapy students: Effect on confidence, knowledge and skills. *Patient Educ Couns*, 102, 694–700.

Hilton C, Trigg R, Minniti A. (2015). Improving the psychological evaluation of exercise referral: Psychometric properties of the Exercise Referral Quality of Life Scale. *Health Psychology Open*, 2, 2055102915590317.

Jackson C. (2015). The Chalder Fatigue scale (CFQ 11): Questionnaire review. *Occupational Medicine*, 65(1), 86.

Jones CJ, Rikli RE, Max J, Noffal G. (1998). The reliability and validity of a chair sit-and-reach test as a measure of hamstring flexibility in older adults. *Research Quarterly Exercise Sport*, 69, 338–343.

Klitzman R. (2006). Improving education on doctor-patient relationships and communication: Lessons from doctors who become patients. *Academic Medicine*, 81, 447–453.

Kovacevic A, Mavros Y, Heisz JJ, Fiatarone Singh MA. (2017). The effect of resistance exercise on sleep: A systematic review of randomized controlled trials. *Sleep Medicine Reviews*, 39, 52–68.

Lederman O, Grainger K, Stanton R, Douglas A, Gould K, Perram A, Baldeo R, Fokas T, Nauman F, Semaan A, Hewavasam J, Pontin L, Rosenbaum S. (2016). Consensus statement on the role of accredited exercise physiologists within the treatment of mental disorders: A guide for mental health professionals. *Australasian Psychiatry*, 24(4), 347–351.

Lohman TG, Roche, AF, Martorell R. (1991). *Anthropometric Standardization Reference Manual*. Champaign, IL: Human Kinetics.

Malone JI, Hansen BC. (2019). Does obesity cause type 2 diabetes mellitus (T2DM)? Or is it the opposite? *Pediatric Diabetes*, 20, 5–9.

McArdle WD, Katch FI, Pechar GS, Jacobson L, Ruck S. (1972). Reliability and interrelationships between maximal oxygen uptake, physical work capacity and step test scores in college women. *Medicine and Science in Sports and Exercise*, 4, 182–186.

Michie S, Abraham C, Whittington C, McAteer J, Gupta S. (2009). Effective techniques in healthy eating and physical activity interventions: A meta-regression. *Health Psychology*, 28, 690–701.

Michie S, van Stralen MM, West R. (2011). The behaviour change wheel: A new method for characterising and designing behaviour change interventions. *Implementation Science*, 6, 42.

Miller WR, Rollinick S. (2012). *Motivational Interviewing: Helping People Change* (3rd Edition). New York: The Guildford Press.

Miller WR, Rose GS. (2009). Toward a theory of motivational interviewing. *The American Psychologist*, 64, 527–537.

Murray CJ, Vos T, Lozano R, Naghavi M, Flaxman AD, Michaud C, Ezzati M, Shibuya K, Salomon JA, Abdalla S, Aboyans V, Abraham J, Ackerman I, Aggarwal R, Ahn SY, Ali MK, Alvarado M, Anderson HR, Anderson LM, Andrews KG, Atkinson C, Baddour LM, Bahalim AN, Barker-Collo S, Barrero LH, Bartels DH, Basáñez MG, Baxter A, Bell ML, Benjamin EJ, Bennett D, Bernabé E, Bhalla K, Bhandari B, Bikbov B, Bin Abdulhak A, Birbeck G, Black JA, Blencowe H, Blore JD, Blyth F, Bolliger I, Bonaventure A, Boufous S, Bourne R, Boussinesq M, Braithwaite T, Brayne C, Bridgett L, Brooker S, Brooks P, Brugha TS, Bryan-Hancock C, Bucello C, Buchbinder R, Buckle G, Budke CM, Burch M, Burney P, Burstein R, Calabria B, Campbell B, Canter CE, Carabin H, Carapetis J, Carmona L, Cella C, Charlson F, Chen H, Cheng AT, Chou D, Chugh SS, Coffeng LE, Colan SD, Colquhoun S, Colson KE, Condon J, Connor MD, Cooper LT, Corriere M, Cortinovis M, de Vaccaro KC, Couser W, Cowie BC, Criqui MH, Cross M, Dabhadkar KC, Dahiya M, Dahodwala N, Damsere-Derry J, Danaei G, Davis A, De Leo D, Degenhardt L, Dellavalle R, Delossantos A, Denenberg J, Derrett S, Des Jarlais DC, Dharmaratne SD, Dherani M, Diaz-Torne C, Dolk H, Dorsey ER, Driscoll T, Duber H, Ebel B, Edmond K, Elbaz A, Ali SE, Erskine H, Erwin PJ, Espindola P, Ewoigbokhan SE, Farzadfar F, Feigin V, Felson DT, Ferrari A, Ferri CP, Fèvre EM, Finucane MM, Flaxman S, Flood L, Foreman K, Forouzanfar MH, Fowkes FG, Fransen M, Freeman MK, Gabbe BJ, Gabriel SE, Gakidou E, Ganatra HA, Garcia B, Gaspari F, Gillum RF, Gmel G, Gonzalez-Medina D, Gosselin R, Grainger R, Grant B, Groeger J, Guillemin F, Gunnell D, Gupta R, Haagsma J, Hagan H, Halasa YA, Hall W, Haring D, Haro JM, Harrison JE, Havmoeller R, Hay RJ, Higashi H, Hill C, Hoen B, Hoffman H, Hotez PJ, Hoy D, Huang JJ, Ibeanusi SE, Jacobsen KH, James SL, Jarvis D, Jasrasaria R, Jayaraman S, Johns N, Jonas JB, Karthikeyan G, Kassebaum N, Kawakami N, Keren A, Khoo JP, King CH, Knowlton LM, Kobusingye O, Koranteng A, Krishnamurthi R, Laden F, Lalloo R, Laslett LL, Lathlean T, Leasher JL, Lee YY, Leigh J,

Levinson D, Lim SS, Limb E, Lin JK, Lipnick M, Lipshultz SE, Liu W, Loane M, Ohno SL, Lyons R, Mabweijano J, MacIntyre MF, Malekzadeh R, Mallinger L, Manivannan S, Marcenes W, March L, Margolis DJ, Marks GB, Marks R, Matsumori A, Matzopoulos R, Mayosi BM, McAnulty JH, McDermott MM, McGill N, McGrath J, Medina-Mora ME, Meltzer M, Mensah GA, Merriman TR, Meyer AC, Miglioli V, Miller M, Miller TR, Mitchell PB, Mock C, Mocumbi AO, Moffitt TE, Mokdad AA, Monasta L, Montico M, Moradi-Lakeh M, Moran A, Morawska L, Mori R, Murdoch ME, Mwaniki MK, Naidoo K, Nair MN, Naldi L, Narayan KM, Nelson PK, Nelson RG, Nevitt MC, Newton CR, Nolte S, Norman P, Norman R, O'Donnell M, O'Hanlon S, Olives C, Omer SB, Ortblad K, Osborne R, Ozgediz D, Page A, Pahari B, Pandian JD, Rivero AP, Patten SB, Pearce N, Padilla RP, Perez-Ruiz F, Perico N, Pesudovs K, Phillips D, Phillips MR, Pierce K, Pion S, Polanczyk GV, Polinder S, Pope CA 3rd, Popova S, Porrini E, Pourmalek F, Prince M, Pullan RL, Ramaiah KD, Ranganathan D, Razavi H, Regan M, Rehm JT, Rein DB, Remuzzi G, Richardson K, Rivara FP, Roberts T, Robinson C, De Leòn FR, Ronfani L, Room R, Rosenfeld LC, Rushton L, Sacco RL, Saha S, Sampson U, Sanchez-Riera L, Sanman E, Schwebel DC, Scott JG, Segui-Gomez M, Shahraz S, Shepard DS, Shin H, Shivakoti R, Singh D, Singh GM, Singh JA, Singleton J, Sleet DA, Sliwa K, Smith E, Smith JL, Stapelberg NJ, Steer A, Steiner T, Stolk WA, Stovner LJ, Sudfeld C, Syed S, Tamburlini G, Tavakkoli M, Taylor HR, Taylor JA, Taylor WJ, Thomas B, Thomson WM, Thurston GD, Tleyjeh IM, Tonelli M, Towbin JA, Truelsen T, Tsilimbaris MK, Ubeda C, Undurraga EA, van der Werf MJ, van Os J, Vavilala MS, Venketasubramanian N, Wang M, Wang W, Watt K, Weatherall DJ, Weinstock MA, Weintraub R, Weisskopf MG, Weissman MM, White RA, Whiteford H, Wiebe N, Wiersma ST, Wilkinson JD, Williams HC, Williams SR, Witt E, Wolfe F, Woolf AD, Wulf S, Yeh PH, Zaidi AK, Zheng ZJ, Zonies D, Lopez AD, AlMazroa MA, Memish ZA. (2013a). Disability-adjusted life years (DALYs) for 291 diseases and injuries in 21 regions, 1990–2010: A systematic analysis for the Global Burden of Disease Study 2010. *The Lancet*, 380(9859), 2197–2223.

Murray J, Craigs CL, Hill KM, Honey S, House A. (2012). A systematic review of patient reported factors associated with uptake and completion of cardiovascular lifestyle behaviour change. *BMC Cardiovascular Disorders*, 12, 120.

Murray J, Fenton G, Honey S, Ara AC, Hill KM, House A. (2013b). A qualitative synthesis of factors influencing maintenance of lifestyle behaviour change in individuals with high cardiovascular risk. *BMC Cardiovascular Disorders*, 13, 48.

Myers J, Prakash M, Froelicher V, Do D, Partington S, Atwood JE. (2002). Exercise capacity and mortality among men referred for exercise testing. *The New England Journal of Medicine*, 346, 793–801.

Myers MG, Godwin M, Dawes M, Kiss A, Tobe SW, Grant FC, Kaczorowski J. (2011). Conventional versus automated measurement of blood pressure in primary care patients with systolic hypertension: Randomised parallel design controlled trial. *British Medical Journal*, 342, d286.

National Centre for Sport and Exercise Medicine (NCSEM) (2010). *A Toolkit for the Design, Implementation & Evaluation of Exercise Referral Schemes*. [Online] Available from: www.ncsem-em.org.uk/resources/exercise-referral-toolkit/.

National Institute for Health and Clinical Excellence (NICE) (2014). *Physical Activity: Exercise Referral Schemes [PH54]*. London: The Stationery Office.

National Institute for Health and Clinical Excellence (NICE) (2019). *Hypertension in Adults: Diagnosis and Management [CG136]*. London: The Stationery Office.

Ntoumanis N, Guerrero MD, Gadeke C, Thøgersen-Ntoumani C. (2018). Do exerciser weight status and perceived motivation predict instructors' motivation and beliefs about the exerciser? A test of motivation contagion effects. *Body Image*, 26, 10–18.

Owen N, Healy GN, Matthews CE, Dunstan DW. (2010). Too much sitting: The population-health science of sedentary behaviour. *Exercise and Sport Science Reviews*, 38(3), 105–113.

Panao I, Carraca EV. (2020). Effects of exercise motivations on body image and eating habits/behaviours: A systematic review. *Nutrition and Dietetics*, 77, 41–59.

Pavey T, Taylor AH, Fox KR, Hillsdon M, Anokye N, Campbell JL, Foster C, Green C, Moxham T, Mutrie N, Searle J, Trueman P, Taylor RS. (2011). Effect of exercise referral schemes in primary care on physical activity and improving health outcomes: Systematic review and meta-analysis. *British Medical Journal*, 343, d6462.

Perk J, De Backer G, Gohlke H, Graham I, Reiner Z, Verschuren M, Albus C, Benlian P, Boysen G, Cifkova R, Deaton C, Ebrahim S, Fisher M, Germano G, Hobbs R, Hoes A, Karadeniz S, Mezzani A, Prescott E, Ryden L, Scherer M, Syvänne M, Scholte op Reimer WJ, Vrints C, Wood D, Zamorano JL, Zannad F. (2012). European Guidelines on cardiovascular disease prevention in clinical practice: The fifth joint task force of the European society of cardiology and other societies on cardiovascular disease prevention in clinical practice (constituted by representatives of nine societies and by invited experts). *Atherosclerosis*, 223, 1–68.

Prochaska JM, Prochaska JO. (2014). A stage approach to enhancing adherence to treatment. In D. I. Mostosky (Ed.), *The Handbook of Behavioural Medicine*. Oxford: John Wiley & Sons.

Rikli RE, Jones CJ. (2013). Development and validation of criterion-referenced clinically relevant fitness standards for maintaining physical independence in later years. *Gerontologist*, 53, 255–267.

Rowley N, Steele J, Mann S, Jimenez A, Horton E. (2021). Delivery approaches within exercise referral schemes: A survey of current practice in England. *Journal of Physical Activity and Health*, 18, 357–373.

Scott SE, Breckon JD, Copeland RJ. (2019). An integrated motivational interviewing and cognitive-behavioural intervention promoting physical activity maintenance for adults with chronic health conditions: A feasibility study. *Chronic Illness*, 15, 276–292.

Steele J, Wade M, Copeland RJ, Stokes S, Stokes R, Mann S. (2021). The National ReferAll Database: An open dataset of exercise referral schemes across the UK. *International Journal of Environmental Research and Public Health*, 18, 4831.

Sykes K, Roberts A. (2004). The Chester step test – a simple yet effective tool for the prediction of aerobic capacity. *Physiotherapy*, 90, 183–188.

Teixeira PJ, Carraça EV, Markland D, Silva MN, Ryan RM. (2012). Exercise, physical activity and self-determination theory: A systematic review. *International Journal of Behavioural Nutrition and Physical Activity*, 9, 78.

Thompson DR, Chair SY, Chan SW, Astin F, Davidson PM, Ski CF. (2011). Motivational interviewing: A useful approach to improving cardiovascular health? *Journal of Clinical Nursing*, 20, 1236–1244.

Verheggen RJ, Maessen MF, Green DJ, Hermus AR, Hopman MT, Thijssen DH. (2016). A systematic review and meta-analysis on the effects of exercise training versus hypocaloric diet: Distinct effects on body weight and visceral adipose tissue. *Obesity Reviews*, 17, 664–690.

Wade M, Mann S, Copeland RJ, Steele J. (2020). Effect of exercise referral schemes upon health and well-being: Initial observational insights using individual patient data meta-analysis from the National Referral Database. *J Epidemiol Community Health*, 74, 32–41.

Waitzkin H. (1984). Doctor-patient communication. Clinical implications of social scientific research. *Journal of the American Medical Association*, 252, 2441–2446.

Wan Y, Heneghan C, Stevens R, McManus RJ, Ward A, Perera R, Thompson M, Tarassenko L, Mant D. (2010). Determining which automatic digital blood pressure device performs adequately: A systematic review. *Journal of Human Hypertension*, 24, 431–438.

Warburton D, Jamnik V, Bredin S, Shephard R, Gledhill N. (2021). The 2021 physical activity readiness questionnaire for everyone (PAR-Q+) and electronic physical activity readiness medical examination (ePARmed-X+): 2021 PAR-Q+. *The Health & Fitness Journal of Canada*, 14(1), 83–87. https://doi.org/10.14288/hfjc.v14i1.351.

Williams GC, Halvari H, Niemiec CP, Sørebø Ø, Olafsen AH, Westbye C. (2014). Managerial support for basic psychological needs, somatic symptom burden and work-related correlates: A self-determination theory perspective. *Work and Stress*, 28, 404–419.

5

PERSONALISING THE EXERCISE REFERRAL EXPERIENCE

Understanding Individual Differences

Zoë Franklin and Dave Thompson

Chapter aims

The aims of this chapter are to:

1. Identify the individual differences that may influence adherence to exercise
2. Identify how different personality types may require different exercise referral processes
3. Analyse the barriers to and facilitators of individuals' exercise referrals and how we can overcome these
4. Recognise how the patient's perceptions of the exercise referral process can influence their goal setting
5. Analyse the role of the exercise specialist in supporting and guiding patients through the referral process to ensure adherence

Introduction

Physical inactivity levels are rising within the UK, although many treatment guidelines are not specific. To effectively enhance individuals' physical activity behaviour, interventions must target the environmental, social and psychological factors underpinning physical activity engagement. While tackling the wider 'environmental' or 'social' constraints on physical activity may be beyond the scope of health and fitness professionals working with patients on a day-to-day basis, addressing and utilising psychological constructs are highly relevant to their role. This chapter will focus on the influence of personality traits on behaviour change and how these traits influence patients' barriers to and facilitators of adherence to exercise.

Personality and individual differences

Researchers have been investigating individual differences relating to personality for decades. McCrae and Costa (1985) identified five core personality traits: 1) extraversion, 2) agreeableness, 3) conscientiousness, 4) neuroticism and 5) openness. One of these 'big five'

DOI: 10.4324/9781315102399-5

factors, neuroticism, has shown consistently strong correlations with measures of trait anxiety (Eysenck, 1997). Trait anxiety is considered an important dimension of personality and is included in most theories as a major personality factor (Digman, 1990). Other theories have primarily focused on the role of the cognitive system (e.g. attentional biases) and trait anxiety when attempting to explain individual differences in the experience of potentially threatening situations (Eysenck, 1992).

Eysenck (1992) proposed a cognitive theory of trait anxiety based on the premise that the function of anxiety is to facilitate the early detection of impending danger in potentially threatening environments. Since it is the attentional system which is involved in threat detection, individuals high and low in trait anxiety should differ in terms of their pre-attentive and attentional functioning. Eysenck proposed that variations in trait anxiety are reflected in a range of 'cognitive biases', which influence processing of ambiguous or threat-related stimuli. These biases include a selective attentional bias, interpretive bias and negative memory bias. It was also assumed that these biases are more evident when situational (e.g. state) anxiety is high. High-anxious individuals are predicted to selectively attend to threat-related stimuli rather than neutral stimuli. They are also more likely to interpret ambiguous stimuli as threatening and to show a negative memory recall bias in explicit memory. Therefore, they are significantly more likely to remember more threat-related than non-threatening events of both a social (e.g. social rejection) and physical (e.g. physical wounds) nature (Eysenck, 1992). Attentional biases have been implicated in both the cause and maintenance of emotional disorders and can cause the exacerbation of anxiety (Koster et al., 2010). Of particular interest to the current research is the finding that an attentional bias to pain-related symptoms in chronic-pain populations may lead to the causation or maintenance of pain. Excessive vigilance may be associated with preoccupation with pain, resulting in a tendency for patients to avoid activities which are deemed threatening to their condition (Schoth et al., 2012).

According to Beck's Schema Theory (Beck et al., 1985), high-anxious individuals have a dysfunctional schema relating to personal harm or threat, resulting in an increased propensity to be distracted by or attend to threat-related stimuli. In particular, this bias may be enhanced when state anxiety is high or when the threat is more personally relevant. The majority of research suggests that high-anxious individuals will demonstrate an attentional bias towards threatening information (Mogg and Bradley, 1998). Some individuals who are part of an exercise referral scheme (ERS) may have negative memories associated with exercise, which may influence their adherence to a programme. In particular, the results suggest that high-anxious individuals have a bias in the processing of threat which facilitates processing of negatively valenced information over pleasant or neutral stimuli (Mogg et al., 2000). This bias towards negative information may influence their cognitions associated with exercise.

Personality types

Individual differences in anxiety and their link to variations in selective attention to threat may be of significance to the treatment and management of chronic pain. Some of the contradictory findings within high- and low-anxious individuals in previous studies suggest there may be an additional cognitive mechanism causing these differences. Subdividing the low-anxious and high-anxious groups based on measures of trait anxiety and defensiveness may provide greater insight into the attentional processes of individuals, thereby influencing an individual's adherence to an exercise referral process.

Differences between individuals in the tendency to experience anxiety appears an important distinction in clinical environments. Weinberger et al. (1979) originally investigated the combination of trait anxiety and defensiveness to explain differences between physiological and behavioural reports of anxiety. These differences reflected variations between individuals in the concordance of different measures of anxiety. Research showed that some individuals reported low levels of self-reported anxiety despite exhibiting elevated levels of physiological anxiety. Defensiveness is regarded as a coping behaviour which causes individuals to avoid negative affect and has been related to emotional and physical health and prevention of threat to self-esteem (Weinberger, 1990). Weinberger et al. (1979) proposed four personality profiles: 1) high-anxious (HA), 2) defensive high-anxious (DHA), 3) low-anxious (LA), and 4) repressor (REP) types. High-anxious individuals score high on trait anxiety and low on defensiveness; defensive high-anxious individuals score high on trait anxiety and defensiveness; low-anxious individuals score low on both trait anxiety and defensiveness; and repressor individuals score low on trait anxiety and high on defensiveness (see Figure 5.1).

The four personality profiles are believed to show different behaviours when confronted with stressful situations (e.g. attending an exercise referral session). Weinberger et al. (1979) reported that although repressors report low levels of distress, their physiological anxiety is similar to that of individuals who have high-anxiety profiles (Fahrenberg, 1992; Gudjonsson, 1981). In contrast, low-anxious individuals do not appear to show any differences between

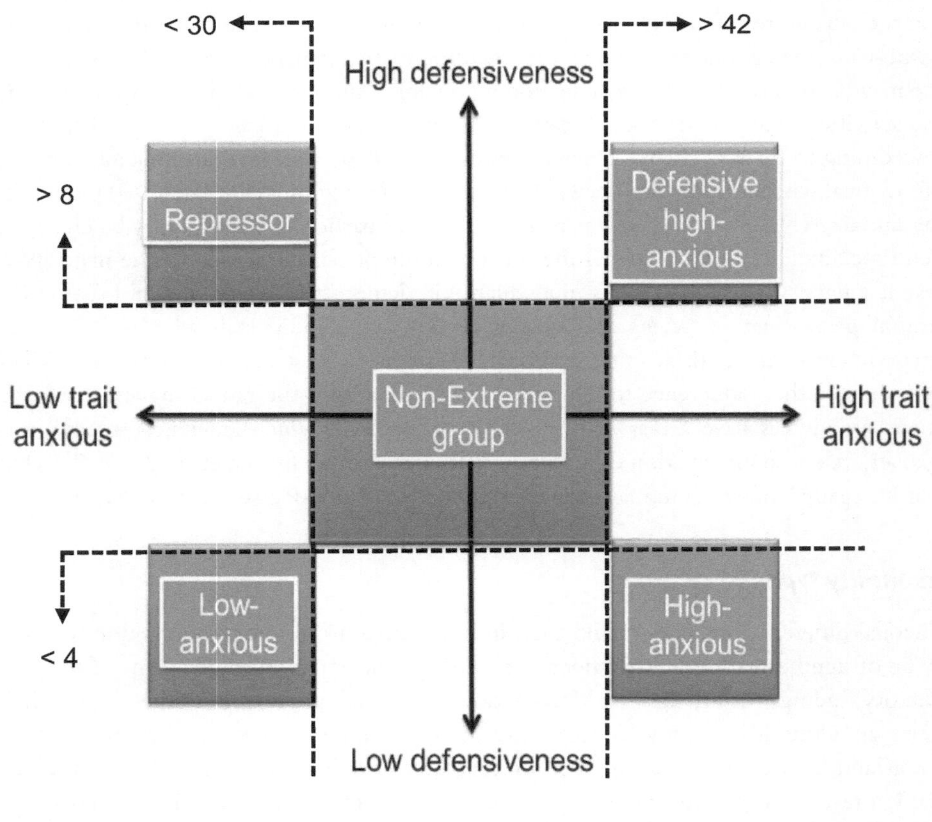

FIGURE 5.1 The four personality types and their cut-off scores for defensiveness and trait anxiety

their self-report measures and physiological measures of anxiety. Weinberger (1990) conducted an extensive review of the repressive personality type and concluded that repressors do not deliberately report low levels of anxiety in order to be considered more socially desirable but because they genuinely believe they are not experiencing negative affect. These findings suggest cognitive factors such as defensiveness can moderate anxiety responses and thus may also influence the individual's response to exercise.

There is a large body of literature investigating the repressive personality type within both the general and chronic pain populations. A relatively high proportion of repressors have been observed within a number of chronic illness populations, such as those with heart disease (20%) and cancer (36%) (Mund and Mitte, 2012; Myers, 2010). Although defensive high-anxious individuals are relatively few in the general population (~7–10%), Creswell and Chalder (2001) found that 46% of chronic fatigue syndrome patients were classified as defensive high-anxious. Lewis et al. (2012) also identified a high prevalence (39%) of the defensive high-anxious personality type within a group of patients with chronic back pain referred to an active rehabilitation programme. It is interesting to note the difference in repressor and defensive high-anxious numbers reported by these studies. For some conditions, repressors may be able to avoid their pain and self-manage treatment, an option not available for conditions with a more clearly defined biomedical diagnosis and treatment pathway. Phipps and Steele (2002) investigated the prevalence of repressors within a population of children with chronic illness (e.g. cancer, juvenile rheumatoid disorders, diabetes mellitus and cystic fibrosis). They found that repressors showed a reluctance to seek social support and engage effectively in psychotherapy. This evidence supports the notion that repressors are more likely to wish to self-manage their condition as they perceive the associated threat of the condition more positively (Eysenck, 2000; Myers, 2010). In addition, they tend to be overly optimistic about their future performance or treatment outcome (Franklin et al., 2015; Jones et al., 2004) and may be more likely to report a negative association with any treatment they receive. This may be particularly important from an exercise referral perspective as some patients may want to do activities away from the exercise referral environment.

Over the past 30 years, there has been substantial research exploring the repressive personality type as they make up approximately 40% of certain populations and are considered an essential group for health psychologists to study (Myers, 2010). Repressors may be better than defensive high-anxious individuals at coping with health behaviours that are perceived to be under their control. Considering the defensive high-anxious group account for up to 46% of a chronic musculoskeletal pain population, it would seem necessary to understand their cognitive responses and individualise their treatment programme to ensure adherence to the exercise programme. Identifying an individual's personality type may give the clinician the ability to increase the number of sessions for a defensive high-anxious individual who requires additional support and to give repressors a series of exercises to be done at home. Ultimately, all patients should be able to self-manage their condition; however, it's essential for the exercise referral practitioner to be able to provide individuals with their own coping mechanisms.

Barriers to and facilitators of adherence

Contributors to an individual's adherence or non-adherence are complex, varied and highly individual. Yet common themes have emerged and show that barriers to and facilitators of adherence occur on multiple levels to include both intrinsic and extrinsic factors. Intrinsic factors define the participants, such as motivation and preferences. Extrinsic factors refer to a participant's environment, such as family or exercise setting. Barriers to attendance include transport problems, cost of attendance, inconvenient times of sessions, dislike of gym environment, travel times and lack of explanation from the clinician. Some predictors of adherence are stable or fixed and must be considered in clinical care delivery, research and policy, while other contributors have the potential to be modified through targeted clinical intervention strategies.

Intrinsic factors

Individualisation

Participants are more trusting and more likely to adhere to the self-management suggestions of health-care professionals (HCP) if they feel they are interested in them and listen to what they say. Some participants, however, can feel as though they have to pester an HCP for an appointment or more information and that their condition is not being taken seriously. It's important to consider the individual's personality type when you are referring someone. Patients can feel throughout a treatment process as though they are passed around to different practitioners, which can lead to a miscommunication, particularly when patients feel their treatment is not progressing. Research has shown that participants understand the time restrictions of different HCP; however, research has identified that they feel treatment sessions are too short. When working with clients, it is important that the patient has substantial communication and contact with the you as the HCP in order to help them better understand their condition and to address any issues that arise. Furthermore, ensuring that your patient understands the reasons they are being referred and does not see the referral as being passed on to another clinician is important.

Goals and motivation

Many pain management programmes are designed to educate patients about their pain and to help them set goals which will improve the areas of their lives on which pain has a significant negative impact. There is good evidence for the efficacy of pain management programmes (Hoffman et al., 2007; Koes et al., 2006; Williams et al., 2012) as they not only give participants the opportunity to find out more about their pain, but they also give them something to look forward to each week: not only having social interactions with people but also feeling involved in their pain management in an active way. Research has identified that when people are part of an ERS, their main aim is not just to lose weight; there are also a range of physical and mental health improvements that they expect to achieve. When participants are referred for exercise interventions, they are encouraged to set goals associated with the intervention; however, a participant's motivation can have an impact on their adherence to the programme. Research studies have demonstrated that participants felt they should exercise but lacked self-motivation (Moore et al., 2011). Furthermore, personal commitments to work, family or social demands made it difficult to find time to exercise. Studies exploring whether the enjoyment of exercise influenced motivation reported that some participants enjoyed the activity itself, whereas others, whilst not enjoying the activity, appreciated the associated benefits such as satisfaction in maintaining the willpower to achieve their goals or the physical benefits (Martin and Woolf-May, 1999; Morgan, 2005).

Extrinsic factors

Support

In order to commit fully to ERS, it is essential that participants have a good support system. This means not just support from the wider medical staff; it is essential that these programmes facilitate the involvement of family, friends and other members of the exercise referral process. Previous research has shown that participants can feel a sense of isolation and that they can be undervalued due to their condition and inability to do certain tasks. In particular, a source of conflict can be when patients feel there is a lack of understanding by family and friends: if participants feel that others think they are 'making it up', and it is 'all in their head', thereby invalidating the pain experience. Several studies have identified that the amount of support they receive from their family is an important factor for them, and it significantly affects their lives, either positively or negatively. As with several long-term conditions, the participant's mood can change daily, depending on how much discomfort they are in, and this can have an impact on their social interactions with family and friends. Support from family and friends is important to how the patients cope on a daily basis. If individuals feel their family and friends understand their condition and how it impacts their ability to complete tasks, it can be easier to be more active and feel less isolated (Franklin et al., 2016). On the other hand, if individuals have little or no family support, this feeling of loneliness is more likely to be associated with participants becoming less active and social, a loss of self-confidence and increased feelings of depression. Previous research has found that cognitive behavioural treatments which include an education element for family are more effective at increasing physical activity (Radojevic et al., 1993). When family members have a better understanding of the condition, the variability in function and the experienced discomfort, individuals feel more supported and better able to manage their condition. However, some individuals can also experience a loss of independence with daily activities, which is evidenced through reliance on family members to complete daily tasks and a role reversal with their children. Previous research has identified a significant impact on the social and family roles for patients. Patients experience significant reductions in parenting, participation in family and social leisure activities and role reversal (e.g. children taking their parents food shopping) (Strumin and Boden, 2004). These factors have also been associated with anxiety and worry about how the individual's pain affects their family (De Souza and Frank, 2011). It is suggested that limitations in fulfilling normal family roles intensifies the negative affect and frustration of role limitations. This highlights the necessity for ERS to include an educational element for family members as they may be unaware of the impact they have on the individual. The provision of clear information about the process, not only to the patient but also to their immediate support networks, is vital to ensuring successful management.

Some studies within other populations have reported how participants benefitted from being able to talk to other patients about their condition and to discuss coping strategies with individuals in a similar situation (Franklin et al., 2016), giving participants the opportunity to have social interactions with people who take them seriously and listen to their concerns about their condition as well as learning new strategies. Such inter-patient sharing of experience and social interaction may offer an effective means to engage with groups of patients and facilitate more self/group help–based approaches. In so doing, it may be possible to facilitate greater opportunity for patients to discuss and learn about their condition without increasing the clinical resource demands of treatment. Although exercise referral sessions should be individualised, giving the patients the opportunities to meet other members on the scheme may enhance both adherence to the scheme and the long-term benefits of exercise.

Session timing and content

Patients like to be given an outline of what is going to happen in the referral process, why that particular intervention is going to be used and how it will influence them. The majority of participants understand that they have a long-term condition and that they should be active in managing it; however, previous research has identified that the treatment process is often more prescriptive than consultative (Franklin et al., 2016). Participants want to have more involvement in planning their treatment so that it addresses their individual needs, and, as a result, they feel they would be more likely to adhere to the advice.

The role of the exercise referral

The relationship between the therapist and patient has been shown to be an important factor in the treatment process, particularly for individuals with chronic pain (Hills and Kitchen, 2007). Satisfied patients have been shown to be more likely to follow their prescribed path of care and have a better relationship with their health-care practitioner (Beattie et al., 2005; Fitzpatrick and Hopkins, 1981). On the other hand, dissatisfied patients perceive their health-care services as less effective and, as a result, have a higher attrition rate from rehabilitative care (Orton et al., 1991).

Communication

Casserley-Feeney et al. (2008) specifically investigated patient satisfaction with physiotherapy care for musculoskeletal pain. They identified greater satisfaction with care that was associated with friendly, polite staff who were professional and knowledgeable and whom the patients thought were approachable and showed that they cared. Other studies have reported the ability of the therapist to communicate effectively as an important factor when rating satisfaction (Cooper et al., 2008; Cousin et al., 2012). This was particularly the case when explaining the condition in more detail and providing self-management strategies (May, 2001; Hills and Kitchen, 2007). Through the use of patient interviews, Cooper et al. (2008) investigated factors which were important to the patient in their physiotherapy care for chronic low-back pain. They identified that the communication of the therapist was a key factor that also influenced other dimensions of care which were important to them (e.g. individual care, decision-making, information and organisation of care). Participants were particularly satisfied with their therapist's communication when treatments, and the reason for these treatments, were explained. Cooper et al. (2008) highlighted the importance of adapting communication styles based on the individual characteristics of the patient. Studies have found that some patients want to be actively involved with their decision-making and treatment planning, whereas others do not want to be involved and would prefer to be prescribed a treatment programme (Chewning et al., 2012). These individual differences may be linked to the personality types of patients and may allow clinicians to tailor their approach, resulting in higher patient satisfaction and possibly better outcome.

Satisfaction

When participants are assessing their satisfaction with treatment, they often consider their health outcomes and their perception of the ER practitioner. Although satisfaction with treatment is not assessed directly within ERS, patients may note this themselves throughout treatment. A patient's adherence to an exercise programme might be increased if they were satisfied with their ER practitioner and achieving their goals for their referred condition. Patients tend to focus their rating of satisfaction with treatment on the final outcome, and as a result, there may be memory bias whereby patients may forget any initial improvements they had at the start of treatment and only focus on their current condition, rather than the whole treatment experience. Towards the end of treatment, patients may have developed effective coping strategies for their condition. Therefore, they may report higher satisfaction if they focus on the outcome and have had a higher level of support from the exercise specialist. Patients who have not seen a change in their condition may be dissatisfied with the outcome, even though the treatment process was good. Patients who do not see a change in their pain may be more likely to drop out at an earlier stage of treatment; this could be due to patient expectations not being met. Research using qualitative methods has highlighted that patient expectations of treatment are not solely based on an improvement in their condition but mainly on the quality of the process and the therapist's characteristics (May, 2001). Less attention has been paid to examining the associations between the satisfaction of psychological needs and exercise.

Adherence

Although not all conditions (e.g. osteoarthritis, chronic musculoskeletal pain etc.) are life threatening, they can significantly affect the individual's quality of life. In particular, the absence of a diagnosis and effective coping strategies can lead to life-changing emotional and social consequences (Bergman et al., 2013). The complex nature of some conditions and the difficulty clinicians face in providing a clear diagnosis present significant challenges as understanding their condition is a critical step for patients to help them engage with the treatment process. Zanini et al. (2014) highlighted that enhancing the communication between patients and clinicians by addressing factors from the patient's perspective helps build a more critical discussion about the treatment options, giving the patient a greater feeling of control and higher overall satisfaction, which is likely to lead to greater adherence. Previous research has found that having a diagnosis for their pain is important for individuals as it gives a feeling of legitimacy to their discomfort. Validation of their condition through diagnosis can help improve their social situations, making patients feel less of a burden on family and friends (Toye and Barker, 2010). Participants reported being more satisfied if their condition had been effectively described to them, particularly if diagrams were used as this gave them a greater understanding of the pain process. Without a valid explanation, patients' belief in the linear diagnosis-treatment-cure model is disturbed, which can cause feelings of worry, depression and anxiety about the future (Campbell and Guy, 2007). This will, in turn, undermine their self-efficacy with daily tasks, thus resulting in higher disability and influencing their adherence to the exercise referral scheme. Self-determination theory (SDT) is uniquely placed among theories of human motivation to examine an individual's characteristics and influence their treatment style to alter behaviour (Deci and Ryan, 2000). SDT distinguishes between intrinsic and extrinsic types of motivation regulating one's behaviour. Intrinsic motivation is defined as doing an activity because of its individual satisfactions. When intrinsically motivated, the person experiences feelings of enjoyment, the exercise of their skills, personal accomplishment and excitement. In contrast to intrinsic motivation, extrinsic motivation refers to doing an activity for instrumental reasons or to obtain some outcome separable from the activity. For example, when a person engages in an activity to gain a tangible or social reward or to avoid disapproval, they are extrinsically motivated. SDT also introduces the concept of basic psychological needs as central to understanding both the satisfactions and supports necessary for high-quality, autonomous forms of motivation. Specifically, SDT argues that there are basic psychological needs for autonomy, competence and relatedness, all of which are essential to psychological health and the development of internal motivation. Satisfaction of these basic needs results in increased feelings of well-being and exercise adherence. Like any other activity, engaging in exercise can be more or less conducive to having one's psychological needs realised. Goal contents have also been explored from an SDT perspective in relation to a range of behaviours, including exercise (Sebire et al., 2009). Specifically, SDT distinguishes intrinsic goals (e.g. seeking affiliation, personal growth or health), as those thought to be more closely related to the fulfilment of the basic psychological needs, from extrinsic goals (e.g. seeking power and influence, wealth or social recognition), which are thought to be associated with 'substitute needs', which are not essential to well-being and personal development. Within the exercise context, extrinsic goals (e.g. when the exercise is performed primarily to improve appearance) or intrinsic goals (e.g. to challenge oneself or to improve health and well-being) can clearly be distinguished. It should be noted that different goals or motives towards a given activity often naturally co-exist in the same person, some being more intrinsic, some less. Identifying participants' motives associated with exercise can influence patient adherence to the exercise and satisfaction of their psychological needs.

Case studies

Presented next are the case studies of two patients who have presented for treatment but are responding to treatment in very different ways and will provide a good insight into people you will support as an ER practitioner:

Case study A

Mary is a 52-year-old lady who works as an NHS manager. She enjoyed exercising when she was younger but now spends a lot of time sitting and leads quite a sedentary lifestyle. Up until a few years ago, she enjoyed going for walks on a weekend with her husband but has now got out of the habit of doing this. She remembers that she used to experience some aching in the knee after longer walks but not to the extent that she gets now. Her pain initially started to deteriorate six months ago after she went on holiday and spent a few days hill walking in the countryside. She initially tried to continue with the walks whilst away but found that they became too painful, and she had to miss the last few days of the walks. On returning from holiday, she tried to continue with all her usual activities but has found that walking any sort of distance significantly increases her pain. She decided that she may need to get fitter so decided to start doing longer walks again. Once her pain settled to some extent, she tried another long walk but found that this again made her pain much worse. She repeated this process a few times, but she has now stopped walking longer distances altogether. This was partly because of the pain but also because she was unsure what was causing her pain and was therefore unsure whether exercise was safe to do or whether it might result in further injury to the knees.

Mary is keen to return to her usual day-to-day activities such as gardening and shopping. However, she also really enjoyed the outdoor part of her holiday and would now like to get back into some regular walks on a weekend. She is keen to engage in active rehabilitation, is willing to engage with supervised sessions and is happy to join a gym to exercise further in her own time if this will help. On further questioning, she was not particularly fearful about exercising but felt that she needed assessing to rule out any serious cause for her pain and check that she was safe to return to longer walks. She also feels that she needs guidance and support to do this in the correct way. She has been assessed by the orthopaedic team and diagnosed with mild to moderate osteoarthritis. She has been advised that she does not need surgery and that the best treatment for this is lower-limb strengthening exercises. She is happy with this suggestion and keen to engage with treatment. She works full time but is able to do some exercise each evening if required. She is happy to do more on a weekend.

Following your initial consultation, she is very enthusiastic to get started and is keen to have a follow-up appointment in the next week to check that she is progressing well and progress on. You agree on a gym programme with her and supervise her performing this. You agree that she will perform this regime four times in total over the week. When you review her at the next session, she was extremely sore after her first unsupervised session and therefore was not able to do any further sessions this week. Despite this, she remains well motivated. On closer questioning, she informs you that she felt extremely happy to be doing something active to help herself after the supervised session. As she did not suffer any adverse reaction after the first session, she spent twice as long in the gym the next day. She agrees to re-commit to the agreed-on programme, regularly attends her follow appointments and continues with her programme in her own time. She still has a tendency to increase her exercises too quickly at times and experiences occasional setbacks.

Case study B

John is a 42-year-old man with long-standing lower-back pain. He works as a self-employed electrician and sometimes has to work up to ten hours per day to 'make ends meet'. He also feels that he cannot afford to turn work down when it is offered and will sometimes work weekends too. His wife also works, and he has two young children whom he drops off at preschool on his way to work. On the days when he can get away from work earlier, he likes to spend time with his children and try and relax. However, he is finding that he is struggling to play with them because he is in so much pain at the end of the day. He is starting to become very frustrated by his worsening pain and is starting to become low in mood and irritable. He worries about the future, particularly whether he will be able to continue to work and support his family. He is having increasing problems at work, particularly when he has to lift heavier objects or get into tight spaces. He reports that it isn't always painful to lift, but occasionally he gets severe pain on these types of activities and therefore tends to avoid doing them as he feels that he is doing further damage to his back.

He has been fully assessed by the orthopaedic team and advised that he has mechanical lower-back pain. No medical intervention is required, and he has been advised that regular exercise recommended by an ER practitioner would be helpful. You discuss his options with him regarding an exercise programme, and he raises several concerns. Firstly, he feels that as he does a physical job and works long hours, he already does enough exercise. He does admit, however, that although some aspects of his job are physically challenging, most of his time is spent in a static position. Furthermore, these are often awkward positions, and he never does any activity that raises his heart rate. Secondly, he does not feel that doing more exercise would be safe for him as he is convinced that he has damaged his back and that doing heavy lifting or impact exercises will cause further injury. Thirdly, he feels that he lacks the time to exercise regularly due to his work and family commitments, which he sees as being more important.

You also discuss which type of exercise he would like to get back to doing. He tells you that he used to play football when he was younger but that it would not be feasible to return to this as he does not have the time to commit to playing for a team. He also feels that he would not be physically able to return to this as it has been so long since he played; he feels that he is too old, and his 'back is too weak'. Other than football, exercise has 'never really been his thing', and there is nothing that he enjoys doing.

He is somewhat reluctant, however, as he has tried this in the past without benefit, and he does not see how exercise can help improve his pain. You agree on a programme with him, and you discuss when he will return for a review. He says that he will not be able to attend regularly due to other demands on his time but agrees to come back to see you in three weeks' time. Unfortunately, he cancels this appointment due to work commitments, so five weeks have passed before you review his progress. He started well with his programme, doing it three times in the first week, although he excluded some of the exercises (deadlifts and shoulder presses) as he felt that these would be harmful to his back. He was quite sore after exercising and felt that he could not work as well because of this. After two weeks, he was not feeling any better, and due to this and the other demands on his time, he has gradually decreased the amount of exercise that he has done. He went to the gym once in his third and fourth week and not at all in his fifth week. He agrees to re-commit and attends his follow up appointments at 3- to 4-week intervals. He does do some exercise at home but not at the agreed-on frequency, and he does not really feel that he is making much progress.

Summary

The NICE guidance on ERS recommends incorporating behaviour change techniques. In order to implement these change, there are certain techniques discussed in this chapter than can be applied. Within the current literature, it's proposed that individualising the treatment experience may lead to improved outcomes including adherence. In particular, addressing the factors that make it more or less likely that participants will make sustained behaviour changes could influence adherence. Firstly, the treatment process and clinician interactions influence the individual's ability to develop effective coping strategies and their satisfaction with treatment. Improving factors surrounding the referral environment may lead to an improved patient experience.

Including a family support day within the referral sessions would give the patient's relatives a better understanding of the effect their condition can have on the patient. Giving relatives an active involvement in the treatment programme may provide more support by relatives as they are made to feel included and given a sense of justification for their input. Practitioners should focus on goals, motivation and enjoyment of exercise. In particular, identifying individuals' preferences on referral setting and the timing and content of activities is valuable background information for agreeing on goals and developing action plans to help behaviour change. Including these factors in an individualised programme could help make exercise a habit after the programme completion and develop coping plans to prevent relapse.

Key points

- In order to provide an individualised programme, practitioners should take into account social and environmental factors which contribute to the individual's programme.
- An individualised programme could help make exercise a habit after the programme completion and develop coping plans to prevent relapse.
- Identifying participants' motives associated with exercise can influence patient satisfaction with both exercise and their own psychological needs.

Study tasks

1. Identify the main barriers to and facilitators of exercise adherence and provide strategies to overcome them.

2. Think of your own example of a person you know who has a condition identified in this book and identify how you might apply self-determination theory to help them become more physically active.
3. Develop an exercise plan for patient A. In particular, you should highlight specific goals that may help their adherence to the plan.
4. For people who do not have a history of physical activity, identify the barriers they might face and the strategies that you would use to modify their perceptions of exercise.
5. Think of your own case study and identify how the individual's motives can influence their satisfaction with exercise.
6. Read the following article and highlight the key points: Gheysen, F. 2018. 'Physical activity to improve cognition in older adults: can physical activity programs enriched with cognitive challenges enhance the effects? A systematic review and meta-analysis'. *International Journal of Behavioural Nutrition and Physical Activity*, 15 (1), 63.
7. Look at the current exercise referral guidelines and identify areas of good practice and guidelines which can be improved.
8. How can the exercise referral specialist influence an individual's adherence to exercise? Identify the factors and how you could apply them.
9. In this chapter, we discussed how personality type can influence a participant's adherence to an exercise referral programme. Demonstrate how you would develop a different programme for each personality type to ensure adherence.
10. Using the case studies provided, discuss how family may influence the participant's adherence. Once you have identified these issues, demonstrate how you could include family in the referral process.

References

Beattie, P., Dowda, M., Turner, C., Michener, L. & Nelson, R. 2005. Longitudinal continuity of care is associated with high patient satisfaction with physical therapy. *Physical Therapy*, 85, 1046–1052.

Beck, A. T., Emery, G. & Greenberg, R. L. 1985. *Anxiety disorders and phobias: A cognitive perspective*. New York: Basic Books.

Bergman, A. A., Matthias, M. S., Coffing, J. M. & Krebs, E. E. 2013. Contrasting tensions between patients and PCPs in chronic pain management: A qualitative study. *Pain Medicine*, 14, 1689–1697.

Campbell, C. & Guy, A. 2007. Why can't they do anything for a simple back problem? A qualitative examination of expectations for low back pain treatment and outcome. *Journal of Health Psychology*, 12, 641–652.

Casserley-Feeney, S. N., Phelan, M., Duffy, F., Roush, S., Cairns, M. C. & Hurley, D. A. 2008. Patient satisfaction with private physiotherapy for musculoskeletal pain. *BMC Musculoskeletal Disorders*, 9, 50.

Chewning, B., Bylund, C. L., Shah, B., Arora, N. K., Gueguen, J. A. & Makoul, G. 2012. Patient preferences for shared decisions: A systematic review. *Patient Education and Counseling*, 86, 9–18.

Cooper, K., Smith, B. H. & Hancock, E. 2008. Patient-centredness in physiotherapy from the perspective of the chronic low back pain patient. *Physiotherapy*, 94, 244–252.

Cousin, G., Schmid Mast, M., Roter, D. L. & Hall, J. A. 2012. Concordance between physician communication style and patient attitudes predicts patient satisfaction. *Patient Education and Counseling*, 87, 193–197.

Creswell, C. & Chalder, C. 2001. Defensive coping styles in chronic fatigue syndrome. *Journal of Psychosomatic Research*, 51, 607–610.

Deci, E. L. & Ryan, R. M. 2000. The" what" and" why" of goal pursuits: Human needs and the self-determination of behavior. *Psychological Inquiry*, 11, 227–268.

De Souza, L. & Frank, A. O. 2011. Patients' experiences of the impact of chronic back pain on family life and work. *Disability and Rehabilitation*, 33, 310–318.

Digman, J. M. 1990. Personality structure: Emergence of the five-factor model. *Annual Review of Psychology*, 41, 417–440.

Eysenck, M. W. 1992. *Anxiety: The cognitive perspective*. London: Lawrence Erlbaum Associates Ltd.

Eysenck, M. W. 1997. *Anxiety and cognition: A unified theory*. Hove: Psychology Press.

Eysenck, M. W. 2000. A cognitive approach to trait anxiety. *European Journal of Personality*, 14, 463–476.

Fahrenberg, J. 1992. Psychophysiology of neuroticism and emotionality. In: Eysenck, M. W., Gale, A. (eds.) *Handbook of individual differences: Biological perspectives*. Chichester: Wiley.

Fitzpatrick, R. M. & Hopkins, A. 1981. Patients' satisfaction with communication in neurological outpatient clinics. *Journal of Psychosomatic Research*, 25, 329–334.

Franklin, Z. C., Smith, N. C. & Fowler, N. E. 2016. A qualitative investigation of factors that matter to individuals in the pain management process. *Disability & Rehabilitation*, 38, 1934–1942.

Franklin, Z. C., Smith, N. C. & Holmes, P. S. 2015. Anxiety symptom interpretation and performance expectations in high-anxious, low-anxious, defensive high-anxious and repressor individuals. *Personality and Individual Differences*, 77, 27–32.

Gudjonsson, G. H. 1981. Self-reported emotional disturbance and its relation to electrodermal reactivity, defensiveness and trait anxiety. *Personality and Individual Differences*, 2, 47–52.

Hills, R. & Kitchen, S. 2007. Satisfaction with outpatient physiotherapy: Focus groups to explore the views of patients with acute and chronic musculoskeletal conditions. *Physiotherapy Theory and Practice*, 23, 1–20.

Hoffman, B. M., Papas, R. K., Chatkoff, D. K. & Kerns, R. D. 2007. Meta-analysis of psychological interventions for chronic low back pain. *Health Psychology*, 26, 1–9.

Jones, K. A., Smith, N. C. & Holmes, P. S. 2004. Anxiety symptom interpretation and performance predictions in high-anxious, low-anxious and repressor sport performers. *Anxiety, Stress & Coping*, 17, 187–199.

Koes, B., Van Tulder, M. & Thomas, S. 2006. Diagnosis and treatment of low back pain. *British Medical Journal*, 332, 1430–1434.

Koster, E. H., Baert, S., Bockstaele, M. & De Raedt, R. 2010. Attentional retraining procedures: Manipulating early or late components of attentional bias? *Emotion*, 10, 230–236

Lewis, S., Fowler, N., Woby, S. & Holmes, P. 2012. Defensive coping styles, anxiety and chronic low back pain. *Physiotherapy*, 98, 86–88.

Martin, C. & Woolf-May, K. 1999. The retrospective evaluation of a general practitioner exercise prescription programme. *Journal of Human Nutrition & Dietetics-Supplement*, 12, 32–42.

May, S. J. 2001. Patient satisfaction with management of back pain. Part 1: what is satisfaction? Review of satisfaction with medical management. Part 2: An explorative, qualitative study into patients' satisfaction with physiotherapy. *Physiotherapy*, 87, 4–20.

McCrae, R. R. & Costa Jr, P. T. 1985. Comparison of EPI and psychoticism scales with measures of the five-factor model of personality. *Personality and Individual Differences*, 6, 587–597.

Mogg, K. & Bradley, B. P. 1998. A cognitive-motivational analysis of anxiety. *Behaviour Research and Therapy*, 36, 809–848.

Mogg, K., Bradley, B. P., Dixon, C., Fisher, S., Twelftree, H. & McWilliams, A. 2000. Trait anxiety, defensiveness and selective processing of threat: An investigation using two measures of attentional bias. *Personality and Individual Differences*, 28, 1063–1077.

Moore, G. F., Moore, L. & Murphy, S. 2011. Facilitating adherence to physical activity: Exercise professionals' experiences of the National Exercise Referral Scheme in Wales. A qualitative study. *BMC Public Health*, 11, 935.

Morgan, O. 2005. Approaches to increase physical activity: Reviewing the evidence for exercise-referral schemes. *Public Health*, 119, 361–370.

Mund, M. & Mitte, K. 2012. The costs of repression: A meta-analysis on the relation between repressive coping and somatic diseases. *Health Psychology*, 31, 640.

Myers, L. B. 2010. The importance of the repressive coping style: Findings from 30 years of research. *Anxiety, Stress & Coping*, 23, 3–17.
Orton, M., Fitzpatrick, R., Fuller, A., Mant, D., Mlynek, C. & Thorogood, M. 1991. Factors affecting women's response to an invitation to attend for a second breast cancer screening examination. *The British Journal of General Practice*, 41, 320.
Phipps, S. & Steele, R. 2002. Repressive adaptive style in children with chronic illness. *Psychosomatic Medicine*, 64, 34–42.
Radojevic, V., Nicassio, P. M. & Weisman, M. H. 1993. Behavioral intervention with and without family support for rheumatoid arthritis. *Behavior Therapy*, 23, 13–30.
Schoth, D. E., Nunes, V. D. & Liossi, C. 2012. Attentional bias towards pain-related information in chronic pain; A meta-analysis of visual-probe investigations. *Clinical Psychology Review*, 32, 13–25.
Sebire, S. J., Standage, M. & Vansteenkiste, M. 2009. Examining intrinsic versus extrinsic exercise goals: Cognitive, affective, and behavioral outcomes. *Journal of Sport and Exercise Psychology*, 31, 189–210.
Strunin, L. & Boden, L. I. 2004. Family consequences of chronic back pain. *Social Science & Medicine*, 58, 1385–1393.
Toye, F. & Barker, K. 2010. 'Could I be imagining this?' – the dialectic struggles of people with persistent unexplained back pain. *Disability and Rehabilitation*, 32, 1722–1732.
Weinberger, D. A. 1990. *The construct validity of the repressive coping style*. Chicago: University of Chicago Press.
Weinberger, D. A., Schwartz, G. E. & Davidson, R. J. 1979. Low-anxious, high-anxious, and repressive coping styles: Psychometric patterns and behavioral and physiological responses to stress. *Journal of Abnormal Psychology*, 88, 369–380.
Williams, A., Eccleston, C. & Morley, S. 2012. Psychological therapies for the management of chronic pain (excluding headache) in adults. *Cochrane Database System Review*, 11, 1–111.
Zanini, C., Sarzi-Puttini, P., Atzeni, F., Di Franco, M. & Rubinelli, S. 2014. Doctors' insights into the patient perspective: A qualitative study in the field of chronic pain. *BioMed Research International*, 514230.

6

BEHAVIOUR CHANGE IN EXERCISE REFERRAL

Paul Gorczynski

Chapter aims

The aims of this chapter are to:

- Support the application of physical activity guidelines
- Introduce individual and environmental factors associated with physical activity
- Present strategies to identify and overcome individual and environmental barriers to physical activity
- Explain how physical activity outcome expectations should be communicated to clients
- Present various behavioural strategies to promote physical activity within exercise referral schemes
- Overview stages of change and goal-setting strategies to promote physical activity
- Suggest strategies to address physical activity relapse

Introduction

The benefits of physical activity are numerous and well documented (Warburton & Bredin, 2016). Extensive, robust evidence has shown that being active can have physical, psychological and social benefits (Warburton, Charlesworth, Ivey, Nettlefold, & Bredin, 2010; Rhodes, Janssen, Bredin, Warburton, & Bauman, 2017; Lubans et al., 2016; Pels & Kleinert, 2016). Physical health benefits can include reduced risk of coronary heart disease, high blood pressure, stroke, metabolic syndrome, type 2 diabetes, breast cancer, colon cancer, falling and all-cause mortality (Lee et al., 2012). Physical activity has been shown to improve cardiorespiratory and muscular fitness, help individuals improve their body mass and composition, strengthen their bone health and increase functional health (Rhodes et al., 2017). Psychological benefits include improvements in cognition, well-being, a sense of self, a sense of independence, self-confidence, self-esteem and symptoms of various mental illnesses, including major depressive disorder, generalised anxiety disorder, stress-related disorders, bipolar disorder, schizophrenia, alcohol use disorder and eating disorders (for a full review, see Stubbs & Rosenbaum, 2018).

DOI: 10.4324/9781315102399-6

With respect to social benefits, people who are active enjoy meeting individuals, sustaining important relationships in their lives, feeling a sense of purpose and pleasure and being active in their communities (Pels & Kleinert, 2016). Being physically active outdoors, be it green or blue physical activity, also brings about several benefits in addition to those physical, psychological and social benefits, like an appreciation for the natural environment, engagement in ecological management and preservation and volunteerism (Dennis & James, 2016). Overall, the evidence to be active is clear and robust.

Despite these benefits, few people engage in sufficient, regular physical activity. A report by Public Health England, showed that 42% of women and 34% of men are not active enough to achieve good health (Office for National Statistics, 2017). These figures show that people in England are inactive when compared to global trends, in which the prevalence of physical inactivity is 27.5% (95% uncertainty interval, 25.0–32.2%; Women, 31.7% (28.6–39.0%); Men, 23.4% (21.1–30.7%)) (Guthold, Stevens, Riley, & Bull, 2018).

Physical activity guidelines

The UK Physical Activity Guidelines provide guidance from the chief medical officer on the amount of physical activity people should do on a daily or weekly basis (Department of Health and Social Care, 2019). The guidelines are age specific: early years (infants under 5 years of age who cannot walk), early years (children under 5 years of age who are capable of walking), children and young people (5 to 18 years), adults (19 to 64 years) and older adults (65+ years). For each age group, guidance is also given to reduce sedentary behaviour, primarily time spent sitting.

For infants and children who cannot walk, the guidelines advocate for physical activity through both floor-based play and water-based activities. Time spent sitting, including time spent in restraints, should be minimised. For children under 5 years of age who are capable of walking, the guidelines encourage the accumulation of 180 minutes of physical activity while also cutting down on sedentary time. Children and young people between 5 and 18 years should get an average 60 minutes of moderate (3–6 Metabolic Equivalents, brisk walking, dancing) or vigorous (> 6 Metabolic Equivalents, running, fast cycling) activity each day. Each week, children and young people are encouraged to engage in a variety of types and intensities of physical activity across the week to develop movement skills, muscular fitness and bone strength. Again, steps should be taken to limit the amount of time spent being sedentary. For adults, over the course of a week, 150 minutes of moderate-intensity activity or 75 minutes of vigorous-intensity activity should be accumulated. Additionally, strength-training exercises should be done at least twice a week. Again, time spent being sedentary should be minimised. Lastly for older adults, 150 minutes of moderate-intensity activity or 75 minutes of vigorous activity should be attained. Twice a week, activities should be engaged in to help with strength training, flexibility and balance. Like all other age groups, time spent being sedentary should be minimised.

Physical activity research frameworks

Epidemiological evidence (Guthold et al., 2018) has shown that being active is not easy and something most people do not do enough of. Research concerning physical activity to date has mostly followed the behavioural epidemiological framework (Sallis & Owen, 1999).

The framework advocates a five-step, non-linear and fluid model set out to establish health outcomes evidence for physical activity behaviour change by better understanding issues of physical activity measurement and determinants of physical activity behaviour change that ultimately lead researchers to design more robust interventions and translate those findings into practice. The framework is non-linear and fluid to allow room for contextual changes over time and adaptability, like new technological advances in physical activity measurement (e.g. mobile phone tracking) or changes in the determinants of physical activity behaviour (e.g. environmental changes including the climate emergency on air quality or temperature). The framework is also inclusive of multiple perspectives toward understanding factors that may influence physical activity behaviour and, ultimately, how physical activity interventions can be designed and delivered. Consequently, the framework acknowledges an ecological perspective towards physical activity (Brofenbrenner, 1979; Sallis, Owen, & Fisher, 2008). The ecological framework is built on an understanding that people operate within both social and physical environments, where multiple factors at multiple levels influence physical activity behaviour. Levels within an ecological framework include intrapersonal (e.g. biological factors, psychological factors), interpersonal (e.g. social relationships), community/organisational (e.g. schools, workplaces), the physical environment (e.g. built and natural) and policy (e.g. regulations, laws) (Sallis et al., 2008). A better understanding of individual and environmental factors that influence physical activity has led to the creation of multi-level interventions that have helped people better identify barriers to and harness facilitators of being active.

Individual and environmental factors

Research that has informed our understanding of factors that influence physical activity behaviour has been derived from both cross-sectional and longitudinal (observational and intervention) studies (Atkin, van Sluijs, Dollman, Taylor, & Stanley, 2016). Cross-sectional studies have shown various relationships between individual and environmental factors and physical activity. These factors are known as correlates. Longitudinal studies have shown various causal inferences between individual and environmental factors and physical activity, or what are known as determinants. Correlates and determinants can be known as mediators when they facilitate a causal relationship between independent and dependent variables, moderators when they determine the strength of a relationship between independent and dependent variables and confounders when they predict the dependent variable and are also associated with the independent variable (Bauman, Sallis, Dzewaltowski, & Owen, 2002; Condello et al., 2017).

For example, there is a causal relationship between a physical activity intervention (independent variable) whereby it leads to improvements in one's physical activity self-efficacy, which leads to an increased amount of time spent being physically active (dependent variable). A causal relationship exists between the intervention, self-efficacy and physical activity. Here, self-efficacy acts as a mediator as it facilitates this causal relationship. To illustrate what a moderator is, consider the variable gender. A physical activity intervention (independent variable) does not affect a person's gender. The time spent being physically active differs between individuals of different genders, with those who identify as men being more physically active than those who identify as women. Here, gender acts as a moderator, where it determines the strength of the relationship between an independent variable and a dependent variable. To explain a confounding variable, consider a person's age. Age may have an impact on the amount of time spent being physically active (dependent variable), where individuals who are older have been shown to be less active. Age may also have an impact on engagement in a physical activity intervention (independent variable), where individuals who are older have been shown to be less willing to enrol in such physical activity interventions or programmes.

Having knowledge of correlates and determinants and their impact on physical activity behaviour is crucial as this knowledge will help develop and advance theories used to underpin physical activity interventions (Biddle, Mutrie, & Gorely, 2015). This knowledge will tell us which groups to target (moderators), how to improve the causal relationship between interventions and physical activity (mediators) and other factors we should be mindful of (confounders). Presented next is a review of some of the current knowledge of some of the most important correlates and determinants and how they have been shown to facilitate physical activity behaviour in adults and older adults.

Correlates and determinants of physical activity

The Lancet Physical Activity Series Working Group (Bauman et al., 2012) examined systematic reviews that explored different correlates and determinants of physical activity. Their review broke down correlates and determinants by demographic and biological factors, psychosocial factors, behavioural factors, social and cultural factors and environmental factors. In each of these categories, they found evidence that either supported or did not support these factors playing a role in influencing physical activity. Many systematic reviews reviewed by the Lancet Group found inconclusive evidence for some factors, meaning it was not certain whether some factors played a role in influencing physical activity. This finding on inconclusive evidence has been supported by Condello and colleagues (2017), who suggested that more rigorous prospective studies be conducted that rely on objective methods of physical activity measurement to understand correlates and determinants.

Demographic and biological factors

Research suggests that as people age, physical activity decreases (Kaewthummanukul & Brown, 2006; Rhodes et al., 1999; Trost, Owen, Bauman, Sallis, & Brown, 2002), with men being more active than women throughout the lifespan (Rhodes et al., 1999; Trost et al., 2002). Physical activity has been shown to increase with income (Plonczynski, 2003; Trost et al., 2002) and health status or one's perceived level of fitness (Rhodes et al., 1999; Trost et al., 2002; Plonczynski, 2003; Allender, Hutchinson, & Foster, 2008; Van Stralen, de Vries, Mudde, Bolman, & Lechner, 2009).

Psychosocial factors

Self-efficacy (i.e. the belief individuals have in their ability to accomplish a task, was one of the strongest correlates and determinants of physical activity (Rhodes et al., 1999; Trost et al., 2002; Plonczynski, 2003; Kaewthummanukul & Brown, 2006; Van Stralen et al., 2009). Intentions to be active were found to be correlated with physical activity (Rhodes et al., 1999; Trost et al., 2002), especially in the beginning stages of becoming active (Van Stralen et al., 2009). Evidence suggests that using a stage approach to becoming active may be beneficial (Trost et al., 2002; Van Stralen et al., 2009), with action planning being most useful in setting intentions in the pursuit of increasing physical activity behaviour (Van Stralen et al., 2009).

Behavioural factors

Some evidence suggests that prior physical activity behaviour plays a role in shaping the physical activity behaviour of adults (Babakus & Thompson, 2012; Barnett, van Sluijs, & Ogilvie, 2012; Trost et al., 2002; Van Stralen et al., 2009; Koeneman, Verheijden, Chinapaw, & Hopman-Rock, 2011). Smoking was also associated with lower levels of physical activity behaviour (Koeneman et al., 2011). Consult these references for further details on behavioural factors influencing physical activity behaviours.

Social and cultural factors

Social support is correlated with physical activity in a range of individuals, particularly from family and peers with similar health concerns (Rhodes et al., 1999).

Environmental factors

Evidence suggests the presence of recreational facilities playing a role in physical activity (Humpel, Owen, & Leslie, 2002; Owen, Humpel, Leslie, Bauman, & Sallis, 2004; Duncan, Spence, & Mummery, 2005; Wendel-Vos, Droomers, Kremers, Brug, & van Lenthe, 2007; Van Stralen et al., 2009), along with effective transportation systems (Humpel et al., 2002; Owen et al., 2004; Duncan et al., 2005; Van Stralen et al., 2009). The aesthetics of an environment also helped individuals become active (Humpel et al., 2002; Cunningham & Michael, 2004; Owen et al., 2004).

Barriers to physical activity

Individual and environmental barriers

The 2007 Health Survey for England (Craig & Shelton, 2008) highlights many individual and environmental barriers to physical activity for women and men. For all adult women, the most cited individual barriers were a lack of time (37%), work commitments (34%), caring responsibilities for children or older individuals (25%), a lack of motivation (25%) and not perceiving oneself as 'sporty' (21%). For women who were older (55–64 years), slightly different barriers existed and were more prominent. For instance, poor health and physical limitations was the most reported barrier (23%), followed by not perceiving oneself as 'sporty' (21%), work commitments (20%), a perception that they didn't need to be any more active (20%) and a lack of time (19%). For women who were younger (16–24 years), the most reported barriers were a lack of time (44%), a lack of motivation (36%), work commitments (35%), a lack of money (34%) and not perceiving oneself as a 'sporty' (27%).

For all adult men, the barriers were work commitments (45%), a lack of time (38%), a lack of motivation (21%), a perception that they don't need to be any more active (17%) and a preference for doing things other than physical activity (15%). For men who were older (55–64 years), the most reported barriers were nearly the same as reported for all adult men, except that poor health and physical limitations was perceived to be a major barrier (21%). For men who were younger (16–24 years), again, the most reported barriers were nearly the same as those reported for all adult men, except that a lack of money was perceived to be a major barrier (23%). For both genders, barriers were relatively similar between the lowest and highest income brackets but with major differences seen in poor health and physical limitations being a problem for both women (lowest = 19%, highest = 9%) and men (lowest = 24%, highest = 5%).

With regard to environmental barriers, results from the Marmot Review 'Fair Society, Healthy Lives' (2010) indicated that improvements in access to good quality open and green space as well as recreation facilities were needed to help individuals become more active. Other research studies have also found that environmental barriers can include the weather, air or noise pollution, safety and a lack of sidewalks (Salmon, Owen, Crawford, Bauman, & Sallis, 2003). Recent research points to poor air quality having a profound impact on levels of physical activity (An, Zhang, Ji, & Guan, 2018). A thorough understanding of barriers to physical activity is key to helping individuals understand what challenges they may encounter that prevent them from being active. This understanding helps shape physical activity interventions at multiple levels and ultimately ensures that such interventions address barriers and take advantage of facilitators that promote activity.

Communicating physical activity guidelines and addressing barriers

Research that has investigated knowledge of the UK Physical Activity Guidelines (Department of Health and Social Care, 2019) by the general public has shown that only 18% of individuals are aware of them, with individuals who are younger, women, employed, have attained higher levels of education and are in good health being more likely to recall them accurately (Knox, Esliger, Biddle, & Sherar, 2013). Only 2% of individuals stated that physical activity should be effortful. Although improvements in knowledge of the guidelines have been seen in recent years (Craig, Mindell, Hirani, Chaudhury, & Esliger, 2009), there are many individuals who are less likely to know what levels and types of physical activity behaviours they should be achieving. For instance, greater efforts to communicate information about the guidelines need to be made to reach older individuals, those who are low-wage workers, those who are unemployed and individuals living with poor health status. Efforts in how information about the guidelines is communicated needs not only to address these demographic factors but also to help individuals identify and overcome barriers to being inactive. Messages need to help individuals recognise discrepancies between their own current behaviours and what the guidelines suggest. By acknowledging and understanding current behaviours, individuals can be better placed to set realistic intentions and set stage-specific goals to become physically active. Messages should also help strengthen self-efficacy and help individuals build beliefs in having the ability to reach their set goals and achieve them in an incremental and sustainable manner. Put simply, messages need to capture an individual's attention, be informative, build confidence and be motivational.

Behavioural theories

Research into the effectiveness of exercise referral schemes has shown that they have not been entirely successful in helping people who are inactive become active (Williams, Hendry,

France, Lewis, & Wilkinson, 2007). A systematic review and meta-analysis of 18 studies showed that exercise referral schemes have a small effect, where 1 person becomes moderately active for every 17 individuals referred to a scheme. Recommendations state that individuals should only be referred to exercise schemes if the schemes are properly designed and consider the readiness for change of individual participants, their levels of self-determination to engage in physical activity and their ability to regulate their physical activity behaviour. Exercise referral schemes also need to help individuals identify and address barriers to becoming active and help them improve low self-efficacy. Such recommendations are in line with research that has explored the correlates and determinants of physical activity (Bauman et al., 2012). But despite the need to help individuals become more active and achieve recommendations as stated in the UK Chief Medical Officer's Guidelines, it should not be forgotten that low levels of activity can have a profound impact on overall health (Warburton & Bredin, 2016). In fact, the greatest impact on decreasing all-cause mortality stems from low levels of activity with only incremental reductions in mortality with increased levels of activity (Lollgen, Bockenhoff, & Knapp, 2009).

For greatest effect, physical activity interventions should be based on sound behaviour change theory (Khan et al., 2002). Next, social cognitive theory (Bandura, 1986) and the transtheoretical model (Prochaska & DiClimente, 1986) are described in detail, along with how they can be applied in a manner to help individuals address important factors associated with physical activity engagement, maintenance and relapse prevention.

Social cognitive theory

Social cognitive theory stipulates that people learn by watching others, with development influenced by their environments (e.g. built, natural), their personal factors (e.g. cognition, mood, attitude) and their behaviours (e.g. frequency, intensity, type, time) (Bandura, 1986). Behaviours, personal factors and environmental factors, referred to as triadic reciprocal causation, are determinants that influence each other and overall learning. Within social cognitive theory, self-efficacy – the beliefs people have about their ability to accomplish particular behaviours – is a central determinant that drives task-oriented behaviour (Bandura, 2004). Self-efficacy can influence multiple factors, including the desired behaviour that is to be accomplished, the goals individuals set for themselves to achieve their desired behaviour, the outcome expectations for their desired behaviour and how they view sociocultural factors that influence their desired behaviour. To date, given the success of social cognitive theory in promoting physical activity, it has been one of the most studied theories in the field (Beauchamp, Crawford, & Jackson, 2019).

With respect to goals, people with greater self-efficacy set more challenging goals for themselves, are more committed to their goals and are more persistent in the face of adversity (Locke & Latham, 2006). Goals provide a great deal of support to an individual trying to achieve a particular desired behaviour. For instance, goals provide structure by focusing one's attention, effort and action toward a particular task. Goals also provide the opportunity for feedback to help individuals ascertain progress with a desired behaviour. In a sense, goals can help individuals know if they've achieved or are on track to achieving their desired behaviour. Goals should be set with the person in mind, meaning there is no one-size-fits-all goal. Goal setting, especially for those who are physically inactive, should be open to recognising a person's learning process, their incremental progress and whether they have adopted their desired behaviour in the form of a habit (McEwan et al., 2016; Swann & Rosenbaum, 2018). Goals should also be stage-of-readiness specific, meaning that they are aligned with the individual's intentions to engage in the desired behaviour.

With respect to outcome expectations, individuals with greater self-efficacy expect various positive outcomes after accomplishing a particular desired behaviour. For instance, individuals who become physically active expect physical (e.g. improved fitness), social (e.g. increased size and depth of social networks) and self-evaluative (e.g. positive assessment of one's own progress) outcomes. With respect to sociocultural factors, individuals with greater self-efficacy are able to identify and overcome barriers that may impede a desired behaviour and identify and make use of individual and environmental facilitators to help achieve a desired behaviour. For instance, an individual with higher levels of self-efficacy who wants to become more active may be able to identify busy times of the week and use a calendar to organise their time in a potentially more efficient manner. Another example may be a person in an environment that is heavily polluted who locates a gym in their community or goes about gaining access to some other indoor facility.

Given the importance of self-efficacy in helping influence desired behaviours, understanding how to strengthen self-efficacy is important (Bandura, 1977). There are four key sources of self-efficacy:

1. Past mastery experiences. Individuals who successfully perform desired behaviours will have the belief that they can successfully perform those behaviours again. The more successful completions of the desired behaviour, the stronger one's self-efficacy. Unfortunately, self-efficacy can be quite fragile, too; failures can undermine an individual's self-efficacy. Setting small steps to achieve a desired behaviour may help strengthen one's self-efficacy.
2. Modelling or vicarious experiences. Watching other individuals successfully complete a desired behaviour may help strengthen an individual's self-efficacy. Similar to past mastery experiences, watching others fail will decrease one's self-efficacy and may discourage an individual from attempting the desired behaviour.
3. Verbal persuasion. Providing individuals with information about how to perform a particular behaviour may strengthen their self-efficacy. Verbal persuasion delivered through positive appraisal can help individuals who believe they have the ability to achieve a desired behaviour.
4. Emotional and physiological states. Positive or negative mood states based on successful or unsuccessful experiences associated with the desired behaviour cognitively prime the individual for the next attempt at the desired behaviour. Memories of previous attempts help influence how an individual feels about a desired behaviour. Physiological states – bodily sensations associated with a desired behaviour – may signal to an individual their level of self-efficacy about a particular desired behaviour. When evaluating emotional and physiological states, a critical appraisal of emotional and physiological information is key.

To help ensure individuals improve their self-efficacy over time and work toward achieving their desired behaviour in a process-oriented manner, the use of a stage-wise model is suggested. Using interventions that rely on the transtheoretical model (Prochaska & DiClimente, 1986) is one strategy.

Transtheoretical model (incorporate relapse)

The transtheoretical model is a set of theories that assess the readiness of individuals to change a desired behaviour and provide a series of cognitive and behavioural strategies, or processes of change, to facilitate adoption of the desired behaviour and prevent relapse (Prochaska & DiClimente, 1986). According to the transtheoretical model, individuals are placed into one of five stages of readiness: precontemplation (a person has no intention of changing a desired behaviour), contemplation (a person intends to change a desired behaviour in the next six months), preparation (a person intends to change a desired behaviour in the next month), active (a person has been engaged in the desired behaviour for between one and six months) and maintenance (a person has been engaged in the desired behaviour for over six months). Within each stage, individuals conduct a decisional balance in which they consider the pros and cons of engaging in a desired behaviour. When individuals identify more cons than pros for engaging in a desired behaviour, they are less likely to change their current behaviour and adopt a desired one. For instance, individuals who identify as being busy and having no time to engage in physical activity are more likely to identify beliefs (cons) that are prevalent amongst individuals who are in the precontemplation and contemplation stages of behaviour change. These individuals believe there are more reasons to not adopt a desired behaviour than to adopt it. It is only when individuals begin to believe there are more pros than cons to adopting a desired behaviour do individuals take active preparatory steps to change their behaviour and move on to another stage of readiness.

To facilitate movement through the stages of readiness, there are five cognitive and five behavioural processes of change. In essence, with stage progression, there is an increase of pros and a decrease in cons (Marshall & Biddle, 2001).

Cognitive processes:

1. Consciousness raising – learning about being physically active and various physical, psychological and social benefits associated with regular activity
2. Dramatic relief – experiencing and recognising feelings associated with being physically inactive and what consequences it may have on one's own health
3. Environmental re-evaluation – becoming aware of how your physical inactivity may have consequences for friends, family and your community
4. Self-re-evaluation – creating a new sense of self by becoming an individual who is active
5. Self-liberation – committing oneself to engaging in regular activity

Behavioural Processes:

1. Counter conditioning – making substitutions for sedentary activity with physical activity
2. Helping relationships – getting social support to become active
3. Social liberation – recognising and taking advantage of social customs to become active (e.g. New Year's resolutions, bicycle-sharing programs, gyms at work)
4. Reinforcement management – rewarding oneself for achieving a desired behaviour
5. Stimulus control – using reminders to remember to engage in regular activity

As individuals move through stages, self-efficacy increases with each successive stage (Marshall & Biddle, 2001). As people begin to believe there are more pros than cons to adopting their desired behaviour, changes are seen in their perspectives towards their own ability to enact a desired behaviour. Self-efficacy is also key to helping individuals overcome physical activity relapse (Marlatt & Gordon, 1985). Specifically, when individuals face high-risk situations, like being busy, they may stop being active and relapse into inactivity. After encountering such a high-risk situation, self-efficacy is key to determining whether someone will cope with the situation in an effective manner and resume the desired behaviour or in an ineffective manner, whereby they grow ever more distant from their desired behaviour. If a person faces a busy situation, choosing an effective coping strategy, like time management and scheduling, may lead to an increase in self-efficacy, where the person will believe in their ability to engage in the desired behaviour because they will have the time to do so. An increase in self-efficacy may lead to an increased chance of becoming active. However, if there is no coping strategy that addresses one's busy schedule, this may have an effect on the individual that results in lower levels of self-efficacy, making the individual less likely to believe they can overcome their sense of being busy and engage in physical activity. Low levels of self-efficacy may lead to negative attributes in the form of self-doubt and self-blame and a higher probability of not resuming in regular activity.

Case study

Stephen is a 65-year-old man with a trans history (pronouns: he, him, his) who works as a union representative for a large trade union in the health-care sector. Stephen has been a union activist for over 40 years and has been heavily involved in fighting for LGBT rights throughout his life. Stephen has always remained active despite having a very busy schedule. Part of his physical activity routine has involved daily runs, which have helped manage his stress. Recently, Stephen was diagnosed with ovarian cancer. Despite successful surgery, chemotherapy and radiation treatment, Stephen doesn't feel like himself. On most days, he can barely get out of bed, let alone go for a walk. Because he is still recovering from his cancer and subsequent treatments, Stephen has been working on a part-time basis until he feels strong enough to return to full-time work. Stephen misses being active and wishes he could get back to running on a daily basis. He feels his inactivity is having a profound impact on his physical and mental well-being.

Referring Stephen to an exercise referral scheme may help him begin to address his inactivity. A step-by-step process, based on exercise counselling, is described next (Gorczynski, Faulkner, Cohn, & Remington, 2014).

Step 1: Information capture

This step includes capturing demographic information on the individual to help better understand contextual factors that may impact levels of physical activity. This can include age, gender identity, race, ethnicity, sexuality, relationship status, health status, working life and housing. All these factors are determinants of physical activity and may play a role in helping someone become and stay active. Information on past and present physical activity behaviours will help the counsellor better plan for the future and what goals to set. Additionally, obtaining information on readiness to be physically active can help place the individual in one of the five different stages of the transtheoretical model (precontemplation, contemplation, preparation, active, maintenance) to better align behavioural strategies with potential goals. Conducting a decisional balance exercise, in which the individual weighs up the pros and cons of changing their physical activity behaviour, will help examine any ambivalence the individual may have towards becoming active and offer further insight into future sessions and how they might be planned.

Stephen is 65 years old, identifies as a man with a trans history and is currently recovering from cancer and various cancer-related interventions. He appears to be gaining strength with each passing day while also being mindful of his very heavy work commitments. He has disclosed working long hours in the past and using running as a source of stress management. He appears to be in the contemplation or preparation stages of the transtheoretical model where he would like to return to running. The information capture stage should be used to better understand exactly how much running Stephen would like to do, and further discussion points may help refine sources of support, should he experience any setbacks.

Step 2: Action planning

This step allows the individual to set future physical activity goals. It calls for a specific, measurable, achievable, relevant and timely goal (Locke & Latham, 2006). Additional information on goal importance and potential barriers to becoming active will establish a clear action plan to help achieve the set goal and address identified barriers. Discussing and identifying a support network – those who may be called upon for assistance with overcoming identified physical activity barriers – will reinforce self-efficacy and motivation to become active.

During this step, Stephen's specific running goal should be established. This would include how far he would like to run and for how long. Additional information on running attire and location may be helpful. A discussion of what may come up in his schedule that could prevent him from running would be useful, as would how he would handle any physical or mental health setbacks.

Step 3: Action plan follow-up

The third step allows the individual to reaffirm their goal and why it's important to them. Recounting steps taken to accomplish their goal in the past week will help identify whether the action plan was followed. If necessary, adjust the goal and scale it to the needs to of the individual. Discussing any barriers that may have come up in the previous week should help identify any unexpected barriers and address whether new strategies are needed to handle future challenges to becoming active. Again, discussing individuals who may be called upon for assistance helps maintain a strong and helpful network of social support. This step can be done as many times as necessary to help ensure the individual is following the action plan and learning to deal with barriers to activity.

In Stephen's case, understanding whether the action plan was followed is key, as is assessing whether the goal is still important to him. Being mindful of both physical and mental health is also important and whether any health challenges have affected the overall physical activity goal.

Conclusion

Overall, the benefits of physical activity are numerous and well documented, and theory-based interventions are needed not only to address barriers to but also to harness facilitators of being active (Warburton & Bredin, 2016). Behavioural strategies used in the context of exercise referral schemes may help individuals gain self-efficacy and set stage-wise goals to become more active. Research shows consistently that any attempt to help individuals become more active needs to be rooted in a sound understanding of behavioural theory.

References

Allender, S., Hutchinson, L., & Foster, C. (2008). Life-change events and participation in physical activity: A systematic review. *Health Promotion International*, 23, 160–172.

An, R., Zhang, S., Ji, M., & Guan, C. (2018). Impact of ambient air pollution on physical activity among adults: A systematic review and meta-analysis. *Perspectives in Public Health*, 138(2), 111–121.

Atkin, A. J., van Sluijs, E. M. F., Dollman, J., Taylor, W. C., & Stanley, R. M. (2016). Identifying correlates and determinants of physical activity in youth: How can we advance the field? *Preventive Medicine*, 87, 167–169.

Babakus, W. S., & Thompson, J. L. (2012). Physical activity among South Asian women: A systematic, mixed-methods review. *International Journal of Behavioral Nutrition and Physical Activity*, 9, 150.

Bandura, A. (1977). Self-efficacy: Toward a unifying theory of behavioral change. *Psychological Review*, 84(2), 191–215. http://dx.doi.org/10.1037/0033-295X.84.2.191

Bandura, A. (1986). *Social foundations of thought and action: A social cognitive theory*. Englewood Cliffs, NJ: Prentice-Hall.

Bandura, A. (2004). Health promotion by social cognitive means. *Health Education & Behavior*, 31(2), 143–164. https://doi.org/10.1177/1090198104263660

Barnett, I., van Sluijs, E. M., & Ogilvie, D. (2012). Physical activity and transitioning to retirement: A systematic review. *American Journal of Preventive Medicine*, 43(3), 329–336. DOI: 10.1016/j.amepre.2012.05.026

Bauman, A., Reis, R. S., Sallis, J. F., Wells, J. C., Loos, R. J. F., Martin, B. W., & the Lancet Physical Activity Series Working Group (2012). *Lancet*, 380, 258–271. DOI: 10.1016/S0140–6736(12)60735-1

Bauman, A. E., Sallis, J. F., Dzewaltowski, D. A., & Owen, N. (2002). Toward a better understanding of the influences on physical activity: The role of determinants, correlates, causal variables, mediators, moderators, and confounders. *American Journal of Preventive Medicine*, 23(2, S1), 5–14.

Beauchamp, M. R., Crawford, K. L., & Jackson, B. (2019). Social cognitive theory and physical activity: Mechanisms of behavior change, critique, and legacy. *Psychology of Sport and Exercise*, 42, 110–117.

Biddle, S., Mutrie, N., & Gorely, T. (2015). *Psychology of physical activity: Determinants, well-being, and interventions*. New York: Routledge.

Bronfenbrenner, U. (1979). *The ecology of human development*. Cambridge, MA: Harvard University Press.

Condello, G., Puggina, A., Aleksovska, K., Buck, C., Burns, C., Cardon, G., . . . DEDIPAC consortium (2017). *International Journal of Behavioral Nutrition and Physical Activity*, 14, 58. DOI: 10.1186/s12966-017-0510-2

Craig, R., Mindell, J., Hirani, V., Chaudhury, M., & Esliger, D. (2009). Accelerometry in adults. In R. Craig, J. Mindell, & V. Hirani (Eds.), *Health survey for England 2008: Volume 1 physical activity and fitness* (pp. 59–88). Leeds, UK: The Health and Social Care Information Centre.

Craig, R., & Shelton, N. (2008). *Health survey for England 2007: Healthy lifestyles: Knowledge, attitudes and behaviour*. Leeds, UK: The NHS Information Centre.

Cunningham, G. O., & Michael, Y. L. (2004). Concepts guiding the study of the impact of the built environment on physical activity for older adults: A review of the literature. *American Journal of Health Promotion*, 18, 435–443.

Dennis, M., & James, P. (2016). Urban participation in urban green commons: Exploring the links between access, volunteerism, biodiversity and wellbeing. *Urban Forestry & Urban Greening*, 15, 22–31.

Department of Health and Social Care (2019). *Physical activity guidelines: UK Chief Medical Officers' report*. Retrieved from https://www.gov.uk/government/publications/physical-activity-guidelines-uk-chief-medical-officers-report

Duncan, M. J., Spence, J. C., & Mummery, W. K. (2005). Perceived environment and physical activity: A meta-analysis of selected environmental characteristics. *International Journal of Behavioral Nutrition and Physical Activity*, 2, 11.

Gorczynski, P., Faulkner, G., Cohn, T., & Remington, G. (2014). Examining the efficacy and feasibility of exercise counseling in individuals with schizophrenia: A single-case experimental study. *Mental Health and Physical Activity*, 7(3), 191–197.

Guthold, R., Stevens, G. A., Riley, L. M., & Bull, F. C. (2018). Worldwide trends in insufficient physical activity from 2001 to 2016: A pooled analysis of 358 population-based surveys with 1·9 million participants. *Lancet Global Health*, 6, e1077–e1086. DOI: 10.1016/S2214-109X(18)30357-7

Humpel, N., Owen, N., & Leslie, E. (2002). Environmental factors associated with adults participation in physical activity: A review. *American Journal of Preventative Medicine*, 22, 58–69.

Kaewthummanukul, T., & Brown, K. C. (2006). Determinants of employee participation in physical activity: Critical review of the literature. *AAOHN Journal*, 54, 249.

Khan, E. B., Ramsey, L. T., Brownson, R. C., Heath, G. W., Howze, E. H., Powell, K. E., . . . Corso, P. (2002). The effectiveness of interventions to increase physical activity. *American Journal of Preventative Medicine*, 22(4, S1), 73–107.

Knox, E. C. L., Esliger, D. W., Biddle, S. J. H., & Sherar, L. B. (2013). Lack of knowledge of physical activity guidelines: Can physical activity promotion campaigns do better? *BMJ Open*, 3, e003633. DOI: 10.1136/bmjopen-2013–003633

Koeneman, M. A., Verheijden, M. W., Chinapaw, M. J., & Hopman-Rock M. (2011). Determinants of physical activity and exercise in healthy older adults: A systematic review. *International Journal of Behavioral Nutrition and Physical Activity*, 8, 142.

Lee, I. M., Shiroma, E. J., Lobelo, F., Puska, P., Blair, S. N., Katzmarzyk, P. T., & Lancet Physical Activity Series Working Group (2012). Effect of physical inactivity on major non-communicable diseases worldwide: An analysis of burden of disease and life expectancy. *Lancet (London, England)*, 380(9838), 219–229. DOI: 10.1016/S0140-6736(12)61031-9

Locke, E. A., & Latham, G. P. (2006). New directions in goal-setting theory. *Current Directions in Psychological Science*, 15(5), 265–268. https://doi.org/10.1111/j.1467-8721.2006.00449.x

Lollgen, H., Bockenhoff, A., & Knapp, G. (2009). Physical activity and all-cause mortality: An updated meta-analysis with different intensity categories. *International Journal of Sports Medicine*, 30(3), 212–224.

Lubans, D., Richards, J., Hillman, C., Faulkner, G., Beauchamp, M., Nilsson, M., . . . Biddle, S. (2016). Physical activity for cognitive and mental health in youth: A systematic review of mechanisms. *Pediatrics*, 138(3), e20161642. DOI: 10.1542/peds.2016-1642

Marlatt, G. A., & Gordon, J. R. (1985). *Relapse prevention: Maintenance strategies in the treatment of addictive behaviors*. New York: Guilford Press.

Marmot, M. (2010). *Fair society, healthy lives: Strategic review of health inequalities in England post-2010*. London: Marmot Review.

Marshall, S. J., & Biddle, S. (2001). The transtheoretical model of behavior change: A meta-analysis of applications to physical activity and exercise. *Annals of Behavioral Medicine*, 23(4), 229–246.

McEwan, D., Harden, S. M., Zumbo, B. D., Sylvester, B. D., Kaulius, M., Ruissen, G. R.,. . Beauchamp, M. R. (2016). The effectiveness of multi-component goal setting interventions for changing physical activity behaviour: A systematic review and meta-analysis. *Health Psychology Review*, 10(1), 67–88, https://doi.org/10.1080/17437199.2015.1104258.

National Statistics (2017, December 13). *Health survey for England, 2016*. Retrieved from https://digital.nhs.uk/data-and-information/publications/statistical/health-survey-for-england/health-survey-for-england-2016

Owen, N., Humpel, N., Leslie, E., Bauman, A., & Sallis, J. F. (2004). Understanding environmental influences on walking: Review and research agenda. *American Journal Preventative Medicine*, 27, 67–76.

Pels, F., & Kleinert, J. (2016). Loneliness and physical activity: A systematic review. *International Review of Sport and Exercise Psychology*, 9(1), 231–260. DOI: 10.1080/1750984X.2016.1177849

Plonczynski, D. J. (2003). Physical activity determinants of older women: What influences activity? *Medsurg Nursing*, 12(4), 213–221.

Prochaska, J. O., & DiClimente, C. C. (1986). Toward a comprehensive model of change. In W. R. Miller & N. Heather (Eds.), *Treating addictive behavior: Processes of change* (pp. 3–27). New York: Plenum.

Rhodes, R. E., Janssen, I., Bredin, S. S. D., Warburton, D. E. R., & Bauman, A. (2017). Physical activity: Health impact, prevalence, correlates and interventions. *Psychology & Health*, 32(8), 942–975. DOI: 10.1080/08870446.2017.1325486

Rhodes, R. E., Martin, A. D., Taunton, J. E., Rhodes, E. C., Donnelly, M., & Elliot, J. (1999). Factors associated with exercise adherence among older adults: An individual perspective. *Sports Medicine*, 28, 397–411.

Sallis, J. F., & Owen, N. (1999). *Physical activity and behavioral medicine*. Thousand Oaks, CA: Sage.

Sallis, J. F., Owen, N., & Fisher, E. B. (2008). Ecological models of health behavior. In K. Glanz, B. K. Rimer, & K. Viswanath (Eds.), *Health behavior and health education: Theory, research, and practice* (4th ed.). San Francisco: Jossey-Bass.

Salmon, J., Owen, N., Crawford, D., Bauman, A., & Sallis, J. F. (2003). Physical activity and sedentary behavior: A population-based study of barriers, enjoyment, and preference. *Healthy Psychology*, 22(2), 178–188.

Stubbs, B., & Rosenbaum, S. (2018). *Exercise based interventions for mental illness: Physical activity as part of clinical treatment*. London, UK: Elsevier.

Swann, C., & Rosenbaum, S. (2018). Do we need to reconsider best practice in goal setting for physical activity promotion? *British Journal of Sports Medicine*, 52, 485–486.

Trost, S. G., Owen, N., Bauman, A. E., Sallis, J. F., & Brown, W. (2002). Correlates of adults' participation in physical activity: Review and update. *Medicine and Science in Sports and Exercise*, 34, 1996.

Van Stralen, M. M., de Vries, H., Mudde, A. N., Bolman, C., & Lechner, L. (2009). Determinants of initiation and maintenance of physical activity among older adults: A literature review. *Health Psychology Review*, 3, 147–207.

Warburton, D. E., Charlesworth, S., Ivey, A., Nettlefold, L., & Bredin, S. S. (2010). A systematic review of the evidence for Canada's physical activity guidelines for adults. *International Journal of Behavioral Nutrition and Physical Activity*, 7, 39. DOI: 10.1186/1479-5868-7-39

Warburton, D. E. R., & Bredin, S. S. D. (2016). Reflections on physical activity and health: What should we recommend? *Canadian Journal of Cardiology*, 32(4), 495–504.

Wendel-Vos, W., Droomers, M., Kremers, S., Brug, J., & van Lenthe, F. (2007). Potential environmental determinants of physical activity in adults: A systematic review. *Obesity Reviews*, 8, 425–440.

Williams, N. H., Hendry, M., France, B., Lewis, R., & Wilkinson, C. (2007). Effectiveness of exercise-referral schemes to promote physical activity in adults: Systematic review. *British Journal of General Practice*, 57(545), 979–986.

7

REACHING HARD-TO-ENGAGE GROUPS WITH PHYSICAL ACTIVITY AND EXERCISE REFERRAL INTERVENTIONS

Andy Pringle, Jason Feavers and Stephen Zwolinsky

Chapter aims

The aims of this chapter are to:

1. Explain hard-to-engage groups and whether they are really hard to reach
2. Discuss the public health case for reaching hard-to-engage groups with PA
3. Consider how we engage hard-to-reach/engage populations in physical activity using ERS
4. Highlight the key implementation characteristics for engaging hard-to-reach/engage male populations using ERS
5. State the key considerations for practitioners working with hard-to-reach/engage groups

Introduction

Exercise referral schemes (ERS) have been one of the most commonly deployed physical activity (PA) interventions over the last 25 years (Department of Health (DoH), 2007); at the height of their popularity, it was estimated that there were somewhere in the region of 800 schemes (although there are far fewer in operation today) (Pringle and Jagroo, 2015). ERS are defined by the National Institute of Health and Care Excellence (NICE) (2014a) as those interventions that seek to increase PA and involve:

- An assessment involving a primary care or allied health professional to determine that someone is sedentary or inactive
- A referral by a primary care or allied health professional to a PA specialist or service
- A personal assessment involving a PA specialist or service to determine what programme of PA to recommend for their specific needs
- An opportunity to participate in a PA programme

This broad and inclusive definition also infers that the uptake of PA opportunities should extend across groups experiencing health inequalities. Indeed, Haskell, Blair and Hill (2009)

DOI: 10.4324/9781315102399-7

outline that data support the need for more comprehensive health-promoting PA policies and programmes, especially for the economically and socially disadvantaged and medically underserved. The NICE review of ERS in 2014 identified 'gaps' in the existing evidence base, including information about the participation levels of under-represented and hard-to-reach groups – such as people with disabilities and those from Black and minority ethnic (BaME)/non-Caucasian backgrounds (NICE, 2014a). Furthermore, data concerning factors that encourage under-represented groups to participate in and complete ERS were also in short supply (NICE, 2014a).

In their review, the NICE (2014a) Public Health Advisory Committee set out to update the *Guidance on Promoting Physical Activity through Exercise Referral* (PH 54) recommended that:

- Policy makers and commissioners should not fund ERS for people who are sedentary or inactive but apparently healthy.
- Primary care practitioners should not refer people who are sedentary or inactive, but otherwise apparently healthy, to ERS.
- Commissioners should only fund ERS for people who are sedentary/inactive and have existing health conditions/other factors that put them at increased risk of ill health.

> As part of the NICE review, it was also reported that 'stakeholders were concerned that the draft recommendations could undermine PA promotion, as they seemed to imply that all ERS are ineffective and that any advice on PA is not valued by NICE'.
>
> Stakeholders felt the recommendations may increase inequalities in health, as many schemes focus on overcoming social isolation and improving people's general participation in the community, versus PA alone. They also noted that those involved in commissioning and delivering ERS believe they are an effective use of public money. This is evident in the number of schemes, the popularity of referrals and anecdotal reports of an increase in PA behaviour and health benefits.
>
> *(NICE, 2014a)*

Indeed, recent evidence suggests 'ERS aligned to the UK best-practice guidelines can positively influence a range of health outcomes, including those associated with lung function and cardiovascular fitness as well as outcomes for functional capacity and mental well-being' (Stewart et al., 2017). Despite the NICE recommendations, ERS are a commonly deployed intervention in the PA promotion landscape (Yang et al., 2017; Din et al., 2015), including their advocacy for so-called hard-to-reach/engage groups, (DoH, 2007; Queen, Crone and Parker, 2015). This chapter therefore considers the promotion of PA for hard-to-reach/engage groups using ERS interventions.

1. Who are hard-to-engage groups, and are they really hard to reach?

Who are the hard to reach/engage?

As we will see later, there is some debate on how the term *hard to reach/engage* accurately relates to unreached groups (Flanagan and Hancock, 2010). Groups so defined have included adult men (Curran et al., 2016; Lewis, Reeves and Roberts, 2017; Grace, Richardson and

Carroll, 2016), indigenous populations (Lévesque, 2017), women (Brook et al., 2017), older adults (Lozano-Sufrategui et al., 2017; Pringle and Zwolinsky, 2017b) and groups whose health needs remain unmet by traditional health services (Edmunds, Roche and Stratton, 2010; Robertson et al., 2013; Grace, Richardson and Carroll, 2016; Lewis, Reeves and Roberts, 2017; Pringle and Zwolinsky, 2017b). This group also includes populations presenting with injurious health conditions and, owing to these, encounter challenges engaging PA services and provision (Mendoza-Vasconez, 2016).

What does hard to reach/engage *really mean?*

As we have seen, the hard-to-reach/engage label has been, and can be, applied to many different groups. Nevertheless, the notional categorisation of individuals to membership of these groups does not automatically mean that individuals are hard to reach/engage. Moreover, there is a danger that such terms can be seen as labels which are unrepresentative. As a result, we need to get a handle on what these terms really mean. Many of these descriptors have emerged out of the inability of PH interventions to engage participants. Indeed Yancey, Ory and Davis (2006) have suggested that

> population groups experiencing disparities in rates of sedentariness and related chronic diseases have generally been considered 'hard to reach' by public health researchers because of their nonresponsiveness to health promotion materials and messages targeting 'general' (i.e. younger, white, urban, affluent) audiences.

Sinclair and Alexander (2012) similarly define 'hard to reach' as a term used to describe a diverse range of groups who often remain unreached by health services.

As health promoters have tried to develop an understanding of what people do not respond and why, their focus has shifted to individual characteristics that make up the profile of the potential non-adopters of health programmes. Freimuth and Mettger (1990) have suggested that 'persons who have a low socioeconomic status (SES), members of ethnic minorities, and persons who have a low level of literacy often are tagged as hard-to-reach'. Descriptors have centred not only on individual determinants, but also on the social and environmental determinants of PA participation (Yancey, Ory and Davis (2006). This should be seen as strength, given the need to consider the determinants of participation in health improvement, including PA interventions, from a holistic or ecological perspective (Bartholomew-Eldredge et al., 2016). Indeed, Mendoza-Vasconez et al. (2016) have reported that underserved populations, including racial/ethnic minorities, individuals with low socioeconomic status and individuals with physical disabilities, are less likely to engage in sufficient moderate to vigorous PA. An ecological definition of *hard to reach* is also provided by Faugier and Sargeant (1997), who refers to people who are difficult to access and/or engage due to specific factors such as accommodation, age, ethnicity, gender, income, language, location and religion. This 'catch-all' description acknowledges the diverse range of factors that impact an individual's PA participation.

Curran and colleagues (2016) have argued that participants from hard-to-reach communities can encounter substantial difficulties when sustaining PA. A reluctance to engage with traditional health services and routes for health improvement exacerbates this issue, meaning individuals do not receive the healthcare and support they require to make meaningful changes to lifestyle behaviours. Curran et al. (2016) refer to the review of the literature by

Collins and Kay (2003) examining sport and social exclusion amongst hard-to-reach populations. Their investigations identified 'social, economic and contextual constraints, lack of structure, income, skills, social capital and a sense of powerlessness) as the major barriers to engagement' in sport and PA. With this in mind, Pringle et al. (2014) defined men engaging in a health improvement programme as hard to engage if they 1) presented multiple CVD risk factors yet did not view their 'risky' health status as problematic and 2) did not engage in primary care health services – such as a GP or health advice service – when they experienced an ailment. Further, Brook and colleagues (2017) defined women as hard to reach with PA interventions if they 1) reported the lowest PA participation rates in the UK and had an increased incidence of stroke, type 2 diabetes, obesity and lower life expectancies and 2) had health needs that were unmet by health campaigns. As seen from the previous section, the terms used have included both behavioural and causal perspectives and frequently centred on the determinants of reach and engagement.

Physical activity interventions

Physical inactivity has been described as a global pandemic (Andersen, Mota and Di Petro, 2016; World Health Organisation, 2018). This concern is centred not only on the population at large (DoH, 2011) but also on those groups defined as 'living less than optimal lifestyles' (Zwolinsky, McKenna and Pringle, 2016), under-represented (Haskell, Blair and Hill, 2009) and hard-to-reach/engage groups (Pringle et al., 2014; Pringle and Zwolinsky 2018). The extent to which groups 'living less than optimal lifestyles' actually engage in PA interventions is an ongoing challenge reflected in the public health literature (Brook et al., 2017; Pringle et al., 2010; Pringle et al., 2014). Indeed, Whitall, Jago and Fox (2011) reported that the Walking the Way to Health Initiative, at the time one of England's most popular PA interventions, was most likely to be taken up by White, middle-class participants. The Local Exercise Action Pilots (LEAP) was a national programme of PA promotion aimed at increasing PA behaviour in the general population and also in hard-to-reach/engage groups (Pringle, McKenna and Zwolinsky, 2018). ERS were widely deployed interventions in this multi-site programme, but the evaluation predominantly recruited participants who were already meeting the PA guidelines (DoH, 2007), endorsing concerns over the extent to which the intervention recruited its target audience. It has been suggested that multi-level approaches are required to make PA accessible to all groups, including those underserved by mainstream health and PA services (Das and Horton, 2016; Reis et al., 2016).

What are the challenges of using the term hard to reach/engage*?*

As we have indicated, there is some debate over the use of the term *hard to reach/engage*. It has been suggested that the term stereotypes people into groups, inferring an inability or reluctance to change health behaviours (Yancey, Ory and Davis, 2006), in some cases suggesting that the unresponsiveness of individuals equates with unworthiness to receive intervention (Whitehead, 1997). Freimuth and Mettger (1990) indicate that 'pejorative labels and preconceptions about various groups may lead to depicting these audiences as powerless, apathetic, and isolated'. Indeed, in some cases, it has been suggested that, in the past, some hard-to-reach/engage audiences have been termed 'obstinate, recalcitrant, chronically uninformed disadvantaged have-nots, illiterate and information poor'. In part, such labels reflect communicators' frustration in trying to reach people unlike themselves and the failure of many campaigns to change high-risk behaviours (Freimuth and Mettger, 1990). It is also important to consider the narrative surrounding the extent to which interventions actually meet the needs of so-called hard-to-engage groups. It is unsurprising that so-called hard-to-reach/engage populations have rejected the label as being unrepresentative (Symons, 2017). Colleagues working in the field of health improvement have also suggested that it is services and interventions that are hard to engage by local groups and communities. That said *hard to reach/engage* remains a commonly used term in the public health (PH) literature. The use of this term is often underpinned by a genuine aspiration to better understand and help those people most in need of health improvement, who face substantial barriers to engage in PA and PH interventions. It is important that this aspiration is not lost in the debate over the use of language whilst at the same time recognising the need to be sensitive regarding the use of language and terminology.

How should we best understand the needs of hard-to-reach/engage groups?

Our examples serve to remind us that we should view people and their health behaviours diversely, holistically and in context (Bartholomew-Eldredge et al., 2016). The factors that result in people being hard to reach/engage or unreached are as diverse as they are complex (Pringle et al., 2014; Pringle and Zwolinsky, 2017a; Yancey, Ory and Davis, 2006). Social ecological perspectives (Chaudhury et al., 2016; Bartholomew-Eldredge et al., 2016; Yancey, Ory and Davis, 2006) remind us that individuals do not live in a vacuum (Curran et al., 2016); moreover, individuals operate within an intrapersonal, social and physical environment, and we should view the determinants for PA participation using these holistic lenses. Further, Yancey and colleagues inform us that 'cultures are not monolithic, and individual differences and subgroup distinctions must also be recognised. There is much within-group variation; such factors as language, income, educational level, and acculturation can also greatly influence responsiveness to different intervention approaches'.

It is therefore important to identify and understand the complex factors that determine why, why not and how groups of individuals engage/might engage PA opportunities (Pringle and Zwolinsky, 2017a). With those thoughts in mind, practitioners should work in partnership with hard-to-reach/engage groups to better understand the multi-level determinants (barriers and facilitators) that determine their engagement in PA and how the associated interventions could be best developed to meet their needs (Bartholomew-Eldredge et al., 2016; Pringle and Zwolinsky, 2018; Yancey, Ory and Davis, 2006). This dialogue should form part of an iterative, bottom-up approach to assessing the PA needs which places individuals at the heart of attempts to understand the issues which result in hard-to-reach/engage groups being unreached (Bartholomew-Eldredge et al., 2016; Kime and Pringle, 2018; Lévesque, 2017; Brook et al., 2017).

2. What is the public health case for reaching hard-to-engage groups?

Although it has been suggested that scarce resources should be invested in those groups most responsive to change (Eyal, 2013), doing so can be turned, for some stakeholders, into a plausible rationale for 'giving up' on the people most resistant and unresponsive to change and most in need of intervention (Whitehead, 1997). What is more, hard-to-reach populations are less likely to engage in sufficient moderate to vigorous physical activity (MVPA) and are therefore at increased risk of morbidity and mortality (Yancey, Ory and Davis, 2006). Left unchecked, these health inequalities will remain unabated (Mendoza-Vasconez et al., 2016). There is a strong PH case for engaging hard-to-reach/engage populations with PA and PH interventions. Arguably, members of our society who have the poorest health and PA profiles and who face the greatest challenges in engaging health improvement services stand to benefit most from interventions that aim to help improve people's health profiles (Mendoza-Vasconez et al., 2016; Pringle et al., 2014; Yancey, Ory and Davis, 2006). Unchecked, their unhealthy behaviours, including physical inactivity, mean individuals are incubating more serious health conditions for later in life (Mendoza-Vasconez et al., 2016; White, 2011), often presenting with reduced treatment options for dealing with emergent health conditions at a later date.

Hard-to-reach/engage groups who remain unreached by PA interventions also delay their opportunity to secure the necessary support to help with changes to their behaviour, including advice and instruction from PA specialists. NICE guidance recommends the use of established behavioural change techniques (BCTs) to promote increased levels of PA (Giné-Garriga et al., 2017). Remaining underserved or unreached also means individuals can encounter a delay in developing and refining the necessary behavioural skills, as well as the social networks and relationships, that support PA participation. These assets are important for establishing the necessary routines for PA to be habitual (Ransdell et al., 2009; Marcus and Forsyth, 2011; Marentes-Castillo et al., 2017). Further, remaining physically inactive poses a significant economic burden (Scarborough et al., 2007), as well as the human and individual cost of suffering from ill health (Yancey, Ory and Davis, 2006). It is unsurprising that Das and Horton (2016) identified physical inactivity as 'a major contributor to death and disability from non-communicable diseases (NCDs) worldwide and confirmed the importance of increasing levels of PA as a priority to combat NCDs' (Dietz et al., 2015). Reaching out to hard-to-engage groups has the potential to reduce inequalities in health by reducing mortality from NCDs (Woringer et al., 2017).

3. How do we engage hard-to-reach populations in physical activity using ERS?

The public health context

Yancey, Ory and Davis (2006) provide a series of case studies to illustrate PA promotion with hard-to-reach/engage populations. Recognising the merits of this approach, we provide our case study focused on PA promotion with hard-to-reach/engage men. Lefkowich, Richardson and Robertson (2017, p. 513) suggest that

> there are two prominent issues that contribute to a lack of health service uptake in hard to reach or hard to engage men: Men are less likely to seek help or take preventative measures, and there are blatant gaps in service availability for men.

It is no surprise that men's health has been highlighted as a concern across Europe (White, 2011) and continues to be an important PH issue. Baker and Shand (2017) report that WHO data show that in 2012, over half of all deaths from NCDs were men. 'Males were more likely than females to die prematurely (under 70 years) from NCDs in almost every country (females were more likely to die prematurely from NCDs in just four countries)'. Major risk factors for men include poor diet, smoking, harmful alcohol consumption and physical inactivity. Further, men do worse than women in respect to all these behaviours (Baker and Shand, 2017).

Men have been shown to demonstrate not only unhealthy lifestyles but also an inaccurate perception of their health and well-being (Lozano-Sufrategui et al., 2017; Pringle et al., 2014). Combined with their non-engagement in traditional health improvement services, this means some men are incubating more serious health consequences for later in life, resulting in higher levels of potentially preventable health conditions and more limited treatment options at a later date (Baker and Shand, 2017; Teo, Ng and White, 2017; White, 2011). It has been suggested that men also face substantial structural barriers to engaging primary health-care services (Baker and Shand 2017; Teo, Ng and White, 2017), as well as the feminisation of health services which are more readily aimed at women, rending services that are less acceptable to men (Lozano-Sufrategui et al., 2017; Pringle et al., 2014). It has also been argued that individualistic approaches to health promotion serve men from economically and socially disadvantaged locations less effectively (Robertson and Baker, 2017). Indeed, Bird et al. (2017) report that 'although more men than women, (65% of men and 58% of women) in England are overweight or obese, more than three times as many women as men have attended local authority funded weight management services'. Further, compared to women, there has been an under-representation of adult men, including males 18 to 49, in major multi-site national PA programmes, including ERS in England (DoH, 2007).

Recognising the non-uptake of health improvement services by men and, on occasion, the poor adoption of national PA programmes (Pringle et al., 2010), it is no surprise that there has been an increased focus on framing men's health improvement opportunities using male-friendly or gender-sensitised approaches (Lefkowich, Richardson and Robertson, 2017). We have witnessed an increased focus on centring PA and PH interventions around the interests of men, including leisure and sporting interests (Grace, Richardson and Carroll, 2016; Hunt et al., 2014; Reddy et al., 2017; Robertson et al., 2016). Our case study emerges from the growing research centred on the use of sport as a channel to reach men with health improvement services (Baker et al., 2016; Curran et al., 2016; Gray et al., 2018; van de Glind et al., 2017; Hargreaves and Pringle, 2018; Lewis, Reeves and Roberts, 2017; Trivedy et al., 2017). In doing so, providing more accessible, affordable and acceptable healthcare to men who would otherwise not engage with traditional health improvement services (Fineberg, 2012), including those provided in primary care.

Case Study: Premier League Health: A National Programme of Men's Health and PA

Intervention context

Government, PH and football leaders have made the case for the power of professional football in connecting previously unresponsive groups to health improvement interventions (Martin et al., 2016; Pringle and Zwolinsky, 2018). With those thoughts in mind, we discuss Premier League Health (PLH) a £1.6 million funded programme of men's health improvement delivered in/by 16 English Premier League football clubs. The outcomes of the programme have been reported elsewhere in more detail within the literature (White et al., 2012; Pringle et al., 2014; Zwolinsky, McKenna and Pringle, 2016). However, we use this example as a case study in this chapter that can be applied to ERS.

In line with contemporary PH guidance (Corbin, Jones and Barry, 2016; Bartholomew-Eldredge et al., 2016) and research (Cade et al., 2017), interventions were supported by local health partners including charities, local authority and the (then) primary care trusts (PCTs). PLH interventions were delivered by the football club community trusts and supervised by health trainers (HTs). HTs are allied health professionals with a background in health promotion (Mathers, Taylor and Parry, 2016), and in this case, HTs received special instruction in men's health improvement (Pringle et al., 2014). HTs were specifically employed by or seconded to the clubs from PCTs (Pringle et al., 2014). In line with guidance (Bartholomew-Eldredge et al., 2016), the programme was made up of a number of interventions, and these fell into three approaches: 1) match day activities, 2) regular classes and groups and 3) outreach work in settings where captive male audiences could be reached, such as workplaces, religious settings, homeless men's centres or working men's clubs and bars, connecting to groups of men who would find it difficult to engage primary health-care services and traditional health improvement provision (Pringle et al., 2014; Zwolinsky, McKenna and Pringle, 2016).

Earlier in this chapter, we highlighted the importance of working with the potential recipients of health improvement programmes to accurately assess the determinants that facilitate/inhibit participation, as well as shaping effective solutions to meet health needs using an iterative approach (Bartholomew-Eldredge et al., 2016). As a result, there was no standardised protocol for the delivery of interventions across the 16 sites. Instead, each club organised its own intervention activities based on local health priorities and needs. Activities reflect the outcomes from each club's needs and community audit assessments, responding to local health priorities while working with available resources and timescales to make interventions operable (Bartholomew-Eldredge et al., 2016; Yancey, Ory and Davis, 2006). Importantly, interventions also reflected ongoing dialogue with key stakeholders, including men, as recommended elsewhere in the literature (Lefkowich, Richardson and Robertson, 2017).

Despite the differences in the interventions, there were a number of common features across the PLH programme and in the 16 clubs. For instance, PLH interventions took place in a combination of football club stadia, training facilities and club-branded/community-based venues. Increasingly, such venues are used for the delivery of health interventions (Hargreaves and Pringle, 2018; Parnell, Curran and Philpott, 2017; Pringle and Zwolinsky, 2018). Under the supervision of the HTs and qualified football coaches, interventions followed a range of modes of PA. These are reported in more detail (Pringle et al., 2014) but included football, group exercise, badminton and gym-based PA twice per week. In doing so, offering a menu of choices to make programmes more adaptable and flexible is important (Yancey, Ory and Davis, 2006; Zwolinsky, McKenna and Pringle, 2016). The ongoing dialogue with men over their PA and health needs was an important feature, recognising that men's health needs change over time, along with individuals' preparedness to address more serious and long-standing health matters that may have been incubating for some time.

A range of channels were used to raise awareness of the programme, including outreach work, football clubs and local media. The most powerful method of letting men know about the programme was word of mouth (Pringle et al., 2014). Men could engage in PA interventions through a range of routes. Reflecting the NICE (2014a) definition of ERS, the most common route was referral by the HTs to the PLH interventions taking place at each club. Referral to PA services by certified exercise professionals and other qualified health-care practitioners can be an important tool to assist individuals (Thornton, 2017). Men attended an initial health assessment in which data was captured on their demographic (age, postcode, nationality, employment status) and pre/post health profile to include, height, weight, BMI, diet, smoking, PA and alcohol behaviours, along with use of primary care and health advice services. As part of the programme, an independent evaluation was commissioned (White et al., 2012).

Key outcomes

Key outcomes have been reported in the peer-review literature and confirm that participants were predominantly white British (70.4%/n = 2669), aged 18–44 (80.2%/n = 3032) and employed (60.7%/n = 1907). One-third (n = 860) 'never' visited their doctor. Over 85% (n = 1428) presented with combinations of lifestyle risk factors. Intention-to-treat analysis showed improvements ($P < 0.001$) in lifestyle profiles. Importantly, given the focus of this chapter on hard-to-reach groups, a third of recruits reported 'never' consulting their GP, and over half 'never' used health advice or health information services. Moreover those hard-to-engage-men who 'never' visited their GP also demonstrated poorer initial health profiles than men who did. These men were more likely to report having three or four lifestyle risk factors, as opposed to those men who did visit their GP (Pringle et al., 2014). Further, dialogue with participants provided explicit accounts supporting the fact that interventions had engaged men described as 'hard to reach/engage' (Robertson et al., 2013; Pringle et al., 2014; White et al., 2012).

Given the suggestion that men are a hard-to-reach group (Hulton et al., 2016; Lozano-Sufrategui et al., 2017; Lewis, Reeves and Roberts, 2017; Teo, Ng and White, 2017; Wohl et al., 2017), recruits of PLH were anything but hard to reach/engage. When provided with affordable, accessible and amenable interventions centred on men's interests and settings and sensitive to men's needs and capacity to respond, men turned up in droves and were hard to avoid! The PLH programme reflected a shift in thinking on how to address men's non-engagement in health improvement and PA provision in the literature (Pringle and Zwolinsky, 2018; Robertson et al., 2016). Outcomes from the evaluation subsequently informed future investments into bespoke men's health interventions delivered in/by professional football clubs (Pringle, McKenna and Zwolinsky, 2018), as well as commercial health-care providers (Lozano-Sufrategui et al., 2017).

4. What are the key implementation characteristics for engaging hard-to-reach male populations using ERS designs?

Research into the key implementation factors was undertaken, involving interviews with men and HTs, and these are more fully reported elsewhere (Pringle et al., 2013; Robertson et al., 2013). We discuss some of the most important considerations for reaching hard-to-engage men in this programme. This list is by no means exhaustive or exclusive to hard-to-engage men, but in the next section, we try to combine outcomes emerging from PLH with the extant literature.

When planning PA-led health improvement interventions in this context:

- Use evidence-based practice and theoretical models/principles to plan, implement and evaluate interventions, such as intervention mapping (Ransdell et al., 2009; Bartholomew-Eldredge, 2016) and theory-based behavioural change methods and applications (Kok et al., 2016; Marcus and Forsyth, 2011; Michie, Van Stralen and West, 2014).
- Understand the needs of men: PA interventions should be built into the philosophies and cultural practices of the communities targeted by interventions (Baker and Shand, 2017; Yancey, Ory and Davis, 2006).
- Identify the determinants at the individual and social-environmental levels and map determinants to evidence-based change methods and their applications (Kok et al., 2016). Adopt and maintain iterative, ongoing and bottom-up approaches to understanding the determinants to PA (Bartholomew-Eldredge et al., 2016).
- Place men at the heart of ongoing conversations when planning and shaping interventions that impact their health and PA.
- Plan and build partnerships with local communities (members of the public) and communities of practice (the professional groups, paid or voluntary, who provide and support PA and PH services) (Mendoza-Vasconez et al., 2016; Kime and Pringle, 2018; Pringle, McKenna and Zwolinksy, 2018).
- Use word of mouth as a powerful tool to raise men's awareness of interventions (Hargreaves and Pringle, 2018): At a number of clubs in PLH, men were told to 'tell their mates' and other like-minded men. In other cases, clubs deployed former programme participants to endorse the programme to other men. Mendoza-Vasconez et al. (2016) have indicated that suggested strategies for the recruitment of underserved populations include the use of multiple recruitment channels and the inclusion of community members in those recruitment strategies. Many of these networks and channels will be unique to these groups of men, so partnering these groups is important.

- Build trust and rapport: Many men have been left disappointed by statutory health services, and for some men, placing trust in yet another 'good idea' or service may be a leap of faith too far. Using the club badge or image, often viewed as a trusted brand by club supporters, can be helpful in making that initial connection (Pringle et al., 2014).
- Use familiar contexts and settings: Proposed interventions must be part of a seamless web of ongoing community practices. In some clubs, PA sessions took place in the football stadia; these were known to men (Pringle and Zwolinsky, 2017b, 2018). Outreach work was conducted with captive audiences such as working men's clubs, mosques, pubs and job centres. At Middlesbrough, HTs gave out beer mats promoting the PLH to men in working men's clubs and pubs. This took the programme to the men, and recruitment took place in a setting they were comfortable with.
- Make it easy to get into the programme: Referral processes should be simple, with few steps to join, and should not take too long (DoH, 2007); those that are overly bureaucratic will deter men from joining.
- Promote flexibility: Providing a menu of PA choices to make programmes more adaptable and flexible is another key implementation factor (DoH, 2007; Yancey, Ory and Davis, 2006). For instance, at Newcastle United, a midnight programme of badminton was offered to fit in with South Asian men who worked as restaurateurs and taxi drivers. A regular 'hop on' point is important for engaging new starters.
- Avoid dictatorial and health-orientated messages: Keep focused on football, sport and/or fitness. For instance, at Hull, a simple strap line – Train like a Tiger – and a picture of a well-known and readily identifiable football player were used to engage men (White et al., 2012).
- Match day and football-themed events have been deployed to raise awareness, and a number of clubs engaged male fans using participatory approaches such as health checks and club-branded materials and competitions (Conrad and Abraham, 2016). However, it is important to note that match day tickets may be beyond the financial capacity of some men (Pringle et al., 2013) while for others, match day events may not be of interest (Dunn and Richardson, 2010).
- Evaluate: van de Glind et al. (2017) have argued that it is important to understand why particular interventions succeed or fail, under which circumstances and whether their effects can be reproduced so that better programmes can be developed and implemented more widely and lessons learned from the process (Pringle, McKenna and Zwolinsky, 2018). Working in partnership with local evaluators including university departments can be a useful alliance to build in this respect. There are good examples of sports and PA providers working in collaboration with their local academic institutions to evaluate programmes (Pringle, McKenna and Zwolinsky, 2018).

5. What are the key considerations for practitioners working with hard-to-engage groups

In terms of ERS for hard-to-reach/engage populations, we have combined our learning from the PLH case study with behaviour change theory to advance understanding of the complex issues that blight reach and engagement. Although it is beyond the scope of this chapter to discuss the detailed theoretical underpinnings of behaviour change that have been discussed elsewhere in this text, we have provided some examples that can be, and have been, applied

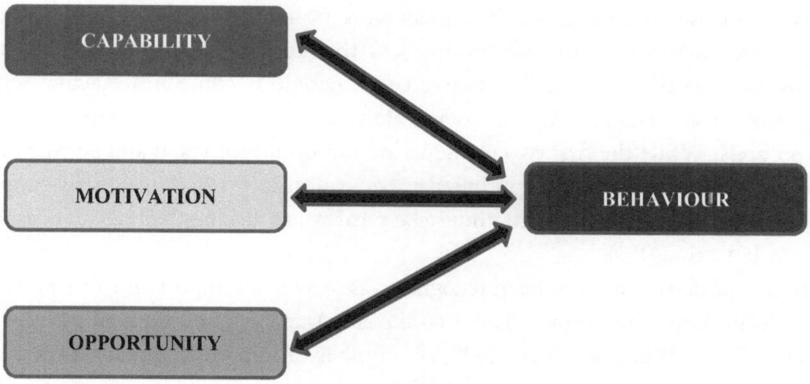

FIGURE 7.1 The COM-B system – a framework for understanding behaviour

Source: Michie, Van Stralen and West, 2011

to implementation science – for example, we refer to COM-B (Figure 7.1). Nevertheless, there are many alternative models and approaches that can be employed with hard-to-reach/ engage populations and ERS. More detail can be found on these (Bartholomew-Eldredge et al., 2016; Kok et al., 2016). To be able to change behaviour, it is useful to have a better understanding of what influences that behaviour in a format that can be applied to a variety of individuals. COM-B is a useful behaviour change model for understanding a range of behaviours (Michie, Van Stralen and West, 2011). At the heart of this model is the understanding that behaviour acts as part of a system involving three conditions: 1) capability, 2) opportunity and 3) motivation.

In a PA context, capability is made up of physical and psychological capability. In relation to participation in an ERS, physical capability would relate to the individual's physical ability to take part in the available physical activities. Medical conditions and disabilities could make some individuals physically incapable of a particular activity, and this would need to be considered alongside participant needs, as discussed earlier. Psychological capability may be a more influential barrier to participation in PA. This would include a person's beliefs about their ability, or self-efficacy, as well as knowledge and beliefs as to the consequences of a particular behaviour. Opportunity relates to the physical and social environment being conducive to the occurrence of the behaviour. Using the holistic lenses we discussed earlier, the physical environment includes access to fitness facilities and services, open spaces or infrastructure which supports PA. The social environment includes the intrapersonal, organisational environment and society, whether the behaviour is considered socially acceptable and whether other similar people behave in that way. Both of these constructs effect motivation, which in itself can be further strengthened or weakened by reflective thought processes and habit (automatic behaviour). Motivation is defined as 'all those brain processes that energize and direct behaviour, not just goals and conscious decision-making. It includes habitual processes, emotional responding, as well as analytical decision-making' (Michie, Van Stralen and West, 2011). Collectively these components impact behaviour. Behaviour change theory can then help in securing a more informed understanding of why people adopt PA interventions or don't.

In principle and practice, these schemes have to 'switch something on' in their participants. Often, this involves some kind of interaction, initially, that is typically better provided by exercise specialists, nurses or health trainers working under the umbrella of the GP, not by primary care doctors who themselves may lack the requisite time, training and, in many cases, skills. Our work has typically observed that people become more active when the following ecological elements exist: 1) social safety, 2) physical safety, 3) enjoyment and 4) personal progress. While the first two elements are important for reach and engagement, the latter two are more important for continued participation in PA. Ensuring that people have the requisite motivation and ability to undertake what we are asking them to do is paramount (Marcus and Forsyth, 2011).

Health-care professionals have been recognised as playing an important role in PA promotion by both the local community (Kime et al., 2018) and communities of practice (Kime and Pringle, 2018; Vishnubala et al., 2020). A number of initiatives are currently underway with the aspiration of promoting PA in healthcare, as well as community settings. Firstly, it has been identified that future medics want to receive more training on PA (Osborne et al., 2017), and we have seen a focus on the inclusion of PA in undergraduate medical school curricula (Gates, 2016). Secondly, the Royal College of General Practice and Public Health England GP Clinical Champion Programme recruits health-care professionals such as GPs, nurses and other allied health professionals to a 'championing' role for PA. As part of the role, 'champions' draw on their local networks and standing and act as advocates for PA, including the provision of training and education to health-care professionals (Public Health England, 2018). Thirdly, Moving Medicine is an interactive, evidence-based web-based tool to support brief advice in PA across a range of diseases and conditions. The intervention includes a series of modules linked to a range of conditions on which PA can have an impact. It offers health-care professionals a number of strategies, time-bound consultations, promotional materials and resources to assist patients in the process of being more physically active (Faculty of Sport and Exercise Medicine and Royal College of General Practitioners, Public Health England, 2018). While GPs and practice nurses may be a first point of contact for many patients, it is important to recognise the contribution of the wider public health force (Centre for Workforce Intelligence and Royal Society for Public Health, 2015).

As we have seen in our case study on hard-to-engage men, primary healthcare was their last point of call, so the role of a broader group of health and social care professionals is also important when promoting PA. This is an important point identified during the updating of the PA guidelines (Mutrie et al., 2018). Recognising the value of 'Making Every Contact Count' (Health Education England, 2018), this group of professionals could include social workers, carers, support workers, community leaders and the health trainers and sports clubs facilitators we witnessed in our case study. It also includes the army of volunteers who give their time to run PA sessions and can signpost individuals to specialist advice and services.

Generally, when deciding what to do – i.e. engaging in an ERS or not – people look and ask 'What will this behaviour yield?' The answer they give themselves to this question generally governs what they do. When they choose one behaviour over another, it is because they are betting that this action will generate the best result. Since action yields a combination of results – some good, some bad – it is the expected sum total of the consequence bundle that drives behaviour (Blue et al., 2016). Therefore, if practitioners want people to act in another way, they have to communicate and demonstrate how a different behaviour would yield better consequences. Importantly, this has to go beyond education and counselling approaches. ERS practitioners need to pay attention to making engagement (DoH, 2007) and PA as easy as possible. One of the main reasons that people are inactive is because they lack the skills/ability to do something different (Robertson et al., 2013; Pringle et al., 2014).

Short term, if PA is undesirable but not impossible – assuming you can reach these people – practitioners can crank up the pressure and get prospective participants active by telling them 'they need to do more' and that 'joining an ERS will be good for them' (Pringle et al., 2010). But in the long run, ERS needs to find a way to remove some of the factors that make this behaviour undesirable, or practitioners will constantly be looking for ways to motivate people to do what they hate doing, and that is never fun! Hard-to reach/engage groups may not know exactly how to have an active lifestyle, but they probably have a good idea about what does not work for them (Pringle et al., 2014). When people are not completely certain about what to do in this situation or it becomes clear that they do not understand how to change it for the better, inactivity is often the logical response. Engaging with our audience to better understand their needs is key, recognising this is an iterative and fluid process which can change as participant needs change (Bartholomew-Eldredge et al., 2016).

The end goal should be to assist and over-determine change by amassing sufficient sources of influence to make the required change inevitable. Part of this requires us to understand the progress that communities – and the individuals within them – are trying to make within their particular circumstances and identify the high-leverage actions that would help lead to change. Delivering any offering within the context of very specific community struggles is the way forward. PLH helps provide a template for effective action and the example that follows shows how this learning can be applied in real-world settings (Jonman, Mackie and Sim, 2013).

Actively engaging a 'reached' hard-to-reach referral:

An example of how PLH can be used to influence individual physical activity behaviour change

In terms of influencing behaviour in relation to PA, the examples that follow are based our work within the PLH programme (Pringle et al., 2014; Zwolinsky, McKenna and Pringle, 2016), our understanding of behaviour change theory and the tacit knowledge and experiential learning from years of working in the field. Our learning in terms of ERS can be interpreted across five areas: 1) assessing current PA levels or other lifestyle risk factors, 2) advising participants to do more PA, 3) agreeing on goals or plans, 4) assisting with the planned course of action or treatment and 5) arranging follow-up. Many programmes actually only deliver on the first two, and that is where they fall short. Although many assess risk factors and may advise better behaviour, change is most likely when we add the next three elements into the mix. That is, agreeing with the participant and establishing some written goals, assisting them with their 'treatment' and arranging follow-up to check and re-assess.

Creating positive PA and lifestyle change, especially for hard-to-reach/engage groups, can be tricky (Yancey, Ory and Davis, 2006). In essence, it needs to be deployed in a way that minimises participant risk and has to be handled with caution, creating motivation and increasing competency in a physically and psychosocially safe environment. By way of example, many participants starting out on the PLH programme asked questions along the lines of how many minutes of exercise or PA they needed to be doing. Typically, they were unsure if it was 30, 60 or 90 minutes a day. They had some idea based on reading papers and listening to the news and other media (Robertson et al., 2013), yet this appeared only to confuse matters and make what they perceived to be the recommended guidelines even less achievable. Participants often made statements like 'The paper says if I'm overweight, I've got to do 90 minutes every day to keep the weight off; is this right?'

The reality is that for many hard-to-reach/engage participants, setting goals for PA or other health behaviours may be unrealistic and discouraging, especially if contemporary guidelines and recommendations appear out of reach. Our own thoughts and bias lead us to believe that contemporary guidelines for PA and lifestyle behaviours can do a big disservice to changing PA behaviours, primarily because they seem unachievable to so many, especially those people who are the most inactive and experience low health literacy (Yancey, Ory and Davis, 2006). Based on our understanding of working with hard-to-reach/engage groups, the 'best' responses to these questions were always variations of 'What are you doing now?' Repeatedly, the response was 'Nothing!' Fundamentally, advising people to do more of anything needs to be handled delicately (Bartholomew-Eldredge et al., 2016; Pringle et al., 2014). When faced with these circumstances and as a starting point for increasing PA levels, suggesting something achievable, such as 10 minutes of MVPA three times a week, has been good starting point for us (DoH, 2011). This approach tries to overcome apathy with downscale goals and the suggestion of small changes. Typically, participants respond to this with 'But that's nowhere near what they say I should be doing'. Nevertheless, the number of times participants came back to the next session and said, 'Hey, I didn't listen to you. The first day I did 12 minutes, next I did 20 and I'm now up to 25'. While the aspiration would be to ideally get participants to meet the recommended guidelines for PA in due course, the reality is that it may take some time to meet this optimal level for health. For some people, the ACSM's 'Start Slow, Progress Slow' is a good starting point (Riebe et al., 2015). Working slowly but steadily towards meeting guidelines provides an opportunity to obtain the health benefits but also practice and learn from the behaviour of being physically active. For some of these individuals, being physically active will be new and may be also be a little strange, and so getting accustomed to performing the PA and the behaviours and routines that support PA, such as planning and time management, will take some time to get used to and to perfect. Therefore, regular practicing is important. Indeed, the NICE guidance on behaviour change (individual approaches) recommends that people are helped to develop routines that support the new behaviour, such as being physically active, recognising that small, manageable changes to daily routines are most likely to be maintained (NICE, 2014b).

The secret is to get them started by giving them simple things that are doable, ideally surrounded by some positive social network, support or any tools they need to get the job done (Pringle and Zwolinsky, 2017a, 2018). Give people the ability and make them feel competent and comfortable (Marcus and Forsyth, 2011), in doing so helping people build their perception that they can plan and perform PA, providing practical hints and tips and strategies for planning and scheduling PA into daily routines.

As we mentioned in Section 4, communication is so important. Convey to the participants – don't criticise (Robertson et al., 2013) – that you understand them (Bartholomew-Eldredge et al., 2016), and use empathy to help the participant identify why they may maintain suboptimal or injurious behaviours (Lozano et al., 2018; White et al., 2012). Help participants become independent and self-motivated (Pringle and Zwolinsky, 2017a). Fundamentally, encourage individuals to understand and accept the need for change; in doing so, understanding change from their perspective is so important (Pringle and Zwolinsky, 2017b). In our experience, the best way to do this is to ask questions and create 'that iterative dialogue' (Zwolinsky, McKenna, Pringle et al., 2016). We have been practicing this for a long time: questions like 'What do you think is the right amount of activity for you?' or 'What do you think is a healthy weight for you?' Even if their answer is only five minutes above or a kilogram below where they are now, we are usually happy with this progress.

During PLH, co-author Stephen Zwolinsky remembers sitting with a male participant who was around six feet tall and 100 kg. Stephen recounts this interaction in the following section:

> I asked him what he thought was an ideal weight? I didn't say to him, 'Your BMI says you ought to weigh between 65–75 kg', I said 'What do you think you should weigh?' He looked at me and said '90 kg maybe 85 kg'. He didn't know this, but I already had some pages marked in my book, one said 95 kg, another 85 kg and the other said 75 kg, so I said 'Wow we're in agreement'. He didn't know I actually had two alternatives. The point here is to agree with people if they are moving in the right direction, we cannot reinforce that enough. Finally, you must advise participants to handle relapse and deal with setbacks and hazards involved in adopting any new health behaviour that typically come with the journey.
>
> *(Pringle and Zwolinsky, 2017b)*

If they relapse one day, all is not lost; it is what they do over the long term! It is important that people can try again.

6. Summary and key points

The summary of the key points emerging from this chapter are as follows:

- *Hard-to-reach/engage* and *unreached* are terms commonly used to describe groups who remain unresponsive or unreached by interventions.
- There exists a strong PH rationale for connecting hard-to-reach/engage groups with PA interventions.
- Hard-to-reach/engage groups face diverse and often complex determinants when adopting PA interventions.
- When attempting to understand the determinants to participation, adopt an ecological and holistic approach.
- Key implementation factors are important considerations when aspiring to connect with hard-to-reach/engage groups; these include:
  - Working with the intended recipients of interventions using a needs-led, bottom-up and iterative approach
  - Developing PA interventions that are flexible, adaptable and based on participant needs
  - Effective communication strategies and choice of language and themes
- Evidence-based practice, theoretical models and principles of behaviour change and PH practice can help explain the complex reasons why hard-to-reach/engage populations adopt/do not adopt PA interventions.

7. Study tasks

We have created 11 study questions relating to this chapter:

1. What is meant by the term *hard-to-reach/engage groups*?
2. What are the issues and difficulties when using the term *hard to reach/engage*?
3. What is the public health case for reaching hard-to-reach/engage groups with PA interventions?
4. What are three key implementation characteristics for reaching hard-to-engage men?
5. What is the NICE definition of ERS?
6. What does the NICE guidance on promoting PA with ERS recommend?
7. What are the different components of COM-B?
8. How can behavioural change theory be helpful to understanding the behaviour of hard-to-reach groups?
9. How can evidence-based practice be deployed to better understand the reasons people adopt/do not adopt PA interventions?
10. Name three examples of theory that can be deployed to understand the behaviour of hard-to-reach/engage groups?
11. What is an ecological approach, and how can this be used to understand determinants of PA participation?

References

Andersen, L.B., Mota, J. and Di Pietro, L., 2016. Update on the global pandemic of physical inactivity. *The Lancet*, 388(1051), pp. 1255–1256.

Baker, C., Loughren, E., Crone, D., Tutton, A. and Aitken, P., 2016. 23 Contemporary lifestyle interventions for public health – Potential roles for professional sports clubs. *Sport and Exercise Psychology: Practitioner Case Studies,* p. 417.

Baker, P. and Shand, T., 2017. Men's health: Time for a new approach to policy and practice? *Journal of Global Health*, 7(1).

Bartholomew-Eldredge, L.K.B., Markham, C.M., Ruiter, R.A., Kok, G. and Parcel, G.S., 2016. *Planning health promotion programs: An intervention mapping approach.* Chichester, John Wiley & Sons.

Bird, L., Cross-Bardell, L., Ward, D. and Kai, J., 2017. *Facilitating access to obesity services for high risk, harder to reach groups: recent learning from the East Midlands region (UK).* Nottingham, East Midlands Academic Health Science Network.

Blue, S., Shove, E., Carmona, C. and Kelly, M.P., 2016. Theories of practice and public health: Understanding (un) healthy practices. *Critical Public Health*, 26(1), pp. 36–50.

Brook, K., Pringle, A., Hargreaves, J. and Kime, N., 2017. Promoting physical activity with Hard-to-Reach women: An iterative and participatory research study. *Perspectives in Public Health*, 137(5), p. 266.

Cade, D., Curran, K., Fuller, A., Hacker, J., Knight, C., Lansley, S., Parnell, D. and Philpott, M., 2017. Perspectives from those involved in healthy stadia. *Sport in Society*, 20(2), pp. 187–201.

Centre for Workforce Intelligence and Royal Society for Public Health, 2015. Understanding the wider public health workforce. Available at: www.cfwi.org.uk/publications/understanding-the-wider-public-health-workforce-in-England/@@publication-detail

Chaudhury, H., Campo, M., Michael, Y. and Mahmood, A., 2016. Neighbourhood environment and physical activity in older adults. *Social Science & Medicine*, 149, pp. 104–113.

Collins, M. and Kay, T., 2003. *Sport and social exclusion*. London, Routledge.

Conrad, D. and Abraham, M., 2016. Sport and public health partnership working. In *Sports-based health interventions* (pp. 77–87). New York, Springer.

Corbin, J.H., Jones, J. and Barry, M.M., 2016. What makes intersectoral partnerships for health promotion work? A review of the international literature. *Health Promotion International* 33(1), pp. 4–26.

Curran, K., Drust, B., Murphy, R., Pringle, A. and Richardson, D., 2016. The challenge and impact of engaging hard-to-reach populations in regular physical activity and health behaviours: An examination of an English Premier League 'Football in the Community' men's health programme. *Public Health*, 135, pp. 14–22.

Das, P. and Horton, R., 2016. Physical activity-time to take it seriously and regularly. *Lancet*, 388(10051), pp. 1254–1255.

Department of Health, 2007. *National evaluation of the local exercise action pilots*. London, Crown. Available at: www.dh.gov.uk/en/Publicationsandstatistics/Publications/PublicationsPolicyAndGuidance/DH_073600 (Accessed 4 April 2016).

Department of Health, 2011. *Start active stay active: A report for the four home countries Medical Officers*. London, Department of Health.

Dietz, W.H., Baur, L.A., Hall, K., Puhl, R.M., Taveras, E.M., Uauy, R. and Kopelman, P., 2015. Management of obesity: Improvement of health-care training and systems for prevention and care. *The Lancet*, 385(9986), pp. 2521–2533.

Din, N.U., Moore, G.F., Murphy, S., Wilkinson, C. and Williams, N.H., 2015. Health professionals' perspectives on exercise referral and physical activity promotion in primary care: Findings from a process evaluation of the National Exercise Referral Scheme in Wales. *Health Education Journal*, 74(6), pp. 743–757.

Dunn, K. and Richardson, D., 2010. I just want to watch the match! A reflective account of men's health themed match day events at an English Premier League Football Club: ISMH World Congress 2010 Abstract 129. *Journal of Men's Health*, 7(3), pp. 323–323.

Edmunds, S., Roche, D. and Stratton, G., 2010. Levels and patterns of physical activity in children and adolescents with type 1 diabetes and associated metabolic and physiologic health outcomes. *Journal of Physical Activity and Health*, 7(1), pp. 68–77.

Eyal, N., 2013. Denial of treatment to obese patients – the wrong policy on personal responsibility for health. *International Journal of Health Policy and Management*, 1(2), p. 107.

Faculty of Sports Medicine, Royal College of General Practitioners and Public Health England, 2018. Moving medicine. Available at: https://movingmedicine.wpengine.com/ (Accessed 16 November 2018).

Faugier, J. and Sargeant, M., 1997. Sampling hard to reach populations. *Journal of Advanced Nursing*, 26(4), pp. 790–797.

Fineberg, H.V., 2012. A successful and sustainable health system – how to get there from here. *New England Journal of Medicine*, 366(11), pp. 1020–1027.

Flanagan, S.M. and Hancock, B., 2010. 'Reaching the hard to reach'-lessons learned from the VCS (voluntary and community Sector). A qualitative study. *BMC Health Services Research*, 10(1), p. 92.

Freimuth, V.S. and Mettger, W., 1990. Is there a hard-to-reach audience? *Public Health Reports*, 105(3), p. 232.

Gates, A.B., 2016. Making every contact count for physical activity – for tomorrow's patients: The launch of the interdisciplinary, undergraduate, resources on exercise medicine and health in the UK. *British Journal of Sports Medicine*. http://dx.doi.org/10.1136/bjsports-2015-095489

Giné-Garriga, M., Coll-Planas, L., Guerra, M., Domingo, À., Roqué, M., Caserotti, P., Denkinger, M., Rothenbacher, D., Tully, M.A., Kee, F. and McIntosh, E., 2017. The SITLESS project: Exercise referral schemes enhanced by self-management strategies to battle sedentary behaviour in older adults: Study protocol for a randomised controlled trial. *Trials*, 18(1), p. 221.

Grace, B., Richardson, N. and Carroll, P., 2016. "If you're not part of the institution you fall by the wayside" Service providers' perspectives on moving young men from disconnection and isolation to connection and belonging. *American Journal of Men's Health*, p. 1557988316634088.

Gray, C.M., Wyke, S., Zhang, R., Anderson, A.S., Barry, S., Brennan, G., Briggs, A., Boyer, N., Bunn, C., Donnachie, C. and Grieve, E., 2018. Long-term weight loss following a randomised controlled trial of a weight management programme for men delivered through professional football clubs: The Football Fans in Training follow-up study. *Public Health Research*, 6(9).

Hargreaves, J. and Pringle, A., 2018. What is it about football? The experiences of football and behaviour change among people with mental health problems. *Mental Health and Physical Activity,* 16, pp. 19–30.

Haskell, W.L., Blair, S.N. and Hill, J.O., 2009. Physical activity: Health outcomes and importance for public health policy. *Preventive Medicine*, 49(4), pp. 280–282.

Health Education England, 2018. Making every contact count. Available at: www.makingeverycontactcount.co.uk/ (Accessed 2 September 2018).

Hulton, A.T., Flower, D., Murphy, R., Richardson, D., Drust, B. and Curran, K., 2016. Effectiveness of a community football programme on improving physiological markers of health in a hard-to-reach male population: The role of exercise intensity. *Soccer & Society*, 17(2), pp. 196–208.

Hunt, K., Wyke, S., Gray, C.M., Anderson, A.S., Brady, A., Bunn, C., Donnan, P.T., Fenwick, E., Grieve, E., Leishman, J. and Miller, E., 2014. A gender-sensitised weight loss and healthy living programme for overweight and obese men delivered by Scottish Premier League football clubs (FFIT): A pragmatic randomised controlled trial. *The Lancet*, 383(9924), pp. 1211–1221.

Jonman, C., Mackie, P. and Sim, F., 2013. The beautiful game. *Public Health*, 127(8), pp. 697–698.

Kime, N. and Pringle, A., 2018. Exercise and physical activity in people with type 1 diabetes: The importance of behaviour change. *Diabetes Research and Clinical Practice*, 138, pp. 282–283.

Kime, N.H., Pringle, A., Rivett, M.J. and Robinson, P.M., 2018. Physical activity and exercise in adults with type 1 diabetes: Understanding their needs using a person-centered approach. *Health Education Research*, 33(5), pp. 375–388.

Kok, G., Gottlieb, N.H., Peters, G.J.Y., Mullen, P.D., Parcel, G.S., Ruiter, R.A., Fernández, M.E., Markham, C. and Bartholomew, L.K., 2016. A taxonomy of behaviour change methods: An intervention mapping approach. *Health Psychology Review*, 10(3), pp. 297–312.

Lefkowich, M., Richardson, N. and Robertson, S., 2017. "If we want to get men in, then we need to ask men what they want": Pathways to effective health programing for men. *American Journal of Men's Health*, 11(5), pp. 1512–1524.

Lévesque, L., 2017. Truth and reconciliation in research physical activity interventions with indigenous communities. *Key Note. International Society of Behaviour Nutrition and Physical Activity Annual Meeting*. Victoria, British Columbia, June 7–11.

Lewis, C.J., Reeves, M.J. and Roberts, S.J., 2017. Improving the physical and mental well-being of typically hard-to-reach men: An investigation of the impact of the Active Rovers project. *Sport in Society*, 20(2), pp. 258–268.

Lozano, L., Pringle, A.R., McKenna, J. and Carless, D., 2018. "There was other guys in the same boat as myself": The role of homosocial environments in sustaining men's engagement in health interventions. *Qualitative Research in Sport, Exercise and Health*, 11(4), pp. 494–509.

Lozano-Sufrategui, L., Pringle, A., Carless, D. and McKenna, J., 2017. 'It brings the lads together': A critical exploration of older men's experiences of a weight management programme delivered through a Healthy Stadia project. *Sport in Society*, 20(2), pp. 303–315.

Marcus, B. and Forsyth, L., 2011. *Motivating people to be physically active*. Champaign, IL, Human Kinetics.

Marentes-Castillo, M., Zamarripa, J., Delgado, M., Ródenas, L. and Álvarez, O., 2017. Decisional balance, self-efficacy and its association to the exercise enjoyment in Mexican population. *Revista de psicología del deporte*, 26(4), pp. 88–92.

Martin, A., Morgan, S., Parnell, D., Philpott, M., Pringle, A., Rigby, M., Taylor, A. and Topham, J., 2016. A perspective from key stakeholders on football and health improvement. *Soccer & Society*, 17(2), pp. 175–182.

Mathers, J., Taylor, R. and Parry, J., 2016. Measuring the impact of Health Trainers Services on health and health inequalities: Does the service's data collection and reporting system provide reliable information? *Journal of Public Health*, 39(1), pp. 139–144.

Mendoza-Vasconez, A.S., Linke, S., Muñoz, M., Pekmezi, D., Ainsworth, C., Cano, M., Williams, V., Marcus, B.H. and Larsen, B.A., 2016. Promoting physical activity among underserved populations. *Current Sports Medicine Reports*, 15(4), pp. 290–297.

Michie, S., Van Stralen, M.M. and West, R., 2011. The behaviour change wheel: A new method for characterising and designing behaviour change interventions. *Implementation Science*, 6(1), p. 42.

Mutrie, N., Standage, M., Pringle, A., Laventure, R., Smith, L., Strain, T., Kelly, P., Dall, P., Milton, K., Chalkley, A., College, N., Foster, C. and Banfield, K., 2018. Expert working group working paper communication and surveillance. *UK Physical Activity Guidelines: Developing Options for Future Communication and Surveillance*. University of Bristol, May 2018.

National Institute of Health and Care Excellence, 2014a. *Promoting physical activity through exercise referral: Partial update*. London, National Institute of Health and Care Excellence.

National Institute of Health and Care Excellence, 2014b. *Behaviour change: Individual approaches*. London, National Institute for Health and Care Excellence. Available at: www.nice.org.uk/guidance/ph49 (Accessed 2 September 2018).

Osborne, S.A., Adams, J.M., Fawkner, S., Kelly, P., Murray, A.D. and Oliver, C.W., 2017. Tomorrow's doctors want more teaching and training on physical activity for health. *British Journal of Sports Medicine*. http://dx.doi.org/10.1136/bjsports-2016-096807

Parnell, D., Curran, K. and Philpott, M., 2017. *Healthy stadia: An insight from policy to practice*. London, Routledge.

Pringle, A. and Jagroo, J., 2015. The impact of exercise referral schemes for hard to reach groups. *Public Health and Primary Care Conference 2015*, Birmingham NEC, Birmingham, UK.

Pringle, A., Marsh, K., Gilson, N., McKenna, J. and Cooke, C., 2010. Cost effectiveness of interventions to improve moderate physical-activity: A study in nine UK sites. *Health Education Journal*, 69(2), pp. 211–224.

Pringle, A., McKenna, J. and Zwolinsky, S., 2018. Linking physical activity & health evaluation to policy: Lessons from UK evaluations. In J. Piggin, L. Mansfield and M. Weed, eds. *Routledge handbook of physical activity policy and practice*. London, Routledge, pp. 411–425.

Pringle, A. and Zwolinsky, S., 2017a. Older people, physical activity and public health. In P. Krustrup and D. Parnell, eds. *Sport and health: Exploring the current state of play*. London, Routledge, pp. 89–110.

Pringle, A. and Zwolinsky, S., 2017b. Investigating key implementation factors for engaging men in health interventions in English Premier League football clubs using Delphi Pol/Card Sort Techniques. In: *ISBNPA, 07 June 2017–10 June 2017*. Victoria, Canada.

Pringle, A. and Zwolinsky, S., 2018. An investigation into the adoption and use of Public Health guidance by professional football club community schemes. *7th International Society of Physical Activity and Health Congress*. London, October 15–17.

Pringle, A., Zwolinsky, S., McKenna, J., Daly-Smith, A., Robertson, S. and White, A., 2013. Delivering men's health interventions in English Premier League football clubs: Key design characteristics. *Public Health*, 127(8), pp. 716–726.

Pringle, A., Zwolinsky, S., McKenna, J., Robertson, S., Daly-Smith, A. and White, A., 2014. Health improvement for men and hard-to-engage-men delivered in English Premier League football clubs. *Health Education Research*, 29(3), pp. 503–520.

Public Health England, 2018. Clinical champions: Embedding physical activity into routine clinical care. Blog June 21. Available at: https://publichealthmatters.blog.gov.uk/2018/06/21/clinical-champions-embedding-physical-activity-into-routine-clinical-care/ (Accessed 2 September 2018).

Queen, M., Crone, D. and Parker, A., 2015. Evaluation of a tactic to engage hard-to-reach patients during the exercise referral process: A longitudinal qualitative study. *European Journal of Person Centred Healthcare*, 3(3), pp. 288–294.

Ransdell, L., Dinger, M., Huberty, J. and Miller, K., 2009. *Planning physical activity programmes. Developing effective physical activity programmes*. Champaign, IL, Human Kinetics.

Reddy, P., Dias, I., Holland, C., Campbell, N., Nagar, I., Connolly, L., Krustrup, P. and Hubball, H., 2017. Walking football as sustainable exercise for older adults – A pilot investigation. *European Journal of Sport Science*, 17(5), pp. 638–645.

Reis, R.S., Salvo, D., Ogilvie, D., Lambert, E.V., Goenka, S., Brownson, R.C. and Lancet Physical Activity Series 2 Executive Committee, 2016. Scaling up physical activity interventions worldwide: Stepping up to larger and smarter approaches to get people moving. *The Lancet*, 388(10051), pp. 1337–1348.

Riebe, D., Franklin, B.A., Thompson, P.D., Garber, C.E., Whitfield, G.P., Magal, M. and Pescatello, L.S., 2015. Updating ACSM's recommendations for exercise preparticipation health screening. *Medicine & Science in Sports & Exercise*, 47(11), pp. 2473–2479.

Robertson, S. and Baker, P., 2017. Men and health promotion in the United Kingdom: 20 years further forward? *Health Education Journal*, 76(1), pp. 102–113.

Robertson, S., Woodall, J., Henry, H., Hanna, E., Rowlands, S., Horrocks, J., Livesley, J. and Long, T., 2016. Evaluating a community-led project for improving fathers' and children's wellbeing in England. *Health Promotion International*, 33(3), pp. 410–421.

Robertson, S., Zwolinsky, S., Pringle, A., McKenna, J., Daly-Smith, A. and White, A., 2013. 'It is fun, fitness and football really': A process evaluation of a football-based health intervention for men. *Qualitative Research in Sport, Exercise and Health*, 5(3), pp. 419–439.

Scarborough, P., Bhatnagar, P., Wickramasinghe, K., Allender, S., Foster, C. and Rayner, M., 2011. The economic burden of ill health due to diet, physical inactivity, smoking, alcohol and obesity in the UK: An update to 2006–2007 NHS costs. *Journal of Public Health*, 4, pp. 527–535.

Sinclair, A. and Alexander, H.A., 2012. Using outreach to involve the hard-to-reach in a health check: What difference does it make? *Public Health*, 126(2), pp. 87–95.

Stewart, L., Dolan, E., Carver, P. and Swinton, P.A., 2017. Per-protocol investigation of a best practice exercise referral scheme. *Public Health*, 150, pp. 26–33.

Symons, J., 2017. 'We're not hard-to-reach, they are! 'Integrating local priorities in urban research in Northern England: An experimental method. *The Sociological Review*, p. 0038026117717432.

Teo, C.H., Ng, C.J. and White, A., 2017. What do men want from a health screening mobile app? A qualitative study. *PloS One*, 12(1), p. e0169435.

Thornton, J., 2017. Physical activity prescription and engaging the entire 'community of practice'. *British Journal of Sports Medicine*, pp. bjsports-2016.

Trivedy, C., Vlaev, I., Seymour, R. and Philpott, M., 2017. An evaluation of opportunistic health checks at cricket matches: The Boundaries for Life initiative. *Sport in Society*, 20(2), pp. 226–234.

van de Glind, I., Bunn, C., Gray, C.M., Hunt, K., Andersen, E., Jelsma, J., Morgan, H., Pereira, H., Roberts, G., Rooksby, J. and Røynesdal, Ø., 2017. The intervention process in the European Fans in Training (EuroFIT) trial: A mixed method protocol for evaluation. *Trials*, 18(1), p. 356.

Vishnubala, D., Pringle, A., Kime, N. and Zwolinksy, S., 2020. The role of general practice nurses in the promotion of physical activity. *Journal of General Practice Nursing*, 6.

Whitall, J., Jago, R. and Fox, K., 2011. Why some do but most don't. Barriers and enablers to engaging low-income groups in physical activity programmes: A mixed methods study. *BMC Public Health*, 11, p. 507.

White, A., 2011. *The state of men's health in Europe. Extended report*. Brussels, European Commission.

White, A., Zwolinsky, S., Pringle, A., McKenna, J., Daly-Smith, A., Robertson, S. and Berry, R., 2012. Premier League Health: A national programme of men's health promotion guidance, good practice and lessons: A toolkit for delivering and evaluating men's health interventions in/by professional football clubs. *Centre for Men's Health & Centre for Active Lifestyles*. Leeds, UK: Leeds Metropolitan University.

Whitehead, M., 1997. How useful is the 'Stages of Change' model? *Health Education Journal*, 56(2), pp. 111–112.

Wohl, A.R., Ludwig-Barron, N., Dierst-Davies, R., Kulkarni, S., Bendetson, J., Jordan, W., Bolan, R., Smith, T., Cunningham, W. and Pérez, M.J., 2017. Project engage: Snowball sampling and direct recruitment to identify and link hard-to-reach HIV-infected persons who are out of care. *JAIDS Journal of Acquired Immune Deficiency Syndromes*, 75(2), pp. 190–197.

Woringer, M., Cecil, E., Watt, H., Chang, K., Hamid, F., Khunti, K., Dubois, E., Evason, J., Majeed, A. and Soljak, M., 2017. Evaluation of community provision of a preventive cardiovascular programme-the National Health Service Health Check in reaching the under-served groups by primary care in England: Cross sectional observational study. *BMC Health Services Research*, 17(1), p. 405.

World Health Organisation, 2018. *Physical activity key facts*. Geneva, World Health Organisation. Available at: www.who.int/news-room/fact-sheets/detail/physical-activity/ (Accessed 1 August 2018).

Yancey, A.K., Ory, M.G. and Davis, S.M., 2006. Dissemination of physical activity promotion interventions in underserved populations. *American Journal of Preventive Medicine*, 31(4), pp. 82–91.

Yang, D.D., Hausien, O., Aqeel, M., Klonis, A., Foster, J., Renshaw, D. and Thomas, R., 2017. Physical activity levels and barriers to exercise referral among patients with cancer. *Patient Education and Counselling*, 100(7), pp. 1402–1407.

Zwolinsky, S., McKenna, J. and Pringle, A., 2016. How can the health system benefit from increasing participation in sport, exercise and physical activity? In *Sports-Based Health Interventions*. New York, Springer, pp. 29–52.

Zwolinsky, S., McKenna, J., Pringle, A., Daly-Smith, A., Robertson, S. and White, A., 2016. Supporting lifestyle risk reduction: Promoting men's health through professional football. *Soccer & Society*, 17(2), pp. 183–195.

8

MAINTAINING EXERCISE BEHAVIOUR FOLLOWING ERS COMPLETION

Michael Eynon, Gill Crowther and Hayley Mills

Chapter aims

By the end of this chapter, you will be able to:

- Contextualise current thinking, evidence and understanding in exercise referral to promote sustained exercise behaviour post ERS completion
- Understand the role of the COM-B model and self-determination theory in encouraging exercise maintenance
- Appraise the practice implications for influencing self-determined motivation during exercise referral to promote sustained exercise behaviour
- Apply behaviour change techniques to effectively enable participants to develop the tools and motivation to sustain exercise behaviour over the longer term
- Gain insight into real-world examples of exercise referral providing a catalyst for exercise maintenance
- Recognise how enablement and exit strategies from exercise referral schemes may facilitate sustained exercise

Introduction

An important part of evaluating exercise referral schemes (ERS) is understanding what happens to patients following the scheme in the short and long term. While the main goal of ERS is to increase physical activity behaviour in an attempt to alleviate health risks, creating an independent, lifelong exerciser should be the overarching objective. The key questions for exercise referral evaluators, therefore, should be whether the schemes are having a positive impact on patient's longer-term behaviour and how sustained exercise behaviour beyond the end of the scheme can be achieved. This chapter seeks to examine the maintenance of behavioural changes as a result of ERS, taking into account appropriate theory, successful interventions and the process of exiting the ERS and applying behaviour change techniques to promote exercise maintenance.

DOI: 10.4324/9781315102399-8

Understanding behaviour and behaviour change

Despite modern day healthcare and advanced technologies, human behaviour with all its complexities plays a critical role in the outcomes and efficacy of interventions (Ryan et al., 2008). See Chapter 6 for details on behaviour change, but a broad understanding of human behaviour and behaviour change techniques is crucial for practitioners delivering ERS if they are going to increase the likelihood of patients maintaining their exercise behaviour once the scheme ends. Behaviour has been defined as:

> Anything a person does in response to internal or external events. Actions may be overt (motor or verbal) and directly measurable, or covert (actions not viewable e.g. physiological responses) and indirectly measurable; behaviours are physical events that occur in the body and are controlled by the brain.
>
> *(Hobbs et al., 2011, p. 31)*

Evidence for the sustainability of behaviours following ERS is limited as very few studies evaluate long-term effects and possibly because effects diminish over time once the intervention ceases (Kwasnicka et al., 2016). Poor adherence to behaviours recommended in lifestyle interventions is widespread, particularly over the longer term (Middleton et al., 2013), which poses a challenge for ERS practitioners. What we do know is that interventions that are most likely to be effective are those that intervene at many levels simultaneously across population (general living and working conditions), community (social and community networks) and individuals (lifestyle factors such as age) (National Institute for Health and Care Excellence [NICE], 2014).

Applying theory to produce longer-term exercise maintenance

To facilitate the maintenance of exercise engagement over the longer term and help offset the risk of developing lifestyle diseases, it is necessary to understand the processes of behavioural change over a prolonged period as a result of ERS engagement. Theories of behaviour change maintenance can provide guidance on interventions promoting sustained change in health behaviours (Kwasnicka et al., 2016). The following section overviews both the COM-B model and self-determination theory in relation to longer-term exercise maintenance, given their relevance and application to exercise referral.

COM-B model

Current guidance on behaviour change interventions in relation to health and well-being recommends use of a model of behaviour change based on capability, opportunity and motivation, known as COM-B (NICE, 2014). COM-B is part of a larger framework, the behaviour change wheel (BCW), which provides a systematic way of depicting and designing behaviour change interventions, drawing together many behaviour change theories and psychological constructs into a single coherent model (Michie et al., 2014). COM-B starts from the premise that, for any behaviour change to occur, a person must:

- Be physically and psychologically *capable* of carrying out the new behaviour
- Have the physical and social *opportunity* to carry out the behaviour
- Be more *motivated* to adopt the new behaviour than the old one

It is the interaction of these three components that promotes the desired behaviour (Michie et al., 2011). Capability can either be physical (e.g. skills and strength) or psychological (e.g. resources and skills, capacity for understanding). Opportunity can also represent physical aspects (e.g. resources, locations or barriers) as well as social (e.g. cultural milieu or exposure to ideas). Motivation is key to the generation of behaviour as it determines what individuals do and how they do it (Michie & West, 2013). It can either be reflective, involving planning (self-conscious intentions) and evaluations (beliefs about what is good and bad), or automatic, involving emotional reactions, drives, impulses and habits (Michie & West, 2013).

A key feature of the COM-B model is that it conceptualises behaviour as a system incorporating context and is designed to capture the range of internal mechanisms (psychological and physical) as well as those relating to the external environment (Michie et al., 2011). It is argued that behaviour can only be truly understood in relation to the context it is performed in (Michie et al., 2011). If the aim of the ERS extends to facilitating exercise maintenance beyond the completion of the scheme, the context of the patient's current lifestyle and situation in terms of social, cultural and economic factors must be recognised and understood.

The application of COM-B to ERS

COM-B provides a practical way of seeing how an ERS can influence future exercise behaviour in individuals. If exercise is to be maintained in the longer term, the three components must exist in sufficient amounts. The behaviour (i.e. exercise) can influence all three components, and capability and opportunity to exercise can both influence motivation (Michie et al., 2011).

In the context of exercise referral, for a person to maintain their exercise behaviour after the scheme ends, they must be motivated to exercise (i.e. want to engage in exercise and enjoy the behaviour), have the capability to exercise (i.e. be competent in exercising) and have the opportunity to exercise (i.e. have feasible access to exercise facilities). Psychological (e.g. increased self-efficacy), social (e.g. exercising with others) and environmental (e.g. having access to exercise) factors have also been associated with long-term exercise behaviour (van Stralen et al., 2009).

In practice, service providers should adopt a person-centred approach in which they work collaboratively with their patients as equal partners to help them establish new exercise habits throughout the duration of the scheme. In this way, they are acting as enablers and maximising likely sustainable change and maintenance of the behaviour in the future.

Self-determination theory

Given that much of the activity that take place in ERS is gym-based and guided by an instructor, it is important to highlight that, for long-term exercise maintenance post ERS, the activities should become more self-determined to the patient. Although there are many competing theories of motivation, the theoretical approach that seeks to explain behaviour through self-determined motivation is Deci and Ryan's (1985, 2000) self-determination theory.

Self-determination theory is a popular theory in explaining the motivational processes influencing exercise participation, particularly over a prolonged period. The theory distinguishes between intrinsic and extrinsic motivation. A person who exercises for intrinsic motives does so for the satisfaction they gain from exercising (e.g. competence, enjoyment).

A person with extrinsic motives exercises in order to obtain rewards or avoid punishments (e.g. lose weight, improve appearance). In order for exercise referral patients to maintain exercise over the longer term, more intrinsic motives should be present.

Influencing self-determined motivation in exercise referral

In order to influence self-determined motivation with patients exercising for intrinsic motives, there are a number of factors that may be useful. The satisfaction of three basic psychological needs for autonomy, relatedness, and competence have been shown to be important for promoting self-determined motivation and exercise behaviour change among exercise referral patients (Edmunds et al., 2007; Eynon et al., 2017; Markland & Tobin, 2010):

- *Autonomy* reflects the need to have choice and be in control of one's own behaviour
- *Relatedness* refers to one's desire to feel connected to and be accepted by peers
- *Competence* involves feelings that one can successfully optimally complete challenging tasks

Exercise referral practitioners should look to target any of these psychological needs in their practices to help patients become more self-determined to exercise. In order to influence autonomy, exercise instructors should seek to provide choice to the patient in their exercise activities. This can be done through offering a range of activity types not limited to the gym environment (e.g. classes, swimming, walking etc.) as well as to offer choice within the specific detail of the programme (i.e. frequency, intensity or timing of sessions). To influence patients' relatedness, practitioners should help them acclimatise to their new exercise environment by introducing them to fellow referrals as well as providing positive experiences on initiation of the scheme. Finally, to influence patients' competence, exercise instructors should ensure that patients 1) are able to perform the exercises prescribed and 2) perceive that they are able to exercise. Also, instructors should try to avoid making assumptions about people's levels and perceived levels of competence.

Self-determination theory-based exercise referral intervention

An ERS based on self-determination theory was produced and assessed in an attempt to enhance long-term exercise behaviour outcomes (Duda et al., 2014). The intervention was aimed at creating an autonomy-supportive climate for exercise referral patients so they could:

1. Be aware of and understand the benefits and risks of increased physical activity and behaviour change
2. Recognise perceived barriers and implement intention(s) to become more active
3. Identify and strengthen sources of social support

The self-determination theory-based ERS was compared with a standard provision ERS. Physical activity improved for patients in both ERS from programme entry to six months later. In addition, autonomy support was related to psychological need satisfaction and self-determined motivation, which served to enhance physical activity engagement at six months. This highlights the effectiveness of both types of ERS in increasing long-term physical activity. Whilst there may be questions around the strength of a self-determination theory-based intervention above a standard-provision ERS, the relationships observed between self-determination theory factors (i.e. need satisfaction and self-determined motivation) and long-term behaviour change indicate potential for self-determination theory-based ERS.

In practice, to enhance the effectiveness of future exercise referral interventions based on self-determination theory, the interventions need to focus on the patients incorporating more self-determined motives to exercise through increasing their perceptions of autonomy, relatedness and competence. This can be achieved through practitioners creating an autonomy-supportive climate in the ERS setting.

Non-adherence, lapse and readoption

In order to gain a comprehensive understanding of behaviour change processes, as well as assessing adoption and adherence behaviours, it is equally important to examine the processes involved in dropout, lapse and relapse behaviour (Prochaska & DiClemente, 1983; Rodgers et al., 2010). Through longitudinal qualitative assessment of inactive women who engaged in a ten-week walking programme, researchers uncovered three separate profiles of ERS patients: non-adherence, lapse and readoption and adherence (Kinnafick et al., 2014). These profiles are outlined next:

Non-adherence: Patients did not continue to exercise following the ten-week programme and exhibited a lack of self-determined motivation whilst also not satisfying the basic psychological needs. In addition, non-adherers did not embrace the support made available to them and viewed the exercise as an inconvenience to their lifestyle.

Lapse and readoption: Patients typically engaged fully with the programme, lapsed on completing it for around two to three months, then readopted physical activity at some stage between six and ten months. During the programme, patients satisfied their psychological needs but also exhibited extrinsic forms of motivation through guilt and obligation to exercise. Upon readoption of exercise, patients had more intrinsic motives to exercise while also satisfying psychosocial needs, which served to foster greater exercise.

Adherence: Patients successfully engaged with the programme and were still exercising at the ten-month follow-up with no experience of lapsing. These patients were exhibited self-determined motivation during the programme as well as satisfying the three basic psychological needs. Enjoyment of exercise was a key factor in adherers' motivation, as well the exercise becoming habitual.

These findings illustrate the role of self-determined motivation in explaining why patients do not sustain exercise beyond the end of the scheme, with a lack of intrinsic motives and need satisfaction fulfilment noted as influential factors. In addition, other influences such as support and lifestyle inconveniences served to influence non-adherers' lack of participation in exercise. Patients who lapsed but then readopted exhibited more intrinsic motives to exercise upon readoption, showing the long-term nature and effect of self-determined motivation on exercise behaviour. Finally, adherence to the scheme and prolonged exercise engagement were very much related to more intrinsic motives and satisfaction of the three basic psychological needs. This shows the reciprocal nature of self-determined motivation and need satisfaction, which has an impact on intentions and attitudes towards being active (Sabiston et al., 2009).

In practice, exercise referral practitioners should seek to enhance patients' self-determined motivation and need satisfaction through the duration of the exercise referral scheme. This should serve to increase the likelihood of prolonged exercise participation once patients have exited the scheme.

Case Study: Maggie – 71 years old, diagnosed with depression

Background

Maggie was referred to an ERS upon being diagnosed with depression whilst also being overweight. Her domestic circumstances meant that she was the main carer for her husband, who is diabetic, and her two brothers, who have both had heart problems. As a result of Maggie attending the ERS, she continues to exercise now.

Outlined next are Maggie's experiences in becoming a long-term exerciser. Attached to her experiences are aspects of concepts that can be applied to help explain how behaviour change can be maintained and serve as a guide for practitioners looking to help ERS patients maintain exercise beyond the end of the scheme.

Maggie's ERS routine

Maggie attended weekly circuit-based exercise classes at the local leisure centre, as well as engaging in gym sessions. She also went swimming early in the morning around two to three times a week.

Maintaining exercise through planning

One of the reasons Maggie has been successful in maintaining physical activity over the long term is that she perceives her exercise behaviour as fitting into her life. For example, she tries to ensure that any personal or medical appointments are arranged at times that do not clash with her exercise regimen. When encountering a potential period of inactivity, such as going on holiday, she recognises the difficulty of getting back into a routine but accepts the challenge of it, aware of the benefits. She said:

> I think when you are constantly doing it [exercising] it's a way of life. It's an automatic thing and I get up and I go. . . . But when you break the pattern then it's mentally harder to get back into it plus you do feel the actual exercise is a bit harder for a while as well.

Enjoyment as motivation

Although Maggie's caring commitments contribute to motivating her exercise behaviour, she also perceives exercise as a form of 'me time'. She said it is 'something for me; it's not for them. It is partly I suppose why I do it for them but no, I go for my own sake as well'. She feels the exercise has helped with her depression and said, 'Well, I don't know how medical this is, but I am sure exercise activates hormones that make you feel better; that's what I wonder'. She also enjoys it:

> I don't know if you could do that sort of thing constantly if you didn't enjoy it. I thoroughly enjoy going. . . . I'm sure I wouldn't be motivated to do it if I was thinking, 'Oh gosh, I can't face that again'.

These aspects of motivation highlight how enjoying exercise can contribute to long-term maintenance of exercise. Practitioners should look to find ways to help patients enjoy exercise or aspects of exercise in order to facilitate long-term behaviour change.

Social network

Maggie also highlighted the importance of a social network that facilitated her engagement with exercise. She said, 'You meet such a lot of nice people, and I always find the staff are really nice. If you didn't get on with the people, then possibly you might not be quite so keen to go'. The exercise classes were supervised, and there was always an instructor available at her gym sessions.

> Just once a week I go. . . . She's [the exercise practitioner] keeping an eye on you and like just lately, or every now and again, she'll change the programme if you feel you're not getting as much benefit out of it. So they are very good at that.

This shows the ongoing role of the practitioner during an ERS patient's exercise journey in continuing to take an interest in them and tailoring the programme to optimise effectiveness.

Enablement and exit strategies

In order for patients to progress from the successful completion of an ERS to the integration of maintaining exercise over the longer term, two key factors may play a role: enablement, including relevant behaviour change techniques, and exit strategies.

Enablement

Professional advice and supervision during an ERS have been identified as key components for success (Mills et al., 2012). This indicates that patients are more likely to engage in and sustain exercise behaviour with professionals present who are knowledgeable and engaged. This support is important in facilitating scheme commitment but brings with it the creation of issues of dependency, whereby patients become dependent on the practitioner in their exercise journey. An emphasis of ERS should be to progressively shift support over the course of the scheme from strategies that can facilitate dependency across to enablement. Enablement is one of the nine intervention functions identified in the BCW (Michie et al., 2011). Within the BCW, the purpose of enablement as an intervention relates to increasing the resources and reducing the barriers to enhance either capability or opportunity.

Exercise referral practitioners therefore need to give patients the tools, the support and the opportunity to enable them to continue with their exercise programmes. They need to target an increase in the knowledge and understanding that patients have in relation to their new behavioural habits. Application of the COM-B model should focus on the drive to move towards enablement, effectively increasing the means and reducing the barriers to increase capability beyond education. This should involve not just providing information to promote the ongoing health benefits of physical activity or imparting the necessary skills required but also providing behavioural support such as ongoing exercise classes for patients to continue exercising.

Enablement and behaviour change techniques (BCTs)

Drawing on the principles of behaviour change, maintenance strategies cannot rely on individual choices and decision-making; they must be based on the environment and making the behaviour automatic through environmental support and prompts, building routine, feedback and reward or incentives (Michie et al., 2014).

A systematic review of studies investigating attendance and completion of referral schemes included factors likely to lead to longer-term physical activity behaviours, which were based on the views of patients themselves (Morgan et al., 2016). The themes identified in the review provide a perspective for practitioners on the BCTs that will lead to longer-term exercise maintenance. Social support, setting goals, motivation, enjoyment, existing health issues and personal commitment all contributed to patients incorporating exercise into their daily lives. Helping patients 'make exercise a habit' once the scheme had formally ended was also identified. A recent review of the psychosocial factors associated with adherence during ERS echoed the importance of motivation, self-efficacy, social support and psychological need satisfaction and noted the importance of exercise identity, self-regulation and realistic expectation for change (Eynon et al., 2019). A review of dietary and physical activity intervention components for adults with an increased risk of diabetes or cardiovascular disease found that the planned use of established BCTs, the mobilisation of social support and having a clear plan for supporting maintenance of behaviour change were more likely to maximise the effectiveness of the interventions (Greaves et al., 2011).

Based on this review-level evidence, with application to long-term maintenance in mind, the following section suggests how BCTs can be utilised in an ERS. BCTs are identified as the smallest 'active' components of an intervention that are likely to lead to its effectiveness: i.e. change behaviour. Practitioners can assist patients to maximise their ability to regulate their own behaviour through techniques such as goal setting, monitoring and feedback as well as action planning. Opportunity to support self-regulation can be maximised through social support, establishing new routines and identifying new environments.

Guidance on how BCTs can be utilised in an ERS is provided next. Practitioners should tailor these techniques throughout the scheme duration to support their patients to maximise capability and confidence in the initial stages and gradually shift this so that patients can utilise these techniques on their own once the scheme ends. The overarching aim is to increase a patient's motivation to maintain exercise behaviour by targeting their capabilities and opportunities. The suggested BCTs are adapted from and advocated via a BCT taxonomy (Michie et al., 2014; Abraham & Michie, 2008). In order to maximise the effectiveness of physical activity interventions, it has been shown that the planned use of established BCTs, the mobilisation of social support and having a clear plan for supporting maintenance of behaviour change are of utmost importance (Greaves et al., 2011).

1. Goals and planning

- Goal setting interventions are generally held to be effective in promoting physical activity behaviour (McEwan et al., 2016). Goals should follow the SMART acronym in that they should be specific, measurable, achievable, realistic and time framed (Stonehouse, 2018). Patients should be prompted to set process goals, such as agreeing to do a daily walk of 30 minutes. Outcome goals based on a desired behaviour that is a reasonable expectation for that individual should be encouraged. For example, setting a date to complete a 5K charity walk or increasing fitness levels enough to reduce the need for medication for a condition such as hypertension.
- Patients should be encouraged to think about planning their future exercise behaviour and should include at least one of context, frequency, duration or intensity: for example, identifying exercise classes in their local community that the patient is happy to and comfortable with committing to attend twice a week. Keeping a diary in which physical activity is planned on a weekly or monthly basis, taking into account other life commitments, may also assist.
- Practitioners should also assist patients with problem solving, such as helping them identify and overcome any barriers and identify facilitative strategies that will influence future behaviour. Discussing how and when breaks in routine might occur is useful when coupled with strategies to prepare for this. For example, first identify those potential breaks, such as holidays or injuries, and prepare with a series of steps and support systems to enable reengagement with activity.
- Assisting the patient in developing explicit 'if-then' coping strategies across a range of these scenarios may also be beneficial as a way of preventing relapse. For example, if a patient is unable to attend exercise classes for a fortnight, they could be encouraged to identify days on which they can go for a walk in their lunch hour.

2. Feedback and monitoring

- Practitioners should monitor and provide feedback on the patient's progress throughout the scheme: for example, taking baseline blood pressure readings and resting heart rates and comparing them as the scheme progresses.
- Encouraging self-monitoring is particularly crucial for long-term exercise maintenance. For example, patients record their exercise behaviour in a daily diary. Other information could also be included, such as weight change, mood states or feelings. This

could be individualised according to the original reason for referral, such as obesity or depression.

- NICE guidance currently recommends that people receive feedback and monitoring at regular intervals for a minimum of one year after the completion of the scheme. Practitioners should, if possible, agree on an appropriate method for contacting the patient to arrange this follow up (e.g. telephone or email).

3. *Social support*

As has been already noted, it has been strongly suggested that social support from practitioners, peers, family and friends is a strong facilitator for adherence to exercise (Morgan et al., 2016).

- Involving family members and partners to discuss ways of increasing physical activity such as walking groups, swimming or other local opportunities based around exercise preferences of the patient is also likely to facilitate long-term maintenance.
- Practitioners are also key providers of social support for their patients. At the beginning of an ERS, patients are likely to rely on this support whilst they increase their confidence and skill set of understanding 'what to do'. As the scheme progresses, social support may come from other sources if viable.
- Verbal persuasion by the practitioner may assuage any self-doubts that the patient may have about exercising: for example, persuading the patient they can successfully increase their physical activity despite their health status and that it will positively help them manage the condition, reduce future risks and lead to a better long-term quality of life.
- Practitioners should also encourage more physical activity over and above that perceived as 'exercise', such as parking away from the supermarket or walking into town instead of getting the bus. This is important as a key aim of an ERS must be to encourage increased physical activity as habitual and normalised behaviour. It is not just about completing the ERS and/or doing an occasional exercise class.

Exit strategies

Finally, there is a need to understand how to provide the best strategies for exercise referral patients to successfully make the transition from the scheme itself to exercising freely on their own. To avoid the longer-term behaviour being contingent on continued high levels of support, the patients must perceive that they are capable of continuing their physical activity without the support and in the face of the challenges that are an inevitable part of lifelong exercise maintenance. The patients would benefit from being encouraged to form their own support systems and coping mechanisms throughout the course of the scheme to ease this transition.

The aim is to facilitate the patient's perception that their ability to remain physically active is not contingent on the scheme-specific support systems, such as the dedicated exercise provider, with whom they are likely to have formed a trusting relationship. It has been previously stated that this concept of 'empowerment' maybe important for supporting success within exercise referral (Mills et al., 2012). An environment during the scheme's duration that fosters this and progressively hands over responsibility to the patient is likely to be beneficial for future behaviour by limiting the potential impact of dependency. Facilitating the patient's ability to develop their own long-term strategies is key as it has been acknowledged that there are high levels of individual variation in what works in changing behaviour (Hutchison & Johnston, 2013). Personalisation in this manner connects the physical activity to the patient's identity (e.g. where they live, what they like and their life stage). We cannot standardise the approach to longer-term exercise maintenance and expect these same strategies to work for all.

Through qualitative assessment of exercise professionals' experiences of the Welsh National ERS, a number of issues were raised regarding the levels of support that should be offered without creating dependence (Moore et al., 2011). Referral patient–only group activities were found to be supportive of adherence through the creation of an empathetic environment and social support and by seeing similar others carrying out the desired behaviours. Cultivating social networks was also identified as a crucial mechanism for lessening dependence and maintaining changes in the longer term. It was also felt that post-scheme maintenance classes should be considered. Some professionals felt the need to balance the benefits of providing interpersonal support in order to maintain motivation and confidence against the risks of patients depending on a level of support that would be unsustainable over the longer term.

Loss of the social aspect of classes was also considered an important reason some people struggled to adhere over the longer term in the Welsh ERS. Some practitioners organise local social events where participants currently engaged in an exercise referral scheme can network with their peers or others who have been through the scheme. Exiting patients from the scheme in clusters and steering them into maintenance classes together have also been shown to encourage peer support. Emerging networks were seen as taking over the role of the ERS in terms of motivating adherence and also providing role models. It may be about the lessening of anxieties and assisting of social assimilation to feel part of a group who are moving forward together.

In practice, successful exit strategies begin whilst in the ERS when there is a progressive handover of the nature of the support systems. During the scheme, the individualised support of the exercise provider could be (where appropriate) progressively decreased, in combination with discussing coping mechanisms and 'what-if' strategies with the individual patients. It is important to remember that there is no one-size-fits-all approach, and ERS practitioners must tailor their approach based on their specialist contextual knowledge and understanding according to the needs of their individual patients. These strategies aim to give the patients the tools to independently establish a positive lifelong relationship with physical activity.

Future recommendations

As we have seen from this chapter, there are a number of facets involved in influencing longer-term exercise maintenance through ERS. In order for ERS to become effective in promoting exercise maintenance over time, we need to be aware of how to move the field forward to promote prolonged exercise behaviour among those who require it most. These are outlined next:

- *Theory-based exercise referral interventions*: Empirical findings have been promising in linking self-determined motivation and psychological need satisfaction with longer-term exercise maintenance. Thus, targeting these factors through exercise referral interventions will help patients incorporate exercise into their lifestyle in the short term to enable sustained exercise through enjoyment, interest and satisfaction over the longer term.

- *Incorporate COM-B into exercise referral practices*: In order to ensure theory-based interventions are effective in promoting longer-term exercise maintenance, services should look to incorporate the COM-B model. Consequently, attention should be paid to exercise referral patients' abilities, opportunities and motivation to exercise in order to facilitate this.
- *Longitudinal follow-up*: The next step in furthering our understanding of longer-term exercise maintenance through exercise referral is to explore what happens to patients following programme exit. This is a period when patients are having to engage in exercise through their own volition (i.e. without supervision or discounted access to facilities etc.). Therefore, contact should remain with individuals who have participated in the scheme to establish their exercise behaviour long after they have completed it. Understanding whether or not they still engage in physical activity months and years later and the reasons behind this would be beneficial in assessing 1) the long-term effects of exercise referral schemes, 2) whether it is useful for long-term health and 3) the psychological mechanisms that contribute to prolonged exercise behaviour.

If future research and specific interventions in exercise referral look to address the recommendations outlined here, then the exercise referral evidence base can continue to grow and strengthen, creating effective theory-driven interventions to enable exercise maintenance over the longer term. The evidence base in exercise referral is not substantial, and as a result, investigations into the long-term behavioural changes of ERS should be welcomed.

Key points

- The BCW and COM-B provide a possible route for policy-makers and exercise referral decision makers to facilitate long-term behaviour change through their programmes' design and delivery.
- Self-determination theory is useful in understanding motivation throughout the duration of and following an exercise referral scheme.
- ERS in general increase adherers psychological need satisfaction and self-determined motivation throughout the scheme, but these reduce in the months that follow it.
- Participants may readopt exercise after dropout following the scheme, with self-determined motives (enjoyment, interest) facilitating continued exercise participation.
- An emphasis of ERS should be to progressively shift support over the course of the scheme from strategies that facilitate dependency across to ones supporting enablement.
- Social support and networks are likely to play an important role in empowering the transition from scheme participation to long-term exercise maintenance
- Assisting the participants in refining their own long-term maintenance strategies is important due to the high levels of individual variation.
- Future recommendations for exercise referral services include 1) embedding theory-based interventions, 2) incorporating the COM-B model into such interventions and 3) providing longitudinal follow-up for greater understanding.

Study tasks

1. Which popular theory has been used to explain motivation in exercise settings?
2. What is the distinction between intrinsic and extrinsic motivation?
3. What do future interventions grounded in self-determination need to elicit for greater intervention effectiveness?
4. Identify and describe the three profiles of exercise referral participants outlined by the work of Kinnafick and colleagues on longer-term exercise maintenance.
5. Identify and describe the key factors of the COM-B model.
6. How could exercise referral schemes facilitate enablement strategies to enhance long-term behaviour change?
7. Describe the exit strategies that could take place to facilitate long-term exercise engagement.
8. Outline what needs to be done to advance exercise referral schemes with respect to long-term behavioural change.

References

Abraham, C., & Michie, S. (2008). A taxonomy of behaviour change techniques used in interventions. *Health Psychology*, *27*(3), 379–387.

Deci, E. L., & Ryan, R. M. (1985). *Intrinsic motivation and self-determination in human behaviour*. New York: Plenum.

Deci, E. L., & Ryan, R. M. (2000). The "what" and "why" of goal pursuits: Human needs and the self-determination of behavior. *Psychological Inquiry*, *11*, 227–268.

Duda, J. L., Williams, G. C., Ntoumanis, N., Daley, A., Eves, F. F., Mutrie, N., . . . Jolly, K. (2014). Effects of a standard provision versus an autonomy supportive exercise referral programme on physical activity, quality of life and well-being indicators: A cluster randomised controlled trial. *International Journal of Behavioral Nutrition and Physical Activity*, *11*, 10.

Edmunds, J., Ntoumanis, N., & Duda, J. L. (2007). Adherence and well-being in overweight and obese patients referred to an exercise on prescription scheme: A self-determination theory perspective. *Psychology of Sport and Exercise*, *8*, 722–740. doi:10.1016/j.psychsport.2006.07.006.

Eynon, M. J., Foad, J., Downey, J., Bowmer, Y., & Mills, H. (2019). Assessing the psychosocial factors associated with adherence to exercise referral schemes: A systematic review. *Scandinavian Journal of Medicine & Science in Sports*, *29*(5), 638–650. doi/abs/10.1111/sms.13403.

Eynon, M. J., O'Donnell, C., & Williams, L. (2017). Assessing the impact of autonomous motivation and psychological need satisfaction in explaining adherence to an exercise referral scheme. *Psychology, Health & Medicine*, *22*(9), 1056–1062. doi:10.1080/13548506.2016.1274041.

Greaves, C. J., Sheppard, K. E, Abraham, C., et al. (2011). Systematic review of reviews of intervention components associated with increased effectiveness in dietary and physical activity interventions. *BMC Public Health*, *11*, 119.

Hobbs, L. J., Campbell, R., Hildon, Z., & Michie, S. (2011). Behaviour change theories across psychology, sociology, anthropology and economics: A systematic review. *Psychology and Health*, *26*(Suppl. 1), 31.

Hutchison, A. J., & Johnston, L. H. (2013). Exploring the potential of case formulation within exercise psychology. *Journal of Clinical Sports Psychology*, *7*, 60–76.

Kinnafick, F. E., Thøgersen-Ntoumani, C., & Duda, J. L. (2014). Physical activity adoption to adherence, lapse, and dropout: A self-determination theory perspective. *Qualitative Health Research*, *24*(5), 706–718. doi:10.1177/1049732314528811.

Kwasnicka, D., Dombrowski, S. U., White, M., & Sniehotta, F. (2016). Theoretical explanations for maintenance of behaviour change: A systematic review of behaviour theories. *Health Psychology Review*, *10*(3), 277–296. doi:10.1080/17437199.2016.1151372.

Markland, D., & Tobin, V. J. (2010). Need support and behavioural regulations for exercise among exercise referral scheme clients: The mediating role of psychological need satisfaction. *Psychology of Sport and Exercise, 11*, 91–99. doi:10.1016/j.psychsport.2009.07.001

McEwan, D., Harden, S. M., Zumbo, B. D., et al. (2016). The effectiveness of multi-component goal setting interventions for changing physical activity behaviour: A systematic review and meta-analysis. *Health Psychology Review, 10*(1). https://doi.org/10.1080/17437199.2015.1104258

Michie, S., Atkins, L., & West, R. (2014). *The behaviour change wheel: A guide to designing interventions*. Surrey, UK: Silverback Publishing.

Michie, S., van Stralen, M. M., & West, R. (2011). The behaviour change wheel: A new method for characterising and designing behaviour change interventions. *Implementation Science, 6*, 42. www.implemetationscience.com/contents/6/1/42.

Michie, S., & West, R. (2013). Behaviour change theory and evidence: A presentation to Government. *Health Psychology Review*, 7(1), 1–22. doi:10.1080/17437199.2011.649445.

Middleton, K. R., Anton, S. D., & Perri, M. G. (2013). Long term adherence to health behaviour change. *American Journal of Lifestyle Medicine*, 7(6), 395–404. doi:10.1177/1559827613488867.

Mills, H., Crone, D., James, D. V. B., & Johnston, L. H. (2012). Exploring the perceptions of success in an exercise referral scheme: A mixed method investigation. *Evaluation Review, 36*(6), 407–429.

Moore, G. F., Moore, L., & Murphy, S. (2011). Facilitating adherence to physical activity: Exercise professionals' experiences of the National Exercise Referral Scheme in Wales. A qualitative study. *BMC Public Health, 11*, 935.

Morgan, F., Battersby, A., Weightman, A. L., Searchfield, L., Turley, R., Morgan, H., . . . Ellis, S. (2016). Adherence to exercise referral schemes by participants – what do providers and commissioners need to know? A systematic review of barriers and facilitators. *BMC Public Health, 16*, 227. doi:10.1186/s12889-016-2882-7.

National Institute for Health and Care Excellence [NICE]. (2014). *Behaviour change: Individual approaches*. www.nice.org.uk/guidance/ph49.

Prochaska, J., & DiClemente, C. (1983). Stages and processes of self-change in smoking: Toward an integrative model of change. *Journal of Consulting and Clinical Psychology, 5*, 390–395.

Rodgers, W. M., Hall, C. R., Duncan, L. R., Pearson, E., & Milne, M. I. (2010). Becoming a regular exerciser: Examining change in behavioural regulations among exercise initiates. *Psychology of Sport and Exercise, 11*, 378–386.

Ryan, R. M., Patrick, H., Deci, L., & Williams, G. C. (2008). Facilitating health behaviour change and its maintenance: Interventions based on self-determination theory. *The European Health Psychologist, 10*, 2–4.

Sabiston, C. M., McDonough, M. H., Sedgwick, W. A., & Crocker, P. R. (2009). Muscle gains and emotional strains: Conflicting experiences of change among overweight women participating in an exercise intervention program. *Qualitative Health Research, 19*(4), 466–480. doi:10.1177/1049732309332782.

Stonehouse, D. P. (2018). How SMART are your patient goals? *British Journal of Healthcare Assistants, 12*(5), 233–235.

Van Stralen, M. M., De Fries, H. D., Mudde, A. N., Bolman, C., & Lechner, L. (2009). Determinants of initiation and maintenance of physical activity among older adults: A literature review. *Health Psychology Review, 3*(2), 147–207.

9

HEALTH COMPLEXITY

Integrating Psychological Skills into Exercise Referral

Charlotte Hilton and Lynne Johnston

Chapter Aims

The aims of this chapter are to:

- Demonstrate the complexity of the interplay between mental and physical illness
- Explore important considerations for the assessment and treatment of illness
- Demonstrate how three psychological approaches – motivational interviewing (MI), formulation and behavioural activation (BA) – can appreciate disease complexity, personalise the exercise referral experience, work from a person-centred perspective and facilitate behaviour change
- Provide practical and feasible examples of how MI, formulation and BA may be utilised in exercise referral schemes (ERS)
- Highlight contemporary issues regarding the complexity of disease within the context of current UK health-care systems and how this impacts ERS

Introduction

The purpose of this chapter is to highlight the disease complexity associated with working in ERS and demonstrate the importance of the personalisation of the exercise referral experience for individual clients. Such clients are commonly referred for exercise for long-term conditions: for example, hypertension, hypercholesterolaemia, impaired glucose tolerance, asthma, arthritis or mental ill health. However, no two people is the same, and therefore a one-size-fits-all approach should be avoided. In this chapter, we describe the complexity and interplay of mental and physical health and demonstrate how a bio-psycho-social approach to understanding health and illness can help address this complexity. Specifically, we make explicit the important distinction between the use of exercise for symptom management and the treatment of underlying causes per se. We also present some practical psychological skills (MI, formulation and BA) to support exercise professionals to contribute to adequately addressing the complex interplay between bio-psych-social causal factors and the presenting

DOI: 10.4324/9781315102399-9

symptoms of illness. With the use of a case study and additional practical learning activities, we demonstrate how health and exercise practitioners might integrate these approaches into routine clinical practice. We argue that the adoption of a bio-psycho-social-driven approach to treatment planning can help exercise professionals more fully integrate the use of exercise as a legitimate symptom treatment option for health improvement.

Treating the Person, Not the Reason for Referral

It is commonly accepted that mental and physical health are intricately inter-related (e.g. British Psychological Society (BPS), 2008; Qin et al., 2014; Rollins et al., 2017). However, reducing this to a simplistic cause-and-effect relationship (i.e. whether it is the mental or physical aspects of health that are causing or maintaining the mental/physical health symptoms) is not helpful when working with clients who have been referred for exercise with long-term, often co-morbid health conditions. For example, the link between psychological stress and physical illness symptoms such as gastrointestinal upsets, dermatitis and hypertension has been widely recognised for many years (e.g. Morgan & Glodston, 1987). Within the area of weight management and diabetes prevention, there is increasing evidence to support the bi-directional relationship between obesity and mental health conditions (e.g. binge eating disorder, major depressive disorder, social anxiety), with an increasing recognition that explanatory models implicate and include a range of biological, social and psychological factors (e.g. National Obesity Observatory, 2011; Johnston et al., 2017b). On this basis, it is more clinically effective to adopt an individualised conceptualisation of an individual's needs, strengths and motivations than one that is more generically defined or one which is reduced to a simplistic cause-and-effect relationship along one dimension (see Hutchinson & Johnston, 2013).

Typical Referrals to Exercise Referral Schemes

The vast majority of patients will be referred with physical and psychological co-morbidities. Thus, the primary reason for referral may be a reflection of a judgement by the referring health-care practitioner rather than the main medical condition per se. Additionally, the commissioning arrangements for a specific service are likely to influence the conditions that are accepted into an ERS (e.g. not accepting 'obesity' as a single reason for referral). With respect to obesity (body mass index (BMI) 40+), within Tier 3 and 4 specialist weight management and bariatric services, the clinical reality is that the majority of those referred to see the clinical (health) psychologist have a long history of underlying (unresolved/undiagnosed) psychological causal factors such as loss, trauma and attachment issues. Unsurprisingly, we know from Tier 2 ERS evaluations that those referred with a diagnosis of obesity/mental health conditions are less likely to complete a referral programme (James et al., 2008). We would strongly suggest that this is often because the obesity/depression/anxiety is a symptomatic consequence of the undiagnosed/untreated loss, trauma and attachment issues. Often at the point of the original referral, these unresolved causal factors can leave the person feeling very low in self-worth/self-care. Commonly, they state that they feel unable to prioritise their own needs over the needs of those around them. Consequently, these clients can find themselves caught up in vicious cycles of dysregulation around lifestyle behaviours (e.g. sleep, eating, activity patterns), which can have a negative co-maintaining impact on the presenting symptoms such as obesity, diabetes and depression. (See Johnston et al., 2017b for more details.)

Given that the majority of people who present with long-term physical health symptoms also present with co-morbid mental health symptoms (e.g. depression and/or anxiety disorder), we must appreciate that individuals referred into a scheme are, in reality, presenting with a complex co-morbid mix of physical and psychological symptoms, such as anxiety and depression. In an evaluation of a multi-site ERS, of the total number referred (N = 278), 33 were specifically referred for depression, with the remainder being referred for physical health conditions: e.g. diabetes (N = 116), obesity (N = 66) (Hilton et al., 2015). Consequently, exercise referral professionals are working with individuals who present with complex disease aetiology. More appropriate stratification of exercise needs and preferences at the point of referral was highlighted as a key recommendation from our earlier work in this area. (See James, et al., 2008, 2009.)

Figure 9.1 provides a simplified visual demonstration of some of the underlying psychological causal factors that could contribute to the experience of symptoms with which an individual is referred into exercise. Typically, it is these symptoms only that are being

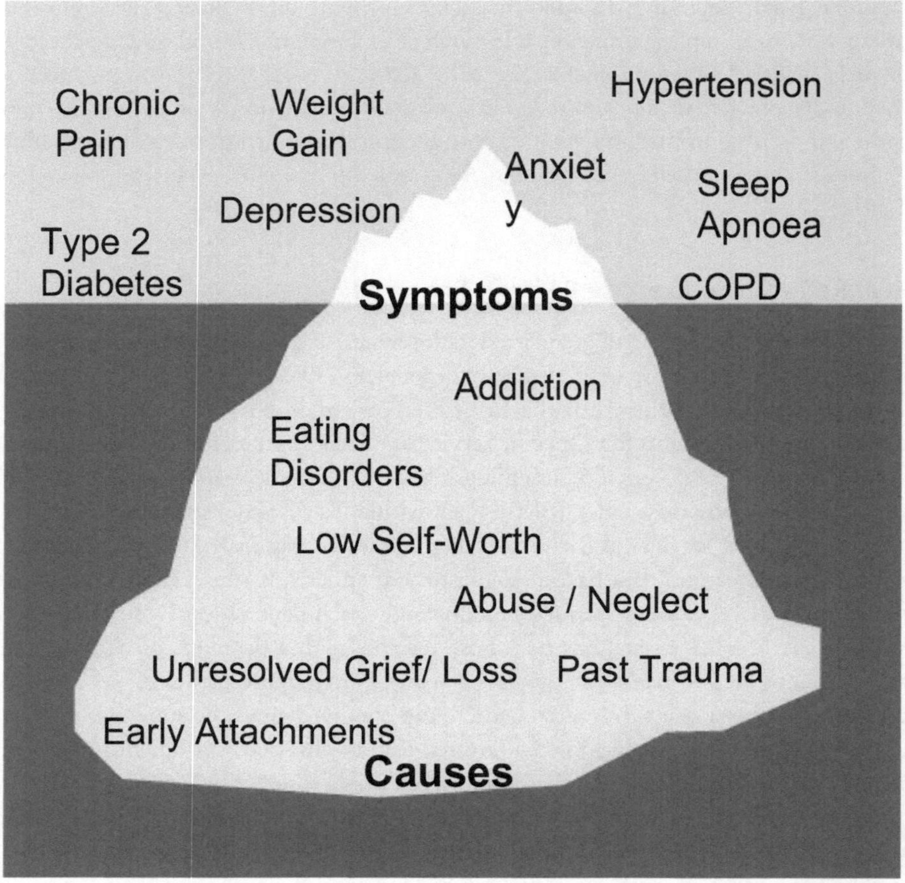

FIGURE 9.1 Symptoms as the Tip of the Iceberg: The Interplay of Causal Factors and Symptoms

addressed within an ERS. Without adjunct psychological treatment, the underlying causal and maintaining factors remain untreated. A further complication is that without adequate psychological assessment and formulation, it is often difficult to disentangle causal and effect factors. Figure 9.1 demonstrates how certain mood states such as anxiety and depression can often be seen as a symptom of various underlying causal factors or they may be a maintaining causal symptom.

Within a clinical exercise psychology context, adequately assessing causal and maintaining factors that contribute to the experience of ill-health symptoms is essential (Hutchinson & Johnston, 2013; Johnston & Hutchinson, 2016; Johnston et al., 2011, 2017b). Specifically, a 5Ps approach to case formulation has been recommended, and the interested reader should review Hutchinson and Johnston (2013), Johnston et al. (2017a), Johnston and Hutchison (2016), Johnston et al. (2011, 2017b) and Johnstone and Dallos (2013) for a more in-depth understanding of this approach. However, in brief, this involves understanding the person's **p**resenting difficulty in relation to their **p**ast life history, the bio-psycho-social factors that **p**recipitated the difficulty (triggering events) and the factors that **p**erpetuate (or maintain) it, as well as any factors that **p**rotect the patient from further deterioration (Johnston & Hutchison, 2016). We will return to case formulation later in the chapter when we present a client case study to exemplify the method.

Understanding the complexity of disease in this way demonstrates how the current provision of ERS is limited to symptom management. Arguably, within the context and service structure of the current provision, ERS are supporting those referred with behavioural activation (BA) (e.g. activity scheduling and reducing avoidant/maladaptive coping behaviours) and mood regulation. We will address BA in more detail later. However, whilst this is a valuable contribution to a more integrated and holistic approach to care, delivered in isolation, this approach is incapable of treating the complexity of multiple morbidity outlined earlier. Theoretical understandings and empirical studies that explore the relationship between exercise and mental health also demonstrate that thus far, exercise and PA have been utilised for the treatment of the symptoms of mental ill health rather than the underlying causes and maintaining factors. However, many authors fail to make this explicit, and the literature has yet to clearly make the distinction between treatment and symptom management. This perpetuates the confusion and lack of clarity regarding the role of exercise for the 'treatment' of mental health disorders (e.g. Dunn et al., 2005).

Important Considerations for the Assessment and Treatment of Referred Conditions

A common approach to the assessment and treatment of both mental and physical illness is known as the medical model (Laing, 1971). Diagnostic assessment tools (e.g. DSM-V, ICD-10) have evolved within this paradigm. Traditionally, this approach assumes that the cause of mental illness is in some way a deficit which may be treated by addressing the specific deficit in question. (Historically, this was viewed as a physical or medical cause.) This is problematic from a strength-based perspective because the implicit message is that the person needs a specific and externally 'prescribed treatment' to address their deficit. When the aforementioned course of prescribed treatment is completed, then the person no longer requires their prescribed medication. Clarke and Eves (1997) exemplified this in an early study when ERS were commonly referred to as 'exercise on prescription'. Part of their scheme evaluation revealed that one 'patient' equated their participation in the programme to a medication prescription. They did not even consider the value in continuing with their exercise because they associated the prescription with completing a course of medication (i.e. without the need to continue as they had not received a repeat prescription). Setting up an ERS within this type of paradigm may have serious unintended consequences with respect to the longer-term impact of the successful maintenance of PA. For example, the emphasis on treatment rather than prevention and the impact of a limited period of reduced fee/free leisure service use (extrinsic reward) upon intrinsic (or internal and personal) motivation challenges long-term PA behaviour change (also see Chapter 8). It has also been previously recognised that ERS fail to account for people's underlying value priorities and that, whilst ERS may recognise behavioural beliefs and attitudes as important determinants of change, there must also be some degree of congruence between those beliefs and a person's more enduring underlying values or priorities (see Chapter 5; Hutchison et al., 2012). Therefore, ERS should be seen as an important part of the PA journey rather than a sole prescription for the 'cure'. This further demonstrates the importance of conducting an enhanced individualised assessment in a manner that includes the client as an active participant in the collaborative assessment and formulation process.

Unless this collaborative process occurs, the medical model and disease classification approach to the assessment and treatment of referred conditions risks employing a reductionist approach to providing exercise to manage the symptoms rather than the underlying causes. The complex combination of relevant biological, psychological and social factors related to the experience of illness are often ignored within a medical model paradigm. The implications of this in terms of 'prescribing' an improved diet and increased physical activity for individuals with obesity has recently been recognised because doing so without a better understanding of the complex (often psychologically driven) causal and co-maintaining factors of obesity reflects a limited one-size-fits-all approach to treatment, which is ineffective for treating the person appropriately and holistically (Johnston et al., 2017b).

Rather than a medical model (deficit treatment) approach, the interplay between physical health and mental health are better reflected by a bio-psycho-social approach to understanding health and illness (Andrasik et al., 2015; Suls & Rothman, 2004). This offers a broader and more inclusive paradigm than the medical model. As the title would suggest, health and disease are understood by considering the dynamic interaction of biological (e.g. genetic and biochemical), psychological (e.g. beliefs, emotional responses, behavioural coping repertoires, attachment styles etc.) and social (e.g. cultural, familial and socioeconomic) factors. It is from this perspective that we present a description of ways in which the exercise referral experience may be personalised and that the all-important interplay and complexity of the relationship between mental and physical health may be better addressed by facilitators. The 'how to' of bio-psycho-social assessment and treatment of illness is perhaps best demonstrated by various counselling approaches. Indeed, there has been a growth in interest in transferring the learning from behaviour change counselling (e.g. MI) to clinical exercise settings. It is in recognition of this and the utility of psychological approaches/skills to address the disease complexity that we have explored thus far that we present three relevant perspectives – person centred/MI, formulation and BA – from a practical perspective for exercise referral.

The Person-Centred Approach and Motivational Interviewing

It is *how* we communicate with clients that is of critical importance (Hilton & Johnston, 2017). Communicating in a manner that demonstrates warmth, empathy, acceptance and trust (often termed therapeutic alliance) has consistently been demonstrated to contribute to favourable outcomes for clients (e.g. Martin et al., 2000; Moyers, 2014). The work of Carl Rogers is commonly associated with a person- (or client-) centred approach. The core values that underpin person centredness are empathy, congruence (warmth and genuineness) and unconditional positive regard (acceptance) (Rogers, 1980). A person-centred approach is often associated with the interpersonal processes between the client and practitioner. There is a greater emphasis on how the practitioner engages with the client than on what specific techniques are used. In therapeutic/behaviour change terms, one person-centred approach that has been utilised across a range of behaviour change settings, including PA and exercise referral, is MI.

MI is a behaviour change counselling method that originated from the field of addictions in the early 1980s. MI builds on the relational components and core values of Carl Rogers, yet MI also has a directional aspect (i.e. to guide the person towards change). One of the key aims of MI is to help an individual resolve their feelings of ambivalence regarding a change in behaviour, attitude or belief. Since its conception, there have been several definitions of MI proposed. However, the originators have most recently defined the approach as 'a collaborative conversation style for strengthening a person's own motivation and commitment to change' (Miller & Rollinick, 2012, p. 12). We have provided detailed accounts of the specific skills associated with MI elsewhere (e.g. Johnston et al., 2017a). We have also provided a critique of some of the more recent developments of the method and approaches to supporting practitioners to develop proficiency, skill assessment and treatment fidelity (Hilton et al., 2016), as well as recommendations for training (Hilton & Johnston, 2017). Of great importance is attention to avoiding an over-reliance on the skills at the expense of how the skills are integrated into a conversation with a client. Ensuring that practitioners maintain acceptance, collaboration and compassion and respect a client's autonomy is considered critical to MI, and these conditions are referred to as the *spirit* of MI (Miller & Rollinick, 2012).

The structure of an MI-consistent conversation is conceptualised by four processes: 1) engaging, 2) focusing, 3) evoking and 4) planning. These processes tend to overlap, and rather than a series of stages that are worked through systematically, it is more useful to consider what the relative emphasis is on each of the processes at a given time within the consult. Figure 9.2 provides a visual representation of the four MI processes.

Central to the MI approach is the importance of working with a client's ambivalence about change. A MI approach would typically encourage the client to consider the relative advantages and disadvantages of change behaviour. For example, there may be aspects to smoking that a client perceives as beneficial and may enjoy whilst also recognising that smoking is detrimental to their health. The process of exploring this ambivalence is referred to as the decisional balance, and the practitioner will skilfully support the client to explore the discrepancy between the current health-reducing behaviour(s) and future goals for health improvement. Crucially, the practitioner will elicit the person's underpinning value/belief system and help them recognise how and why certain behaviours are consistent/inconsistent with this. Typically, this will support the client to increase their motivation to change and thereby resolve their internalised ambivalence. During this process, the client may provide reasons not to change (sustain talk) or examples of change talk. Change talk is integral to MI and refers to any statements a client may make that suggests they have the desire, ability, reasons and/or need to change their behaviour. For example, you may hear a client say, 'I really want to get my diabetes under better control, and I'm going to exercise'. Table 9.1 presents a visual representation of the decisional balance appropriate to PA/exercise. Examples of sustain and change talk that might be heard are also provided.

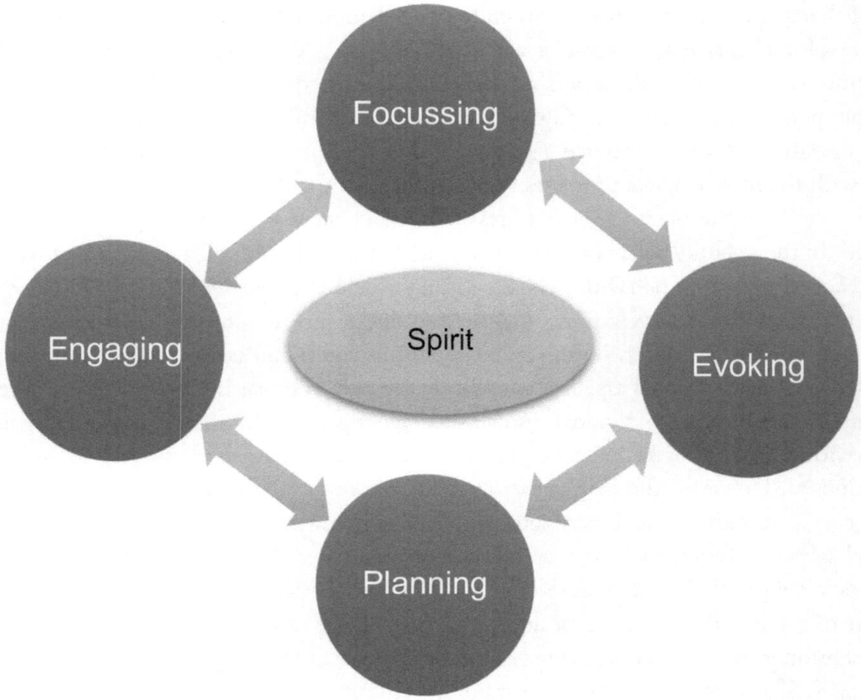

FIGURE 9.2 The Four Processes of Motivational Interviewing

TABLE 9.1 Motivational Interviewing Decisional Balance

	Advantages	*Disadvantages*
Change	Improve my fitness Increase my confidence Improve my breathing May socialise more Make my family proud Make new friends Time for myself **Example of change talk:** 'I know that I need to get more active. I want to; I do think that I would feel much better'.	Lack of time Fear of failure Fear of unknown Potential embarrassment Lots of effort needed Potential cost **Example of sustain talk:** I'm not sure I have enough time to be more active, and I don't really know what exercises to do. I've never really been a sporty person'.
No Change	More free time No worry about failing No worry about pain I might feel while exercising Don't have to give up my TV viewing in the evening Don't have to spend money on gym membership/activity clothing/footwear **Example of sustain talk:** 'I'm worried that being more active will be painful for me because my joints often hurt'.	Health conditions could worsen Gain more weight Disappoint my family Worried about what my GP will say Be a burden on others as I get older **Example of change talk:** 'If I don't become more active, then I'm worried that my health could deteriorate, and I'll just be even more of a burden on my family'.

MI also includes some important terminology. The acronym OARS referrers to the use of **o**pen questions, **a**ffirmations, **r**eflective listening and **s**ummaries. Reflections/reflective listening is a method of checking that the practitioner has understood the client accurately; they invite the client to elaborate and demonstrate empathic listening. They range from a simple repetition of things that the client may have said to more complex reflections of the emotion and underpinning meaning behind the client's words. Box 9.1 provides some examples.

BOX 9.1 EXAMPLES OF REFLECTIVE LISTENING

Client: 'My weight has been a problem for a long time now; it's affecting my health, and I'm worried'.

Simple reflection response: **'You're concerned'.**

Complex reflection: **'This has now got to a point where things need to change'.**

OR

'You're concerned about the impact of your weight on your health and what that may mean for you in the future'.

The righting reflex refers to the desire to 'fix a problem'. Within an MI-consistent conversation, this should be avoided. Similarly, if it is felt that a person would benefit from being provided with some information, we always ask permission. A useful strategy to avoid assuming that information is needed/wanted/relevant is elicit, provide, elicit (EPE). Firstly, elicit permission by asking if the client agrees to talk about something you feel might be helpful to them, then provide the information in a neutral way. For example, you might suggest that 'some people find it helpful if . . .', then always ask the client how the information you have provided is relevant to them or something that allows the client to personalise the information you have shared with them.

There are additional useful strategies that help the practitioner better understand the client's specific circumstances and to enhance engagement. For example, a typical-day strategy invites a client to describe their day but with a focus on the change behaviour (e.g. physical activity [PA]). Also, agenda setting can help avoid prematurely focusing on an area of importance that the practitioner may deem important for the client, rather than inviting the client to determine the focus of the conversation. For example, you may describe some of the common topics of conversation to a client (e.g. exercise, PA, weight management, blood sugars) and invite the client to choose which of those they would like to focus on or if there is something else that is more important to them. It may also be useful to assess a client's perceived readiness to change behaviour using scaling questions. Within an MI context, a person's perception of readiness to change is best understood by an assessment of their perceived 1) importance and 2) confidence to make behaviour changes. A person's perception of their importance and confidence to change behaviour are key indicators of readiness to change, and there is a direct relationship between the two. Therefore, we ask both scaling questions so that we can assess perceived readiness. Box 9.2 provides examples of how these scaling questions may be asked and some follow-up questions the practitioner may ask to elicit further change talk.

BOX 9.2 EXAMPLE SCALING QUESTIONS

Practitioner: On a scale of 1 to 10, with 1 being not at all important and 10 being extremely important, how important is it to you to become more active?

Client: Perhaps about a 5.

Practitioner: Why a 5 and not a lower number, say a 1 or 2? (This response invites the client to justify and elaborate on their answer, which can often result in further change talk.)

Practitioner: On a scale of 1 to 10, with 1 being not at all confident and 10 being extremely confident, how confident are you that you can become more active?

Client: Perhaps about a 3/

Practitioner: What would help you move the 3 up to a 3.5? (This response invites the client to imagine factors that may make them increase their confidence and elaborate on their answer, which can often result in further change talk.)

Change talk is an important aspect of MI. The acronym DARN-CAT is often used to help identify client language that may indicate their **d**esire, **a**bility, **r**eason and **N**eed to change behaviour and whether there are any signs of **c**ommitment to change or indications of behaviour change **a**ctivation or if the client is already **t**aking steps to change. The acronym EARS is used to identify how the practitioner might respond to change talk with the intention of strengthening a client's commitment to change. Responses might include invitations for **e**laboration, providing **a**ffirmations, **r**eflective listening and **s**ummaries in response to any change talk that they may hear.

Developing Proficiency in Motivational Interviewing

The quality and duration of MI training and opportunities for skill development via ongoing coaching, for example, are important considerations for supporting people to develop proficiency in MI. An initial three-day programme of training appears to be sufficient as an introduction to the method (Miller & Moyers, 2006). However, as experienced trainers and long-established members of the international network of MI trainers (MINT), we would always recommend opportunities for follow-up supervision and support to develop skills through both qualitative (see Hilton et al., 2016) and quantitative (e.g. the Motivational Treatment Integrity Scale [MITI]) (Moyers et al., 2015) assessment and feedback. A list of trainers who are members of the Motivational Interviewing Network of Trainers (MINT) can be found here: www.motivationalinterviewing.org. Trainers who are members of MINT have had to demonstrate a competent level of proficiency and understanding of the method and have attended a Training New Trainers (TNT) event facilitated by MINT members in order to be listed as a trainer by MINT.

Box 9.3 details a useful activity that is intended to help exercise professionals consider how they might integrate MI into a routine conversation with a client. In response to each of the questions, try to identify the MI skills that are most appropriate. Some suggestions are provided.

BOX 9.3 MOTIVATIONAL INTERVIEWING SKILLS ACTIVITY

Activity: Consider the information you might commonly see included in an exercise referral form or think of a client you may have worked with recently. Ask yourself the following:

1. How could you start the conversation with the client in an MI-consistent way?
Thank the client for coming to the appointment (affirmation). Avoid checking the details of the referral form or suggesting that they have attended for help with the conditions provided on the form. Instead try asking 'What brings you here today?' or something similar (open question).

2. What open questions might you ask to elicit details from the client regarding their experience of illness and how it affects them?
Introduce a range of questions that start with 'what', 'when', 'why', 'where' or 'how'. For example, you may ask, 'Tell me about how the breathlessness affects you'.

3. How would you demonstrate to the client that you are listening carefully, check that you have understood them accurately and invite them to elaborate on important things that they have said?
Ensure that you listen reflectively throughout the conversation. Regularly repeat back to the client information they have provided to you. Ensure that you integrate both complex and simple reflections into your conversation. Try to couple your reflections with an open question. For example: Client: 'I'd like to lose weight'. Practitioner: 'Lose weight' (simple reflection). 'Why is that important to you?' (open question).

4. How might you assess how ready the client is to change their exercise behaviour?
Ensuring that you introduce plenty of open questions and reflections into your consultation should help you establish client readiness. However, the importance and confidence scaling questions may also be useful.

5. If you felt that the client would benefit from some information about the benefits of physical activity and/or exercise, how would you share this with them in an MI-consistent way?
Always ask permission before providing information. (See EPE strategy.)

6. How might you end the conversation in an MI-consistent way?
Summarise the consultation, ensuring that you include any change talk you may have heard, and invite the client to confirm the accuracy of what has been presented to them and elaborate further. Ask if there is anything important to them that you haven't had the opportunity to discuss yet or that you may have missed.

Case Formulation

Case formulation – often simply referred to as formulation – involves a process between the client and the practitioner of mutually generating and exploring plausible explanations for the problems experienced (Johnston & Hutchison, 2016). As mentioned earlier, one approach to formulation is described as the 5 Ps. Whilst it has not been recognised within the MI literature as yet, arguably, when we are 'focusing' in MI, we are very much formulating in this regard. To help demonstrate how we would formulate in an ERS context, we present a case study of a female who has been referred for exercise. The case study is detailed to reflect the disease complexity that we have highlighted throughout this chapter and to exemplify the level of detail that may have been generated because of an MI-consistent consultation. Read the case study carefully:

Case Study

Sonya is a 42-year-old recently divorced woman. Her husband left her three years ago to begin a new life with a younger woman; he now has a young daughter aged 2 years. Sonya has two sons (18 and 13 years). Her elder son left home three months ago to attend university. Her younger son spends the vast majority of his (non-school) waking hours 'gaming' or socialising with friends. Sonya has worked as a secretary in a local law firm for the last 20 years.

Sonya has always struggled to maintain a healthy weight and has a history of attempting various diets and commercial weight loss programmes in an effort to maintain weight loss. She recalls her mother having a history of 'yo-yo dieting' and remembers her own first 'proper diet' at the age of 12 years. Dieting has resulted in her weight fluctuating throughout her life, and weight gain has followed each failed diet. Sonya has internalised the failed diets as part of her and views many aspects of her life as a 'failure'. She is highly self-critical and adopts an 'all or nothing' approach to her eating/activity patterns, and over the years, this has gradually led her to believe that she is 'not worth much'.

Over the last three years in particular, Sonya has gradually become more and more socially avoidant. Her husband's 'rejection and betrayal' has hurt her deeply. She worried that their mutual friends would judge her for being 'not good enough to keep him' and/or feel pity for her and reinforce her anger towards him. It felt easier to avoid, and as time has gone on, it has become more difficult to reconnect. Many of their mutual friends have continued to socialise with her ex-husband and his new wife. Her children are becoming increasingly independent, and this has left her more and more lonely, socially isolated and feeling that she is 'surplus to requirements'. Her mother lives locally but is starting to become somewhat frail, and Sonya is worried about her memory problems and a couple of recent falls. She does not speak with her brother (who lives abroad) due to a long-standing family feud which occurred over her father's funeral arrangements.

Sonya is aware of her low mood and knows she 'should' make the effort to socialise, but she just feels nobody would want to spend any time with her because she is 'so boring'. Her body mass index (BMI) is 43.9 $kg \cdot m^{-2}$, and she has just been advised by her GP that she has 'borderline' type 2 diabetes. This has made her even more upset as her maternal grandmother had diabetes, and she is aware of the various complications that her grandmother experienced before she died.

Sonya enjoyed playing netball during her senior school years but has never considered herself an active or 'sporty' person. The thought of attending a leisure centre or community group-based exercise is extremely daunting to her. Consequently, Sonya has never attempted to increase her physical activity via the means of structured exercise. Her concerns about attending a structured exercise programme are further aggravated by her social anxiety and low mood, for which she has been prescribed medication (Citalopram 20 mg daily). Sonya describes herself as someone who has always been lacking in confidence. However, since the breakdown of her marriage and subsequent divorce (12 months ago), she has noticed a steady decline in her mood and an increase in her anxiety levels. She has gained 10 kg in the last three years and, other than her secretarial work, has now withdrawn socially almost completely. Sonya describes a feeling of loss, redundancy and helplessness. She reports that she has a very low opinion of herself, but she is keen to try to improve her mental and physical health.

Complete the study task that follows described in Box 9.4.

BOX 9.4 FORMULATION STUDY TASK

Study task: Use the blank copy of the formulation diagram in Figure 9.3 to identify what Sonya's presenting difficulties are, relevant past life history, the bio-psycho-social factors that precipitated the difficulties (triggering events), the factors that perpetuate (or maintain) them and any factors that protect the Sonya from further deterioration.

Figure 9.4 presents a populated formulation diagram with some exemplar answers.

Whilst formulation is a useful approach to integrate with the focusing process of MI, BA is ideally suited to help the client and practitioner in the planning process of MI. Formulating as a method of focusing the consultation avoids a premature focus (termed the premature focus trap in MI) on an aspect of a client's life that the practitioner may deem key to behaviour change without fully exploring all the factors (e.g. 5 Ps) that contribute to a person's current PA/exercise behaviour. Similarly, behaviour therapy (BT) and BA are particularly pertinent to exercise referral and PA behaviour change because the approach supports the identification and appropriate planning of activities that are likely to contribute to the reduction of

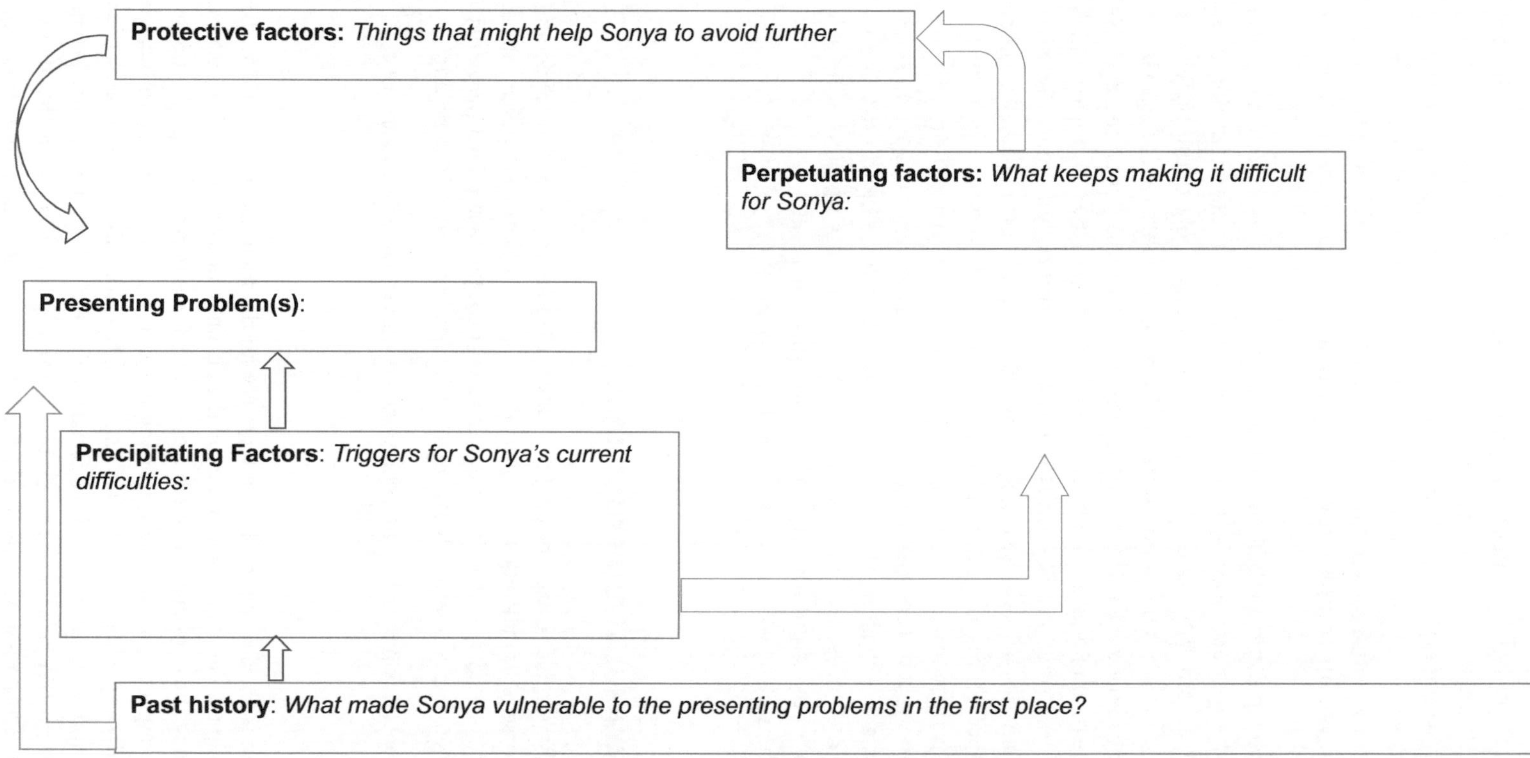

FIGURE 9.3 Blank Formulation Diagram for Sonya Case Study

Source: Adapted from Johnston L. H., Hilton, C. E., & Lane, C. (2017). Psychological management in bariatric surgery. In Weaver (Ed.), Practical guide to obesity medicine. London: Elsevier.

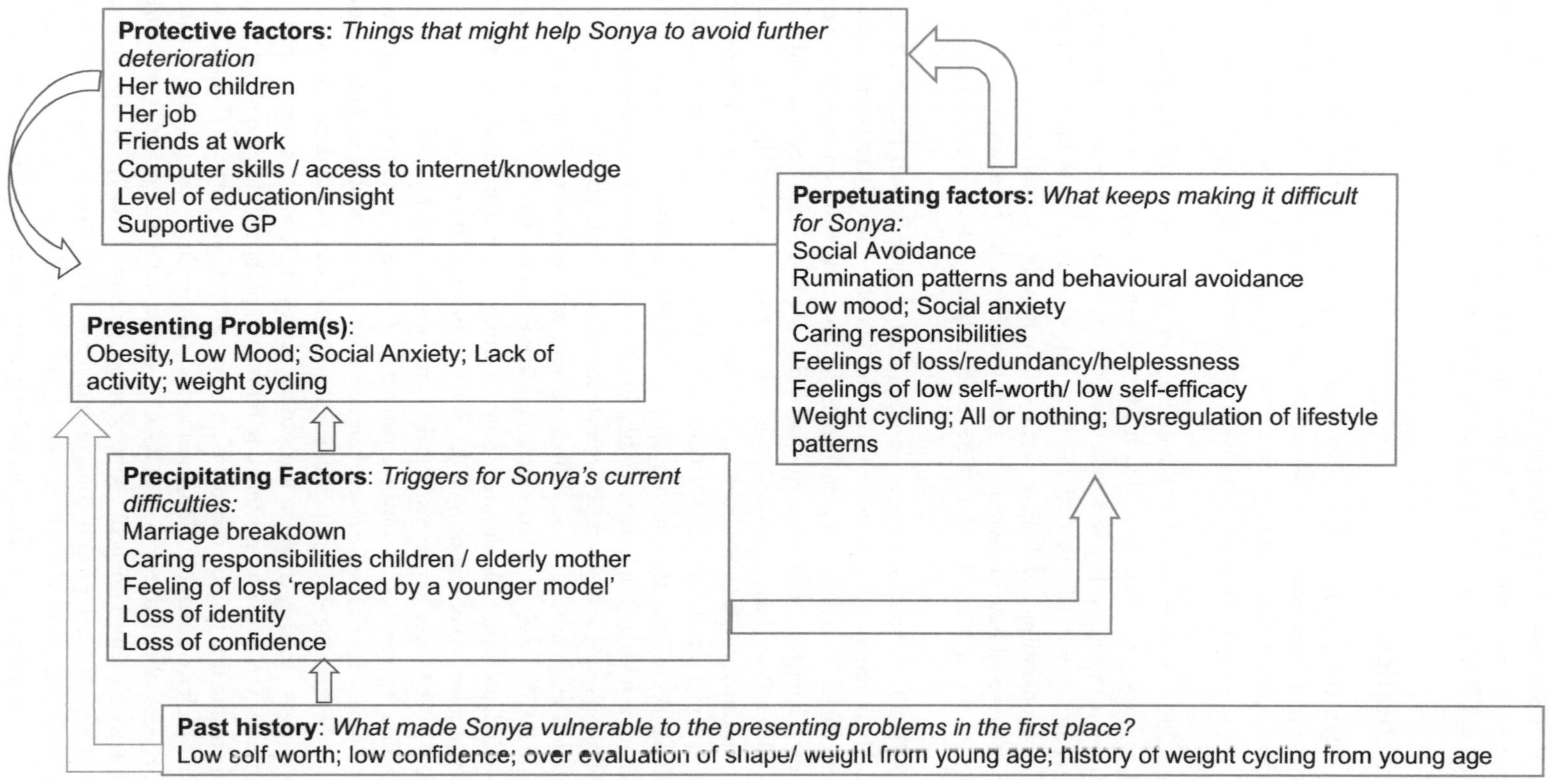

FIGURE 9.4 Populated Formulation Diagram for Sonya Case Study

Source: Adapted from Johnston L. H., Hilton, C. E., & Lane, C. (2017). Psychological management in bariatric surgery. In Weaver (Ed.), Practical guide to obesity medicine. London: Elsevier.

unhealthy behaviour patterns. What follows is a summary of the key aspects of BT and BA with a specific focus on the treatment of major depressive disorder (MDD) as a common reason for referral to ERS. We also identify how BA fits with the planning process of MI.

Behavioural Activation

Contextualism views the person-environment relationship as one rather than something residing within the individual (e.g. thoughts, beliefs, inner conflicts) (Jacobson, 2001). This contrasts with the cognitive approach (e.g. Beck et al., 1979), which views the environment as a contextual influence which shapes an individual's perceptions and beliefs (see Martell et al., 2001, p. 15).

Martell et al. (2001) describe five key assumptions in their conceptualisation of BA for depression: not to view depression as a 'deficit'; to view depression as an 'understandable' response to context; to work on behavioural changes to help develop new 'behaviour-context interactions'; and to view the practitioner as an 'expert coach, consultant and personal trainer'. In BA, the practitioner and client work collaboratively to scrutinise behaviours in their context to understand how behavioural avoidance patterns have become reinforcing via a depression loop (Addis & Martell, 2004). Clients are helped to develop alternative ways of responding.

Jacobson (2001) emphasise clear steps in communicating their model. First, they discuss the vicious cycles between mood, activity and context, then the role of behavioural activation in breaking these cycles. Crucially, they challenge the notion that mood change is needed prior to behaviour change; instead, they emphasise the need for BA to be goal rather than mood directed. This is described as an 'outside-in' rather than 'inside-out' approach. Second, they highlight the need for individualised 'focused activation' that is genuinely positively reinforcing for that individual, not simply random activities that are presumed enjoyable. Therefore, utilising BA within the planning process of MI enhances this person-centred approach to activity planning. Third, they emphasise the importance of expressing empathy and optimism whilst also providing a clear rationale for 'directed activation'. After presenting the model, Jacobson et al. advocate a collaborative approach to detect 'secondary problem behaviours' (Figure 9.5) as well as the precipitating life events that have led to, and are maintaining, the client's depression. The distinguishing feature of BA is that behaviours and their consequences are studied in context using a detailed functional analysis.

Jacobson (2001) used three acronyms to help communicate the principles of BA treatment to clients. **T**rigger, **r**esponse, **a**voidance **p**attern (TRAP) is used to help clients understand how their avoidance patterns maintain their depression. Triggers may include situations, events or people; they can be historical or current, internal, external and/or interpersonal. The depressive response to triggers often leads to avoidant behavioural patterns which may offer short-term relief yet, in the longer term, reinforce the problem. Helping people understand both the form and function of their behavioural response is a key part of therapy. Avoidance patterns can include procrastination, rumination, complaining etc. (Addis & Martell, 2004). **T**rigger, **r**epose, **al**ternative **c**oping (TRAC) is used to help understand how to change avoidance by replacing it with a (graded) **a**ctive **c**oping alternative. Finally, the third acronym, ACTION, summarises the key process components for change – **a**ssess function of behaviour, **c**hoose to avoid or activate, **t**ry out chosen behaviour **i**ntegrate new behaviours/develop routines, **o**bserve form/function of outcome, **n**ever give up (or **n**ow Evaluate) – emphasising

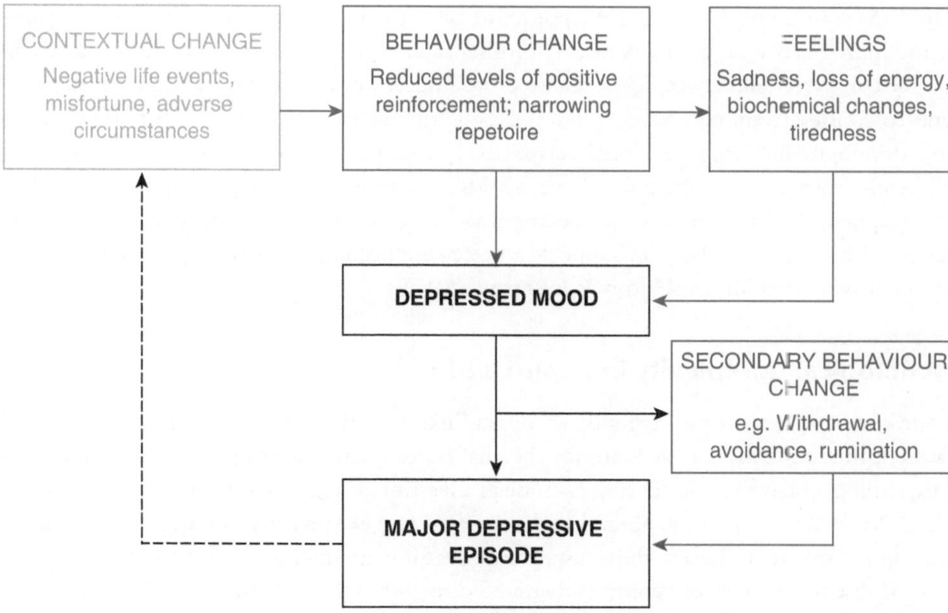

FIGURE 9.5 Behavioural activation model of depression with secondary behaviour change

Source: Personal communication

the importance of reflection/repetition. Practically, a practitioner may invite the client to generate a list of activities/positive behaviours that they might be interested in undertaking (e.g. go for a walk, call a friend). These activities and behaviours can then be graded in terms of ease and reward (1–10) with 1 being very difficult or not at all rewarding and 10 being very easy and very rewarding). A further strategy involves the client and practitioner collaboratively developing a weekly activity schedule in which the activities/behaviours identified as most rewarding and achievable are mapped across the morning, afternoon and evening, thereby developing a behavioural activation plan.

Dimidjian et al. (2011) point to the renewed interest in BA approaches over the last 20 years, including complex and co-morbid physical health conditions. Given the high levels of co-morbidity between obesity and depression (Pagoto et al., 2013), evidence for the use of BA to treat both conditions is emerging. There is an increasing evidence base for its use generally, and with co-morbid obese and depressed women specifically. When we consider BA for depression and increased PA in the context of an ERS, the utility of this approach is clear. From a BA perspective, a person who is caught up in patterns of overthinking and a behavioural avoidance cycle would be assisted in stopping the avoidance and activating alternative coping strategies. The mental and physical benefits of PA mean that if one approach to activation was increased activity, then there is amplified benefit to this change process. In pharmacological terms (if, for this context, we assume that stronger doses lead to better treatment outcomes), approaches to BA activation more generally may reflect a weaker dose, whereas BA that includes PA would reflect a stronger dose. However, a critical consideration for this process is the experience of feeling undecided about behaviour change (ambivalence), and thus, this exemplifies a further opportunity for combining BA with the MI approach.

Indeed, combining MI with BA appears to be a particular promising approach to supporting individuals with complex disease profiles such as those referred into ERS (e.g. Balán et al., 2016). We would encourage exercise professionals working in clinical exercise environments to consider training opportunities for these methods as part of their continued professional development. From a national perspective, adopting these approaches to personalising the exercise referral experience for clients avoids standardisation, embraces individual differences (Ogden, 2016), addresses the specific psychological processes associated with exercise referral (Hilton et al., 2016) and supports a better understanding of what works, for whom and under what conditions (Hilton & Johnston, 2017).

Psychological Complexity in Health and ERS

To our knowledge, there are currently no direct links with ERS in the UK and psychological treatment models. This may account for the challenges mental health professionals and clinical psychologists have in considering exercise as a legitimate adjunct to treatment (Faulkner & Biddle, 2001). Fox (2000) purports that the reasons why exercise is not routinely considered as an adjunct treatment for conditions such as depression are unclear. However, the complexity of the disease, the lack of genuine integrated care within the UK, the lack of clarity within the exercise science literature regarding the treatment of mental health causes and symptoms and the absence of treatment models as an integral part of exercise/ERS, we argue, would account for this. Therefore, in the current chapter, the combination of 1) a critique of current health-care systems within the UK, with a particular emphasis on the limitations of such for routinely prescribing exercise, and 2) practical psychological skills for health and leisure professionals is intended to support improved exercise care pathways. For the majority of those referred into ERS, if the exercise is not maintained, the symptoms associated with their mental health will return upon cessation of activity. We recognise that not all those referred have co-morbid disease mechanisms such as loss, trauma and attachment issues. However, for the majority of those for whom this is relevant, the lack of inclusion of ERS within an integrated multidisciplinary service means that individuals are not holistically assessed. Arguably, this may have implications for the ability of practitioners to adequately formulate the patient's difficulties and to engage in a meaningful treatment planning process early enough in the treatment pathway.

This may also account for the high volume of complex patients with co-morbid (untreated) conditions that are referred into specialist services (e.g. specialist weight management services, bariatric services). We know from personal clinical experiences (totalling hundreds of clinical hours) that these patients often report a long history of a failure of services to address these crucial factors. It is important to note that the measures often employed to assess depression within PA and exercise studies (e.g. Beck's Depression Inventory [BDI]; Beck et al. (1961)) are measures of symptomatology. The clinical reality is that in practice, psychometric assessments such as the BDI are only used as part of a more complete assessment that comprises a more detailed history, clinical interview and, most importantly, a bio-psycho-social formulation of the individuals presenting difficulties, maintaining factors and underlying causes. Unlike clinical practice, academic studies typically do not include a structured clinical interview and formulation. Consequently, one could argue that the academic literature (and subsequent policy literature) is developing the 'evidence base' grounded in clinical indications of symptomatology rather than a full clinical assessment of a specific psychological disorder (e.g. major depressive disorder, binge eating disorder, post-traumatic stress disorder, emotionally unstable personality disorder). This further complicates the development of the evidence base, policy and subsequent practice. It is clear that there is benefit from exploring a new way of working in this regard, and this is steadily being recognised (e.g. DH, 2011c; Roth & Pilling, 2015).

However, to date, health-care services are not organised in a manner such that they can deliver genuine integrated care that considers the whole person or addresses the broad bio-psycho-social factors that influence the person's experience of illness, wellness and treatment. This has implications for ERS because schemes are functioning within the same limitations, and this impacts what leisure professionals do and how they do it. As we outlined earlier (and in Figure 9.1), the most common difficulties that a person referred for exercise may be presenting with include several undiagnosed co-maintaining disorders (e.g. social anxiety, reactive depression, binge eating disorder). Further information regarding the co-maintaining cycles associated with these presentations within the context of an obesity referral can be found in our recent chapter elsewhere (Johnston et al., 2017b). The interested reader will also find greater detail regarding the application of appropriate psychological skills for the assessment and treatment of obesity.

The value of enhancing the psychological skills of exercise and allied health professionals (e.g. health psychologists) through training in a 5 Ps approach to case formulation (described earlier) has already been proposed (Hilton & Johnston, 2017; Hutchinson & Johnston, 2013; Johnston et al., 2017a). However, Hutchinson and Johnston (2013) recognise some of the practical implications of enhancing the clinical skills of exercise professionals: namely, that this method of working may uncover underlying clinical issues that an exercise professional may not be trained to identify, assess, formulate and treat. Consequently, Hutchinson and Johnston (2013) proposed that better links between ERS and Improving Access to Psychological Therapy (IAPT) services may have the scope to formulate appropriate treatment plans that have PA/exercise as an integral part of the treatment model (e.g. depression). However, thus far, ERS have been slow to respond to this proposal.

Whilst there is a government commitment to support and expand IAPT services (NHSE, 2016), even the high-intensity service (Step 3) tends to be symptom focused and concentrates on the treatment of a specific condition in relative isolation. Therefore, we would recommend that ideally, a psychology-led ERS pathway be coordinated by a clinical health psychology service. Doing so would allow for clinical health psychologists to assess whether IAPT support would be sufficient to address the psychological aspects of a patient's referral for exercise. If not, it may be more appropriate for support to be provided directly by the clinical health psychology service. We recognise that, with the increased focus on investing in IAPT, there has been less emphasis on clinical health psychology services, and, as mentioned earlier, regrettably, core training for health psychologists (see BPS, 2015) means that they may lack the clinical skills required to assess and treat patients who would be suitable for a psychology-led ERS service (Hilton & Johnston, 2017). Therefore, within the current NHS service provision, clinical health psychologists have the training and skills required to formulate and develop a treatment plan for someone with a very complex bio-psycho-social disease profile. Previous qualitative work that sought to investigate clinical psychologists' views on the utility of exercise as adjunct therapy identified such clinicians as key stakeholders in this regard (Faulkner & Biddle, 2001). However, looking forward, we would encourage policy-makers and training/education providers to respond to the growth in the recognition of working from a bio-psycho-social perspective – one that considers mental and physical health inseparable – by tailoring services and training accordingly. This would include a greater emphasis on clinical skills for trainee health psychologists, enhanced knowledge regarding the benefits of PA and exercise for trainee clinical psychologists, a lesser emphasis on condition-specific psychological treatment and a greater emphasis on formulation skills for IAPT services and enhanced psychological skills (e.g. BA, MI) for exercise professionals. For example, integrating MI into the exercise referral care pathway would help avoid common assumptions of readiness to change and a premature focus on exercise planning/behavioural activation by instructors and allied health professionals. Integrating MI into ERS is also likely to impact retention and long-term behaviour change because MI creates opportunities to explore a person's desires, abilities, reasons, needs and readiness to change from a person-centred perspective. Working in this way contributes to enhancing a person's intrinsic motivation to change and avoids a one-size-fits-all approach that would otherwise challenge the change process.

There is a growing interest in opportunities to integrate exercise professionals into the wider public health workforce (Royal Society for Public Health, 2018). There is an equal interest in MI training for the therapy sector as well as the leisure industry. This may reflect an increased awareness of the importance of engagement and behavioural change processes (alongside psychological factors) within ERS and also within services such as IAPT. Training in psychological skills (such as MI) or psychological treatment models more generally (e.g. BA) is currently unavailable through the usual leisure industry training pathways; therefore, increasing these opportunities or linking with the British Psychological Society (BPS) or the British Association for Behavioural and Cognitive Psychotherapies (BABCP) training workshops (see continued professional development [CPD] opportunities online) would support the development of exercise professionals in this regard.

Summary

The health conditions with which individuals are referred for exercise reflect an interplay between mental and physical ill health, in which we cannot have physical wellness without mental wellness and vice versa (e.g. Department of Health, 2011). There are added limitations regarding the duration of referral programmes, and the notion of short-term prescription periods that, even despite the efforts of schemes that are more long-term behaviour-change focused, create a conflicting message for those referred. The integration of ERS into multidisciplinary health services that have the capacity to address any underlying causal and maintaining psychological factors associated with physical ill health will better support ERS, the exercise professionals who deliver them and those referred.

Whilst there is a growing recognition of the need to adequately address psychological health within the context of long-term illness, the current organisation of health-care service is far from ideal. IAPT practitioners would benefit from being skilled in formulation because the current approach to service delivery is somewhat manualised and symptom focused, rather than formulating a complex co-morbid condition (see 5 Ps earlier). Arguably, the health and leisure industry would be better delivered by a clinical health psychology-led long-term-condition (LTC) service that genuinely integrates psychologists, dieticians, ERS and exercise professionals (e.g. Watt et al., 2016). However, given the current limitations of UK health service delivery, in the current chapter we have provided some pragmatic and feasible solutions to support the personalisation of the exercise referral experience within the context of disease complexity.

Finally, to support the consolidation of the skills associated with MI, formulation and BA that we presented in Figure 9.4: our initial thoughts on a skills summary guide that utilises MI and the four processes as the primary approach to supporting an individual through PA behaviour change. The rationale for this is that 1) MI is an effective evidence-based approach to supporting people through feelings of ambivalence about PA/exercise; 2) a MI approach supports practitioners to work from a person-centred perspective and avoid premature focus; and 3) training opportunities for MI are relatively easy to access. Figure 9.5 also maps formulation and BA onto the relevant MI processes such that how the three approaches may be combined can be represented visually. It is also noteworthy that BA has traditionally adopted a more directive stance than MI. Thus, BA may involve the practitioner making suggestions for changes without asking permission per se. To date, there appears to be less emphasis in BA on the importance of changes being generated by the client (in MI terms, change talk). Clearly, from an MI point of view, the adoption of a directive approach with unsolicited advice giving risks falling into the trap of the righting reflex (and thus resistance from the client). We believe that there is enormous scope to combine these approaches with MI as the guiding foundation for interpersonal process factors which can then maximise the likelihood of more helpful conversations about BA. The value of combining MI and BA is being recognised (e.g. Balán et al., 2016), in addition to MI and cognitive behavioural approaches more generally (e.g. Westra & Norouzian, 2018). We specifically believe that both approaches can be integrated within the context of exercise and PA behaviour change and that this is a particularly timely integration within the context of the disease complexity that we have highlighted in the current chapter. It should be stressed that a skills guide such as this should not be used during a conversation with a client so as to avoid a heavily scripted, manualised or mechanistic approach to the consultation, which would be damaging to MI spirit and the client experience. This is merely an aide-mémoire to guide the integration of the three approaches which we have discussed in this chapter.

Key Points

- Mental and physical health are inseparable, and therefore, ideally, ERS need to sit within an integrated model of care to respond to this adequately.
- Within the current UK health-care provision, links between primary care, exercise referral, IAPT, clinical psychology and dietetics may offer a pragmatic and feasible solution to ensuring that PA/exercise is considered as part of a broader treatment plan. However, both health practitioners and ERS professionals require training to deliver these services adequately.
- Motivational interviewing, formulation and behavioural activation approaches offer pragmatic and feasible solutions to personalising the exercise referral experience and facilitating behaviour change.

Study Task Questions

1. Discuss the relative advantages/disadvantages of a bio-psycho-social approach to understanding complex co-morbid presentations within an ERS.

2. What are the key ingredients of motivational interviewing (MI)?
3. What do we mean by change talk, sustain talk and ambivalence within MI?
4. What are the four processes within MI?
5. What do we mean by TRAP, TRAC, action within behavioural activation?
6. Why would we use a combination of BA and MI to treat a co-morbid presentation of reactive depression and obesity?
7. Is obesity a physical or psychological condition?
8. What is your understanding of the bio-psycho-social relationship between physical and mental health?
9. Is formulation a process or a product?
10. What role does motivational interviewing have in ERS?
11. How can we make better use of psychological models and skills within ERS and an integrated model of care?

References

Addis, M.E. and Martell, C.R. 2004. *Overcoming depression one step at a time*. Oakland, CA: New Harbinger.

Andrasik, F., Goodie, J. and Peterson, A. 2015. *Biopsychosocial assessment in clinical health psychology*. 1st ed. London: Guilford Press.

Balán, I.C., Lejuez, C.W., Hoffer, M. and Blanco, C. 2016. Integrating motivational interviewing and brief behavioural activation therapy: Theoretical and practical considerations. *Cognitive Behavioural Practice* 23(2), pp. 205–220.

Beck, A.T., Rush, A., Shaw, B. and Emery, G. 1979. *Cognitive therapy of depression*. London: Guilford Press.

Beck, A.T., Ward, C.H., Mendelson, M., Mock, J. and Erbaugh, J. 1961. An inventory for measuring depression. *Archives of General Psychiatry* 4, pp. 561–571.

British Psychological Society. 2008. *Briefing paper no. 27. Clinical health psychologists in the NHS*. Leicester: The British Psychological Society.

British Psychological Society. 2015. *Qualification in health psychology stage 2: Candidate handbook*. Available from: www.bps.org.uk/system/files/Public%20files/qhp_ stage_2_candidate_handbook_jan_2015.pdf [accessed 14 January 2018].

Clarke, P. and Eves, F. 1997. Applying the transtheoretical model to the study of exercise prescription. *Journal of Health Psychology* 2(2), pp. 195–207.

Department of Health. 2011. *No health without mental health a cross-government mental health outcomes strategy for people of all ages*. Available from: www.gov.uk/government/uploads/system/uploads/attachment_data/file/213761/dh_124058.pdf [accessed 6 March 2018].

Dimidjian S., Barrera M. Jr, Martell C., Muñoz R.F. and Lewinsohn P.M. 2011. The origins and current status of behavioral activation treatments for depression. *Annual Review of Clinical Psychology* 7, pp. 1–38.

Dunn, A.L., Trivedi, H.T., Kampert, J.B., Clark, C.G. and Chambliss, H.O. 2005. Exercise treatment for depression. *American Journal of Preventative Medicine* 28(1), pp. 1–8.

Faulkner, G. and Biddle, S. 2001. Exercise and mental health: It's just not psychology! *Journal of Sports Science* 19(6), pp. 433–444.

Fox, K.R. 2000. Self-esteem, self-perceptions and exercise. *International Journal of Sport Psychology* 31(2), pp. 228–240.

Frankl, V.E. 1997. *Man's search for meaning*. Mass market paperback. New York: Simon & Schuster.

Hilton, C.E. and Johnston, L.H. 2017. Health psychology: It's not what you do, it's the way that you do it. *Health Psychology Open*. Available from: http://journals.sagepub.com/doi/pdf/10.1177/2055102917714910 [Accessed 5 March 2018].

Hilton, C.E., Lane, C. and Johnston, L.H. 2016. Has motivational interviewing fallen into its own premature focus trap? *International Journal for the Advancement of Counselling* 38(2), pp. 145–158.

Hilton, C.E., Trigg, R. and Minitti, A. 2015. Improving the psychological evaluation of exercise referral: Psychometric properties of the exercise referral quality of life scale. Available from: http://journals.sagepub.com/doi/pdf/10.1177/2055102915590317 [accessed 13 October 2017].

Hutchinson, A.J. and Johnston, L.H. 2013. Exploring the potential of case formulation within exercise psychology. *Journal of Clinical Sport Psychology* 7, pp. 60–76.

Hutchison, A.J., Johnston, L.H. and Breckon, J.D. 2012. A grounded theory of successful physical activity behaviour change. *Qualitative Research in Sport, Exercise and Health* 5(1), pp. 109–126.

Jacobson, S. 2001. Contextualism and global doubts about the world. *Synthese* 129(3), pp. 381–404.

James, D.V.B., Johnston, L.H., Crone, D., Sidford, A.H., Gidlow, C., Morris, C. and Foster, C. 2008. Factors associated with physical activity referral uptake and participation. *Journal of Sports Sciences* 26, pp. 217–224.

James, D.V.B., Mills, H., Crone, D., Johnston, L., Morris, C. and Gidlow, C. 2009. Factors associated with physical activity referral completion and health outcomes. *Journal of Sport Science* 27(10), pp. 1007–1017.

Johnston, L. and Dallos, R. 2013. *Formulation in psychology and psychotherapy: Making sense of people's problems*. 2nd ed. London: Routledge.

Johnston, L.H., Hilton, C.E. and Lane, C. 2017a. Motivational interviewing and mindfulness in weight management. In Weaver, J. ed. *Practical guide to obesity medicine*. London: Elsevier, pp. 193–214.

Johnston, L.H., Hilton, C.E. and Lane, C. 2017b. Psychological management in bariatric surgery. In Weaver, J. ed. *Practical guide to obesity medicine*. London: Elsevier, pp. 299–313.

Johnston, L.H. and Hutchinson, A.J. 2016. Influencing health behaviour: Applying theory to practice. In Scott, A. and Gidlow, C. eds. *Clinical exercise science*. London: Routledge, pp. 224–247.

Johnston, L.H., Hutchison, A.J. and Ingham, B. 2011. The utility of biopsychosocial models of clinical formulation within stress and coping and applied practice. In Devonport, T. ed. *Managing stress from theory to application*. New York: Nova Science Publishers, pp. 261–291.

Laing, R. 1971. *The politics of the family and other essays*. London: Routledge.

Martell, C.R., Addis, M.E. and Jacobson, N.S. 2001. *Depression in context*. Norton: London.

Martin, D.J., Garske, J.P. and Davis, K.M. 2000. Relation of the therapeutic alliance with outcome and other variables. A meta analytic review. *Journal of Consulting and Clinical Psychology* 68, pp. 438–450.

Miller, W.R. and Moyers, T.B. 2006. Eight stages in learning motivational interviewing. *Journal of Teaching in the Addictions* 5(1), pp. 3–17.

Miller W.R. and Rollinick S. 2012. *Motivational interviewing: Helping people change*. 3rd ed. New York: The Guildford Press.

Morgan, W.P. and Glodston, S.E. (1987). *Exercise and mental health*. London: Taylor Francis.

Moyers, T.B. (2014). The relationship in motivational interviewing. *Psychotherapy Theory Research Practice Training* 51(3), pp. 358–363.

Moyers, T.B., Manuel, J.K. and Ernst, D. 2015. *Motivational interviewing treatment integrity coding manual 4.1.2*. Available from: www.motivationalinterviewing.org/sites/default/files/miti4_2.pdf [accessed 27 April 2017].

National Health Service England. 2016. *The five year forward view for mental health*. Available from: www.england.nhs.uk/wp-content/uploads/2016/02/Mental-Health-Taskforce-FYFV-final.pdf [accessed 5 March 2018].

National Obesity Observatory. 2011. *Obesity and mental health*, March. www.noo.org.uk/uploads/doc/vid_10266_Obesity%20and%20mental%20health_FINAL_ 070311_MG.pdf [accessed 12 August 2018].

Ogden, J. 2016. Celebrating variability and a call to limit systematization: The example of the behaviour change technique taxonomy and the behaviour change wheel. *Health Psychology Review*. Available from: http://dx.doi.org/10.1080/17437199.2016.1190291 [accessed 17 July 2017].

Pagoto, S., Schneider, K., Jojic, M., DeBiasse, M. and Mann, D. 2013. Evidence-based strategies in weight-loss mobile apps. *American Journal of Preventive Medicine* 45(5), pp. 576–582.

Qin, P., Horton, K., Mortensen, P.B., et al. 2014. Combined effects of physical illness and comorbid psychiatric disorder on risk of suicide in a national population study. *The British Journal of Psychiatry* 204(6), pp. 430–435.

Rogers, C. 1980. *A way of being*. Boston: Houghton Mifflin Company.

Rollins, A.L., Wright-Berryman, J., Henry, N.H., Quash, A.M., Benbow, K., Bonfils, K.A., Hedrick, H., Miller, A.P., Firmin, R. and Salyers, M.P. 2017. Managing physical and mental health conditions: Consumer perspectives on integrated care. *Social Work in Mental Health* 15(1), pp. 66–79.

Roth, A.D. and Pilling, S. 2015. *A competence framework for psychological interventions with people with persistent physical health conditions*. Available from: www.ucl.ac.uk/pals/research/cehp/research-groups/core/pdfs/Physical_Health_Problems/Physical_Background_Doc.pdf [accessed 6 March 2018].

Royal Society for Public Health. 2018. *Going the distance: Exercise professionals in the wider public health workforce*. Available from: www.rsph.org.uk/uploads/assets/uploaded/14e49b8d-73e5-4a29-be661 69ec1a38a71.pdf [accessed 23 July 2018].

Suls, J. and Rothman, A. (2004). Evolution of the biopsychosocial model: Prospects and challenges for health psychology. *Health Psychology* 23(2), pp. 119–125. doi:10.1037/0278-6133.23.2.119.

Watt, A., Johnston, L.H. and Wells, T. 2016. Sticky plasters and septic wounds: One dietician's journey in weight management (Part 1 & 2). *Complete Nutrition* 16(1 & 2), pp. 60–62.

Westra, H.A. and Norouzian, N. (2018). Using motivational interviewing to manage process markers of ambivalence and resistance in cognitive behavioural therapy. *Cognitive Therapy and Research* 42(2), pp. 193–203.

10
OBESITY

Louisa Herring and David Broom

Chapter aims

The aims of this chapter are to support you to:

- Define obesity and have an awareness of the prevalence data
- Understand the obesity treatment pathway in the UK
- Evaluate the various methods and approaches to obesity management
- Recognise the benefits of physical activity and exercise in the treatment of obesity
- Appreciate the complexity of exercise programming for obesity and its associated co-morbidities
- Confidently recommend exercise for varying levels of obesity that is client centred and compile a 12-week programme

Introduction

Obesity prevalence worldwide has more than doubled since 1980 and is now recognised as a 'chronic, relapsing, progressive disease process' needing immediate action to manage the global epidemic (Bray et al., 2017; World Health Organisation, 2015). Adult and childhood obesity incidence in the United Kingdom (UK) are among the highest in the developed world (Royal College of Physicians (RCP), 2013). England's overweight and obesity prevalence accounts for around 62% of the adult population, of which 25% are categorised as being with obesity; this is a 10% increase since 1993 (Public Health England, 2014; Welbourne et al., 2014).

Obesity is defined as 'abnormal or excessive fat accumulation that may impair health' and is often attributed to low levels of physical activity and a disproportionate energy intake (Hill et al., 2012; World Health Organisation, 2017). Obesity is classified following prolonged excessive weight gain when the body's energy stores of fat exceed those that are expended. The main cause of overweight and obesity is physical inactivity, excessive sedentary behaviour and/or increased calorie consumption. Weight gain can be a result of medical conditions (e.g. endocrine disorders, hyperthyroidism) or a side effect of medications and smoking cessation.

DOI: 10.4324/9781315102399-10

It can also be the result of genetic disorders e.g. Prader-Willi syndrome, and whilst genes play a role in the development of obesity, the gene pool has not changed that significantly in recent decades to be the main contributing factor.

The current universal body mass measurement is body mass index (BMI), which is a simple calculation derived from stretch stature and body mass (World Health Organisation, 2017). BMI allows the calculation and comparison of national and international prevalence rates for each classification listed in Table 10.1 (James et al., 2001). The equation used to derive BMI is body mass in kilograms (kg) divided by stretch stature in metres (m) squared [(2)] (BMI = kg/m^2) (World Health Organisation, 2017).

Despite the prevalence of obesity in black, Asian and other minority ethnic groups being similar to or lower than that of white European populations, the prevalence of co-morbidities such as type 2 diabetes mellitus (T2DM) and cardiovascular diseases (CVD) is greater amongst black, Asian and other minority ethnic groups. It must therefore be noted that at lower BMI classifications, people of black, Asian and other minority ethnic groups are at an increased risk of chronic health conditions over that of white European populations (Corazon Barba et al., 2004; National Institute for Health and Care Excellence (NICE), 2013b). (See Table 10.2.)

The rising prevalence of obesity is contributing to significant cardio-metabolic complications and higher rates of obesity-related diseases (Vinciguerra et al., 2013), such as T2DM, CVD, dyslipidemia, hypertension, obstructive sleep apnoea, arthritis and non-alcoholic fatty liver disease (Colquitt et al., 2009; Nguyen & Lau, 2012).

Morbid obesity also contributes to reductions in physical function, walking speed and further increases the occurrence of disability (Herring et al., 2016; Lyytinen et al.,

TABLE 10.1 BMI classifications and associated co-morbidity risks

Classification	*BMI ($kg \cdot m^2$) (General guidelines)*	*Risk of associated co-morbidities (e.g. T2DM and CVD)*
Underweight	**< 18.5**	
Normal weight	**18.5–24.9**	**Acceptable**
Pre-obesity	25.0–29.9	Increased risk
Obesity	**≥ 30.0**	**High risk**
Obesity class I	30.0–34.9	
Obesity class II	35.0–39.9	
Obesity class III	≥ 40.0	

KEY: $kg \cdot m^2$: kilogram per metre squared; T2DM: Type 2 diabetes mellitus
Source: National Institute for Health and Care Excellence (NICE), 2013a; World Health Organisation, 2017

TABLE 10.2 BMI and associated co-morbidity risks for Asian populations

BMI ($kg \cdot m^2$) (General guidelines)	*Risk of associated co-morbidities (e.g. T2DM and CVD)*
< 18.5	Underweight
18.5–23.0	Acceptable
23.0–27.5	Increased risk
≥ 27.5	High risk

KEY: $kg \cdot m^2$: kilogram per metre squared; T2DM: Type 2 diabetes mellitus; CVD: cardiovascular diseases
Source: Corazon Barba et al., 2004; National Institute for Health and Care Excellence (NICE), 2013

2013; Miller et al., 2009). These mobility limitations negatively affect the ability to perform activities of daily living (ADLs) such as walking, stair climbing, transitioning from a seated to standing position, housework and dressing due to musculoskeletal conditions (Capodaglio et al., 2010; Sainio et al., 2007). All the above factors associated with obesity lead to a reduction in health-related quality of life (HRQoL) domains, specifically activity/mobility, symptoms, personal hygiene/clothing, emotions, social interactions, sexual life and eating behaviour.

(Duval et al., 2006)

Public Health England (PHE) reported that UK wide, overweight and obesity-related ill health cost the National Health Service (NHS) an estimated £6.1 billion in 2014–2015, with economic development being compromised due to obesity-related costs of £27 billion on wider society. By 2050 these costs are projected to reach £9.7 billion and £49.9 billion, respectively (Public Health England, 2017). The Royal College of Physicians (RCP) published 'The Action on Obesity: Comprehensive Care for All' report in January 2013 and reported similar cost prediction figures by 2050 if the obesity epidemic is not addressed appropriately (Royal College of Physicians, 2013). Commercial profit-making weight loss programmes (e.g. Weight Watchers [WW] and Slimming World) are growing in popularity in an attempt to prevent and treat obesity and its associated co-morbidities, although long-term weight maintenance in such programmes is unclear (Truby & Bonham, 2011). The RCP have highlighted the importance of multidisciplinary team (MDT) services to reduce the obesity burden and its associated diseases and co-morbidities (Royal College of Physicians, 2013). The NHS has therefore developed a tiered approach to MDT weight-management services nationwide, depending on the severity of obesity; however these services vary nationwide, and no standardised guidelines exist (National Institute for Health and Care Excellence (NICE), 2014a). NICE (2014c) define the tiers of weight management as follows:

Tier 1 covers universal services (such as health promotion or primary care)
Tier 2 covers lifestyle interventions
Tier 3 covers specialist weight management services
Tier 4 covers bariatric surgery
(National Institute for Health and Care Excellence (NICE), 2014b)

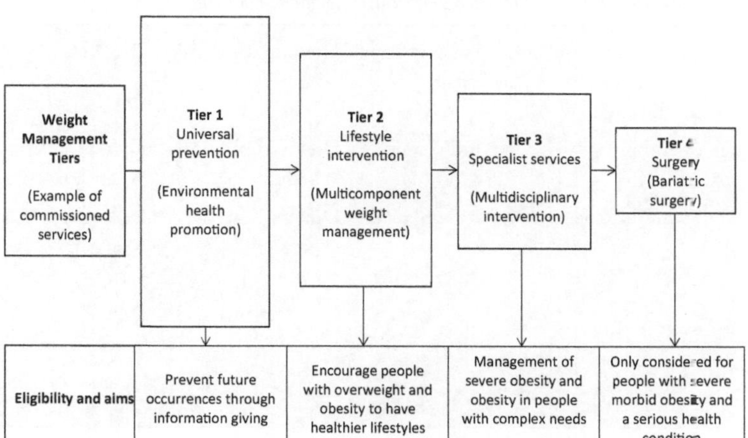

FIGURE 10.1 The UK Obesity Care Pathway

Source: Adapted from Department of Health, 2013

The management of obesity and current treatment pathways

Guidelines for managing people with overweight or obesity within the NHS have been established by the National Institute for Health and Care Excellence (NICE) (National Institute for Health and Care Excellence, 2014a). Concerns regularly arise over the validity of BMI alone due to muscle being more dense than fat; as a result, those with a mesomorph body profile (e.g. bodybuilders) would be classified as being with obesity. Consequently, BMI is acceptable for population-level monitoring, but in terms of individual classification, both BMI and waist circumference (WC) have been incorporated in these guidelines. The presentation of co-morbidities has also been incorporated because presentation of these means a patient is likely to be at greater risk at a lower BMI classification. Table 10.3 illustrates the NHS guidelines for the management of overweight and obesity.

General advice

Routine identification of overweight and obesity typically occurs in primary care as general practitioners (GP) see three-quarters of patients at least once per year, with individuals with obesity attending more regularly (McLaughlin et al., 2017). Therefore, advice on healthy weight and lifestyle is typically provided by a GP or a health-care professional (HCP), as suggested for individuals who are overweight in Table 10.3. A cross-sectional survey was undertaken by Jackson et al. (2013) on 810 UK adults with overweight and obesity to examine the influence of HCPs' advice on motivation to lose weight and attempts to lose weight. Participants were asked three questions, one of which was if they had ever received advice to lose weight. Only 17% of people with overweight and 42% of people with obesity responded

TABLE 10.3 NICE guidelines for the management of overweight and obesity

BMI classification	*Waist circumference*			*Co-morbidities present*
	Low (males ≤94 cm; females ≤80 cm)	*High (males 94–102 cm; females 80–88 cm)*	*Very high (males ≥ 102 cm; females ≥ 88 cm)*	
Overweight	General advice on healthy weight and lifestyle	Diet and physical activity	Diet and physical activity	Diet and physical activity; consider drugs
Obesity I	Diet and physical activity	Diet and physical activity	Diet and physical activity	Diet and physical activity; consider drugs
Obesity II	Diet and physical activity; consider drugs	Diet and physical activity; consider drugs	Diet and physical activity; consider drugs	Diet and physical activity; consider drugs; consider surgery
Obesity III	Diet and physical activity; consider drugs; consider surgery	Diet and physical activity; consider drugs; consider surgery	Diet and physical activity; consider drugs; consider surgery	Diet and physical activity; consider drugs; consider surgery

KEY: BMI: body mass index

Source: National Institute for Health and Care Excellence (NICE), 2014a

that they could remember having received weight-loss advice from a HCP, highlighting the need for better HCP training (Jackson et al., 2013). The choice of weight management intervention should be discussed on an individual basis to identify personal preference, taking into consideration their lifestyle, health status (co-morbidities), fitness, ability to undertake activities of daily living and willingness to change (NICE, 2021). Being pregnant and living with obesity should be recognised and the appropriate pathway followed (NICE, 2021).

Diet and physical activity

If a person presents with overweight or obesity, one of the first approaches is dietary advice and/or exercise referral if the HCP and patient believe this is the route needed to optimise the individual's care (NICE, 2014a; NICE, 2021). NICE (2014b) have identified that the prevention and management of obesity can be facilitated by physical activity; hence, obesity is incorporated into exercise referral schemes (ERS). The success and adherence of people with obesity partaking in ERS can be attributed to the motivational skills and professional, supportive and friendly nature of the instructor (Herring et al., 2014; Williams et al., 2007).

Diet advice should be offered and varies depending on the individual; it can be delivered through their GP or practice nurse or via referral to a dietetic service. The target is to tailor dietary changes to food preferences and allow for a flexible and individual approach to reducing calorie intake whilst avoiding restrictive and nutritionally unbalanced diets due to their ineffectiveness in the long term (NICE, 2014a). It is well noted that a combination of dietary and physical activity intervention results in significant and clinically meaningful (5%) initial weight loss compared to diet alone in people with obesity (Curioni & Lourenco, 2005). The extensive heterogeneity of obesity lifestyle services offered by multiple local authorities and clinical commissioning groups (CCGs) makes it difficult to develop an individual and universal model (Hassan et al., 2016). Hassan et al. (2016) undertook a systematic review and reported wide variations in the approaches, methods and tools used in the 17 included studys. They concluded that weight loss was greater in individuals receiving a lifestyle programme than those receiving standard care, and those who encompassed both diet and exercise components exhibited the superior weight loss.

Tier 2 weight management services

Primary care providers are more readily referring people with overweight and obesity to Tier 2 weight management lifestyle services with the aim of weight loss and increasing physical activity to reduce the risk of obesity-related diseases through public, private and voluntary sectors (National Institute for Health and Care Excellence, 2014b). NICE (2014c) recommend that commissioners commission lifestyle weight management programmes that address multiple components (diet, physical activity and behaviour change) developed by specialists in each area. They should entail weekly or fortnightly sessions for three months, set achievable goals to promote lifelong lifestyle change and prevent weight regain (National Institute for Health and Care Excellence, 2014b). For long-term benefits, more than the clinically meaningful 5% weight loss is required with lifelong maintenance; however, on average, this level of weight loss is not achieved in such services (Welbourne et al., 2014). Optimising and sustaining weight loss through conventional methods and commercial weight-loss programmes is challenging, emphasising why the demand for drug therapy and more invasive weight loss techniques such as bariatric surgery is increasing (see Tier 3 weight management services section) (Steinbrook, 2004; Welbourne et al., 2014). Lv et al.'s (2017) systematic review reports modest clinically significant weight loss when undertaking comprehensive and intensive behavioural interventions, but these may not significantly improve cardio-metabolic risk factors associated with obesity. However, evidence of the effectiveness of behavioural interventions versus pharmacological or surgical treatment is currently limited (Lv et al., 2017).

Drug therapy

Orlistat is currently licensed for prescription in the UK (Booth et al., 2015; NHS Choices, 2016a; Yanovski & Yanovski, 2014). Pharmacotherapy through the administration of Orlistat is designed as an adjunct to lifestyle change in the form of dietary restriction and exercise and does result in long-term sustained moderate weight loss (Jain et al., 2011; Linne et al., 2003). It is recommended that Orlistat be used to facilitate weight loss in adults who have a BMI of ≥ 30 kg.m^2 (≥ 28 kg.m^2 with associated risk factors) (NICE, 2021). Its primary function is preventing the absorption of fats from the human diet by acting as a lipase inhibitor.

It stops the absorption of approximately one-quarter of ingested fat, which passes in the patient's stools, thus indicating why dietary change is important, and regular GP monitoring is needed to reduce the risk of side effects (flatulence, with or without oily spotting; sudden bowel movements; and fatty, oily or soft stools) (Medicines and Healthcare Products Regulatory Agency, 2014). Clinical trials of this anti-obesity drug concur with guidelines and conclude that it is well tolerated and effective when utilised in combination with positive lifestyle change to help attain and maintain optimal weight loss (Jain et al., 2011). However, it should not be taken for longer than six months (Medicines and Healthcare Products Regulatory Agency, 2014). NICE guidance suggest orlistat therapy should only be continued beyond three months if the individual has lost at least 5% body weight since starting the medication (NICE, 2021). See Table 10.4 for the effect of orlistat on the exercise response.

Liraglutide is another drug used in the management of obesity alongside increased physical activity and a reduced calorie diet (NICE, 2021). Liraglutide is typically prescribed in secondary care Tier 3 weight management services for individuals with a BMI of ≥ 35 kg.m^2 (≥ 32.5 kg.m^2 for members of minority ethnic groups), with non-diabetic hyperglycaemia or a fasting plasma glucose level of 5.5 to 6.9 mmol/L and at a high risk of cardiovascular disease (NICE, 2021). Liraglutide is a GLP-1 derivative which suppresses appetite and delays gastric emptying, making it effective for weight loss (Mehta et al., 2017).

Tier 3 weight management services

People with obesity progress to Tier 3 weight management if they have a complex disease status, if conventional treatment has been unsuccessful, if drug therapy is being considered (specifically for a higher BMI statuses [≥ 50 kg.m^2]), if a very low-calorie diet (VLCD) is necessary or if bariatric surgery is being considered (Blackshaw et al., 2014; National Institute for Health and Care Excellence, 2014a). VLCDs are diet plans that involve eating ~800 kilo calories or less, using clinically supervised meal replacement techniques for weight loss (NHS Choices, 2016b).

Tier 3 weight management services are designed to meet the needs of people with obesity who have a BMI of ≥ 40 kg.m^2 or ≥ 35 kg.m^2 with co-morbidities that cannot be adequately

TABLE 10.4 Medication considerations for exercise for people with obesity

Class name	*Generic name*	*Brand name*	*Indication*	*Action*	*Side effects*	*Exercise considerations*
Orlistat	Orlistat	Xenical Alli	Orlistat is used to facilitate weight loss in overweight and obesity.	Orlistat acts as a lipase inhibitor preventing the absorption of fats from the human diet therefore reducing caloric intake.	Changes in bowel function due to unabsorbed fat. These can include: • Fatty/oily stools • Oily spotting • Flatulence • Intestinal gas with discharge • Urgent need to pass a bowel movement • Increased number of bowel movements • Poor bowel control • Diarrhea • Clay-coloured stools • Rectal pain • Stomach pain • Nausea • Vomiting • Weakness • Dark urine • Itching • Loss of appetite • Jaundice • Teeth or gum problems • Cold symptoms • Headache • Back pain • Skin rash • Allergic reaction	Undertaking exercise is recommended when taking Orlistat. Due to faecal urgency, it is important the participant has an awareness of where the toilets are. They are encouraged to wear dark clothing and have a change of clothes in case accidents occur.

managed in Tier 2 services (National Institute for Health and Care Excellence, 2014a). Tier 3 typically adopts a MDT approach, comprising a specialist physician, specialist nurse, specialist dietitian, psychologist, psychiatrist and physiotherapist or exercise specialist (Blackshaw et al., 2014). The service is designed to assess obesity-associated co-morbidities and obtain indicative measurements (blood pressure, lipid profile, liver function, endocrine function, fasting insulin concentration, fasting glucose concentration and oral glucose tolerance test (OGTT)) (National Institute for Health and Care Excellence, 2014a).

Tier 3 service provision is variable nationwide and in many areas is unavailable due to times of austerity and local authority funding cuts. Without Tier 3 services, it is challenging for individuals to access bariatric surgery (Tier 4 services) (National Institute for Health and Care Excellence, 2014a). It is recognised that those people with obesity who proactively manage their diet and exercise as a result of attending a Tier 3 service are more likely to optimise their post-surgical outcome as they have the skills necessary for the lifestyle changes needed to promote weight loss and prevent weight regain (National Institute for Health and Care Excellence, 2014a). Furthermore, people who are being considered for bariatric surgery 'should undergo a service based weight loss programme (non-surgical tier 3/4) for a duration of 12–24 months', thus indicating the challenge that occurs if an area does not provide Tier 3 services (National Institute for Health and Care Excellence, 2014a). This is an opportunity for exercise referral services to work with other allied health-care professionals (AHPs) to develop Tier 3 services if none are available.

Tier 4 weight management service: Bariatric surgery and specialist complex obesity service

Currently, the most effective and sustainable method of weight loss for people with morbid obesity (BMI ≥ 40 kg/m^2 or ≥ 35 kg/m^2 when presenting co-morbidities) is bariatric surgery combined with long-term lifestyle modification (Madura & Dibaise, 2012). Bariatric surgery, or weight loss surgery, is defined as surgery on the stomach and/or intestines to facilitate weight loss (MedicineNet, 2016). The type of bariatric surgery procedure performed and the lifestyle adaptations individuals make and maintain dictate the rate and sustainability of weight loss (Jassil et al., 2015; Papalazarou et al., 2010). The three main surgical techniques currently used in the UK are 1) laparoscopic adjustable gastric banding, 2) vertical sleeve gastrectomy (restrictive procedures), and 3) roux-en-Y gastric bypass (malabsorptive and restrictive procedure) (Dent et al., 2010; Madura & Dibaise, 2012; Welbourne et al., 2014).

The expertise of the surgical department as well as the preference of the individual dictate the type of procedure performed. Multidisciplinary support is also recommend after bariatric surgery to optimise the concomitant lifestyle changes essential for weight loss and maintenance (nutritional, psychological, physical activity and exercise education) (Royal College of Physicians, 2013). Post-operative weight regain is likely to occur if such advice is not available or adhered to post surgery (Odom et al., 2010). Dietetic monitoring is the only discipline consistently offered nationwide due to the important dietary changes necessary after bariatric surgery. Dietetic monitoring is offered for two years after surgery as part of NHS standard care, whilst physical activity, exercise and psychological support are not routinely available, even though post-operative weight loss can be influenced positively by individuals' increasing their physical activity behaviour (Colquitt et al., 2009; Egberts et al., 2012; Livhits et al., 2010). Egberts et al. (2012) undertook a meta-analysis and concluded that a greater mean weight loss of 3.62 kg was seen in physically active patients following bariatric surgery than in their physically inactive counterparts.

Physical activity and exercise for obesity management

Physical activity and exercise are often overlooked in routine overweight and obesity care, possibly due to poor portrayal in the mainstream media due to research findings being misinterpreted. One common misconception is that exercise can make you eat more however, despite there being some compensation, exercise can induce energy deficits without eating more at the next meal (Dorling et al., 2018). As research evolves, the importance of physical activity for optimising weight loss outcomes in people with obesity is gaining greater recognition and policy-makers and national organisations with a remit for health promotion have recognised the importance of promoting physical activity as part of a healthy lifestyle, regardless of one's BMI and independent of weight loss (Coen & Goodpaster, 2015; Foster-Schubert et al., 2012; Herring et al., 2017; Hills & Byrne, 2004; Livhits et al., 2010; National Institute for Health and Care Excelence, 2013a). Research suggests that in MDT services for obesity, an educational exercise element alone is insufficient for enhancing physical activity participation (Herring, Stevinson et al., 2017; Herring, Wagstaff et al., 2014). This therefore highlights the importance of supervised and structured exercise support in such services and official guidelines to aid people's understanding of what is needed for their weight loss or maintenance goal. Although currently there are no implemented guidelines relating to physical activity for weight loss and maintenance, an accumulating body of evidence supports the argument that development of formal recommendations is required for all tiers of weight management.

Response to exercise

The following describes how the body responds to exercise in a person with obesity.

Cellular interactions between exercise and obesity

The cellular interaction between exercise and obesity is complex; exercise aids the increase of free fatty acid (FFA) oxidation to meet the increased lipolysis demands of obesity. Exercise also alters the production of cell-signalling proteins; cytokines, specifically adipokine (fat); and myokine (muscle) hormones. Exercise-induced myokine release through muscular activity provides beneficial metabolic effects through the stimulation of glucose uptake, glucose tolerance, fat oxidation and regulating skeletal muscle regeneration (So et al., 2014). When proinflammatory adipokine secretion increases, this can lead to insulin resistance and/or glucose intolerance as a result of a chronic inflammatory state. Exercise alters the adipokine profile by increasing anti-inflammatory adipokine secretion and reduces proinflammatory cytokines (Golbidi & Laher, 2014). Research suggests that both adipokines and myokines contribute to the facilitation of exercise-induced health benefits, and their profiles are down regulated by physical inactivity.

Exercise and adiposity

The increased accumulation of excess body fat and central adiposity in obesity is the main contributing factor to all obesity-related complications (e.g. metabolic, co-morbidities). Body fat distribution is important, where visceral and upper body (android) adipose tissue accumulation is linked with metabolic complications rather than lower body (gynoid) adiposity, increasing the risk of insulin resistance and T2DM along with other co-morbidities. Both physical inactivity and sedentary behaviour contribute to the increased accumulation of visceral adipose tissue and total body fat; aerobic exercise of sufficient frequency, duration and intensity to increase energy expenditure contributes to body fat and visceral fat reduction

(Goedecke & Micklesfield, 2014). However, a combination of aerobic and resistance training is the optimal type of exercise as aerobic exercise facilitates fat-mass reduction while resistance training increases fat free mass (FFM), which helps increase resting metabolic rate (RMR) (see next section) (Willis et al., 2012). Previous research confirms this by demonstrating that multi-modal exercise programmes lead to decreased abdominal subcutaneous and visceral fat compared with aerobic training alone (Park et al., 2003).

Metabolic rate

RMR is typically associated with the amount of FFM. A common misconception is that people with obesity have a 'slower metabolic rate', but this is not the case. Research has shown that people with obesity have a higher energy expenditure and resting metabolic rate because of the increased cost of moving a greater body mass (Ravussin et al., 1982). Also, adipose tissue is not an insert substance, and energy is expended to undertake various metabolic processes such as secretion of the hormone leptin.

Weight loss encompasses a combination of both fat mass and FFM reduction, in which the reduction in FFM negatively affects RMR and hinders weight loss. It is therefore desirable for weight loss interventions to promote fat mass loss while maintaining RMR through the preservation of FFM. It is well documented that both fat mass and FFM reduce when weight loss is initiated via hypocaloric diets. Nevertheless, the addition of exercise to hypocaloric diets –predominantly resistance exercise – can attenuate this reduction in lean mass–making exercise, an important component for weight loss. However, research has found that low-intensity aerobic exercise (walking and arm cranking) during energy deficit also preserves FFM (Calbet et al., 2017). Consequently, conserving FFM during weight loss is important to maintain RMR in people with obesity, and exercise, regardless of type, needs to be incorporated into the weight loss programmes.

In addition to these factors associated with obesity and the body's response to exercise, it is important to acknowledge variations in fluid. During prolonged moderate-intensity aerobic exercise (progressing from 14.0^{0} C to 25.0^{0} C), people with obesity display higher sweat rates, lower urine outputs and greater fluid intake than lean counterparts (Eijsvogels et al., 2011). This could increase the risk of developing sodium and fluid imbalances, highlighting the importance of exercising in appropriate environmental conditions and the need for increased fluid consumption.

Exercise versus dietary restriction for improving body composition in obesity

Fundamentally, and you cannot defy the laws of physics, a reduction in body mass can only occur when energy expenditure outweighs energy intake over a given time frame (Hill et al., 2012). To lose one pound of fat, it is necessary to expend 3,500 kcal (American College of Sports Medicine, 2010). How such a deficit is created should be the sole preference of the person wanting to lose weight and can be achieved via exercise, dietary restriction or a combination of the two. Variations in body mass are concomitant with increases and decreases in energy expenditure, which are mainly dictated by changes in FFM, the main metabolically active component of the body (Muller et al., 2016). Obesity treatments' main goal is to preserve FFM whilst maximising fat-mass loss (Heymsfield et al., 2014).

Research has investigated different dietary methods on body composition change, with a systematic review of this research concluding that a hypocaloric model induces a larger effect relative to any other dietary methods of body mass, fat mass and FFM retention (Clark, 2015). A 12-month hypocaloric diet (700 kcal daily deficit) in those with a mean BMI of 36 kg.m^2 elicits weight loss (−2.6 kg) and improved physical function (Kaukua et al., 2004). Research in a female-only cohort with obesity found an 8.5% weight loss, 4.4 cm reduction in waist circumference and 4.2% reduction in percentage body fat through caloric restriction, compared to a 2.4%, 2.0 cm and 1.6% reduction, respectively, through exercise alone (Imayama et al., 2012). Clark et al. (2015), however, report that body composition change (both fat-mass reduction and FFM preservation) is more effective than any diet intervention when undertaking an exercise intervention and is a more effective stimulus to reverse hormone and adipokine/cytokine signals to healthy ranges. Weiss et al. (2007) found in response to 12 months of calorific restriction, FFM and physical capacity decreased; this, however, was not shown in a similar weight loss induced through exercise. Research also shows FFM and aerobic capacity reduce when weight loss is induced through hypocaloric diets alone, as well as a reduction in fat mass and strength (Heymsfield et al., 2014; Weiss et al., 2007). Energy restriction alone also had either a neutral or negative influence on cardiorespiratory fitness and muscular strength in the absence of exercise training and instigated greater FFM loss (Miller et al., 2013). Research has found that exercise also helps preserve FFM during excessive weight loss initiated through bariatric surgery (Huck, 2014).

It is the heterogeneity of participants, study designs and the outcomes and the means by which they are measured that contribute to the efficacy of findings between diet and exercise in the treatment of obesity; however, initiating the energy imbalance needed for weight loss strongly points to a combined intervention of diet with any type of exercise rather than either diet or exercise alone. A combination of exercise and caloric restriction can initiate up to 20% more weight and fat loss, improved function and reduced FFM loss than modification of diet alone (Rankin, 2013).

Combined exercise and dietary restriction for improving body composition in obesity

A combination of dietary restriction and physical activity is recommended to stimulate the required 3,500 kcal energy deficit for meaningful weight loss (American College of Sports Medicine, 2010; Hill et al., 2012). Therefore, expending 250 kcal through physical activity and/or exercise and limiting dietary intake by 250 kcal daily would enable a weight loss of one pound per week (American College of Sports Medicine, 2010). Imayama et al. (2012) found superior results in those undertaking a combined intervention than a diet or exercise intervention alone, leading to a 10.8% weight loss, 7.0 cm reduction in waist circumference and 5.9% reduction in percentage body fat.

Miller et al. (2013) systematically reviewed 14 studies and looked at the effects of exercise training in addition to energy restriction on functional capacities and body composition in adults with obesity during weight loss; they concluded that energy restriction with the addition of exercise training improves body composition and fitness. It is clear that the inclusion of exercise is important to accompany hypocaloric diets to aid improvements in body composition specifically limiting FFM loss. Research has examined specific types of exercise and dietary adjustment and identified a significant increase in FFM when combining resistance exercise with a high protein diet, as opposed to implementing both factors independently (Verreijen, 2017). When using diet and exercise as a means to lose weight, it is important to set realistic and attainable goals to ensure the weight loss is maintainable, prevent injury and prevent relapse. Clark et al. (2015) report that dietary restriction alone, without either resistance or endurance training, is less effective than a combination of both at inducing the energy deficit important for body composition improvements in people with overweight and obesity in both sexes.

Exercise and obesity-related co-morbidities

Apart from the increased morbidity and mortality risk associated with obesity, the accumulation of excess body fat and central adiposity contribute to common co-morbidities (Jarolimova et al., 2013). Common obesity-related co-morbidities includes T2DM, CVD, hypertension, dyslipidaemia, osteoarthritis, obstructive sleep apnoea, non-alcoholic fatty liver disease and depression (Colquitt et al., 2009; Nguyen & Lau, 2012). Weight loss can improve general health by reversing and preventing these obesity-associated co-morbidities (Welbourne et al., 2014). Research shows lifestyle interventions with a physical activity component or structured exercise programme in classes I, II and III obesity improves co-morbidities in adults with obesity, specifically T2DM, hypertension, hyperlipidemia, sleep apnoea, osteoarthritis, asthma and depression (Baillot et al., 2015; Freitas et al., 2018).

When considering the four-tiered approach to obesity, bariatric surgery combined with long-term lifestyle modification is currently the most effective and sustainable method of weight loss for people with morbid obesity, improving co-morbidities and mortality, and has been readily researched (Madura & Dibaise, 2012). A systematic review of 136 studies (22,094 participants) examined co-morbidity resolution or improvement as a result of weight loss induced by bariatric surgery, concluding that 86% of people with T2DM, 70% of those with hyperlipidaemia, 79% of hypertensive patients, and 8% of sleep apnoea sufferers experienced improvement or complete resolution (Buchwald et al., 2004). Therefore, if exercise facilitates weight loss and maintenance regardless of the weight loss method undertaken, it is an important factor in the resolution of co-morbidities. However, considerations must be made when exercising with co-morbidities and medications, especially those that may affect vision, sensation, heart rate, blood pressure and blood glucose levels (McQueen, 2009).

Recommendations for fitness testing and exercise programming for people with obesity

Risk assessment and medical history

It is essential to follow due diligence in terms of risk assessment and medical history prior to any fitness testing or exercise programming, in particular for obesity. This is because there may be other medicated and/or non-medicated co-morbidities that may affect what exercise to prescribe. Here are some examples;

Example 1: An individual is referred for supervised exercise because of they are with obesity. After assessing their medical history, taking their blood pressure and discussing their medications, it becomes apparent that they have hypertension, yet they have not been prescribed any related medications. If this individual were to exercise before their blood pressure was well managed/stable, this could increase the risk of a cardiovascular-related incident. In this case, the individual should be referred back to the GP and re-referred to the ERS when blood pressure– associated risks are mitigated.

The individual is re-referred back to the ERS and deemed safe to exercise. However, due to their hypertension, heavy weight lifting, over gripping and breath holding (Valsalva) would be avoided, and dynamic exercises using large muscle groups would be recommended.

Example 2: An individual with T2DM (which regularly accompanies obesity) is referred for supervised exercise. The exercise instructor was made aware of this after discussing their medical history and recording medications. With T2DM comes additional complications, such as diabetic neuropathy; in this case, the exercise programming should avoid increasing the individual's blood pressure too high initially, therefore avoiding high-intensity exercise.

Example 3: An individual presenting with morbid obesity has diagnosed osteoarthritis in both knees. They would like their exercise programme to help them lose weight and help alleviate their osteoarthritis symptoms. To begin with, it would be more suitable to perform aerobic exercise on a recumbent bike than a treadmill, whilst light resistance exercises would be used to improve muscle strength and range of movement around the arthritic joints.

Exercise testing and assessment in people with obesity

It is important that measurements of physical function (e.g. cardiorespiratory fitness and muscle strength) are determined at the beginning of any exercise prescription, firstly to gain an idea of the individual's starting ability and secondly to set a starting benchmark that can be improved on or checked for regressions. These measurements should be repeated regularly, typically midway and after completion of an exercise programme, as the feedback can be used as a motivational tool and tangible functional measurement for the individual to see their progress.

Aerobic fitness testing

If the equipment and facilities are available, an aerobic fitness test to determine oxygen consumption should be undertaken for screening purposes, as well as a baseline indication of cardiorespiratory fitness. VO_2max is the maximum rate of oxygen consumption measured during incremental exercise. For people with obesity and morbid obesity, it is vital that the protocol and exercise equipment be chosen carefully since treadmills dedicated to undertaking VO_2max tests usually have greater weight limits than bikes.

There are different graded treadmill exercise tests such as the Balke, Bruce, Ellestad and modified Astrand (Beltz et al., 2016; Bryant et al., 2014). The two commonly used protocols in healthcare are outlined next.

1. The Balke protocol maintains a constant treadmill speed and increases the gradient every minute for males or every three minutes for females.

   Male – Treadmill speed set at 3.3 mph; treadmill gradient start point is 0%. After one minute, the gradient is raised to a 2% incline and is increased by 1% each minute thereafter.

Female – Treadmill speed set at 3.0 mph; treadmill gradient start point is 0%. After one minute, the gradient is raised to a 2.5% incline and is increased by 2.5% every three minutes thereafter.

Maximum oxygen uptake value (ml/min):
Men $VO_2max = 1.444$ (time) + 14.99
Women $VO_2max = 1.38$ (time) + 5.22

2. The Bruce protocol increases gradient and speed every three minutes, regardless of gender.

   Stage 1 = 1.7 mph at 10% gradient
   Stage 2 = 2.5 mph at 12% gradient
   Stage 3 = 3.4 mph at 14% gradient
   Stage 4 = 4.2 mph at 16% gradient
   Stage 5 = 5.0 mph at 18% gradient
   Stage 6 = 5.5 mph at 20% gradient
   Stage 7 = 6.0 mph at 22% gradient
   Stage 8 = 6.5 mph at 24% gradient
   Stage 9 = 7.0 mph at 26% gradient

Previous exercise intervention research has used the Balke protocol and electrocardiogram (ECG) monitoring for screening people with morbid obesity before undertaking combined aerobic and resistance supervised and structured exercise training (Herring et al., 2017). Although maximal exercise testing is limited by availability of equipment as well as willingness of the individual, the Balke protocol is likely the best option as it maintains a constant speed (typically walking). The impact of walking exercise is less than that of jogging, thus allowing the individuals to get as close to maximal exercise as possible. The Balke protocol can also be adapted and performed on a cycle ergometer if necessary.

Maximum oxygen uptake value (L/min):

Men $VO_2max = 14.8 - (1.379 \times T) + (0.451 \times T^2) - (0.012 \times T^3)$
Women $VO_2max = 4.38 \times T - 3.9$
*T = Total time on the treadmill measured as a fraction of a minute (e.g. a test time of 9 minutes 30 seconds would be written as T = 9.5).

Limitations of VO_2max testing include the incremental exercise protocol not being a familiar form of physical activity for the individual as well as the individual's willingness to exercise to max, particularly if they are inactive and with high sedentary behaviour. Having appropriately trained individuals to conduct the test, motivate the individual and interpret the results is essential (Lewis et al., 2001).

Incremental Shuttle Walk Test (ISWT)

As a safe alternative to treadmill testing, the ISWT is a valid symptom-limited maximal and progressive test of functional capacity that correlates strongly with VO_2max values attained during cardiorespiratory testing on a treadmill and is used across different clinical populations. Cardiac and respiratory specialisms use this test as part of exercise rehabilitation services

(Lewis et al., 2001; Revill et al., 1999; Singh et al., 1994). The test involves walking consecutive ten-metre shuttles in time with an audible beep that becomes progressively faster until the participant is no longer able to maintain the required pace.

The test has a total of 12 one-minute levels (total distance: 1,020 metres). Individuals should perform a practice ISWT before the 'true test' to minimise the influence of learning effects. Individuals are asked to walk for as long as possible until reaching the test termination criteria whilst the assessor records the number of shuttles performed (Lewis et al., 2001; Revill et al., 1999). The termination criteria include failure to reach the cone in the allocated time (more than 0.5m away from the cone when the beep sounds), if oxygen saturation (SpO_2) falls below 80%, if the individual is unable to continue, excessive dyspnea, fatigue and pain).

The individual should remain in the clinical area for at least 15 minutes following the test, when measures of blood pressure, oxygen saturation, rating of perceived exertion (RPE Borg scale) and breathlessness (the modified Borg dyspnoea scale) are taken. The ISWT is not currently validated in people with obesity, but it is being used successfully in this population, and systematic reviews report the ISWT as a valid and reliable test to assess exercise capacity in clinical populations (Herring, Stevinson et al., 2017; Herring, Stevinson, Davies et al., 2016; Herring, Wagstaff et al., 2014; Parreira et al., 2014). The ISWT in clinical populations has been validated against VO_2max and VO_2peak (MacSween et al., 2001; Parreira et al., 2014). Clinical populations also show a linear relationship between the number of shuttles completed and functional capacity (MacSween et al., 2001).

The limitations of the ISWT include finding a big enough space for the test to be conducted over the ten-metre course. It must be conducted twice the first time it is completed, and the individual supervising should have conducted the appropriate training before completing it. The advantages do, however, outweigh the limitations in people with obesity; the ISWT is easily undertaken in the field and is a more familiar form of physical activity if the person can do so as it reflects walking, an activity required for ambulation. The ISWT test is cheap in application, does not require much equipment and requires no face mask; its result is ready immediately after completion; and the general population can understand the outcome as the performance in the test is reported as a distance in metres.

Unfortunately, VO_2max testing is expensive and rarely available in the field where exercise programmes may be delivered. Therefore, there are equations for estimating VO_2max in the absence of available equipment (Bryant et al., 2014), and other alternatives are provided hereafter.

Sit-to-stand test

The five times sit-to-stand test is an objective measurement indicative of functional lower limb muscle strength, dynamic balance and functional mobility (Goldberg et al., 2012; Whitney et al., 2005). This test also reflects common activities of daily living and has previously been used in people with obesity before and after prescribed exercise (Herring et al., 2017).

Participants should start seated on a standard chair with their arms folded across their chest. They are then instructed to stand up and sit down five times as quickly as they can upon the command 'Go'. If the individual achieves all five sit-to-stand movements, record the time this was achieved in. If the individual did not manage five, how many they completed should be recorded as well as the duration taken.

The testing chair should remain at a consistent height at each assessment and be appropriate for people with obesity (e.g. check weight restrictions; chair height should ensure a 90° angle at the knee when in a seated position and no lower). The advantages of this measurement are that it is familiar to transitioning in and out of a chair for those who can do so, it can be undertaken in the field and it is cheap to perform with minimal equipment.

Handgrip strength test

Grip strength, another low-cost indicator of muscle strength and function which focuses on the upper body, has been shown to change as a result of exercise (Roberts et al., 2011). Grip strength has been shown to improve as a result of combined aerobic and resistance programmes as well as resistance exercise interventions initiated in people with obesity (Huck, 2014; Stegen et al., 2011).

When performing this functional measurement, participants should stand with their arms down by their sides with a slight bend at the elbow and, when directed, squeeze the grip strength dynamometer with as much force as possible. The score in kilograms (kg) should be noted after each measurement. A pause of 10 to 20 seconds should occur between repetitions, and the test should be repeated three times on both sides in order to calculate an average score.

The advantages include its straightforward nature and the minimal equipment required; it can be undertaken anywhere and is cheap to perform after a one-off payment for the dynamometer.

Physical activity and exercise programming in people with obesity

The FITT (frequency, intensity, time and type of exercise) principal should be considered when exercise programming for people with obesity, thus outlining how often one should exercise, how long for, the type of exercise to undertake and at what intensity this exercise should be performed in order to encourage engagement and adherence with the programme. If the volume or intensity is too high, this can lead to fatigue, soreness and dropout. If too low, then the programme may not stimulate changes to weight loss–related or other health outcomes, which can be demotivating.

Physical activity volume

It is suggested that all adults should aim to meet current general physical activity guidelines of 150 minutes of moderate-intensity (or 75 minutes of vigorous-intensity) physical activity weekly, undertake muscle strengthening exercises on at least two days weekly and reduce sedentary time for health benefits (Department of Health, 2019). Unfortunately there are no globally recognised physical activity guidelines for weight loss and weight maintenance for people with overweight and obesity, although the American College of Sports Medicine (ACSM) (2010) has published some.

To the authors' knowledge, there are no structured and consistent physical activity/exercise guidelines for weight loss programmes for differing levels of obesity or across the four levels of the treatment pathway previously mentioned. Nor are there any official physical activity guidelines for before or after undergoing bariatric surgery for weight loss maintenance.

In the UK, official guidelines are needed to standardise the care provided nationwide across the four tiers of obesity to optimise body composition outcomes at varying levels of obesity. Recommendations and advice for such services and weight loss exist; however, these vary depending on the institution and can be very vague (American College of Sports Medicine, 2010; National Institute for Health and Care Excellence, 2014a, 2014b).

NICE guidance for people with overweight or obesity reports limited physical activity instruction or direction for multicomponent lifestyle services (typically Tiers 2 and 3 weight management and sometimes Tier 4 support pre-/post-surgery); such advice includes discussing the importance and benefits of incorporating physical activity long term, teaching safe physical activity and behaviour-change strategies, promoting the sustainability of increased physical activity (e.g. walking) and reduced sedentary behaviour and signposting to local services. Collecting a physical activity outcome should be considered, ensuring any supervised physical activity is supervised by an appropriately qualified individual and taking medical conditions into consideration. Donnelly et al. (2009) reports a dose-response relationship between physical activity and both weight loss and weight loss maintenance, inferring that the more physical activity undertaken, the better the weight loss outcome (American College of Sports Medicine, 2010; Donnelly et al., 2009).

NICE currently recommends that health professionals 'advise people who have been obese and have lost weight to perform 60–90 minutes of moderate intensity activity a day to avoid regaining weight' (National Institute for Health and Care Excelence, 2014), whilst the ACSM have more specific recommendations, suggesting varying amounts of moderate-intensity physical activity, depending on an individual's weight- or health-related goal (Donnelly et al., 2009; Haskell et al., 2007). These weekly recommendations include 150 minutes for maintaining and improving health, 150 to 250 minutes for the prevention of weight gain, 200 to 300 minutes to prevent weight gain after weight loss and 225 to 420 minutes to promote clinically significant weight loss (American College of Sports Medicine, 2010; Donnelly et al., 2009).

It would be beneficial for the UK to develop standardised guidelines for the delivery of multicomponent/multidisciplinary weight management services which incorporate supervised and structured physical activity based on currently availible evidence and best practice of what works. Current national recomendations need to recognise that exercise advice alone is insufficient for improving health-related fitness parameters for optimising body composition (Herring, Stevinson et al., 2017; Herring, Wagstaff et al., 2014; Royal College of Physicians, 2013).

The following ACSM recommendations for supervised moderate-intensity physical activity durations could be incorporated into the UK's four-tiered approach to weight management:

Tier 1–150–250 minutes per week for the prevention of weight gain
Tier 2–225–420 minutes per week to promote clinically significant weight loss
Tier 3–225–420 minutes per week to promote clinically significant weight loss
Tier 4 – Pre-surgery – 225–420 minutes per week to promote clinically significant weight loss

Post-surgery – 200–300 minutes per week to prevent weight gain after weight loss.

To maintain motivation, it is important when recommending physical activity to start at a realistic level (frequency and duration of the exercise session) and gradually progress the frequency of activity. Hence, starting at the lower end of the recommended duration is important (5 * 30 minute exercise sessions). However, for some with obesity, this is still unrealistic and unattainable, so just building more low-intensity physical activity into daily life, such as moving around the house more, standing instead of sitting and walking around the garden, are important to start at a realistic, participant-specific duration and frequency and work towards any recommendations.

Warm up and cool down

A progressive warm up should always precede the main body of an exercise programme and last a minimum of five to ten minutes. The warm-up should progress from a low to moderate intensity to prevent overexertion, followed by flexibility exercise and preparing the body for the main part of the session (American College of Sports Medicine, 2011). A cool-down should be undertaken at the end of every session for a minimum duration of five to ten minutes, to gradually return the body and heart rate back to pre-exercising levels (American College of Sports Medicine, 2011).

Exercise intensity

Moderate-intensity aerobic and resistance exercise can be performed and is tolerable by people with obesity due to its safe nature, its ability to be performed in different environments and the increased likelihood of it being sustainable whilst helping promote exercise self-management.

According to the ACSM (2010) moderate-intensity aerobic exercise is expressed as between 64% and 77% of maximum heart rate (12–14 RPE on the 6–20 Borg scale). Moderate intensity for resistance exercises is expressed as 60% of the participant's estimated one-repetition maximum. The resistance for this relative intensity can be identified by performing the exercise at a weight where 17 repetitions are possible as 17 repetitions equate to 60% of the one-repetition maximum (Williams et al., 2007). Eight to twelve repetitions equate to 70% to 80% of one repetition maximum (Williams et al., 2007).

Exercise intensity monitoring

Exercise intensity can be expressed either as a percentage of maximum heart rate (%HRmax), as a percentage of heart rate reserve (%HRR)/VO_2reserve) or as a rating of perceived exertion (RPE). These can all be estimated using predetermined equations and imputing certain variables measured directly from the individual. Alternatively, and more accurately, %HRmax can be accurately derived from the successful completion of an aerobic fitness test and is the desired measurement for monitoring exercise intensity if facilities for monitoring heart rate are available.

If heart rate measurements are used, it is important for the individuals undertaking exercise to also understand the equivalent rating of perceived exertion level. This will help them understand at what level to exercise once the supervised and prescribed exercise is completed. Therefore, using an exercise intensity chart such as Figure 10.2 can be useful.

Example client
Age of client = 30
Age-predicted HR_{max} (220- 30) = 190 bpm

% HR_{max}	Beats per minute (bpm)	Rating of perceived exertion (RPE)
		7 Very, very light
		8
		9 Very light
57%	108	10
		11 Fairly Light
64%	122	12
70%	133	13 Somewhat hard
77%	146	14
		15 Hard
84%	160	16
91%	173	17 Very hard
		18
96%	182	19 Very, very hard
100%	190	20

Adapted from (American College of Sports Medicine (ACSM), 2010)

FIGURE 10.2 An example exercise intensity chart for exercise prescription: A visible comparison of heart rate boundaries and RPE to promote self-management

Source: Adapted from American College of Sports Medicine, 2010)

Practitioners need to be mindful, if a client is taking HR-lowering medication because one of their co-morbidities is hypertension, that RPE must be used. RPE can also be used when undertaking any form of physical activity incorporated into daily living, enabling individuals to self-manage their physical activity when not supervised, notwithstanding the importance of 'feeling OK'. If the end user doesn't feel 'OK', then they will get little out of the session.

It is important to start at a lower level if moderate intensity is not achievable, then gradually build up. However, increases in duration or frequency should always precede increases in intensity (McQueen, 2009).

Type

Selecting the type of exercise is important when prescribing exercise for people with obesity to encourage body composition improvements. Exercise type and mode are important predictors of fat-mass loss and FFM gain in obesity-related exercise intervention research

(Hansen et al., 2007). There is an increasing amount of research investigating aerobic and resistance exercise training on body composition in people with obesity.

Aerobic versus resistance exercise

Regardless of type whether it's aerobic or resistance training, compared to exercise education alone, research shows the addition of supervised and structured exercise to a MDT weight management programme significantly improves anthropometric, functional and psychological measures in people with obesity with a BMI ≥ 35 kg·m^2 (Herring et al., 2014). However, contrary to this, another study found that aerobic exercise contributes more to weight loss and improved cardiopulmonary fitness in individuals with obesity than anaerobic exercise (Al Saif & Alsenany, 2015). Both research studies completed different type of anaerobic training, with Al Saif and Alsenany (2015) getting participants to undertake anaerobic training on the treadmill, whereas Herring et al. (2014) got participants to complete a resistance training programme in a local gym to mimic a real-life setting. Regardless, the improvements in muscular strength, power and endurance caused by resistance exercise positively affect the functional tasks of daily living (C. T. Miller et al., 2013).

Herring et al. (2014) undertook a RCT investigating the efficacy of a 12-week supervised and structured aerobic versus resistance training programme in people with obesity referred to a multidisciplinary weight management service for morbid obesity. They found that after undertaking a 12-week supervised training programme, both aerobic and resistance training positively affected health-related fitness parameters. Furthermore, they reported that previously untrained individuals undertaking a resistance exercise programme experience early adaptations typically associated with aerobic training, such as an increase in aerobic fitness and functional capacity.

When recommending a combined aerobic and resistance training exercise programme, a warm-up, cool down and flexibility exercises should also be incorporated. The types of exercise being performed should be appropriate for the individual's size and co-morbidity status to ensure that motivation is maintained. The last repetition of each set (between 8 and 15 repetitions for two or three sets) should result in volitional fatigue to achieve these benefits (McQueen, 2009). For superior results, resistance exercises that target large muscle groups should be the main focus in this population. Functional capacity and any relevant co-morbidities should also be taken into consideration.

Adapting exercise for people with obesity

There are few obesity-related contraindications for exercise; the predominant contraindications arise depending on the severity of obesity and when individuals present one or more co-morbidities associated with obesity (Table 10.5).

Exercise supervision

It is well noted that supervised exercise has superior outcomes to non-supervised exercise in people with obesity, and exercise education alone is insufficient to prevent declines in health-related fitness parameters indicative of tasks for daily living (Herring et al., 2014; Nicolai et al., 2009). All weight management or weight loss services should incorporate a supervised

TABLE 10.5 The main considerations to be aware of when prescribing exercise for people with obesity

Areas of consideration	*Obesity considerations for exercise*
Functional/ physiological	Avoid high-impact exercises
	Full weight-bearing activities should be carefully considered*
	Take careful consideration when prescribing floor exercise*
	Thermoregulation difficulties
	Avoid agility exercises*
	Caution to avoid overuse injuries
Motivational	Avoid starting at a higher level than necessary
	Agree on realistic SMART goals
	Vary the exercises and exercise sessions
	Incorporate activity into lifestyle and make it convenient for the individual
Safety	Supportive clothing and footwear
	Check equipment weight restrictions
	Prescribe the correct exercise intensity
	Prevent exacerbating any current or previous injuries
	Take into consideration any co-morbidities
	Ensure an appropriate exercise environment

Key: *Take into consideration the individual's size and co-morbidity status

and structured physical activity element to optimise their participants' health-related outcomes and provide a more effective holistic approach to weight loss. During supervised exercise, the motivational skills and professional, supportive and friendly nature of the instructor contribute to the success, adherence and improved motivation of the participant (N. H. Williams et al., 2007). It is unclear how or if exercise is maintained after such programmes, and long-term maintenance for continued participation is important. Consequently, it is important to supervise and progress the programme in a way that individuals learn and prepare to self-manage their exercise.

Case study

A 55-year-old lady attends an appointment with her GP as a result of excessive weight gain, increased knee pain and wanting to discuss bariatric surgery. Approximately two years ago, she was diagnosed with T2DM and categorised as being with obesity (BMI 34 $kg.m^2$), which she wanted to self-manage. Other co-morbidities included depression, hypercholesterolemia and stable hypertension. She was inactive due to not meeting the physical activity guidelines, sat for more than ten hours per day and had a high calorific diet.

On the recent visit, the GP checked her BMI, fasting blood glucose, glycated hemoglobin (HbA_{1c}), blood pressure and full lipid profile. The lady's BMI had increased to 42 $kg.m^2$, and all blood-related markers had worsened. Consequently, the GP adjusted her medications accordingly and wanted to refer her to a weight management programme.

The lady has previously attended numerous commercial weight loss services, losing significant amounts of weight but with weight regain occurring within six months every time. Taking these factors into consideration, her GP refers her to the local multidisciplinary NHS Tier 3 weight management service, which includes the supervision and provision of a structured physical activity programme.

This NHS Tier 3 weight management service is one of few that offers supervised and structured physical activity programmes combined with a medical assessment, psychological support and dietary advice. Focusing solely on physical activity, an initial assessment was undertaken by the exercise specialist. This assessment is designed to assess risk, obtain a medical history and current medication, take necessary measurements and discuss the participant's expectations (goals), confidence and readiness to participate in such a programme.

As the lady had shown a willingness to participate in supervised and structured exercise, baseline physical functional measurements were obtained and an exercise programme developed. The exercise programme will last for 12 weeks and will be supervised in a community gymnasium with standard equipment.

TASK – State the fitness assessment you will undertake as well as the timing and develop the 12-week exercise programme.

When developing an exercise programme for this individual, please consider the following:

- You should select which functional measurements are most appropriate and when they will be assessed.
- You should write an exercise programme using the FITT principle, taking into consideration her size, co-morbidities, goals, current ability level and facilities available.
- You should outline how this will be monitored and progressed throughout the 12-week programme.

Important considerations for physical activity and exercise programming in weight management interventions for people with obesity

The following are examples of key considerations when trying to increase physical activity and exercise in people with obesity as part of weight management interventions:

- Assess readiness to be more active and use a variety of behaviour change techniques.
- Identify barriers and any anxiety or body image issues and support your client to overcome them.
- Identify any previous negative experiences and raise confidence as demanded.
- If possible, minimise sensations of displeasure – adherence is a prerequisite for success, and people usually avoid activities they find overly aversive.

- Understand that intermittent activity may be more manageable for those with a very high BMI even if it is of low intensity and sporadic throughout the day.
- Undertake appropriate fitness testing and assessment of functional performance at baseline to inform goal setting. Repeat regularly to monitor changes and make suitable adaptions to the programme.
- Identify and work with the client's own goals, not what you think they should be.
- Start simple, progress gradually and safely, but do not stereotype into gentler activities to avoid stigma.
- Clients may have low physical work capacity due to excess weight as well as poor joint mobility and balance.
- Consider how having co-morbidities such as joint pain, hypertension and type 2 diabetes can influence the physical activity programme.
- Use non-weight-bearing activities if impact is an issue and have an injury prevention strategy.
- Consider if the exercise equipment available is fit for purpose due to body size and shape. Modify the equipment or avoid fixed resistance machines if needed.
- Have a good understanding of the client's medications (e.g. orlistat) and side effects that may lead to flatulence and/or faecal urgency. Openly discuss these in preparation for any events.
- Total energy expenditure is key, and how the client achieves this is largely up to them. Asking the question 'Tell me about the physical activities or sports you currently or used to enjoy' will encourage discussion.
- Support clients to understand their responses to physical activity and exercise – what is 'normal' for them?
- To manage expectations, make it clear that everyone is different, and responses will vary.
- Inform your client it is likely that other health outcomes will be improving, even in the event of no weight loss.

Summary

Obesity is a complex 'chronic, relapsing, progressive disease process' which needs immediate action to manage the global epidemic. Increasing obesity and morbid obesity levels are contributing to significant cardio-metabolic complications, higher rates of obesity-related diseases, reductions in HRQOL and reductions in physical function. The importance of and need for MDT services for reducing the obesity burden and its associated co-morbidities are increasing. A four-tiered obesity care pathway has been developed to manage the differing levels of overweight and obesity in the UK, but unfortunately, physical activity and exercise are often overlooked in such services, possibly due to misrepresentation in mainstream media and research findings being taken out of context.

Physical activity and exercise should be important parts of any weight loss journey. The main objective in the treatment of obesity is to increase energy expenditure during the normal daily routine. A combined moderate-intensity aerobic and resistance training programme facilitates fat-mass reduction and helps preserve FFM, ultimately helping sustain RMR (important for weight loss). It is important to start at a lower level if moderate intensity is not achievable.

Before beginning any exercise programme, it is important to have an initial session to assess risk, obtain a medical history and current medication, take necessary measurements and discuss the participant's expectations (goals), confidence and readiness to participate in such a programme. The exercises and activities selected should be chosen carefully to ensure they are appropriate for the individual's ability, size and co-morbidity status, but fundamentally, they should reflect the client's personal preference. Contraindications of exercise for obesity and any relevant co-morbidities also need to be taken into consideration and are important to progress supervised exercise programmes in a way that individuals learn and prepare to self-manage their exercise and maintain it long term.

Key points

- There are numerous interventions and different services available throughout the UK to manage obesity. These services, however, vary nationwide, and there are no standardised guidelines for the promotion of physical activity in these services.
- Research shows that fat mass, FFM, strength and aerobic capacity reduce when weight loss is induced through hypocaloric diets alone. Therefore, preservation of FFM whilst maximising fat-mass loss is a goal of obesity treatments, which can be achieved with the inclusion of exercise as part of a weight management programme.
- The severity of obesity, previous weight loss attempts and type of weight loss intervention accompanying the exercise performed are some factors that may dictate how the body responds to exercise.
- It is suggested that for clinically significant weight loss (5%), 225 to 420 minutes of moderate-intensity physical activity should be undertaken weekly. To maintain motivation, it is important, when deciding on the initial dose, to start at a realistic patient-specific level regardless of recommendations and gradually build up. Increases in duration or frequency should precede increases in intensity.
- There are few obesity-related contraindications for exercise, with the predominant contraindications depending on the severity of an individual's obesity or the presentation of one or more obesity-related co-morbidities.

TABLE 10.6 At-a-glance summary guide to exercise considerations for people with obesity

Pathophysiology summary	Obesity occurs as a result of excessive weight gain when the body's energy store of fat exceeds its expenditure. The main causes of overweight and obesity are inactivity, increased sedentary behaviour and/or increased calorie consumption.
Aims of exercise	The aim of exercise in the treatment of obesity is to expend more calories than one would in their normal daily routine and increase total daily energy expenditure. Increasing physical activity positively affects energy balance when avoiding the ingestion of additional calories to compensate for those expended. A combination of aerobic and resistance training is the optimal type of exercise to facilitate fat-mass reduction and increase fat free mass, respectively.

Exercise considerations (including contraindications)	There are few obesity-related contraindications for exercise or factors to consider. The predominant contraindications arise depending on the severity of obesity (e.g. increased risk of joint injury), environmental conditions (e.g. an increased risk of dehydration) and when individuals present one or more co-morbidities associated with obesity.
Frequency	Frequency of exercise depends on the individual's ability, severity of obesity and co-morbidity status, but the end goal is to be active every day and to break up sedentary behaviour often. It is very important to maintaining motivation in this population when prescribing exercise to start at a realistic level (frequency and duration of the exercise session) and gradually progress.
Intensity	Moderate-intensity exercise is recommended, but low-intensity physical activity can also lead to beneficial health and fitness outcomes in those who are severely deconditioned. People with obesity should not be stereotyped into doing gentler activities, and high intensity is safe as long as appropriate risk assessment and screening has taken place.
Time	Duration of exercise depends on the individual's ability, severity of obesity and co-morbidity status. Hence, starting at the lower end of the recommended duration is important. 225 to 420 minutes per week is suggested to promote clinically significant weight loss. A starting point of 5 * 45 minute exercise sessions for some individuals with obesity is still unrealistic and unattainable; it is therefore important to start at a realistic, participant-specific duration and frequency and work towards the 225- to 420-minute-per-week recommendation.
Type	Aerobic and resistance exercise
Common medications associated	Orlistat.
Key safety considerations	Orlistat can cause faecal urgency.
Effect of exercise on conditions	A combination of both moderate-intensity aerobic and resistance exercise of sufficient frequency contributes to the following aspects of obesity: • Increases the energy expenditure necessary for reducing body fat • Decreases abdominal, subcutaneous and visceral fat • Preserves/increase FFM for optimising RMR • Improves psychological parameters and quality of life Conserving FFM during weight loss is important to maintain RMR in people with obesity, and exercise, regardless of type, needs to be incorporated into the weight loss programmes.

References

Al Saif, A., & Alsenany, S. (2015). Aerobic and anaerobic exercise training in obese adults. *Journal of Physical Therapy Science*, *27*(6), 1697–1700. doi: 10.1589/jpts.27.1697.

American College of Sports Medicine (ACSM). (2010). *ACSM's resource manual for guidelines for exercise testing and prescription* (6th ed.). Baltimore: Lippincott Williams & Wilkins.

American College of Sports Medicine (ACSM). (2011). *Complete guide to fitness & health* (B. Bushman, Ed.) Physical Activity and Nutrition Guidelines for Every Age. Champaign, IL: Human Kinetics.

Baillot, A., Romain, A. J., Boisvert-Vigneault, K., Audet, M., Baillargeon, J. P., Dionne, I. J., . . . Langlois, M. F. (2015). Effects of lifestyle interventions that include a physical activity component in class II and III obese individuals: A systematic review and meta-analysis. *PLoS One, 10*(4), e0119017. doi: 10.1371/journal.pone.0119017.

Barba, C., Cavalli-Sforza, T., Cutter, J., Darnton-Hill, I., Deurenberg, P., Deurenberg-Yap, M., . . . Zimmet, P. (2004). Appropriate body-mass index for Asian populations and its implications for policy and intervention strategies. *The Lancet, 363*(9403), 157–163. doi: 10.1016/S0140-6736(03)15268-3.

Beltz, N. M., Gibson, A. L., Janot, J. M., Kravitz, L., Mermier, C. M., & Dalleck, L. C. (2016). Graded exercise testing protocols for the determination of VO2max: Historical perspectives, progress, and future considerations. *British Journal of Sports Medicine (Hindawi Publ Corp), 2016*, 3968393. doi: 10.1155/2016/3968393.

Blackshaw, J., Montel, S., King, S., Jarvis, A., & Valabhji, J. (2014). *Report of the working group into: Joined up clinical pathways for obesity*. NHS England Publications. Retrieved from www.england.nhs.uk/wp-content/uploads/2014/03/owg-join-clinc-path.pdf.

Booth, H. P., Prevost, A. T., & Gulliford, M. C. (2015). Access to weight reduction interventions for overweight and obese patients in UK primary care: Population-based cohort study. *British Medical Journal Open, 5*(1), 1–7. doi: 10.1136/bmjopen-2014-006642.

Bray, G. A., Kim, K. K., & Wilding, J. P. H. (2017). Obesity: a chronic relapsing progressive disease process. A position statement of the world obesity federation. *Obesity Reviews, 18*(7), 715–723. doi: 10.1111/obr.12551.

Bryant, C. X., Newton-Merrill, S., Green, D. J., & American Council on Exercise (Eds.). (2014). *ACE personal trainer manual* (5th ed.). San Diego, CA: American Council on Exercise.

Buchwald, H., Avidor, Y., Braunwald, E., et al. (2004). Bariatric surgery: A systematic review and meta-analysis. *The Journal of the American Medical Association, 292*(14), 1724–1737. doi: 10.1001/jama.292.14.1724.

Calbet, J. A. L., Ponce-Gonzalez, J. G., Calle-Herrero, J., Perez-Suarez, I., Martin-Rincon, M., Santana, A., . . . Holmberg, H. C. (2017). Exercise preserves lean mass and performance during severe energy deficit: The role of exercise volume and dietary protein content. *Front Physiol, 8*, 483. doi: 10.3389/fphys.2017.00483.

Capodaglio, P., Castelnuovo, G., Brunani, A., Vismara, L., Villa, V., & Capodaglio, E. M. (2010). Functional limitations and occupational issues in obesity: A review. *International Journal of Occupational Safety and Ergonomics, 16*(4), 507–523.

Clark, J. E. (2015). Diet, exercise or diet with exercise: Comparing the effectiveness of treatment options for weight-loss and changes in fitness for adults (18–65 years old) who are overfat, or obese; systematic review and meta-analysis. *Journal of Diabetes and Metabolic Disorders, 14*, 31. doi: 10.1186/s40200-015-0154-1.

Coen, P. M., & Goodpaster, B. H. (2015). A role for exercise after bariatric surgery? *Diabetes, Obesity and Metabolism*. doi: 10.1111/dom.12545.

Colquitt, J. L., Picot, J., Loveman, E., & Clegg, A. J. (2009). Surgery for obesity. *Cochrane Database of Systematic Reviews, 15*(2), 1–243.

Curioni, C. C., & Lourenco, P. M. (2005). Long-term weight loss after diet and exercise: A systematic review. *International Journal of Obesity and Related Metabolic Disorders, 29*(10), 1168–1174.

Dent, M., Chrisopoulos, S., Mulhall, C., & Ridler, C. (2010). *Bariatric surgery for obesity*. Oxford: National Obesity Observatory.

Department of Health. (2013). *Developing a specification for lifestyle weight management services: Best practice guidance for tier 2 services*. London: Department of Health, Retrieved from www.gov.uk/government/uploads/system/uploads/attachment_data/file/142723/Weight_Management_Service_Spec_FINAL_with_IRB.pdf.

Department of Health. (2019). *UK Chief medical officers' physical activity guidelines*. London: TSO.

Donnelly, J. E., Blair, S. N., Jakicic, J. M., Manore, M. M., Rankin, J. W., & Smith, B. K. (2009). American college of sports medicine position stand. Appropriate physical activity intervention strategies for weight loss and prevention of weight regain for adults. *Medicine & Science in Sports & Exercise, 41*(2), 459–471. doi: 10.1249/MSS.0b013e3181949333.

Dorling, J., Broom, D. R., Burns, S. F., Clayton, D. J., Deighton, K., James, L. J, . . . Stensel, D. J. (2018). Acute and chronic effects of exercise on appetite, energy intake, and appetite-related hormones: The modulating effect of adiposity, sex, and habitual physical activity. *Nutrients, 10*(9). doi: 10.3390/nu10091140.

Duval, K., Marceau, P., Lescelleur, O., Hould, F. S., Marceau, S., Biron, S., . . . Lacasse, Y. (2006). Health-related quality of life in morbid obesity. *Obesity Surgery, 16*(5), 574–579.

Egberts, K., Brown, W. A., Brennan, L., & O'Brien, P. E. (2012). Does exercise improve weight loss after bariatric surgery? A systematic review. *Obesity Surgery, 22*(2), 335–341.

Eijsvogels, T. M., Veltmeijer, M. T., Schreuder, T. H., Poelkens, F., Thijssen, D. H., & Hopman, M. T. (2011). The impact of obesity on physiological responses during prolonged exercise. *International Journal of Obesity (Lond), 35*(11), 1404–1412. doi: 10.1038/ijo.2010.277.

Foster-Schubert, K. E., Alfano, C. M., Duggan, C. R., Xiao, L., Campbell, K. L., Kong, A., . . . McTiernan, A. (2012). Effect of diet and exercise, alone or combined, on weight and body composition in overweight-to-obese post-menopausal women. *Obesity (Silver Spring, Md.), 20*(8), 1628–1638. doi: 10.1038/oby.2011.76.

Freitas, P. D., Silva, A. G., Ferreira, P. G., da Silva, A., Salge, J. M., Carvalho-Pinto, R. M., . . . Carvalho, C. R. F. (2018). Exercise improves physical activity and comorbidities in obese adults with asthma. *Medicine & Science in Sports & Exercise*. doi: 10.1249/mss.0000000000001574.

Goedecke, J. H., & Micklesfield, L. K. (2014). The effect of exercise on obesity, body fat distribution and risk for type 2 diabetes. *Medicine & Science in Sports & Exercise, 60*, 82–93. doi: 10.1159/000357338.

Golbidi, S., & Laher, I. (2014). Exercise induced adipokine changes and the metabolic syndrome. *Journal of Diabetes Research, 2014*, 16. doi: 10.1155/2014/726861.

Goldberg, A., Chavis, M., Watkins, J., & Wilson, T. (2012). The five-times-sit-to-stand test: Validity, reliability and detectable change in older females. *Aging Clinical and Experimental Research, 24*(4), 339–344.

Hansen, D., Dendale, P., Berger, J., van Loon, L. J., & Meeusen, R. (2007). The effects of exercise training on fat-mass loss in obese patients during energy intake restriction. *Sports Medicine, 37*(1), 31–46.

Haskell, W. L., Lee, I. M., Pate, R. R., Powell, K. E., Blair, S. N., Franklin, B. A., . . . Bauman, A. (2007). Physical activity and public health: Updated recommendation for adults from the American college of sports medicine and the American heart association. *Medicine & Science in Sports & Exercise, 39*(8), 1423–1434. doi: 10.1249/mss.0b013e3180616b27.

Hassan, Y., Head, V., Jacob, D., Bachmann, M. O., Diu, S., & Ford, J. (2016). Lifestyle interventions for weight loss in adults with severe obesity: A systematic review. *Clinical Obesity, 6*(6), 395–403. doi: 10.1111/cob.12161.

Herring, L. Y., Stevinson, C., Carter, P., Biddle, S. J. H., Bowrey, D., Sutton, C., & Davies, M. J. (2017). The effects of supervised exercise training 12–24 months after bariatric surgery on physical function and body composition: A randomised controlled trial. *International Journal of Obesity (Lond), 41*(6), 909–916. doi: 10.1038/ijo.2017.60.

Herring, L. Y., Stevinson, C., Davies, M. J., Biddle, S. J., Sutton, C., Bowrey, D., & Carter, P. (2016). Changes in physical activity behaviour and physical function after bariatric surgery: A systematic review and meta-analysis. *Obesity Reviews, 17*(3), 250–261. doi: 10.1111/obr.12361.

Herring, L. Y., Wagstaff, C., & Scott, A. (2014). The efficacy of 12 weeks supervised exercise in obesity management. *Clinical Obesity, 4*(4), 220–227.

Heymsfield, S. B., Cristina Gonzalez, M. C., Shen, W., Redman, L., & Thomas, D. (2014). Weight loss composition is one-fourth fat-free mass: A critical review and critique of this widely cited rule. *Obesity Reviews: An Official Journal of the International Association for the Study of Obesity, 15*(4), 310–321. doi: 10.1111/obr.12143.

Hill, J. O., Wyatt, H. R., & Peters, J. C. (2012). Energy balance and obesity. *Circulation, 126*(1), 126–132. doi: 10.1161/CIRCULATIONAHA.111.087213.

Hills, A. P., & Byrne, N. M. (2004). Physical activity in the management of obesity. *Clinics in Dermatology, 22*(4), 315–318.

Huck, C. J. (2014). Effects of supervised resistance training on fitness and functional strength in patients succeeding bariatric surgery. *Journal of Strength and Conditioning Research, 29*(3), 589–595.

Imayama, I., Ulrich, C. M., Alfano, C. M., Wang, C., Xiao, L., Wener, M. H., . . . McTiernan, A. (2012). Effects of a caloric restriction weight loss diet and exercise on inflammatory biomarkers in overweight/obese postmenopausal women: A randomized controlled trial. *Cancer Research, 72*(9), 2314–2326. doi: 10.1158/0008-5472.CAN-11-3092.

Jackson, S. E., Wardle, J., Johnson, F., Finer, N., & Beeken, R. J. (2013). The impact of a health professional recommendation on weight loss attempts in overweight and obese British adults: A cross-sectional analysis. *BMJ Open, 3*(11). doi: 10.1136/bmjopen-2013-003693.

Jain, S. S., Ramanand, S. J., Ramanand, J. B., Akat, P. B., Patwardhan, M. H., & Joshi, S. R. (2011). Evaluation of efficacy and safety of orlistat in obese patients. *Indian Journal of Endocrinology and Metabolism, 15*(2), 99–104. doi: 10.4103/2230-8210.81938.

James, P. T., Leach, R., Kalamara, E., & Shayeghi, M. (2001). The worldwide obesity epidemic. *Obesity Research, 9*(4), 228S–233S.

Jarolimova, J., Tagoni, J., & Stern, T. A. (2013). Obesity: Its epidemiology, comorbidities, and management. *The Primary Care Companion for CNS Disorders, 15*(5), PCC.12f01475. doi: 10.4088/PCC.12f01475.

Jassil, F. C., Manning, S., Lewis, N., Steinmo, S., Kingett, H., Lough, F., . . . Batterham, R. L. (2015). Feasibility and impact of a combined supervised exercise and nutritional-behavioral intervention following bariatric surgery: A pilot study. *Journal of Obesity, 2015*, 1–12.

Kaukua, J. K., Pekkarinen, T. A., & Rissanen, A. M. (2004). Health-related quality of life in a randomised placebo-controlled trial of sibutramine in obese patients with type II diabetes. *International Journal of Obesity and Related Metabolic Disorders, 28*(4), 600–605. doi: 10.1038/sj.ijo.0802591.

Lewis, M. E., Newall, C., Townend, J. N., Hill, S. L., & Bonser, R. S. (2001). Incremental Shuttle Walk Test in the assessment of patients for heart transplantation. *Heart, 86*(2), 183–187. doi: 10.1136/heart.86.2.183.

Linne, Y., Rooth, P., & Rossner, S. (2003). Success rate of Orlistat in primary-care practice is limited by failure to follow prescribing recommendations: The referral letter content vs clinical reality. *International Journal of Obesity and Related Metabolic Disorders, 27*(11), 1434–1435. doi: 10.1038/sj.ijo.0802401.

Livhits, M., Mercado, C., Yermilov, I., Parikh, J. A., Dutson, E., Mehran, A., . . . Gibbons, M. M. (2010). Exercise following bariatric surgery: Systematic review. *Obesity Surgery, 20*(5), 657–665.

Lv, N., Azar, K. M. J., Rosas, L. G., Wulfovich, S., Xiao, L., & Ma, J. (2017). Behavioral lifestyle interventions for moderate and severe obesity: A systematic review. *Preventive Medicine, 100*, 180–193. doi: 10.1016/j.ypmed.2017.04.022.

Lyytinen, T., Liikavainio, T., Paakkonen, M., Gylling, H., & Arokoski, J. P. (2013). Physical function and properties of quadriceps femoris muscle after bariatric surgery and subsequent weight loss. *Journal of Musculoskeletal and Neuronal Interactions, 13*(3), 291–300.

MacSween, A., Brydson, G., Creed, G., & Capell, H. A. (2001). A preliminary validation of the 10-metre Incremental Shuttle Walk Test as a measure of aerobic capacity in women with rheumatoid arthritis. *Physiotherapy, 87*(1), 38–44.

Madura, J. A., & Dibaise, J. K. (2012). Quick fix or long-term cure? Pros and cons of bariatric surgery. *F1000 Medicine Reports, 4*(19), 1–9.

McLaughlin, J. C., Hamilton, K., & Kipping, R. (2017). Epidemiology of adult overweight recording and management by UK GPs: A systematic review. *The British Journal of General Practice, 67*(663), e676–e683. doi: 10.3399/bjgp17X692309.

McQueen, M. A. (2009). Exercise aspects of obesity treatment. *The Ochsner Journal, 9*(3), 140–143.

MedicineNet. (2016). *Medical definition of bariatric surgery*. Retrieved from www.gov.uk/government/uploads/system/uploads/attachment_data/file/142723/Weight_Management_Service_Spec_FINAL_with_IRB.pdf.

Medicines and Healthcare Products Regulatory Agency (MHRA). (2014). *Public assessment report – decentralised procedure – Orlistat Mylan 60mg capsules, hard (Orlistat)*. (Medicines and Healthcare Products Regulatory Agency, Ed.). London: Medicines and Healthcare Products Regulatory Agency.

Mehta, A., Marso, S. P., Neeland, I. J. 2017. Liraglutide for weight management: A critical review of the evidence. *Obesity Science & Practice*, *3*(1), 3–14. doi: 10.1002/osp4.84.

Miller, C. T., Fraser, S. F., Levinger, I., Straznicky, N. E., Dixon, J. B., Reynolds, J., & Selig, S. E. (2013). The effects of exercise training in addition to energy restriction on functional capacities and body composition in obese adults during weight loss: A systematic review. *PLoS One*, *8*(11), e81692. doi: 10.1371/journal.pone.0081692.

Miller, G. D., Nicklas, B. J., You, T., & Fernandez, A. (2009). Physical function improvements after laparoscopic Roux-en-Y gastric bypass surgery. *Surgery for Obesity and Related Diseases*, *5*(5), 530–537.

Muller, M. J., Enderle, J., & Bosy-Westphal, A. (2016). Changes in energy expenditure with weight gain and weight loss in humans. *Current Obesity Reports*, *5*(4), 413–423. doi: 10.1007/s13679-016-0237-4.

National Institute for Health and Care Excelence (NICE). (2013a). *Physical activity: Brief advice for adults in primary care*. London: National Institute for Health and Care Excelence (NICE) Retrieved from www.nice.org.uk/guidance/ph44/resources/physical-activity-brief-advice-for-adults-in-primary-care-pdf-1996357939909.

National Institute for Health and Care Excellence (NICE). (2013b). BMI: Preventing ill health and premature death in black, Asian and other minority ethnic groups. *Public Health Guideline*. Retrieved 20 November 2017, from www.nice.org.uk/guidance/ph46/resources/bmi-preventing-ill-health-and-premature-death-in-black-asian-and-other-minority-ethnic-groups-pdf-1996361299141.

National Institute for Health and Care Excellence (NICE). (2014a). Obesity: Identification, assessment and management. *Clinical Guideline*. Retrieved from National institute for Health and Care Excellence website: www.nice.org.uk/guidance/cg189/resources/obesity-identification-assessment-and-management-pdf-35109821097925.

National Institute for Health and Care Excellence (NICE). (2014b). *Weight management: lifestyle services for overweight or obese adults (PH53)*. Retrieved from www.nice.org.uk/guidance/ph53/resources/weight-management-lifestyle-services-for-overweight-or-obese-adults-pdf-1996416726469.

National Institute for Health and Care Excellence (NICE). (2014c). Obesity: Identification, assessment and management of overweight and obesity in children, young people and adults. *NICE Clinical Guideline 189*. Retrieved 11 May 2015, from www.nice.org.uk/guidance/cg189/resources/guidance-obesity-identification-assessment-and-management-of-overweight-and-obesity-in-children-young-people-and-adults-pdf.

National Institute for Health and Care Excellence (NICE). (2021). Obesity management in adults. *Clinical Guideline*. Retrieved from National Institute for Health and Care Excellence website: https://pathways.nice.org.uk/pathways/obesity#path=view%3A/pathways/obesity/obesity-management-in-adults.xml&content=view-node%3Anodes-assess-lifestyle-comorbidities-and-willingness-to-change.

Nguyen, T., & Lau, D. C. (2012). The obesity epidemic and its impact on hypertension. *The Canadian Journal of Cardiology*, *28*(3), 326–333.

NHS Choices. (2016a). *Obesity*. Retrieved 11 November 2017, from www.nhs.uk/conditions/obesity/treatment/#medication.

NHS Choices. (2016b). *Very low calorie diets*. Retrieved 14 May 2018, from www.nhs.uk/Livewell/loseweight/Pages/very-low-calorie-diets.aspx.

Nicolai, S. P., Kruidenier, L. M., Leffers, P., Hardeman, R., Hidding, A., & Teijink, J. A. (2009). Supervised exercise versus non-supervised exercise for reducing weight in obese adults. *The Journal of Sports Medicine and Physical Fitness*, *49*(1), 85–90.

Odom, J., Zalesin, K. C., Washington, T. L., Miller, W. W., Hakmeh, B., Zaremba, D. L., . . . McCullough, P. A. (2010). Behavioral predictors of weight regain after bariatric surgery. *Obesity Surgery*, *20*(3), 349–356.

Papalazarou, A., Yannakoulia, M., Kavouras, S. A., Komesidou, V., Dimitriadis, G., Papakonstantinou, A., & Sidossis, L. S. (2010). Lifestyle intervention favorably affects weight loss and maintenance following obesity surgery. *Obesity*, *18*(7), 1348–1353.

Park, S. K., Park, J. H., Kwon, Y. C., Kim, H. S., Yoon, M. S., & Park, H. T. (2003). The effect of combined aerobic and resistance exercise training on abdominal fat in obese middle-aged women. *Journal of Physiological Anthropology and Applied Human Science*, *22*(3), 129–135.

Parreira, V. F., Janaudis-Ferreira, T., Evans, R. A., Mathur, S., Goldstein, R. S., & Brooks, D. (2014). Measurement properties of the Incremental Shuttle Walk Test: A systematic review. *Chest*, *145*(6), 1357–1369.

Public Health England. (2014). *Adult weight data factsheet*. Public Health England. Retrieved from www.noo.org.uk/securefiles/150915_1027//AdultWeight_Aug2014_v2.pdf.

Public Health England. (2017). *Health matters: obesity and the food environment*. England: Public Health England. Retrieved from www.gov.uk/government/publications/health-matters-obesity-and-the-food-environment/health-matters-obesity-and-the-food-environment – 2.

Rankin, J. W. (2013). Effective diet and exercise interventions to improve body composition in obese individuals. *American Journal of Lifestyle Medicine*, *9*(1), 48–62. doi: 10.1177/1559827613507879.

Ravussin, E., Burnand, B., Schutz, Y., & Jéquier, E. (1982). Twenty-four-hour energy expenditure and resting metabolic rate in obese, moderately obese, and control subjects. *The American Journal of Clinical Nutrition*, *35*(3), 566–573.

Revill, S. M., Morgan, M. D. L., Singh, S. J., Williams, J., & Hardman, A. E. (1999). The endurance shuttle walk: A new field test for the assessment of endurance capacity in chronic obstructive pulmonary disease. *Thorax*, *54*(3), 213–222. doi: 10.1136/thx.54.3.213.

Roberts, H. C., Denison, H. J., Martin, H. J., Patel, H. P., Syddall, H., Cooper, C., & Sayer, A. A. (2011). A review of the measurement of grip strength in clinical and epidemiological studies: Towards a standardised approach. *Age Ageing*, *40*(4), 423–429. doi: 10.1093/ageing/afr051.

Royal College of Physicians (RCP). (2013). *Action on obesity: Comprehensive care for all Report of a working party*. London: RCP.

Sainio, P., Martelin, T., Koskinen, S., & Heliövaara, M. (2007). Educational differences in mobility: The contribution of physical workload, obesity, smoking and chronic conditions. *Journal of Epidemiology and Community Health*, *61*(5), 401–408. doi: 10.1136/jech.2006.048306.

Singh, S. J., Morgan, M. D., Hardman, A. E., Rowe, C., & Bardsley, P. A. (1994). Comparison of oxygen uptake during a conventional treadmill test and the shuttle walking test in chronic airflow limitation. *European Respiratory Journal*, 7(11), 2016–2020.

So, B., Kim, H-J., Kim, J., & Song, W. (2014). Exercise-induced myokines in health and metabolic diseases. *Integrative Medicine Research*, *3*(4), 172–179. doi: 10.1016/j.imr.2014.09.007.

Stegen, S., Derave, W., Calders, P., Van Laethem, C., & Pattyn, P. (2011). Physical fitness in morbidly obese patients: Effect of gastric bypass surgery and exercise training. *Obesity Surgery*, *21*(1), 61–70.

Steinbrook, R. (2004). Surgery for severe obesity. *The New England Journal of Medicine 350*(11), 1075–1079.

Truby, H., & Bonham, M. (2011). What makes a weight loss programme successful? *British Medical Journal*, *343*. doi: 10.1136/bmj.d6629.

Verreijen, A. M., Engberink, M. F., Memelink, R. G., van der Plas, S. E., Visser, M., Weijs, P. J. (2017). Effect of a high protein diet and/or resistance exercise on the preservation of fat free mass during weight loss in overweight and obese older adults: A randomized controlled trial. *Nutrition Journal*, *16*(1).

Vinciguerra, F., Baratta, R., Farina, M. G., Tita, P., Padova, G., Vigneri, R., & Frittitta, L. (2013). Very severely obese patients have a high prevalence of type 2 diabetes mellitus and cardiovascular disease. *Acta Diabetologica*, *50*(3), 443–449.

Weiss, E. P., Racette, S. B., Villareal, D. T., Fontana, L., Steger-May, K., Schechtman, K. B., . . . Washington University School of Medicine, Calerie Group. (2007). Lower extremity muscle size and strength and aerobic capacity decrease with caloric restriction but not with exercise-induced weight loss. *Journal of Applied Physiology (Bethesda, Md.: 1985)*, *102*(2), 634–640. doi: 10.1152/japplphysiol.00853.2006.

Welbourne, R., Small, P., Finlay, I., Sareela, A., Somers, S., Mahawar, K., . . . Kingsman, R. (2014). The NBSR National Bariatric Surgery Registry of the British Obesity & Metabiolic Surgery Society – second registry report (Second Registry Report ed.). Oxfordshire, England.

Whitney, S. L., Wrisley, D. M., Marchetti, G. F., Gee, M. A., Redfern, M. S., & Furman, J. M. (2005). Clinical measurement of sit-to-stand performance in people with balance disorders: Validity of data for the five-times-sit-to-stand test. *Physical Therapy, 85*(10), 1034–1045.

Williams, M. A., Haskell, W. L., Ades, P. A., Amsterdam, E. A., Bittner, V., Franklin, B. A., . . . Stewart, K. J. (2007). Resistance exercise in individuals with and without cardiovascular disease: 2007 update: A scientific statement from the American heart association council on clinical cardiology and council on nutrition, physical activity, and metabolism. *Circulation, 116*(5), 572–584. doi: 10.1161/circulationaha.107.185214.

Williams, N. H., Hendry, M., France, B., Lewis, R., & Wilkinson, C. (2007). Effectiveness of exercise-referral schemes to promote physical activity in adults: Systematic review. *The British Journal of General Practice, 57*(545), 979–986.

Willis, L. H., Slentz, C. A., Bateman, L. A., Shields, A. T., Piner, L. W., Bales, C. W., . . . Kraus, W. E. (2012). Effects of aerobic and/or resistance training on body mass and fat mass in overweight or obese adults. *Journal of Applied Physiology, 113*(12), 1831–1837. doi: 10.1152/japplphysiol.01370.2011.

World Health Organisation. (2015, March 2013). Obesity and overweight. *Fact Sheet N°311*. Retrieved 01 September 2017, from www.who.int/mediacentre/factsheets/fs311/en/.

World Health Organisation. (2017). *BMI classification*. Retrieved 01 September 2017, from http://apps.who.int/bmi/index.jsp?introPage=intro_3.html.

Yanovski, S. Z., & Yanovski, J. A. (2014). Long-term drug treatment for obesity: A systematic and clinical review. *The Journal of the American Medical Association, 311*(1), 74–86. doi: 10.1001/jama.2013.281361.

11

TYPE 1 DIABETES

Richard Bracken, Mary Finn, Jane Yardley and Othmar Moser

Chapter aims

The aims of this chapter are to:

- Explore the management of type 1 diabetes (T1DM) around exercise
- Detail the importance of regular physical activity in improving functional ability and cardiovascular and metabolic health
- Outline guidelines for adjusting exogenous insulins and carbohydrates around exercise to facilitate regular participation in physical activity
- Provide an insight into real-life clinical case studies that detail prudent adjustments made by patients as they strive to engage in physical activity for different outcomes, like weight management, hypoglycaemia avoidance and/or performance

Overview of type 1 diabetes

Type 1 diabetes (T1DM) is characterised by an absolute or relative lack of insulin due to autoimmune destruction of the insulin-secreting β-cells within the pancreas. The resultant loss of pancreatic ß-cell function means a dependency on exogenous insulin therapy to regulate circulating blood glucose. Too little injected insulin can result in 'hyperglycaemia': that is, high blood glucose (> 10 mmol/L (180 mg/dL)) whilst, conversely, too much injected insulin may result in 'hypoglycaemia', or low blood glucose (< 3.9 mmol/L (70 mg/dL)).

An acute bout of exercise increases the risk of hypoglycaemia due to increased glucose disposal into working muscle by insulin independent and dependent pathways. To counteract exercise-induced hypoglycaemia, people with T1DM must alter exogenous insulin and/or consume additional carbohydrates, depending on the volume (intensity and duration) and type of exercise (Moser *et al.*, 2020). Factors such as injection site, body temperature, time of day, blood flow and previously administered insulin, pharmacokinetics of specific insulins (e.g. basal or prandial insulin) and antecedent hypoglycaemia will also impact blood glucose concentrations (Pitt *et al.*, 2020).

DOI: 10.4324/9781315102399-11

Mild hypoglycaemic episodes frequently occur in people with T1DM, even in people with good glycaemic control. Although this may translate to low glycosylated haemoglobin (HbA_{1c})concentration, tight therapy management must also be balanced against the long-term negative consequences of hyperglycaemia and risk of long-term complications like microvascular complications, such as retinopathy and nephropathy (albuminuria), and neuropathy and macrovascular problems, such as coronary heart disease, cerebrovascular disease and peripheral artery disease (Chiang *et al.*, 2014). Physical activity can decrease mortality risk caused by micro- and macrovascular complications and is associated with the volume and frequency of physical activity (Tikkanen-Dolenc *et al.*, 2016, 2017).

Management and medications

Insulin therapy

Most people with T1DM are treated with multiple-dose insulin injections (MDII) or continuous subcutaneous insulin infusion (CSII) to achieve near-physiological blood glucose concentration (Yeh *et al.*, 2016) (see Table 11.1). Insulin analogues (laboratory grown and genetically altered) are now used over human insulin as they decrease variability in insulin action. The choice of adopting MDII or CSII is individual and will depend on a person's lifestyle choices, amongst other factors. CSII is preferable over MDII for the improvement of long-term glycaemic control in paediatric and adult people (measured via HbA_{1c}) (Jeitler *et al.*, 2008; Misso Marie *et al.*, 2010). HbA_{1c} represents the percentage of glucose attached to haemoglobin molecules with long-term blood glucose over the preceding 8 to12 weeks correlating to higher HbA_{1c} values. There is no clear evidence of a reduction in incidence of mild or severe hypoglycaemia between CSII and MDII, with some studies showing no (Pozzilli *et al.*, 2014) or lower risk in CSII over MDII therapy (Misso Marie *et al.*, 2010; Pickup and Sutton, 2008). From a practical point of view, CSII therapy allows the flexibility of basal-insulin profiles and the ability to painlessly inject rapid-acting insulin, allowing a tailored therapy according to the patient's needs. These factors may also contribute to observed improvements in health-related quality of life and patient satisfaction.

Dose adjustment for normal eating

Besides exogenous insulin therapy, people with T1DM should participate in educational programmes that match prandial rapid-acting insulin dose to an amount of carbohydrate intake and target pre- and post-prandial blood glucose levels, as well as how to handle exercise and stress levels. Two different strategies have been defined to avoid a mismatch between carbohydrate intake and insulin dose (Schmidt and Nørgaard, 2014; Walsh *et al.*, 2011):

1. Carbohydrate factor (CarbF)

   The CarbF is the amount of carbohydrates (g) that needs to be consumed per injecting 1 unit (U) of bolus insulin. For example, a person with T1DM has a CarbF of 10 g carbohydrates and eats a meal with 50 g carbohydrates, then a total of 5 U bolus insulin will be injected (50 g carbs divided by a CarbF of 10 g carbs = 5 U bolus insulin).

TABLE 11.1 Medication considerations for exercise for people with type 1 diabetes

Class name	*Generic name*	*Brand name*	*Indication*	*Action*	*Side effects*	*Exercise considerations*
Insulin analogue (bolus insulin)	insulin aspart faster- acting aspart insulin lyspro insulin glulisine	NovoRapid/ Fiasp NovoLog Humalog Apidra	Diabetes mellitus	Onset of action of 5 to 15 minutes, peak effect in 1 to 2 hours and duration of action of 4 to 6 hours	Fat hypertrophy at injection site; local reactions at injection site; transient oedema; overdose causes hypoglycaemia	Needs to be adapted for pre-exercise meal and post-exercise meal, depending on volume and type of exercise (-25% to -75% of regular pre-meal insulin dose)
Insulin analogue (basal insulin)	Insulin Glargine U100	Lantus	Diabetes mellitus	Onset of insulin effect in 3 to 4 hours; the insulin effect plateaus over the next few hours and is followed by a relatively flat duration of action that lasts 24 hours	Fat hypertrophy at injection site; local reactions at injection site; transient oedema; overdose causes hypoglycaemia	Needs to be reduced if exercise is performed over consecutive days by around 25% of regular basal insulin dose
Insulin analogue (basal insulin)	Insulin Detemir	Levemir	Diabetes mellitus	Onset of insulin effect in 3 to 4 hours; the insulin effect plateaus over the next few hours and is followed by a relatively flat duration of action that lasts 12 to 24 hours	Fat hypertrophy at injection site; local reactions at injection site; transient oedema; overdose causes hypoglycaemia	Needs to be reduced if exercise is performed over consecutive days by around 25% of regular basal insulin dose
Insulin analogue (basal insulin)	Insulin Degludec	Tresiba	Diabetes mellitus	Onset of insulin effect in 3 to 6 hours; the insulin effect plateaus over the next few hours and is followed by a relatively flat duration of action that lasts 42 hours	Fat hypertrophy at injection site; local reactions at injection site; transient oedema; overdose causes hypoglycaemia	N/A
Insulin analogue (basal insulin)	Insulin Glargine U300	Toujeo	Diabetes mellitus	Onset of insulin effect in 3 to 6 hours; the insulin effect plateaus over the next few hours and is followed by a relatively flat duration of action that lasts 36 hours	Fat hypertrophy at injection site; local reactions at injection site; transient oedema; overdose causes hypoglycaemia	N/A

2. Correction factor (CorrF)

The CorrF is the expected decrease in blood glucose concentration when a person with T1DM injects 1 U of bolus insulin without consuming any carbohydrates. This is mainly used when patients are running on a high blood glucose concentration. For example, if a patient is running on 15 mmol/L (260 mg/dL) blood glucose, has a CorrF of 3 mmol/L (54 mg/dL) and aims to go down to a blood glucose concentration of 6 mmol/L (108 mg/dL), then a bolus insulin dose of 3 U will be injected (expected decrease of 9 mmol/L is three times the CorrF of 3 mmol/L (54 mg/dL).

The following calculations might be easily performed by people with T1D autonomously (Walsh *et al.*, 2011):

$$\text{CarbF} = \frac{2.6\,x\,Weight\,(lb)}{Total\,daily\,insulin\,dose} \text{ or } \frac{5.7\,x\,Weight\,(kg)}{Total\,daily\,insulin\,dose}$$

$$Carb = \frac{5.7\,x\,75kg\ bodyweight}{20U\ bolus\ insulin + 35U\ basal\ insulin\ perday}$$

$$= 7.8\,grcarbs\ are\ covered\ by\ 1\ U\ of\ bolus\ insulin$$

$$CorrF = \frac{1960\,mg\,/\,dL}{Total\,daily\,insulin\,dose} \text{ or } \frac{109\,mmol\,/\,L}{Total\,daily\,insulin\,dose}$$

$$e.g.:\ CorrF = \frac{109\,mmol\,/\,L}{20U\ bolus\ insulin + 35U\ basal\ insulin\ per\ day}$$

$= 3.1$ *mmol/L is the expected blood glucose decrease by 1 U of injected bolus insulin*

CarbF and CorrF calculations should be carefully applied and adapted in relation to current guidelines from the American Diabetes Association (ADA) when dealing with stress, physical activity and exercise training (Colberg *et al.*, 2016).

Targets for blood glucose control

Therapy targets should be in accordance with the recommendations of the ADA, notably HbA_{1c} concentration below 7.0% (53 mmol/mol), pre-prandial capillary plasma glucose concentration ranging from 4.4 to 7.2 mmol/L (80 to 130 mg/dL) and peak post-prandial capillary plasma glucose concentration below 10.0 mmol/L (180 mg/dL) (Chamberlain *et al.*, 2016). A low HbA_{1c} concentration might be associated with a higher number of hypoglycaemic episodes and longer time spent in hypoglycaemia. Success in achieving pre- and post-prandial target blood glucose concentration is accomplished by frequent self-monitoring of blood glucose (SMBG). SMBG should be dictated by the patient's individual needs, and this may require testing six to ten times daily and even more in case of exercise training or illness (Chiang *et al.*, 2014).

The advent of new technologies such as intermittently scanned glucose monitoring (isCGM) systems and continuous glucose monitoring (CGM) systems (e.g. combined with CSII) might reduce the risk of hypoglycaemia through real-time displays of glucose dynamics and/or alarms to alert people with T1DM to falling glucose. CGM and isCGM are devices that monitor glucose concentration continuously and offer opportunities for painless observations of interstitial glucose concentrations. A sensor is inserted in the interstitium and measures glucose continuously (every five minutes or less) or whenever the person with T1DM swipes a reader within close proximity of the sensor. Glucose concentration are displayed on a reader or mobile device (Moser *et al.*, 2018). Newer devices utilise algorithms to 'close the gap' between known differences in blood and interstitial glucose compartments.

People with T1DM should strive to achieve as 'normal' a blood glucose concentration similar to that of healthy individuals in daily living. However, daily routines are necessary to control large swings in blood glucose concentration, and the individual should try to establish standardised routines that they stick to. On the other hand, focusing excessively on routines may result in a cognitive discord. Significant depressive symptoms affect approximately one in four adults with diabetes, and therapy goals should be administered carefully in conjunction with the person living with the condition and in accordance with actual living conditions (Holt, 2015). A peak post-prandial blood glucose concentration below 10.0 mmol/L (180 mg/dL) can often only be achieved when leaving a time gap between rapid-acting insulin injection and carbohydrate ingestion (which may conversely increase the risk of early hypoglycaemia), ingesting mainly low–glycaemic index carbohydrates and splitting carbohydrates over at least one hour. A further problem is that the intra-individual requirements for exogenous insulin may vary by ~30% overnight and by 20% during waking hours, due to factors such as meal composition, differences in glucose turnover, alterations in physical activity and changes in insulin sensitivity (Thabit and Hovorka, 2016).

Basal and bolus insulin should be injected into the subcutaneous tissue of the abdomen, lateral region of the thigh or anterior buttocks. It should be ensured that the insulin is not injected intramuscularly due to accelerated insulin absorption. (This increases the risk of hypoglycaemia.) Systematic rotating of injection sites within one area is recommended to prevent lipohypertrophy or lipoatrophy (American Diabetes Association, 2002). An additional factor which increases insulin absorption is the higher temperature on the surface of the skin altering subcutaneous microcirculation, resulting in a lower dose of insulin required (Pfützner *et al.*, 2015). This should be considered when dealing with exercising patients who are regularly physically active and/or in warm environments.

The future of diabetes management is promising with respect to novel insulins (e.g. once-weekly basal insulins, faster-acting bolus insulins) and new technologies (artificial pancreas technology). Overall, diabetes management is highly individualised and should be established after a clear assessment of the patient's needs, lifestyle and psychological status, to strive towards the achievement of a lifelong tight glucose control.

Effect of type 1 diabetes on the acute exercise response

Exercise elevates metabolic rate and increases the rate of glucose entry into skeletal muscle independent of, but in addition to, insulin-mediated glucose uptake. This additional uptake can mean a rapid loss of glucose from the circulation. Exercise also flushes out exogenous insulin from subcutaneous depots into the circulation (Pitt *et al.*, 2020), resulting in an inhibition of hepatic glucose output, further predisposing to hypoglycaemia. In the pancreas of the individual with T1DM, ß-cell impairment results in a gradual loss of α-cell glucagon secretion that reduces a counter-regulatory response to falling blood glucose. Furthermore, previous bouts of hypoglycaemia and/or exercise within the previous 24 hours desensitise patients' awareness of falling glucose concentrations and impair counterregulatory responses to exercise (Galasetti *et al.*, 2003). Consequently, hypoglycaemia may become a frequent occurrence during exercise. The increased risk of developing hypoglycaemia during exercise is a major concern for patients and may act as a barrier for T1DM individuals wishing to exercise (Brazeau *et al.*, 2008).

Blood glucose responses to physical activity in individuals with T1DM are greatly impacted by using insulin analogues. Regardless of how insulin is administered, most individuals with T1DM will be hyperinsulinaemic when they undertake exercise. Naturally produced insulin has a half-life of approximately five minutes (Sönksen *et al.*, 1973), and insulin concentration drops when physical activity starts, dependent on exercise intensity and duration. Fast-acting synthetic insulin preparations peak after ~45 minutes and may take several hours to fully clear the system (McGibbon *et al.*, 2013). During moderate-intensity (aerobic) exercise, this results in amplified glucose uptake as muscles take in glucose by both insulin-independent (contraction-mediated) and insulin-dependent routes, alongside a potentially reduced glucagon response.

Furthermore, having higher-than-desired circulating insulin will suppress the release of glucagon that should take place during physical activity (Mallad *et al.*, 2015). With insufficient glucagon secretion, access to glucose stores (glycogen) in liver and muscle cells is reduced. Thus, moderate aerobic activity often results in an initial decline in blood glucose concentration. For this reason, a reduction in injected insulin may need to be made either hours before exercise if on MDI or 60 to 90 minutes before activity if using an insulin pump to lower the risk of hypoglycemia. Physical activity can also increase the appearance of insulin from subcutaneous depots to circulation (Mallad *et al.*, 2015; Admon *et al.*, 2005), making the timing of administration even more important. In consideration of this, carbohydrate supplementation may also be required (Moser *et al.*, 2020).

High-intensity activities, which include sustained high-intensity aerobic exercise, short sprints, heavy weight lifting and several competitive sports, stimulates the sympathetic nervous system, resulting in counter-regulatory hormone (adrenaline, noradrenaline, cortisol, glucagon) release. As part of the fight-or-flight response, catecholamines (adrenaline and noradrenaline) cause several systemic changes, including elevations in heart rate and blood pressure, and augmented blood flow to exercising muscles. They also ensure that fuel is made available to the muscles by releasing large amounts of stored glucose from the liver (hepatic glycogenolysis). This response causes an increase in blood glucose concentration proportional to the intensity of the exercise stimulus (McMurray *et al.*, 1987). For example, a study in young adults with T1DM demonstrated that the rate of glucose appearance increases with increasing exercise intensity until it matches the rate of glucose disappearance at an intensity of 80% of maximal aerobic rate (Shetty *et al.*, 2016). For activities at an intensity greater than this, the rate of glucose appearance exceeds glucose uptake, resulting in hyperglycemia (Mitchell *et al.*, 1988). Consequently, high-intensity intervals can be used as a strategy to slow or decrease the reduction in blood glucose concentrations during physical activity in individuals with T1DM (Bally *et al.*, 2016; Iscoe and Riddell, 2011; Guelfi *et al.*, 2005) when exercise is performed post-prandially. Performing a ten-second maximal sprint after moderate-intensity exercise can acutely oppose a further fall in glycemia (Bussau *et al.*, 2006), an improvement in post-exercise glycemia attributed to increased levels of catecholamines, growth hormone and cortisol.

The time of day that physical activity is performed may also impact the blood glucose responses. While studies are sparse, there is evidence to indicate that morning physical activity, even performed in a fasting state, is associated with lower (if any) declines in blood glucose when compared to afternoon activity (Ruegemer *et al.*, 1990; Yamanouchi *et al.*, 2002; Gomez *et al.*, 2015). This trend has been found with aerobic exercise (Yamanouchi *et al.*, 2002; Gomez *et al.*, 2015; Ruegemer *et al.*, 1990), resistance exercise (Toghi-Eshghi and Yardley, 2019) and high-intensity intermittent exercise (Yardley, 2020). This may be due to lower levels of circulating insulin resulting from the absence of recent meal-related boluses or higher levels of growth hormone (Perriello *et al.*, 1990; Boyle *et al.*, 1992) and cortisol (Kanaley *et al.*, 2001). With these hormones elevated, free fatty acids and hepatic glucose are more readily available for use, thereby sparing blood glucose. A recent study using CGM also found that morning exercise could be beneficial for blood glucose control for up to 24 hours compared to days when no exercise was performed, as morning exercise (and not afternoon exercise) resulted in more CGM readings in near-euglycaemic range on the subsequent day (Gomez *et al.*, 2015). This finding may be limited to aerobic exercise as Toghi-Eshghi and Yardley (2019) found more post-exercise hyperglycemia after morning resistance exercise than after the same protocol performed in the afternoon.

Regardless of the type or duration of activity performed, the risk of hypoglycaemia remains for several hours following exercise in individuals with type 1 diabetes (Davey *et al.*, 2013; McMahon *et al.*, 2007). While aerobic activities have been associated with rebound hyperglycaemia within three hours of termination (Yardley *et al.*, 2012, 2013; Zaharieva and Riddell, 2015), they have also been associated with increases in insulin sensitivity (Hamrin and Henriksson, 2008) and an elevated risk of nocturnal hypoglycaemia (Admon *et al.*, 2005; Davey *et al.*, 2013; McMahon *et al.*, 2007). The latter is believed to be the result of both increased insulin sensitivity and the replenishment of glycogen stores in the liver and skeletal muscles (Maehlum *et al.*, 1978). This risk seems to be greater when activity is performed later in the day as compared to the morning (Gomez *et al.*, 2015). While higher-intensity activities are associated with less risk of hypoglycaemia during exercise, the risk of post-exercise hypoglycaemia with these types of activities is still uncertain, with some studies showing little or no hypoglycemia after high-intensity exercise sessions (Bally *et al.*, 2016; Iscoe and Riddell, 2011; Yardley *et al.*, 2012), while others show an increase in the frequency of hypoglycaemia (Maran *et al.*, 2010; Wilson *et al.*, 2015). This phenomenon may be related to the intensity of the exercise performed as Rempel *et al.* (2018) only found an increase in post-exercise nocturnal hypoglycemia after the most intense (i.e. one-minute intervals at 80% of aerobic rate) high-intensity intermittent exercise session in their study.

Effects of exercise training

People with T1DM can expect to obtain the health benefits and improvements in functional capacity that people without the condition stand to gain from regular physical activity. The reader is referred to some recent reviews of the effects of regular physical activity in people with T1DM (Kennedy *et al.*, 2013; Quirk *et al.*, 2014; Yardley, Hay, *et al.*, 2014; Tonoli *et al.*, 2012; Chimen *et al.*, 2012; Röhling *et al.*, 2016). Regular exercise improves body composition, triglycerides, total cholesterol, blood pressure and BMI in both children and adults with T1DM (Bohn *et al.*, 2015; Quirk *et al.*, 2014; Riddell *et al.*, 2017). Aerobic fitness, muscular strength, cardiorespiratory capacity, micro- and macro-vascular improvements and reductions in some cardiovascular disease risk factors have been shown to improve with regular exercise training. However, the longer-term glycaemic changes in regularly exercising individuals with T1DM are more difficult to discern, possibly due to the need for extra carbohydrate around exercise.

Recommendations for fitness testing and exercise programming

Good clinical management for people with T1DM should incorporate regular physical activity. Unfortunately, many people fail to reach minimum physical activity guidelines (Plotnikoff *et al.*, 2006) due to fears of poor blood glucose control around activities (Brazeau *et al.*, 2008) and a failure to appreciate how different forms of exercise have different metabolic impacts. This combination results in poor confidence in managing blood glucose appropriately during and after exercise and discourages longer-term involvement in physical activity. Learning how to adjust diet and insulin to endurance or strength activities can help form an individualised 'acute exercise management strategy' that helps patients overcome barriers to obtaining the physical and psychological health benefits of being regularly active. If people with T1DM have been appropriately assessed and have minimal complications, they should be encouraged to start a regular physical activity programme and embark on the development of a safe regimen themselves (Colberg *et al.*, 2016).

General considerations for increasing physical activity

Several points need to be considered when increasing physical activity in people with T1DM:

- Performing unfamiliar exercise can cause glucose fluctuations that will differ when the same exercise is performed regularly.
- Different types of activity like aerobic or resistance exercise and different exercise intensities can alter glucose differently.
- Intermittent exercise such as soccer and child's play can cause different glucose responses, given the unpredictable nature of the activity.
- Exercise in the morning rather than the afternoon or evening may have different glucose responses, given the different amounts of on-board insulin and diurnal hormone variation.
- Always have water and some carbohydrate available during exercise.
- Never advocate exercise within 24 hours of severe hypoglycaemia.
- Wear comfortable clothing and footwear.
- Inspect feet regularly for signs of irritation, broken skin or infection.

Complications

Given the well-reported elevated risk of cardiovascular disease in people with diabetes, it is advisable to refer the individual for a graded exercise test to exclude underlying significant heart disease. If the patient has significant proliferative diabetic retinopathy or nephropathy, it is recommended they engage in low-impact cardiovascular activities such as swimming, aqua-aerobics, yoga, Pilates, walking or cycling. Activities that involve high-intensity elements, such as team sports, or encourage competition and heavy-resistance exercise should be avoided. If the patient has peripheral or autonomic neuropathy or ulcers, check feet before activity and recommend non-weight-bearing aerobic activities such as swimming, aqua-aerobics, cycling or chair or arm exercises and avoid prolonged walking, step aerobics or jogging. The ADA adopted guidelines for exercise pre-participation health screening from the American College of Sports Medicine (ACSM). The model for exercise pre-participation health screening is based on (Colberg *et al.*, 2016):

- Current physical activity level (low, moderate or high)
- Presence of signs or symptoms and/or known cardiovascular, metabolic or renal disease
- The expected exercise intensity

Exercise pre-participation health screening is not necessary for asymptomatic individuals who wish to begin low- or moderate-intensity physical activity and exercise. However, if exercise intensity is high in asymptomatic individuals (e.g. sports competitions) or in general in symptomatic patients, we recommend performing a pre-exercise medical clearance.

Insulin and carbohydrate adjustments for aerobic exercise

See Figure 11.1 for insulin and CHO adjustments around exercise.

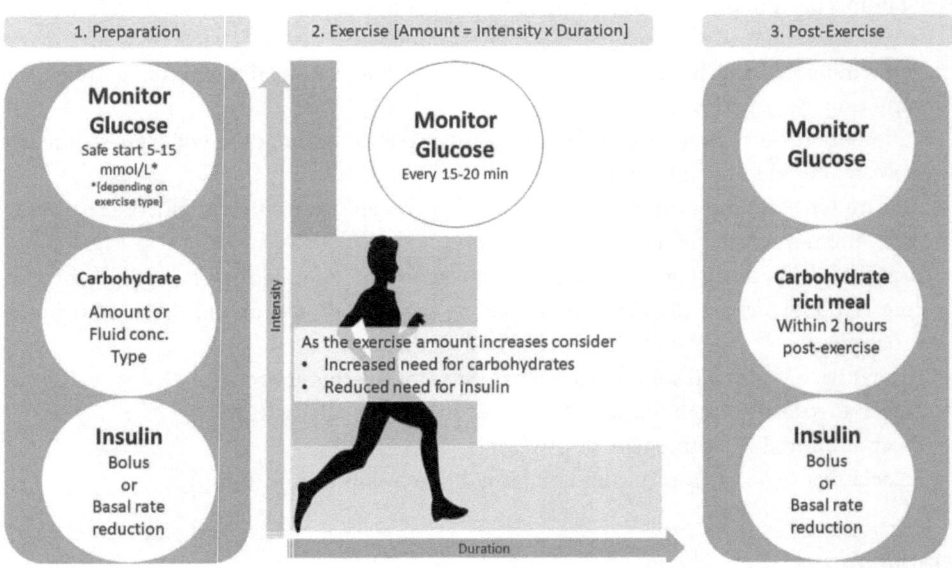

FIGURE 11.1 A schematic to represent some important factors to consider in the planned integration of exercise into the daily management of a person with T1DM performing aerobic exercise

Safe blood glucose ranges around exercise

If not using CGM devices, a one-hour and immediate pre-exercise capillary blood glucose sample will provide important information on the stability and direction of blood glucose changes. Immediate pre-exercise blood glucose concentration should be > 5 mmol/L and < 15 mmol/L, but if > 15 mmol/L and in the presence of raised blood ketones, exercise should be delayed until values decline and ketones dissipate (International Diabetes Federation – Education, 2011). Blood glucose responses should be checked every 15 to 20 minutes in the initial familiarisation to regular exercise and serve as a learning strategy. Check blood glucose at one hour after exercise to ensure maintenance of euglycaemia.

Basal-bolus insulin reduction for aerobic exercise?

Research demonstrates protection against nocturnal hypoglycaemia when basal insulin is reduced on the day of exercise (Campbell *et al.*, 2015). Reductions to pre-exercise rapid-acting (bolus) insulin of 50% of usual rapid-acting insulin made one hour before physical activity is prudent (West *et al.*, 2011b). If patients are on CSII therapy (continuous subcutaneous insulin infusion) using pumps, bolus insulin should be reduced by 25% to 75% at the pre-exercise meal, depending on the type, intensity and duration of exercise. Especially if bolus insulin is on board, basal insulin rates can be reduced by 50% to 80% up to 90 minutes prior to the start of exercise for exercise duration longer than 30 minutes. Alternatively, suspending basal insulin can be considered at the start of exercise for a duration of 60 minutes (Zaharieva *et al.*, 2020). Importantly, basal perfusion must be continued immediately after the end of exercise. Additional carbohydrates (5–30 g/h) may be needed based on blood glucose and/or interstitial glucose monitoring (Riddell *et al.*, 2017). Lower basal rates can also be considered overnight post-exercise, especially if the exercise session was performed later in the day (Riddell *et al.*, 2017). See Table 11.1 for the effects of medications on the exercise response in people with T1D.

Carbohydrate ingestion for aerobic exercise

For regular physical activity, individuals should ensure adequate amounts of carbohydrate the day of exercise to counteract heightened insulin sensitivity in regularly exercising tissue and provide the necessary glucose for skeletal muscle and liver glycogen resynthesis before the next exercise session.

In an exercise session, a reduction in rapid-acting insulin is usually administered alongside carbohydrate consumption. Low–glycaemic index (GI) carbohydrates (or foods that are low GI) are associated with lower glycaemic fluctuations without detriment to exercise performance (West *et al.*, 2011a; West *et al.*, 2011b). Current recommendations suggest ingestion of carbohydrate per kilogram of body mass per planned duration of exercise and recognition of the amount of on-board insulin (Riddell *et al.*, 2017; Moser *et al.*, 2020). As the patient progresses with training, ongoing refinement of ingested amounts will be needed as improved metabolic regulation and insulin sensitivity occur.

Following exercise, there is a need to reduce insulin and increase carbohydrate to account for an increased organ sensitivity to insulin and greater rate of muscle and liver glucose replenishment. Therefore, consumption of a low–GI carbohydrate–rich meal and a 50% reduction in usual rapid-acting insulin one hour after exercise can reduce glycaemic fluctuations and protect patients against hypoglycaemia for up to eight hours (Campbell *et al.*, 2014, 2015).

Insulin and carbohydrate adjustments for strengthening exercises

Strengthening exercises cause counter-regulatory hormone (catecholamines, growth hormone) responses that may increase blood glucose concentrations, in particular when performed in a fasted state (Turner *et al*, 2015; Toghi-Eshghi and Yardley, 2019). The amount of weight lifted in a session can determine the degree of hyperglycaemia, and (for morning exercise, at least), there is less need to consume carbohydrates for strength exercise lasting ~15 to 45 minutes. Beyond this duration, the increase in muscle glucose uptake tempers the exercise-induced hyperglycaemia (Turner *et al.*, 2015). Moreover, if exercise-induced hyperglycaemia occurs, a small rapid-acting insulin dose immediately after exercise can help reduce blood glucose to euglycaemic levels (Turner *et al.*, 2016). Alternatively, individuals can be encouraged to perform aerobic exercise (Yardley, Sigal, *et al.*, 2014) after resistance exercise to counteract increases in blood glucose. Strength exercises performed in the afternoon and lasting longer than 30 minutes may require carbohydrate intake, albeit in much smaller amounts than with aerobic exercise (Yardley *et al.*, 2012).

Case studies

Case study 1 Weight loss

Sarah is 35 years old and has had T1DM for 31 years. She is on a basal-bolus injection regimen of once-daily glargine insulin (19 units) and 1 unit of bolus insulin per 12 grams carbohydrate. She presented to the dietitian looking for advice on weight loss. Her weight was 82 kg, BMI 28.2 kg/m^2. Her most recent HbA$_{1c}$ was 7.1% (54 mmol/mol). However, her glucose meter downloads revealed significant blood glucose variability and frequent hypoglycaemic episodes. She has a background history of moderately increased albuminuria.

We began initially by asking Sarah to complete a seven-day food, blood glucose and physical activity diary, and we booked a follow-up appointment to review this. The diary helped Sarah identify some poor dietary habits. It also highlighted her lack of physical activity. In the first collaborative consultation, we set achievable goals with an aim to review in one month and set further targets/progress towards higher goals.

Initial goals set:

1. We explored possible barriers to exercise. She reported that exercising with T1DM was very difficult, and she struggled with motivation. She identified fear of hypoglycaemia as her main barrier. We discussed ways to avoid hypoglycaemia: e.g. planning exercise, insulin adjustments in preference to carbohydrate supplementation (thus avoiding additional calorie intake) and

timing of exercise (exercise in the morning, which will result in lower declines in blood glucose than afternoon exercise).

We agreed on a gradual increase, starting initially with two 10-minute bouts of moderate-intensity walking every second day and increasing gradually, with a goal of at least 30 minutes most days, with no more than two consecutive days without exercise.

2. Sarah identified two main areas in her diet to target initially: 1) reduce alcohol intake to < 11 units per week and 2) choose high fibre carbohydrate choices at meals (e.g. oats, pulses, whole-wheat pasta, brown rice) over current alternatives.
3. We encouraged continued self-monitoring through the use of an online or paper diary and also a pedometer, using an initial daily steps goal of > 5,000 steps (aiming over time for ~10,000 steps per day).

On review after one month, Sarah had managed to achieve a weight loss of 2.3 kilograms, which was meeting her target weight loss of 0.5 to 1.0 kilogram per week. This weight loss was mainly through dietary changes as Sarah was still struggling with motivation to exercise. Therefore, the aim was to focus over the next two months on continuing to achieve her exercise goals.

Case study 2 Hypoglycaemia avoidance

Kate is 30 years of age and has had T1DM for 14 years. She was referred to the diabetes team as she had recently started exercising but was experiencing frequent hypoglycaemic episodes during and after exercise. Her weight is 64.1 kg; BMI 24 kg/m^2. Her most recent HbA1c was 7.4% (57 mmol/mol). She was on a basal-bolus insulin regimen (detemir insulin 10 units twice daily and 2–5 units of aspart insulin). Kate was very motivated to get fit, but due to difficulty managing her blood glucose around exercise, she reported being very close to giving up.

Her exercise was mainly aerobic (jogging between 7–12 km per week), along with two resistance training sessions (free weights and resistance machines) per week. She usually exercised one or two hours after her breakfast or lunch. We reviewed Kate in clinic with a seven-day food, exercise and blood glucose diary.

Issues identified from diary:

- She was exercising with too much active insulin on board. She did not reduce her insulin bolus with her meal one or two hours before exercise. Also, following exercise, she tended to make small reductions to her usual bolus insulin (-25%) with her next meal. She was experiencing hypoglycaemia during exercise and in the post-exercise period (five to six hours after).

- She tended not to eat anything after exercise until her next meal approximately two hours later, which may contribute to poor recovery and exacerbate hypoglycaemia.
- Her basal insulin (detemir) was too high as her blood glucose dropped overnight by approximately 4–6 mmol/L. Due to her exercise volume, her insulin detemir needed to be reduced overall.

Suggested changes:

1. After consultation with her diabetes team, we recommended a reduction in basal insulin detemir by 20%.
2. Trial a 50% reduction in bolus insulin aspart one to two hours before exercise and a 50% reduction in bolus insulin aspart with her post-exercise meal.
3. Aim for pre-exercise starting blood glucose of between > 5–10 mmol/L.
4. Choose a post-exercise recovery snack providing carbohydrate and protein. She opted for a low-calorie option (low-fat milk/low-fat yoghurt).
5. Consider morning exercise, doing her resistance session immediately before her aerobic training or trial a ten-second maximal intensity sprint after aerobic training to help reduce hypoglycaemia.
6. Trial changes and email a further food, exercise and blood glucose diary for review.

On review of Kate's diary there was a significant reduction in hypoglycaemic episodes during and following exercise. She reported that since making reductions to her insulin around exercise, along with incorporating some resistance training in advance of her aerobic workouts, her blood glucose management around exercise had greatly improved.

Case study 3 Glucose management around extreme endurance events

David is aged 22 years and was diagnosed with T1DM 2 years ago. His weight is 70 kg; BMI 22.3 kg/m^2. His most recent HbA_{1c} was 6.5% (48 mmol/mol). His diabetes is managed with insulin pump therapy (CSII) and continuous glucose monitoring (CGM). David is extremely active. He trains daily (either swimming, biking or running) and also does one brick session (bike/run) per week. He competes in triathlons (sprint and Olympic distance) and is hoping to complete a half Ironman (expected duration of competition: five to six hours).

He was referred with difficulty managing his blood glucose around exercise as his duration and intensity of training had recently increased. Despite this excellent

HbA1c, his CGM downloads showed significant blood glucose variability, and he experienced frequent hypoglycaemia. We reviewed him in clinic with a food and exercise diary (one week) and his CGM downloads. Overall, he had an excellent diet, making very healthy choices at meals and snacks.

Issues identified from diary:

- During long duration sessions (1.2 km open-water swim and 9 km trail run [1hr 45 min duration] and bike/run combination sessions [2 hr duration]), his blood glucose was dropping by an average of 5 mmol/L, and he was experiencing hypoglycaemic episodes up to six hours post-exercise.
- With his meal 1.5 to 2 hours before these sessions, he was doing a 50% decrease in bolus insulin. He was reducing his basal rate at the start of his session by only 25% and returning to normal basal on finishing. His intake of carbohydrate was insufficient at 20 g per hour during exercise.
- Following exercise sessions, he would delay his next meal, which could be two hours after training.

Suggested changes:

1. After consultation with his diabetes team, we recommended reducing basal insulin to 50% 60 minutes before the start of training, during training and 60 minutes after.
2. Ensure his blood glucose at the start of exercise is between > 5–10 mmol/L.
3. Increase carbohydrate intake to 50 grams per hour during exercise (mixture of sports drinks and carbohydrate gels).
4. Recovery is critical to replenish his glycogen stores, repair any muscle damage and avoid hypoglycaemia. Therefore, introduce a low glycaemic snack immediately post-training/competition consisting of approximately 70 grams carbohydrate and 20–25 g protein (500 ml Nesquik chocolate milk/2 Weetabix and a yoghurt). With this snack, he was advised to only take 50% of his bolus insulin.
5. To avoid hypoglycaemia following evening training, David was advised to reduce his basal insulin by 10% for at least seven hours post-training and to consume a low– glycaemic index snack (glass of milk and yoghurt) before bed.
6. Plan: Review trialled changes in two weeks with food and exercise diary and CGM data.

David went on to successfully complete his first half Ironman two months after our review. Reviewing his CGM data during and following the half Ironman showed that he managed to maintain his blood glucose close to target throughout the event, without any hypoglycaemic episodes.

Summary

Type 1 diabetes is a complex metabolic condition that necessitates a lifelong dependency on exogenous insulin and careful adjustment of carbohydrate intake to control blood glucose concentrations. Notwithstanding this, regular physical activity should be encouraged as evidence supports cardiovascular, respiratory, metabolic and quality of life benefits. Developing good glycaemic control and healthy amounts of physical activity takes time but results in an ability for lifelong involvement in sports and exercise for the individual with T1DM.

Key points

- Physical activity should be promoted to all people with T1DM with consideration of background fitness, complications and goals.
- Carbohydrate and exogenous insulins may need to be adjusted to facilitate safe participation in an acute bout of exercise.
- Regular physical training can improve many physiological systems in the body, but improvements in glycaemic control may be more difficult to demonstrate so should not be the sole focus.

Study tasks

1. What does HbA1c represent?
2. How do we characterise type 1 diabetes?
3. Define hyperglycaemia.
4. Define hypoglycaemia and state the potential factors that contribute to its development.
5. State where a person with diabetes should avoid insulin injections and why.
6. State a HbA1c, fasting or post-prandial indicator of good glycaemic control.
7. How does circulating glucose enter the tissue cells?
8. Explain how high-intensity activities increase blood glucose concentrations.
9. State what activities a person with significant proliferative diabetic retinopathy or nephropathy should engage in and avoid.
10. What checks should a person with diabetes make if they have peripheral or autonomic neuropathy or ulcers?

TABLE 11.2 At-a-glance summary guide to exercise considerations for people with type 1 diabetes

Condition name	Type 1 diabetes mellitus (T1DM)
Pathophysiology summary	Type 1 diabetes mellitus is characterised by an absolute or relative lack of insulin due to autoimmune destruction of the insulin-secreting β-cells in the pancreas. The resultant loss of pancreatic ß-cell function means a dependency on exogenous insulin therapy to regulate circulating blood glucose.
Aims of exercise	To improve glycaemic control, insulin sensitivity, glucose variability, body composition, lipid profiles, blood pressure and BMI; reduce the risk of micro- and macrovascular complications.

Exercise considerations (including contraindications)	Unfamiliar exercise can cause unexpected glucose fluctuations. Exercise types (endurance, resistance, intermittent) alter glucose concentration differently. Exercise in the morning rather than the afternoon or evening may induce different glucose responses. Always have water and some carbohydrate available during exercise; wear comfortable clothing and footwear.
Frequency	Three days per week with no more than two consecutive days without activity for adults. Shorter durations (minimum 75 minutes per week) of high-intensity or interval training may be sufficient for younger and more physically fit individuals with T1DM. Children and adolescents with T1DM should engage in 60 minutes or more per day of moderate vigorous-intensity physical activity, with vigorous and muscle-strengthening activities included at least three days per week.
Intensity	Moderate to high.
Time	50 minutes.
Type	All types of exercise, depending on personal preference.
Common medications associated	Exogenous insulin administered via bolus-basal regimen (MDI) or insulin pump therapy (CSII).
Key safety considerations	High risk of glycaemic disturbances; most common is hypoglycaemia during and after exercise.
Effect of exercise on conditions	The main effect of low- to moderate-intensity exercise is to lower blood glucose significantly within a short period of time. Higher exercise intensities may lead to an increase in blood glucose concentration during exercise and lead to a larger decrease in circulation glucose post-exercise. Regular exercise increases insulin sensitivity, which translates to reduction in total daily insulin. Insulin therapy adaptation needs to be discussed with diabetes consultant.

References

Admon, G., Weinstein, Y., Falk, B., Weintrob, N., Benzaquen, H., Ofan, R., Fayman, G., Zigel, L., Constantini, N. and Phillip, M. (2005) 'Exercise with and without an insulin pump among children and adolescents with type 1 diabetes mellitus', *Pediatrics*, 116(3), pp. e348–e355. doi: 10.1542/peds.2004-2428.

American Diabetes Association. (2002) 'Insulin administration', *Diabetes Care*, 25(Supplement 1), pp. S112–115. doi: 10.2337/diacare.25.2007.S112.

Bally, L., Zueger, T., Buehler, T., Dokumaci, A. S., Speck, C., Pasi, N., Ciller, C., Paganini, D., Feller, K., Loher, H., Rosset, R., Wilhelm, M., Tappy, L., Boesch, C. and Stettler, C. (2016) 'Metabolic and hormonal response to intermittent high-intensity and continuous moderate intensity exercise in individuals with type 1 diabetes: A randomised crossover study', *Diabetologia*, 59(4), pp. 776–784. doi: 10.1007/s00125-015-3854-7.

Bohn, B., Herbst, A., Pfeifer, M., Krakow, D., Zimny, S., Kopp, F., Melmer, A., Steinacker, J. M. and Holl, R. W. (2015) 'Impact of physical activity on glycemic control and prevalence of cardiovascular risk factors in adults with type 1 diabetes: A cross-sectional multicenter study of 18,028 patients', *Diabetes Care*, 38(8), pp. 1536–1543. doi: 10.2337/dc15-0030.

Boyle, P. J., Avogaro, A., Smith, L., Shah, S. D., Cryer, P. E. and Santiago, J. V. (1992) 'Absence of the dawn phenomenon and abnormal lipolysis in type 1 (insulin-dependent) diabetic patients with chronic growth hormone deficiency', *Diabetologia*, 35(4), pp. 372–379.

Brazeau, A.-S., Rabasa-Lhoret, R., Strychar, I. and Mircescu, H. (2008) 'Barriers to physical activity among patients with type 1 diabetes', *Diabetes Care*, 31(11), pp. 2108–2109. doi: 10.2337/dc08-0720.

Bussau, V. A., Ferreira, L. D., Jones, T. W. and Fournier, P. A. (2006) 'The 10-s maximal sprint: A novel approach to counter an exercise-mediated fall in glycemia in individuals with type 1 diabetes', *Diabetes Care*, 29(3), pp. 601–606. doi: 10.2337/diacare.29.03.06.dc05-1764.

Campbell, M. D., Walker, M., Bracken, R. M., Turner, D., Stevenson, E. J., Gonzalez, J. T., Shaw, J. A. and West, D. J. (2015) 'Insulin therapy and dietary adjustments to normalize glycemia and prevent nocturnal hypoglycemia after evening exercise in type 1 diabetes: A randomized controlled trial', *BMJ Open Diabetes Research & Care*, 3(1), pp. e000085–e000085. doi: 10.1136/bmjdrc-2015-000085.

Campbell, M. D., Walker, M., Trenell, M. I., Stevenson, E. J., Turner, D., Bracken, R. M., Shaw, J. A. and West, D. J. (2014) 'A low-glycemic index meal and bedtime snack prevents postprandial hyperglycemia and associated rises in inflammatory markers, providing protection from early but not late nocturnal hypoglycemia following evening exercise in type 1 diabetes', *Diabetes Care*, 37(7), pp. 1845–1853. doi: 10.2337/dc14-0186.

Chamberlain, J. J., Rhinehart, A. S., Shaefer, C. F. and Neuman, A. (2016) 'Diagnosis and management of diabetes: Synopsis of the 2016 American Diabetes Association standards of medical care in diabetes', *Annals of Internal Medicine*, 164(8), pp. 542–552. doi: 10.7326/M15-3016.

Chiang, J. L., Kirkman, M. S., Laffel, L. M. B. and Peters, A. L. (2014) 'Type 1 diabetes through the life span: A position statement of the American Diabetes Association', *Diabetes Care*, 37(7), pp. 2034–2054. doi: 10.2337/dc14-1140.

Chimen, M., Kennedy, A., Nirantharakumar, K., Pang, T. T., Andrews, R. and Narendran, P. (2012) 'What are the health benefits of physical activity in type 1 diabetes mellitus? A literature review', *Diabetologia*, 55(3), pp. 542–551. doi: 10.1007/s00125-011-2403-2.

Colberg, S. R., Sigal, R. J., Yardley, J. E., Riddell, M. C., Dunstan, D. W., Dempsey, P. C., Horton, E. S., Castorino, K. and Tate, D. F. (2016) 'Physical activity/exercise and diabetes: A position statement of the American Diabetes Association', *Diabetes Care*, 39(11), pp. 2065–2079. doi: 10.2337/dc16-1728.

Davey, R. J., Howe, W., Paramalingam, N., Ferreira, L. D., Davis, E. A., Fournier, P. A. and Jones, T. W. (2013) 'The effect of midday moderate-intensity exercise on postexercise hypoglycemia risk in individuals with type 1 diabetes', *The Journal of Clinical Endocrinology & Metabolism*, 98(7), pp. 2908–2914. doi: 10.1210/jc.2013-1169.

Galasetti, P., Tate T., Neill, R. A., Morrey, S., Wasserman, D. H. and Davis, S. N. (2003 July) 'Effect of antecedent hypoglycemia on counterregulatory responses to subsequent euglycemic exercise in type 1 diabetes', *Diabetes*, 52(7), pp. 1761–1769. doi: 10.2337/diabetes.52.7.1761.

Gomez, A. M., Gomez, C., Aschner, P., Veloza, A., Muñoz, O., Rubio, C. and Vallejo, S. (2015) 'Effects of performing morning versus afternoon exercise on glycemic control and hypoglycemia frequency in type 1 diabetes patients on sensor-augmented insulin pump therapy', *Journal of Diabetes Science and Technology*, 9(3), pp. 619–624. doi: 10.1177/1932296814566233.

Guelfi, K. J., Jones, T. W. and Fournier, P. A. (2005) 'The decline in blood glucose levels is less with intermittent high-intensity compared with moderate exercise in individuals with type 1 diabetes', *Diabetes Care*, 28(6), pp. 1289–1294. doi: 10.2337/diacare.28.6.1289.

Hamrin, K. and Henriksson, J. (2008) 'Interstitial glucose concentration in insulin-resistant human skeletal muscle: Influence of one bout of exercise and of local perfusion with insulin or vanadate', *European Journal of Applied Physiology*, 103(5), pp. 595–603. doi: 10.1007/s00421-008-0753-3.

Holt, R. I. G. (2015) 'Diabetes and depression', 14(6). doi: 10.1007/s11892-014-0491-3.Diabetes.

International Diabetes Federation – Education. (2011) *Online diabetes education modules Section 2. Diabetes and lifestyle intervention*. Belgium: International Diabetes Federation.

Iscoe, K. E. and Riddell, M. C. (2011) 'Continuous moderate-intensity exercise with or without intermittent high-intensity work: Effects on acute and late glycaemia in athletes with type 1 diabetes mellitus', *Diabetic Medicine*, 28(7), pp. 824–832. doi: 10.1111/j.1464-5491.2011.03274.x.

Jeitler, K., Horvath, K., Berghold, A., Gratzer, T. W., Neeser, K., Pieber, T. R. and Siebenhofer, A. (2008) 'Continuous subcutaneous insulin infusion versus multiple daily insulin injections in patients with diabetes mellitus: Systematic review and meta-analysis', *Diabetologia*, 51(6), pp. 941–951. doi: 10.1007/s00125-008-0974-3.

Kanaley, J. A., Weltman, J. Y., Pieper, K. S., Weltman, A. and Hartman, M. L. (2001) 'Cortisol and growth hormone responses to exercise at different times of day 1', *The Journal of Clinical Endocrinology & Metabolism*, 86(6), pp. 2881–2889. doi: 10.1210/jcem.86.6.7566.

Kennedy, A., Nirantharakumar, K., Chimen, M., Pang, T. T., Hemming, K., Andrews, R. C. and Narendran, P. (2013) 'Does exercise improve glycaemic control in type 1 diabetes? A systematic review and meta-analysis', *PLoS One*, 8(3). doi: 10.1371/journal.pone.0058861.

Maehlum, S., Felig, P. and Wahren, J. (1978) 'Splanchnic glucose and muscle glycogen metabolism after glucose feeding during postexercise recovery', *The American Journal of Physiology*, 235(3), pp. E255–E260.

Mallad, A., Hinshaw, L., Schiavon, M., Dalla Man, C., Dadlani, V., Basu, R., Lingineni, R., Cobelli, C., Johnson, M. L., Carter, R., Kudva, Y. C. and Basu, A. (2015) 'Exercise effects on postprandial glucose metabolism in type 1 diabetes: A triple-tracer approach', *American Journal of Physiology. Endocrinology and Metabolism*, 308(12), pp. E1106–E1115. doi: 10.1152/ajpendo.00014.2015.

Maran, A., Pavan, P., Bonsembiante, B., Brugin, E., Ermolao, A., Avogaro, A. and Zaccaria, M. (2010) 'Continuous glucose monitoring reveals delayed nocturnal hypoglycemia after intermittent high-intensity exercise in nontrained patients with type 1 diabetes', *Diabetes Technology & Therapeutics*, 12(10), pp. 763–768. doi: 10.1089/dia.2010.0038.

McGibbon, A., Richardson, C., Hernandez, C., Dornan, J. and Dornan, J. (2013) 'Pharmacotherapy in type 1 diabetes', *Canadian Journal of Diabetes*, 37, pp. S56–S60. doi: 10.1016/j.jcjd.2013.01.020.

McMahon, S. K., Ferreira, L. D., Ratnam, N., Davey, R. J., Youngs, L. M., Davis, E. A., Fournier, P. A. and Jones, T. W. (2007) 'Glucose requirements to maintain euglycemia after moderate-intensity afternoon exercise in adolescents with type 1 diabetes are increased in a biphasic manner', *Journal of Clinical Endocrinology and Metabolism*, 92(3), pp. 963–968. doi: 10.1210/jc.2006-2263.

McMurray, R. G., Forsythe, W. A., Mar, M. H. and Hardy, C. J. (1987) 'Exercise intensity-related responses of beta-endorphin and catecholamines', *Medicine and Science in Sports and Exercise*, 19(6), pp. 570–574.

Misso Marie, L., Egberts Kristine, J., Page, M., O'Connor, D. and Shaw, J. (2010) 'Continuous subcutaneous insulin infusion (CSII) versus multiple insulin injections for type 1 diabetes mellitus', *Cochrane Database of Systematic Reviews*, 51(1), pp. 941–951. doi: 10.1007/s00125-008-0974-3.

Mitchell, T. H., Abraham, G., Schiffrin, A., Leiter, L. A. and Marliss, E. B. (1988) 'Hyperglycemia after intense exercise in IDDM subjects during continuous subcutaneous insulin infusion', *Diabetes Care*, 11(4), pp. 311–317. doi: 10.2337/diacare.11.4.311.

Moser, O., Riddell, M. C., Eckstein, M. L., Adolfsson, P., Rabasa-Lhoret, R., van den Boom, L., Gillard, P., Nørgaard, K., Oliver, N. S., Zaharieva, D. P., Battelino, T., de Beaufort, C., Bergenstal, R. M., Buckingham, B., Cengiz, E., Deeb, A., Heise, T., Heller, S., Kowalski, A. J., Leelarathna, L., Mathieu, C., Stettler, C., Tauschmann, M., Thabit, H., Wilmot, E. G., Sourij, H., Smart, C. E., Jacobs, P. G., Bracken, R. M. and Mader, J. K. (2020 December) 'Glucose management for exercise using continuous glucose monitoring (CGM) and intermittently scanned CGM (isCGM) systems in type 1 diabetes: Position statement of the European association for the study of diabetes (EASD) and of the international society for pediatric and adolescent diabetes (ISPAD) endorsed by JDRF and supported by the American s(ADA)', *Pediatr Diabetes*, 21(8), pp. 1375–1393. doi: 10.1111/pedi.13105. Epub 2020 Oct 13. PMID: 33047481; PMCID: PMC7702152.

Moser, O., Yardley, J. and Bracken, R. (2018) 'Interstitial glucose and physical exercise in type 1 diabetes: Integrative physiology, technology, and the gap in-between', *Nutrients*, 10(1), p. 93. doi: 10.3390/nu10010093.

Perriello, G., De Feo, P., Torlone, E., Fanelli, C., Santeusanio, F., Brunetti, P. and Bolli, G. B. (1990) 'Nocturnal spikes of growth hormone secretion cause the dawn phenomenon in type 1 (insulin-dependent) diabetes mellitus by decreasing hepatic (and extrahepatic) sensitivity to insulin in the absence of insulin waning', *Diabetologia*, 33(1), pp. 52–59.

Pfutzner, A., Raz, I., Bitton, G., Klonoff, D., Nagar, R., Hermanns, N. and Haak, T. (2015) 'Improved insulin absorption by means of standardized injection site modulation results in a safer and more efficient prandial insulin treatment. A review of the existing clinical data. [Review]', *Journal of Diabetes Science & Technology*, 9(1), pp. 116–122. doi: 10.1177/1932296814555400.

Pickup, J. C. and Sutton, A. J. (2008) 'Severe hypoglycaemia and glycaemic control in type 1 diabetes: Meta-analysis of multiple daily insulin injections compared with continuous subcutaneous insulin infusion', *Diabetic Medicine*, 25(7), pp. 765–774. doi: 10.1111/j.1464-5491.2008.02486.x.

Pitt, J. P., McCarthy, O. M., Hoeg-Jensen, T., Wellman, B. M. and Bracken, R. M. (2020 October 21) 'Factors influencing insulin absorption around exercise in type 1 diabetes', *Front Endocrinol (Lausanne)*, 11, pp. 573275. doi: 10.3389/fendo.2020.573275. PMID: 33193089; PMCID: PMC7609903.

Plotnikoff, R. C., Taylor, L. M., Wilson, P. M., Courneya, K. S., Sigal, R. J., Birkett, N., Raine, K. and Svenson, L. W. (2006) 'Factors associated with physical activity in Canadian adults with diabetes', *Medicine and Science in Sports and Exercise*, 38(8), pp. 1526–1534. doi: 10.1249/01.mss.0000228937.86539.95.

Pozzilli, P., Battelino, T., Danne, T., Hovorka, R., Jarosz-Chobot, P. and Renard, E. (2014) 'Continuous subcutaneous insulin infusion in diabetes: Patient populations, safety, efficacy, and pharmacoeconomics', *Diabetes/Metabolism Research and Reviews*, 32(30), pp. 13–23. doi: 10.1002/dmrr.

Quirk, H., Blake, H., Tennyson, R., Randell, T. L. and Glazebrook, C. (2014) 'Physical activity interventions in children and young people with type 1 diabetes mellitus: A systematic review with meta-analysis', *Diabetic Medicine*, 31(10), pp. 1163–1173. doi: 10.1111/dme.12531.

Rempel, M., Yardley, J. E., MacIntosh, A., Hay, J. L., Bouchard, D., Cornish, S., Marks, S. D., Hai, Y., Gordon, J. W. and McGavock, J. (2018 October 26) 'Vigorous intervals and hypoglycemia in type 1 diabetes: A randomized cross over trial', *Scientific Reports*, 8(1), p. 15879. doi: 10.1038/s41598-018-34342-6. PMID: 30367116; PMCID: PMC6203731.

Riddell, M. C., Gallen, I. W., Smart, C. E., Taplin, C. E., Adolfsson, P., Lumb, A. N., Kowalski, A., Rabasa-Lhoret, R., McCrimmon, R. J., Hume, C., Annan, F., Fournier, P. A., Graham, C., Bode, B., Galassetti, P., Jones, T. W., Millán, I. S., Heise, T., Peters, A. L., Petz, A. and Laffel, L. M. (2017) 'Exercise management in type 1 diabetes: A consensus statement', *The Lancet Diabetes & Endocrinology*, 8587(17), pp. 1–14. doi: 10.1016/S2213-8587(17)30014-1.

Röhling, M., Herder, C., Roden, M., Stemper, T. and Müssig, K. (2016) 'Effects of long-term exercise interventions on glycaemic control in type 1 and type 2 diabetes: A systematic review', *Experimental and Clinical Endocrinology & Diabetes*, 124(8), pp. 487–494. doi: 10.1055/s-0042-106293.

Ruegemer, J. J., Squires, R. W., Marsh, H. M., Haymond, M. W., Cryer, P. E., Rizza, R. A. and Miles, J. M. (1990) 'Differences between prebreakfast and late afternoon glycemic responses to exercise in IDDM patients', *Diabetes Care*, 13(2), pp. 104–110.

Schmidt, S. and Nørgaard, K. (2014) 'Bolus calculators', *Journal of Diabetes Science and Technology*, 8(5), pp. 1035–1041. doi: 10.1177/1932296814532906.

Shetty, V. B., Fournier, P. A., Davey, R. J., Retterath, A. J., Paramalingam, N., Roby, H. C., Cooper, M. N., Davis, E. A. and Jones, T. W. (2016) 'Effect of exercise intensity on glucose requirements to maintain euglycemia during exercise in type 1 diabetes', *The Journal of Clinical Endocrinology and Metabolism*, 101(3), pp. 972–980. doi: 10.1210/jc.2015-4026.

Sönksen, P. H., Tompkins, C. V., Srivastava, M. C. and Nabarro, J. D. (1973) 'A comparative study on the metabolism of human insulin and porcine proinsulin in man', *Clinical Science and Molecular Medicine*, 45(5), pp. 633–654.

Thabit, H. and Hovorka, R. (2016) 'Coming of age: The artificial pancreas for type 1 diabetes', *Diabetologia*, 59(9), pp. 1795–1805. doi: 10.1007/s00125-016-4022-4.

Tikkanen-Dolenc, H., Wadén, J., Forsblom, C., Harjutsalo, V., Thorn, L. M., Saraheimo, M., Elonen, N., Rosengård-Bärlund, M., Gordin, D., Tikkanen, H. O., Groop, P.-H. and FinnDiane Study

Group (2016) 'Frequent and intensive physical activity reduces risk of cardiovascular events in type 1 diabetes', *Diabetologia*. doi: 10.1007/s00125-016-4189-8.

Tikkanen-Dolenc, H., Wadén, J., Forsblom, C., Harjutsalo, V., Thorn, L. M., Saraheimo, M., Elonen, N., Tikkanen, H. O., Groop, P.-H. and FinnDiane Study Group (2017) 'Physical activity reduces risk of premature mortality in patients with type 1 diabetes with and without kidney disease', *Diabetes Care*, 40(12), pp. 1727–1732. doi: 10.2337/dc17-0615.

Toghi-Eshghi, S. R. and Yardley, J. E. (2019 November 1) 'Morning (Fasting) vs afternoon resistance exercise in individuals with type 1 diabetes: A randomized crossover study', *The Journal of Clinical Endocrinology and Metabolism*, 104(11), pp. 5217–5224. doi: 10.1210/jc.2018-02384. PMID: 31211392.

Tonoli, C., Heyman, E., Roelands, B., Buyse, L., Cheung, S. S., Berthoin, S. and Meeusen, R. (2012) 'Effects of different types of acute and chronic (training) exercise on glycaemic control in type 1 diabetes mellitus: A meta-analysis', *Sports Medicine*, 42(12), pp. 1059–1080. doi: 10.2165/11635380-000000000-00000.

Turner, D., Luzio, S., Gray, B. J., Bain, S. C., Hanley, S., Richards, A., Rhydderch, D. C., Martin, R., Campbell, M. D., Kilduff, L. P., West, D. J. and Bracken, R. M. (2016) 'Algorithm that delivers an individualized rapid-acting insulin dose after morning resistance exercise counters post-exercise hyperglycaemia in people with type 1 diabetes', *Diabetic Medicine*, 33(4), pp. 506–510. doi: 10.1111/dme.12870.

Turner, D., Luzio, S., Gray, B. J., Dunseath, G., Rees, E. D., Kilduff, L. P., Campbell, M. D., West, D. J., Bain, S. C. and Bracken, R. M. (2015) 'Impact of single and multiple sets of resistance exercise in type 1 diabetes', *Scandinavian Journal of Medicine & Science in Sports*, 25(1), pp. e99–109. doi: 10.1111/sms.12202.

Walsh, J., Roberts, R. and Bailey, T. (2011) 'Guidelines for optimal bolus calculator settings in adults', *Journal of Diabetes Science and Technology (Online)*, 5(1), pp. 129–135. doi: 10.1177/193229681100500118.

West, D. J., Morton, R. D., Stephens, J. W., Bain, S. C., Kilduff, L. P., Luzio, S., Still, R. and Bracken, R. M. (2011a) 'Isomaltulose improves postexercise glycemia by reducing CHO oxidation in T1DM', *Medicine and Science in Sports and Exercise*, 43(2), pp. 204–210. doi: 10.1249/MSS.0b013e3181eb6147.

West, D. J., Stephens, J. W., Bain, S. C., Kilduff, L. P., Luzio, S., Still, R. and Bracken, R. M. (2011b) 'A combined insulin reduction and carbohydrate feeding strategy 30 min before running best preserves blood glucose concentration after exercise through improved fuel oxidation in type 1 diabetes mellitus', *Journal of Sports Sciences*, 29(3), pp. 279–289. doi: 10.1080/02640414.2010.531753.

Wilson, D. M., Calhoun, P. M., Maahs, D. M., Chase, H. P., Messer, L., Buckingham, B. A., Aye, T., Clinton, P. K., Hramiak, I., Kollman, C., Beck, R. W. and In Home Closed Loop Study Group (2015) 'Factors associated with nocturnal hypoglycemia in at-risk adolescents and young adults with type 1 diabetes', *Diabetes Technology & Therapeutics*, 17(6), pp. 385–391. doi: 10.1089/dia.2014.0342.

Yamanouchi, K., Abe, R., Takeda, A., Atsumi, Y., Shichiri, M. and Sato, Y. (2002) 'The effect of walking before and after breakfast on blood glucose levels in patients with type 1 diabetes treated with intensive insulin therapy', *Diabetes Research and Clinical Practice*, 58(1), pp. 11–18.

Yardley, J. E. (2020, December) 'Fasting may alter blood glucose responses to high-intensity interval exercise in adults with type 1 diabetes: A randomized, acute crossover study', *Can J Diabetes*, 44(8), pp. 727–733. doi: 10.1016/j.jcjd.2020.09.007. Epub 2020 Sep 14. PMID: 33160882.

Yardley, J. E., Hay, J., Abou-Setta, A. M., Marks, S. D. and McGavock, J. (2014) 'A systematic review and meta-analysis of exercise interventions in adults with type 1 diabetes', *Diabetes Research and Clinical Practice*. Elsevier Ireland Ltd, 106(3), pp. 393–400. doi: 10.1016/j.diabres.2014.09.038.

Yardley, J. E., Iscoe, K. E., Sigal, R. J., Kenny, G. P., Perkins, B. A. and Riddell, M. C. (2013) 'Insulin pump therapy is associated with less post-exercise hyperglycemia than multiple daily injections: An observational study of physically active type 1 diabetes patients', *Diabetes Technology & Therapeutics*, 15(1), pp. 84–88. doi: 10.1089/dia.2012.0168.

Yardley, J. E., Kenny, G. P., Perkins, B. A., Riddell, M. C., Malcolm, J., Boulay, P., Khandwala, F. and Sigal, R. J. (2012) 'Effects of performing resistance exercise before versus after aerobic exercise on glycemia in type 1 diabetes', *Diabetes Care*, 35(4), pp. 669–675. doi: 10.2337/dc11-1844.

Yardley, J. E., Sigal, R. J., Riddell, M. C., Perkins, B. A. and Kenny, G. P. (2014) 'Performing resistance exercise before versus after aerobic exercise influences growth hormone secretion in type 1 diabetes', *Applied Physiology, Nutrition, and Metabolism*, 39(2), pp. 262–265. doi: 10.1139/apnm-2013-0329.

Yeh, H., Brown, T. T., Maruthur, N., Ranasinghe, P., Berger, Z. and Golden, S. H. (2016) 'Comparative effectiveness and safety of methods of insulin delivery and glucose monitoring for diabetes mellitus', *Annals of Internal Medicine*, 157(5), 336–347.

Zaharieva, D. P., Cinar, A., Yavelberg, L., Jamnik, V. and Riddell, M. C. (2020, March) 'No disadvantage to insulin pump off vs pump on during intermittent high-intensity exercise in adults with type 1 diabetes', *Canadian Journal of Diabetes*, 44(2), pp. 162–168. doi: 10.1016/j.jcjd.2019.05.015. Epub 2019 Jun 7. PMID: 31416695.

Zaharieva, D. P. and Riddell, M. C. (2015) 'Prevention of exercise-associated dysglycemia: A case study-based approach', *Diabetes Spectrum. American Diabetes Association*, 28(1), pp. 55–62. doi: 10.2337/diaspect.28.1.55.

12

TYPE 2 DIABETES

Joseph Henson, Oluwaseun Anyiam and Dane Vishnubala

Chapter aims

The aims of this chapter are to:

- Outline the mechanisms underlying the development of type 2 diabetes, making specific reference to the terms *insulin resistance*, *relative insulin deficiency* and *pancreatic β cell dysfunction*
- Describe the different treatment options for managing glycaemic control in type 2 diabetes
- Highlight the importance of optimising cardiovascular risk factors and the approaches for managing complications
- Explain the effects type 2 diabetes and its associated complications can have on an individual's ability to exercise
- Outline the effects of exercise on insulin resistance and the potential benefits on glycaemic control and cardiovascular risk factor modification
- List the main recommendations for safe prescription of exercise in type 2 diabetes

Introduction

Type 2 diabetes mellitus (T2D), is a complex heterogeneous disease which affects around 90% of those individuals with diabetes; type 1 diabetes and gestational diabetes mainly make up the remaining 10% (International Diabetes Federation 2019). In 2019, the global prevalence of diabetes was estimated to be 463 million (1 in 11 adults aged 20–79 years), with this figure expected to rise to more than 592 million by 2035 (International Diabetes Federation 2019).

In England and Wales, diabetes is one of the most common chronic illnesses, accounting for one in ten of all hospital admissions and causing approximately 15% of all deaths per year (Hex et al. 2012). T2D consumes approximately 10% of the total National Health Service

DOI: 10.4324/9781315102399-12

budget for England and Wales, which equates to £1.5m an hour, with this figure is likely to rise to 17% by 2035 (Hex et al. 2012).

People with T2D have a significantly lower life expectancy than those without. Gu et al. found that the life expectancy of people with diabetes between 55 and 64 is eight years less than their non-diabetic equivalents, and younger participants (aged 25 to 44) were more than three times more likely to die prematurely (Gu et al. 1998).

The dramatic reduction in life expectancy observed in patients with type 2 diabetes is largely the result of concomitant cardiovascular disease. Cardiovascular complications are the leading cause of death in people with diabetes, with over 50% of deaths attributable to heart disease (Einarson et al. 2018). Furthermore, these complications can cause a considerable impact on the well-being of patient, with blindness, heart failure, kidney failure and leg amputations being much more common in patients with diabetes.

Consequently, management of the condition is not just focused around optimisation of glycaemic control; the modification of cardiovascular risk factors plays a critical role. The ultimate aim of T2D management is to minimise the risk of cardiovascular morbidity (Davies et al. 2018a).

Overview of pathology

Although type 1 and type 2 diabetes manifest in similar ways, resulting from the presence of chronic hyperglycaemia, the underlying mechanisms are very different. Type 1 diabetes is characterised by the presence of an absolute insulin deficiency; however, the situation with T2D is far more complex. T2D is described as a disorder primarily of insulin resistance, which in the latter stages can result in a relative insulin deficiency. This (in)ability to secrete adequate amounts of insulin depends on beta-cell function and mass. Chronic hyperglycaemia is detrimental to pancreatic beta-cells, causing impaired insulin secretion and playing an essential role in the regulation of beta-cell turnover. Note this deficiency is relative, not absolute as in the case of type 1 diabetes, and it is this distinction that underlies the subtle differences in the symptoms and management approaches of the two types. The most obvious example of this is the fact that whilst the majority of patients with T2D can be managed without insulin therapy, insulin is essential for the management of type 1 diabetes.

Insulin is an important hormone in the human body which regulates the metabolism of carbohydrates, lipids and amino acids. Its specific effects are listed next (Dimitriadis et al. 2011):

- Increased glucose uptake into muscle and adipose tissue
- Increased rate of glucose metabolism and glycogen production in muscle and adipose tissue
- Inhibition of glycogen breakdown and gluconeogenesis in the liver and muscle cells
- Simulation of fatty acid synthesis in tissues (from glucose metabolism)
- Increased triglyceride uptake and reduced rate of lipolysis in adipose tissue, resulting in increased fat storage
- Increased rate of cholesterol and very low-density lipoprotein synthesis in the liver
- Increased rate of amino acid transport and protein synthesis, primarily in muscle (also adipose tissue and liver)

It is secreted from β cells located in the pancreas in response to increased blood glucose concentration. In the fasted state – when there is no digestion occurring – insulin secretion is low, and at these low concentrations, it is mainly interacting with the liver to regulate the amount of gluconeogenesis occurring to maintain normal blood glucose levels (Hatting et al. 2018). Following food ingestion, insulin is secreted in response to rising blood glucose concentrations and acts primarily on muscle and adipose tissue with the overall aim of maintaining blood glucose concentrations between the normal physiological range (3.5–8.0 mmol/L) (Rizza 2010).

The majority of insulin action occurs on muscle cells; indeed, skeletal muscle is the largest insulin-sensing organ of the body and is responsible for 85% of whole body glucose uptake (Dimitriadis et al. 2011). There is a consensus that it is resistance to insulin within skeletal muscle is the primary pathology that ultimately results in T2D (DeFronzo 2010; Wilcox 2005) (although differing opinions do exist in the literature), indicating the importance of exercise in its management.

Several studies have proposed impaired glycogen synthesis within muscle cells as the initial defect leading to skeletal muscle insulin resistance, and this has been shown to have a strong genetic component (DeFronzo 2009a). Impaired glycogenesis disrupts insulin-signalling pathways within the muscle cell, eventually attenuating the cell's response to insulin. Insulin signalling may also be aggravated by elevated levels of fatty acids (Sears 2015), thus providing some explanation for the link between obesity and insulin resistance. It is likely that there is interplay between a number of mechanisms that result in disrupted insulin signalling; however, the combined effect is an impaired ability of the muscle cell to increase glucose uptake and metabolism.

The reduced response of muscle cells to insulin results in a compensatory adaptation by pancreatic β cells to increase insulin secretion in order to maintain normal blood glucose concentration (Cerf 2013). Initially, this compensation is adequate; however, as the insulin resistance progresses, the β cells become incapable of secreting enough insulin. Once this point is reached, hyperglycaemia ensues, which exacerbates the situation by further impairing insulin secretion and causing damage and destruction of β cells (Cerf 2013). The overall resultant effect is chronic progressive hyperglycaemia and the onset of T2D.

Other mechanisms may also be contributing to the development of hyperglycaemia. Hepatic insulin resistance is well known to be associated with T2D (Shulman 2014). Hepatic insulin resistance results in elevated fasting blood glucose concentration as the liver produces excessive levels of glucose in the fasted state due to the impaired response to insulin. Furthermore, hepatic insulin resistance strongly correlates with visceral fat content and fatty acid levels, again providing a link between obesity and T2D (Kirchhoff et al. 2007). Elevated free fatty acids can also cause direct damage to β-cell function in a similar way to chronic hyperglycaemia (Robertson et al. 2004).

As stated previously, T2D results from an interplay of insulin resistance and a relative insulin deficiency. Several mechanisms are present which can result in either of these phenomena, and the contribution of each likely differs among individual patients. Methods to improve insulin sensitivity are well known to improve blood glucose concentrations and may even cause complete reversal of T2D (Hallberg et al. 2019). Thus, the role of insulin resistance is of crucial importance, and the effects of exercise in improving this will be discussed later in the chapter.

Management and medications

The association between hyperglycaemia and cardiovascular disease is well documented (Laakso 1999; Selvin et al. 2004). Haemoglobin A1c (HbA1c) is reflective of the average blood glucose concentrations for the last two to three months and is a common marker for monitoring glycaemic control that also serves as an indicator for diabetes-related diseases (National Institute for Health and Care Excellence[NICE] 2019a). For example, in the 1990s, the pioneering Diabetes Control and Complications Trial (DCCT) study demonstrated that in people with 'insulin-dependent' diabetes, a 2% reduction in HbA1c decreased the rate of development of retinopathy, microalbuminuria (> 30 to < 300 mg/d) and frank albuminuria (> 300 mg/d) by 54%, 39% and 54%, respectively (Diabetes Control and Complications Trial Research Group, Nathan et al. 1993).

The same group proceeded to show that after 6.5 years of follow-up, this 2% reduction in HbA1c also reduced the risk of severe cardiovascular events (nonfatal myocardial infarction, stroke or death from cardiovascular disease) by 57% (Nathan et al. 2007). These findings were since replicated by other groups, such as the United Kingdom Prospective Diabetes Study (UKPDS) (Holman et al. 2008), and as a consequence, optimisation of glycaemic control has been of paramount importance in the management of patients with diabetes.

Current NICE guidance for T2D states that patients should be supported to achieve a target HbA1c of 48 mmol/mol (6.5%) (National Institute for Health and Care Excellence 2019). However, this target may vary, depending on a patient's circumstances, and an individualised approach to target setting is recommended. Methods of achieving this target differ from those in type 1 diabetes and are discussed next.

Management of glycaemic control

First-line therapy for those with T2D includes metformin and a comprehensive lifestyle evaluation (including weight management and physical activity) (Davies et al. 2018b). Depending on the HbA1c concentration, the management of glycaemic control follows a step-wise approach and a number of factors must be considered. These include:

- Symptoms at presentation
- Pre-existing co-morbidities
- Patient preference
- Tolerability

Importantly, a patient who is symptomatic at presentation – polyuria, thirst, weight loss – necessitates immediate initiation of insulin (or a sulphonylurea in mild cases). Otherwise, treatment should follow the NICE algorithm, which is summarised in Figure 12.1 (National Institute for Health and Care Excellence 2019a).

Management of complications

Blood pressure

Hypertension affects the vast majority of patients with diabetes and is associated with a higher risk of both cardiovascular disease and progressive renal dysfunction (de Boer et al.

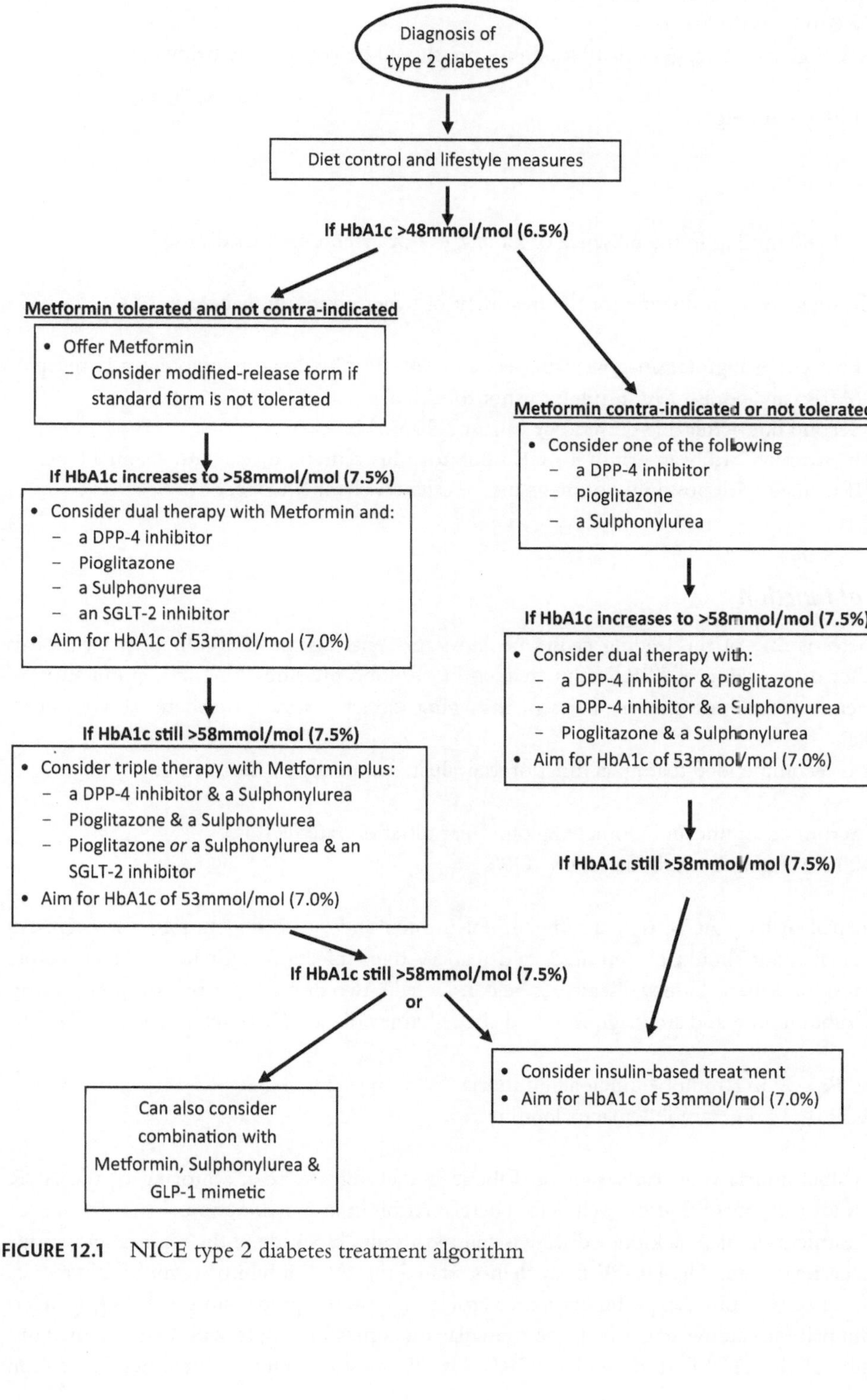

FIGURE 12.1 NICE type 2 diabetes treatment algorithm

2017). There has been much debate about optimal blood pressure targets, and whilst there is agreement that a systolic blood pressure less than 140 mmHg is beneficial, studies like the ACCORD study suggest that the benefits of aiming for lower targets are minimal (ACCORD Study Group et al. 2010).

NICE guidance suggests that blood pressure should be consistently below:

- 140/80 mmHg

or

- 130/80 mmHg in the presence of kidney, eye or cerebrovascular disease

NICE suggests the following for the treatment of hypertension in diabetes:

- First line – angiotensin-converting-enzyme (ACE) inhibitor (or angiotensin II-receptor (AIIR) antagonist if ACE inhibitor not tolerated)
- Second line – thiazide diuretic **or** calcium channel blocker
- If African-Caribbean origin – ACE Inhibitor **plus** diuretic **or** calcium channel blocker
- If woman with possibility of pregnancy – calcium channel blocker

Renal function

Diabetes is one of the leading causes of end-stage renal disease (ESRD). Hypertension is another major cause of ESRD; thus reduction of blood pressure alongside optimisation of glycaemic control are the priorities in managing kidney disease in diabetes (Davies et al. 2018a).

It is recommended that renal function is evaluated annually by measuring:

1. Serum creatinine and estimated glomerular filtration rate (eGFR)
2. Urine albumin:creatinine ratio (ACR)

A normal urinary ACR is < 2.5 mg/mmol in men and < 3.5 mg/mmol in women. An abnormal result should be repeated, and urinary tract infection must be excluded before diagnosis of diabetic kidney disease can be considered – two or more positive samples confirm microalbuminuria and are diagnostic of diabetic kidney disease (Gross et al. 2005).

ACR ≤ 30 mg/mmol = microalbuminuria
ACR > 30 mg/mmol = macroalbuminuria

Microalbuminuria is an early sign of diabetic kidney disease, so monitoring of the ACR allows for early identification well before deterioration in kidney function.

Treatment of diabetic kidney disease is centred around blockade of the renin-angiotensin-aldosterone system. The HOPE study demonstrated that ACE inhibitors significantly reduce the level of albuminuria/proteinuria and, crucially, slow the progression to ESRF ('Effects of ramipril on cardiovascular and microvascular outcomes in people with diabetes mellitus: Results of the HOPE study and MICRO-HOPE substudy. Heart Outcomes Prevention

Evaluation Study Investigators 2000). AIIR antagonists are recommended if ACE inhibitors are not tolerated. A recent meta-analysis showed no superiority of one over the other and no benefit in combining the two to treat diabetic nephropathy (Bangalore et al. 2016). If the ACE inhibitor/AIIR-antagonist has been titrated up to the maximum dose and target blood pressure has still not been achieved, then alternative antihypertensives will be added.

Referral to a renal specialist is generally considered in the following situations:

- eGFR < 30
- Rapid deterioration in eGFR
- Haematuria (dipstick or frank)

Lipid profile

In conjunction with glycaemic control and blood pressure, optimisation of lipids is vital to facilitate improvement in overall cardiovascular disease risk. It has been suggested that control of lipids in patients with diabetes might even be more beneficial for reducing cardiovascular risk than tight glycaemic control (Gaede et al. 2008).

As a consequence, it is recommended that the full lipid profile (total cholesterol, HDL cholesterol, LDL cholesterol and triglycerides) is checked annually. Although NICE do not specify absolute targets for lipid control, it is generally accepted that the following should be aimed for:

- Total cholesterol < 4.0 mmol/L
- LDL cholesterol < 2.0 mmol/L
- HDL cholesterol > 1.0 mmol/L
- Triglycerides < 1.7 mmol/L

The treatment of choice is statins, which have demonstrated a 13% and 21% reduction in mortality and major vascular events, respectively, per every 1 mmol/L reduction in LDL concentration (Cholesterol Treatment Trialists' (CTT) Collaboration et al. 2010).

Foot-related complications

Foot related complications can be caused by diabetic neuropathy (nerve damage), peripheral vascular disease or a combination of the two. NICE estimate that up to 10% of people with diabetes will have a foot ulcer at some point (National Institute for Health and Care Excellence 2019b). Not only is it prevalent, but it is also an important cause of serious morbidity and mortality. Diabetes is responsible for more than 80% of non-traumatic limb amputations, and up to 70% of these patients will then die within five years of their amputation (National Institute for Health and Care Excellence 2019b).

NICE recommend the following foot examination is performed annually, assessing specifically for presence or risk of foot disease:

- Inspection for:
    - Ulceration
    - Infection/inflammation

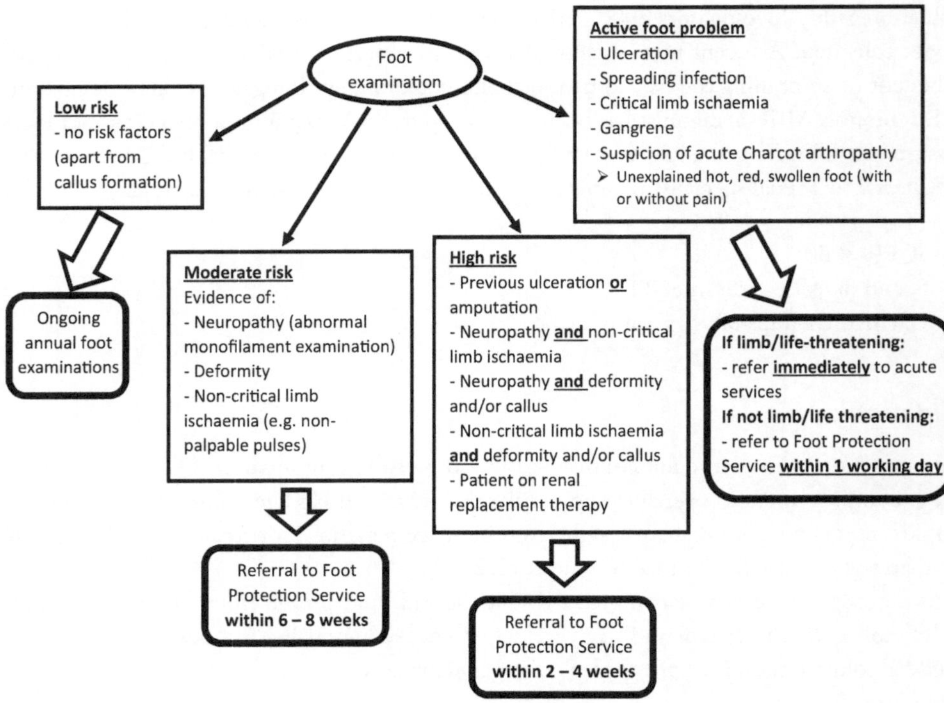

FIGURE 12.2 Foot health risk assessment

    - Gangrene
    - Callus formation
    - Deformity (including Charcot's arthropathy)
- Examination for neuropathy using a 10 g monofilament
- Examination of pulses (dorsalis pedis and posterior tibial)

Note that feet should also be examined any time a patient presents with a foot problem or on any admission to hospital. The examination should be performed with a view to identifying and managing the risk of developing further foot disease. Once this risk is identified, patients should be referred to the appropriate management pathway, as summarised in Figure 12.2.

The foot protection service is a multidisciplinary team that is led by a podiatrist with specialist training in diabetic foot problems. It also involves input from diabetologists, diabetes specialist nurses, vascular surgeons, orthopaedic surgeons, microbiology, biomechanics and orthotics.

Retinopathy

Eye disease is another common complication of diabetes which can have major consequences. Diabetic retinopathy is present in around 40% of patients with diabetes and is the leading cause of blindness in patients aged 20 to 74 (Cheung et al. 2010). The onset and progression of retinopathy is closely associated with glycaemic control, and the ACCORD trial demonstrated that intensive glycaemic control can reduce the risk of retinopathy (ACCORD Study Group, ACCORD Eye Study Group et al. 2010).

All patients with diabetes should be incorporated into an annual eye-screening programme involving digital retinal photography (National Institute for Health and Care Excellence 2019) so patients at risk of disabling eye disease can be identified early and preventative measures can be taken to avoid significant morbidity. Retinal photographs are reviewed by trained retinal screeners who assess both the peripheral retina and the macula and assign a grade against the criteria in Table 12.1 (National Institute for Health and Care Excellence 2019).

Once a grade has been determined for the extent of both retinopathy and maculopathy, patients are managed accordingly (National Institute for Health and Care Excellence 2019). Patients with no evidence of maculopathy (M0) remain in the annual screening programme; however, if there is any evidence of maculopathy (M1), they are referred to the hospital eye service.

Retinopathy is managed in the following way:

- Patients with grades R0 and R1 remain in the annual screening programme.
- Patients with grade R2 are referred to the hospital eye service.
- Patients with grade R3 receive a fast-track referral to the hospital eye service for immediate review (i.e. within 24 hours).

In addition to referral for specialist ophthalmological review upon the development of retinopathy or maculopathy, it is also imperative to identify and address any cardiovascular disease risk factors. This includes improvement of glycaemic control and tight control of blood pressure and cholesterol (as well as smoking cessation). Patients should be educated regarding the risks of worsening eye disease if these issues are not addressed.

TABLE 12.1 Eye health assessment grading criteria

Retinopathy	
R0	No abnormalities
R1 (Background)	Microaneurysms
	Retinal haemorrhages ± exudate
R2 (Pre-proliferative)	Multiple blot haemorrhages
	Venous beading
	Venous loop or reduplication
R3 (Proliferative)	New vessel formation
	Pre-retinal/vitreous haemorrhage
	Pre-retinal fibrosis ± tractional retinal detachment
Maculopathy	
M0	No abnormalities
M1	Exudate or retinal thickening within 1 disc diameter of the centre of the fovea
	Group of exudates within the macula
	Microaneurysm or haemorrhage within 1 disc diameter of the centre of the fovea if associated with visual impairment

Management of lifestyle factors

Smoking and alcohol

Smoking significantly increases the risk of cardiovascular disease, particularly in the presence of diabetes. As a result, NICE guidelines stipulate that patients with diabetes who smoke should be given advice about smoking cessation and use of cessation services (National Institute for Health and Care Excellence 2019). This is particularly important for those who have developed early cardiovascular complications (e.g. microalbuminuria or pre-proliferative retinopathy), and patients should be advised that stopping may reduce the risk of progression to more severe disease.

The risks of excessive alcohol intake are well documented, and patients with diabetes should be given the same advice as any person regarding this. In addition, patients need to be made aware of the increased risk of hypoglycaemia with excessive alcohol intake when taking insulin or sulphonylurea medication.

Autonomic neuropathy

Autonomic neuropathy occurs when the nerves that control involuntary bodily functions are damaged. Although a less commonly recognised complication of diabetes, it can still lead to significant negative effects on the well-being of patients. The manifestations of autonomic neuropathy include:

- Orthostatic hypotension
- Resting tachycardia
- Gastroparesis (bloating, early satiety, nausea, vomiting, post-prandial hypoglycaemia)
- Diarrhoea/gut bacterial overgrowth
- Constipation
- Faecal incontinence
- Erectile dysfunction
- Female sexual dysfunction
- Neurogenic bladder
- Gustatory sweating/anhidrosis
- Argyll-Robertson pupil

Manifestations such as gastroparesis, orthostatic hypotension and erectile dysfunction may well improve with appropriate management; therefore, it is important to screen for these regularly and consider pharmacological options where possible.

Effect of type 2 diabetes on the exercise response

T2D and its associated complications can affect the physical well-being of patients in a variety of ways which can have associated effects on their physical ability to perform exercise.

Chronic hyperglycaemia significantly reduces the size and strength of muscle, resulting in a discernible reduction in exercise tolerance (Kalyani et al. 2015, Gulsin et al. 2020). Additionally, it may accelerate the decline in muscle strength and functional status observed with advancing age (Bianchi 2016). Chronic hyperglycaemia also leads to impaired joint mobility, likely due to the formation of metabolites that interact with the collagen in the joint surfaces (Abate et al. 2013).

The combination of reduced muscle strength, exercise tolerance and mobility will undoubtedly affect the ability of patients with T2D to engage in specific forms of exercise. Although high-intensity aerobic training or resistance training may be the most beneficial form of exercise required to improve the health of patients with T2D, the presence of these factors may render them physically incapable to perform such exercise and realise their benefits. For this reason, aerobic exercise of lower or moderate intensity is often the most appropriate approach.

The presence of complications will also affect exercise response, and the complication which is likely to have the most significant affect is cardiovascular disease. Cardiovascular disease is caused by impaired blood supply resulting from atherosclerosis, which is also accelerated by T2D (DeFronzo 2010). This can directly affect the vascular supply to muscle, further impacting muscle function. However, one important manifestation of atherosclerosis is ischaemic heart disease, which can lead to impaired cardiac function and consequently reduced whole-body exercise tolerance. In the presence of ischaemic heart disease, the concern of precipitating an acute cardiac event whilst exercising is an important one, and patients may well avoid exercise because of this.

The other common manifestation is peripheral vascular disease, which can result in a range of additional problems, from exercise-induced limb pain to limb amputations. In particular, the presence of limb amputations will obviously affect the type of exercise a patient can participate in. Furthermore, it signifies a high risk of precipitating an acute cardiovascular event, even in the absence of other cardiovascular disease.

Neuropathy is another complication of T2D that can have an impact on exercise participation, particularly autonomic neuropathy. The autonomic nervous system mediates the 'stress response' to physical activity. Patients with autonomic dysfunction suffer from chronotropic incompetence (inability to elevate the heart rate in response to physical activity), heat-related illness (due to an impaired sweating response) and postural hypotension. These symptoms could also reduce the patient's ability to engage in exercise safely, particularly the more vigorous or high-intensity forms.

The effects of prescribed medications on the exercise response are described in Table 12.2.

Effects of exercise training

The effects of exercise on patients with T2D demonstrate a considerable amount of individual variation. There are a wide range of exercise options available, and different individuals may respond more positively to one type than another. In addition, T2D is a disorder of impaired glucose control which is strongly associated with obesity and predisposes to a high risk of cardiovascular disease. Therefore, one must consider these three parameters when discussing the potential effects of exercise on improving the health of patients with T2D. An individual may have a dramatic improvement in HbA1c with high-intensity training but may notice significant weight loss with moderate-intensity continuous training, both of which will improve health.

This demonstrates the crucial importance of identifying the key motivators underlying the individual's desire to engage in exercise to improve their health, particularly highlighting which aspects of their health they are most interested in improving. Additionally, an exercise

TABLE 12.2 Medication considerations for exercise for people with type 2 diabetes

Class name	*Generic name (Brand name)*	*Action*	*Side effects*	*Exercise considerations and safety/dose adjustments*
Biguanides	**metformin** (Bolamyn, Diagemet, Glucient, Glucophage and Metabet)	Increases insulin sensitivity and reduces hepatic gluconeogenesis; maximum plasma concentration is reached in ~2.5 hours; steady-state plasma concentrations are reached within 24 to 48 hours	**Common** Abdominal pain; decrease in appetite; diarrhoea; gastrointestinal disorder; nausea; alterations in taste; vomiting **Uncommon** Hepatitis; lactic acidosis (discontinue); skin reactions; reduced vitamin B12 absorption	• Generally safe; no dose adjustment for exercise
Dipeptidyl peptidase-4 inhibitors (DPP-4i)*	**alogliptin** (Vipidia) **linagliptin** (Trajenta) **sitagliptin** (Januvia) s**axagliptin** (Onglyza) **vildagliptin** (Galvus)	Inhibits DDP-4 to increase insulin secretion and lower glucagon secretion; the effect may begin quickly, within the first one to two weeks; blood glucose may begin to drop after just a few doses; weight neutral	**Common** Headache **Uncommon** Constipation; dizziness; skin reactions	• Generally safe; no dose adjustment for exercise • Slight risk of congestive heart failure with saxagliptin and alogliptin
Glucagon-like peptide-1 receptor agonists (GLP-1RA)	**dulaglutide** (Trulicity) **exenatide** (Byetta) **liraglutide** (Saxenda) **lixisenatide** (Lyxumia)	Binds to and activates the GLP-1 receptor to increase insulin secretion; suppresses glucagon secretion and slows gastric emptying, thus encouraging weight loss; it takes about two weeks to lower blood glucose levels	**Common** Decrease in appetite; lack of energy; burping; constipation; diarrhoea; dizziness; dry mouth; gallbladder disorders; gastrointestinal discomfort; headache; increased risk of infection; insomnia; nausea; skin reactions; alterations in taste; toothache; vomiting **Uncommon** Dehydration; malaise; pancreatitis; renal impairment; tachycardia	• Generally safe; no dose adjustment for exercise but may need to lower insulin or sulfonylurea dose • May increase risk of hypoglycaemia when used with insulin or sulfonylureas but not when used alone

Sodium-glucose transporter 2 inhibitors (SGLT2i)	**canagliflozin** (Invokana) **dapagliflozin** (Forxiga) e**mpagliflozin** (Jardiance)	Reversibly inhibits SGLT2 in the renal proximal convoluted tubule to reduce glucose reabsorption and increase urinary glucose excretion; associated with weight loss and significantly improves cardiovascular risk; starts to work after ~2 hours to reduce blood glucose levels, but it may take a week for it to take full effect	<u>Common</u> Back pain; diabetic ketoacidosis; dizziness; dyslipidaemia; hypoglycaemia (in combination with insulin or sulfonylurea); increased risk of infection; rash; urinary disorders. <u>Uncommon</u> Constipation; dry mouth; genital pruritus; hypovolaemia; thirst; vulvovaginal pruritus	• Generally safe; no dose adjustment for exercise • May increase risk of hypoglycaemia when used with insulin or sulfonylureas but not when used alone
Sulfonylureas	**ginenclamide** (Amglidia) **gliclazide** (Diamicron among others) **glimepiride** (Amaryl) **glipizide** (Glucotrol) **tolbutamide** (Orinase)	Acts via augmentation of secretion of insulin from pancreatic beta-cells; sulphonylureas may also cause a reduction in serum glucagon and potentiate the action of insulin at the extrapancreatic tissues; associated with weight gain; duration of action ranges from 6 to 24 hours	<u>Common</u> Abdominal pain; diarrhoea; hypoglycaemia; nausea. <u>Uncommon</u> Hepatic disorders; vomiting	• Generally safe; no specific dosing adjustments for acute exercise • May require downward dose titration in response to regular exercise training if an increase in the frequency of hypoglycemia occurs
Thiazolidinediones	**pioglitazone** (Actos and Glidipion)	Reduces peripheral insulin resistance, leading to a reduction of blood-glucose concentration; associated with weight gain In the fasting state, first measurable in serum within 30 minutes, with peak concentrations observed within two hours; food slightly delays the time to peak serum concentration to three to four hours but does not alter the extent of absorption	<u>Common</u> Bone fractures; increased risk of infection; numbness; visual impairment <u>Uncommon</u> Bladder cancer; insomnia	• Generally safe; no dose adjustment for exercise • Fluid retention
Insulin	**See Chapter 11**			

* For DPP-4i and SGLT2i medication, the brand name changes when combined with metformin

practitioner must also maintain flexibility in their approach to exercise recommendation and be willing to consider an alternative approach if a recommendation does not produce the desired results. An individual's lack of response to an exercise intervention is not always caused by a fundamental inability to respond to exercise; it may not be the correct exercise modality for them.

Overall effects of exercise on type 2 diabetes outcomes

A number of large-scale meta-analyses have consistently demonstrated an improvement in glycaemic control following a long-term exercise intervention, with a reduction in HbA1c in the region of around 0.6 to 0.7% (Umpierre et al. 2011; Boule et al. 2001). At first glance, this may seem like a minimal improvement; however, considering the UKPDS group findings of a 1% rise HbA1c representing a 21% increased risk of death (Stratton et al. 2000), a 0.6% improvement has some clear clinical significance.

Exercise interventions can also reduce the risk of developing T2D in people who are at high risk, with efficacy trials demonstrating that lifestyle interventions (where physical activity is a core component) can reduce the risk of T2D by 30 to 60% (Gillies et al. 2007). These landmark studies have also been shown to yield benefits after the cessation of the initial intervention. For example, the Da Qing Diabetes Prevention Programme demonstrated that a relative risk reduction of 45% was maintained at 23 years (17 years after the intervention ended) (Li et al. 2014). Furthermore, within-trial data of the Finnish Diabetes Prevention Programme shows that the rate of progression to T2D at follow-up (7 years) was dramatically reduced (to almost zero) for those who made five modest lifestyle changes. These included a reduction in weight, increase in physical activity, increase in fibre intake and reduction in total fat and saturated fat intake (Lindstrom et al. 2006). It is important to note that the success of such prevention programmes is largely underpinned by reductions in body weight and increasing levels of physical activity. As described previously, the risk of fatal cardiovascular events is much higher in individuals with type 2 diabetes than in the normal population; therefore, the ultimate aim of T2D management is to reduce this risk as much as possible. It is important to elucidate the effect of any management intervention on reducing this risk, and exercise treatment is no exception.

Although prospective studies investigating the benefits of long-term exercise interventions on cardiovascular outcomes are limited, there is strong evidence that exercise interventions improve a wide range of risk factors associated with cardiovascular disease (Snowling, Hopkins 2006). Balducci et al. (2010) examined people living with obesity and T2D who were previously sedentary and were enrolled to a 12-month exercise programme. They demonstrated significant improvements across almost all risk factors for cardiovascular disease, as well as overall cardiovascular risk scores.

The Look AHEAD Study (Look AHEAD Research Group et al. 2013) investigated the effects of intensive lifestyle modifications on the occurrence of serious cardiovascular events (myocardial infarction, stroke, hospitalisation from angina, heart failure or peripheral vascular disease and fatal myocardial infarction) in older adults with T2D over a period of approximately ten years. These results were compared to a diabetes support and education control group. Somewhat disappointingly, the study reported no significant difference in serious cardiovascular events between the groups. This may have been driven by the greater use of medications known to induce cardiovascular benefits in the diabetes support and education group. It is also important to note that the main aim of the lifestyle modification was achievement of 7% weight loss rather than participation in a formalised exercise programme. (The aim was 175 minutes per week.) As a result, the goal of increased physical activity was primarily to assist with weight maintenance efforts. In addition, the exercise was predominantly unsupervised and home based. Therefore, the results appear to be largely dependent on adherence to the intervention content and delivery

In summary, participation in exercise has been consistently shown to cause clinically significant improvements in glycaemic control in individuals with type 2 diabetes. This, along with improvement in other parameters related to cardiovascular disease, does lead to a reduction in overall risk of cardiovascular disease, although there is an absence of prospective data demonstrating a reduction in cardiovascular events. The next section discusses the specific mechanisms involved in the improvement in glycaemic control and cardiovascular risk factors.

Mechanism of exercise-induced improvement in glycaemic control

As described previously, T2D is primarily a disorder of increased insulin resistance, which eventually results in the development of β cell dysfunction, leading to a relative deficiency in insulin. It is this relative insulin deficiency that results in hyperglycaemia and the consequent physical manifestations of type 2 diabetes.

Skeletal muscle is the largest insulin-sensing organ in the human body and is reported to be responsible for 80 to 90% of body glucose uptake (DeFronzo, Tripathy 2009b). Thus, it is of no surprise that a reduced response to insulin in skeletal muscle is likely to be the initial pathology leading to the development of T2D (Wilcox 2005). The improvement in glycaemic control seen with exercise is largely attributed to improvement in insulin sensitivity (Colberg et al. 2016). To understand the mechanisms of this, one must first consider the mechanisms of glucose uptake induced by muscle contraction.

Muscle contraction–induced glucose uptake

It is well established that muscle contractions result in increased uptake of glucose into the contracting muscle cells (Richter, Hargreaves 2013). This is a physiologically necessary action as contracting muscles require energy, which is provided in the form of glucose. Thus, during physical activity, energy (i.e. glucose) requirements in the active muscle cells increase dramatically and this is met by an increase in glucose uptake. Importantly, the mechanism by which contracting muscles increase their glucose uptake does not require the presence of insulin (non-insulin-mediated glucose uptake) (Baron et al. 1988).

In active muscles, a number of physiological changes occur to augment the increase of glucose uptake into muscle cells and provide them with the energy needed to function effectively. Firstly, blood flow to the skeletal muscles increases up to a magnitude of 20-fold compared to resting conditions (Sarelius, Pohl 2010). This dramatically elevated blood flow leads to increased delivery of glucose to the muscle cells and is thought to be the largest contributor to the increase in glucose uptake seen with physical activity (Sarelius, Pohl 2010).

In addition to these vascular effects, mechanisms at the cellular level also act to facilitate increased glucose uptake. Skeletal muscle contraction acutely results in increased presence of glucose transporter type 4 (GLUT4) to the surface of muscle cells. Glucose diffuses into muscle cells primarily through these GLUT4, so their increased presence in the cell membranes, along with the increased glucose delivery to the muscle cells, ultimately results in an elevated rate of glucose diffusion into the contracting cells. Studies in mice that genetically lack the GLUT4 receptor show a vastly reduced change in glucose uptake in response to exercise, demonstrating the importance of GLUT4 in this process (Howlett et al. 2013, Wojtaszewski et al. 1999).

Once glucose enters the muscle cell, it is incorporated into a chain of reactions which eventually lead to the generation of energy, and it has been suggested that this process also improves in response to muscle contraction. The first step of glucose metabolism is its conversion to glucose-6-phosphate (G-6-P) via the enzyme hexokinase (HK). In normal conditions, G-6-P exhibits negative feedback on HK in order to control its activity and prevent excessive metabolism of glucose (Calmettes et al. 2013). In contracting muscle cells, the influx of glucose reduces the concentration of G-6-P, thus removing the inhibition of HK and increasing its activity.

Thus, there are three main mechanisms acting synergistically to increase glucose delivery, uptake and metabolism in active muscle cells. Whilst these mechanisms are independent of insulin, there is a high degree of overlap between them and the mechanisms responsible for insulin-stimulated glucose uptake into muscle cells. It is important to note that as exercise and insulin work via different pathways, stimulation of both can lead to an excessive response, explaining the increased risk of hypoglycaemia in individuals who take insulin when exercising.

Mechanisms of improved insulin sensitivity

Insulin also promotes glucose uptake into muscle cells by stimulating an increased presence of GLUT4 on the cell membranes of muscle cells to promote uptake of glucose into cells. Repeated bouts of exercise have been shown to cause a prolonged increase in the GLUT4 content of muscles in patients with type 2 diabetes (Zierath et al. 2000). Thus, following repeated bouts of exercise, less insulin is required to produce the same amount of glucose uptake into cells, indirectly resulting in improved insulin sensitivity.

Exercise may also exhibit positive effects directly on the intracellular pathways stimulated by insulin. Exercise has been noted to increase the concentration of the insulin receptor and its binding of insulin and improve downstream signalling (Roberts et al. 2013). Other effects of exercise include reduction in inflammatory cytokines that disrupt insulin-signalling pathways (Roberts et al. 2013) and increased expression of hexokinase genes, potentially resulting in an increased rate of glucose metabolism stimulated by insulin (Harrington, Bush 2003).

Arguably most significantly, exercise has been suggested to improve the function of insulin-secreting β cells. Recently, Madsen et al. reported an increased pancreatic β-cell function in individuals with type 2 diabetes following an eight-week high-intensity interval training programme (Madsen et al. 2015). Slentz et al. reported similar findings following vigorous and moderate-intensity exercise, albeit via different mechanisms (Slentz et al. 2009).

Similarly, resistance training is known to facilitate physiological adaptations in those with T2D. Broadly, these include beneficial changes in insulin sensitivity through increased skeletal muscle mass, glucose storage, enhanced glucose clearance and improved mitochondrial oxidative capacity (Pesta et al. 2017). These systemic factors may contribute to synergistically ameliorate HbA1c in patients with T2D.

In summary, muscle is the largest organ in the human body responsible for glucose homeostasis. Exercise causes increases of glucose uptake via physiological mechanisms which are related to the pathways mediated by insulin. Chronic increases in GLUT4 presence in muscle cell membranes are seemingly the most pertinent mechanism by which exercise improves insulin resistance; however, other intracellular mechanisms undoubtedly exist. Exercise may even lead to improvements in pancreatic β-cell function, although further research into this area is required.

Mechanisms of exercise-induced reductions in cardiovascular risk factors

Chronic hyperglycaemia is a major risk factor for cardiovascular disease and the effects of exercise in ameliorating this were discussed in the previous section. Exercise also leads to improvements in other risk factors associated with cardiovascular disease, and these are outlined next.

Blood pressure – Vascular endothelial dysfunction is a common consequence of type 2 diabetes (Avogaro et al. 2011). This results in hypertension, as well as contributing to several other complications of type 2 diabetes. Vascular endothelial function can be improved and restored with exercise, resulting in an improvement in blood pressure (Lee et al. 2018). Although beneficial effects on blood pressure are not always demonstrated in clinical trials, a large meta-analysis of 54 trials with a total of 2,419 participants conclusively demonstrated that exercise interventions induce a modest but significant reduction in both systolic and diastolic blood pressure (Whelton et al. 2002).

Myocardial function – Myocardial function is impaired in individuals with T2D. Vascular endothelial dysfunction contributes to this, and exercise-induced improvements in endothelial function will facilitate restoration of cardiac function. However, participation in exercise also induces direct effects on cardiac function. For example, Cassidy et al. reported a 12% relative increase in left ventricular wall mass and a consequent increase in both stroke volume and ejection fraction after 12 weeks of high-intensity interval training (Cassidy et al. 2016). More recently, a 12-week programme of supervised aerobic training (three sessions per week at a moderate intensity) has also been shown to improve diastolic function in working-age adults with T2D (Gulsin et al. 2020).

Dyslipidaemia – An abnormal lipid profile is closely associated with T2D, and the combination of both dramatically increases the risk of cardiovascular disease. Exercise of sufficient intensity or duration has been shown to increase activity of lipoprotein lipase and cholesteryl ester transfer protein which both improve the body's lipid profile (Mann et al. 2014). Typically, most individuals experience modest short-term changes, on the order of 2 to 5% (Mora et al. 2007).

Physical fitness – Although impaired physical fitness is associated with the presence of risk factors for cardiovascular disease, it has been shown that low physical fitness is itself an independent risk factor for cardiovascular disease (Gupta et al. 2011). Thus, the improvements in physical fitness seen with exercise of all modalities improves this risk and may lead to an observable increase in survival.

Recommendations for fitness testing & exercise programming

Exercise modality

Several studies have investigated the benefits of both aerobic and resistance training in the management of T2D. It is well known that aerobic exercise increases overall cardiorespiratory

TABLE 12.3 Summary of physical activity guidelines for people with type 2 diabetes

Moderate-intensity exercise	A minimum of 150 minutes per week, not allowing more than two days to elapse between exercise sessions.
Vigorous-intensity exercise, including vigorous-intensity continuous exercise as well as high-intensity interval training (HIIT)	Potential to be used as an alternative to moderate-intensity aerobic exercise provided a minimum of 75 minutes per week is undertaken. This may be more relevant in younger and more active individuals.
Light-intensity physical activity, including tasks of daily living and low-intensity structured exercise	Increasing active tasks of daily living should be recommended to all. This intensity of exercise may also be used as the initial focus or as an introduction to exercise in previously inactive individuals.
Resistance exercise	Two to three sessions per week performed on non-consecutive days, with eight to ten exercises per session. One to three sets of each exercise should be performed, reaching 'near-fatigue' by the end of each set.
Flexibility training	Two to three sessions per week focusing on major muscle-tendon groups. Strongly recommended for patients aged > 50 years and those with poor physical function and/or peripheral neuropathy.
Sedentary behaviour	All patients should reduce their daily levels of sedentary behaviour. In particular, prolonged sitting should be interrupted at least every 30 minute with either light or moderate activity.

Source: Adapted from ADA Guidelines for Adults with Type 2 Diabetes (Colberg et al. 2016)

fitness whilst resistance training improves muscle strength and endurance, both of which contribute to overall physical fitness.

Consequently, the current guidance recommends that patients with T2D participate in both aerobic and resistance training A summary of these guidelines is provided in Table 12.3.

Given the relative equivalency of metabolic benefits across different modalities (aerobic and resistance), individual preferences, motivations and circumstances should inform choice. Therefore, any exercise prescription should combine a clinical evaluation with the individual's personal preference. This is important as patients with T2D are likely to exhibit multi-morbidity, which may synergistically impair their physical capabilities. For example, resistance training in combination with aerobic exercise may be encouraged in those with sarcopenia/frailty/poor physical function, given their higher risk of falling and potential peripheral limitations.

Exercise intensity

The effect of exercise intensity has been extensively investigated, with beneficial effects evident across the continuum of human movement (from light activity through to high-intensity interval training [HIIT]). Therefore, in order to provide a frame of reference, the definitions are discussed here. A brief summary can also be found in Table 12.4.

Light-intensity physical activity

The implementation of lower-intensity exercise (corresponding to approximately 40% $\dot{V}O_2$ peak [rate of perceived exertion (RPE) 9–11]), at least during the early stages of a new exercise programme, may lower the risk of adverse events and reduce reliance on risk stratification

TABLE 12.4 Categories of exercise intensity across the continuum of human movement

Exercise intensity	*% $\dot{V}O_2$ peak*	*% HR max*	*Borg rating of perceived exertion (RPE)*	*% 1-RM*
Light	37–40	57–63	9–11	30–49
Moderate	46–63	64–76	12–13	50–69
Vigorous	64–90	77–95	14–17	70–84
Near-maximal	≥ 91	≥ 96	≥ 18	≥ 85

% $\dot{V}O_2$ peak – percentage of peak oxygen consumption
% HR max – percentage of maximal heart rate
RPE – Rating of perceived exertion (Borg 1982)
% 1-RM – percentage of one-repetition maximum
Source: Adapted from (Garber et al. 2011)

and monitoring. This is particularly pertinent in previously inactive individuals, those with multi-morbidity, older adults and those with physical limitations.

Moderate- to vigorous-intensity aerobic exercise

Continuous moderate- to vigorous-intensity aerobic exercise (50–80% $\dot{V}O_2$ peak) remains the most prevalent form of training. This is largely due to its well-demonstrated efficacy and safety in those with T2D. Typically, it is characterised by steady-state moderate- to vigorous-intensity exercise (50–80% $\dot{V}O_2$ peak), with the ultimate aim of enabling individuals to perform training sessions lasting between 45 and 60 minutes.

High-intensity interval training

As previously discussed, low adherence to exercise training programmes remains a major concern in epidemiological studies. Consequently, HIIT has been proposed as an alternative to more traditional forms of exercise. HIIT is typically divided into aerobic and sprint forms (Wisloff et al. 2007, Little et al. 2011), with the latter seldom used in clinical populations due to its demanding workload (characterised by very short bursts [10–30s] of maximal activity). Alternatively, aerobic HIIT protocols offer a more practical alternative for patients with type 2 diabetes. However, caution is still warranted, and progression should be driven by patient tolerance. Low-volume HIIT (LV-HIIT) and aerobic interval training (AIT) are the most widely reported in the literature. LV-HIIT consists of ten one-minute intervals performed at near-maximal aerobic capacity (80–95% $\dot{V}O_2$ peak), which are alternated with one-minute periods of low-intensity active recovery. AIT is characterised by four four-minute bouts at 85 to 95% of maximal heart rate, alternated with three-minute recovery intervals at 50 to 75% HR max (Wisloff et al. 2007, Little et al. 2011).

Resistance exercise

Whilst improving endurance capacity in patients with T2D is paramount, this form of exercise alone does not address the multi-domain deficits present in this population. Those with

T2D are also at increased risk of sarcopenia, impaired balance and reduced flexibility (Collamati et al. 2016), all of which may limit functional capacity and quality of life. Initiating exercise training of any kind without addressing these deficits may also increase risk of injury and aggravate outcomes. Therefore, the inclusion of resistance training is now accepted practice when designing an exercise programme for patients with T2D, as outlined in the American Diabetes Association (ADA) guidelines. (See Table 12.3.)

Exercise volume

As well as the specific recommendations for patients with T2D highlighted in Table 12.3, it is also important to note that any increased movement is likely to induce some form of cardiometabolic benefit. For example, epidemiological and experimental evidence is beginning to emerge demonstrating that breaking up prolonged bouts of sitting with standing, slow walking or other forms of light-intensity physical activity (e.g. walking, simple resistance exercises) elicits substantial, acute improvements in post-prandial glucose metabolism in individuals with established (or at high risk of) T2D (Henson et al. 2016; Dempsey et al. 2016; McCarthy et al. 2017; Henson et al. 2016).

Chronic interventions have also shown that when matched for energy expenditure, prolonged, continuous light-intensity exercise training is as effective as continuous moderate- to high-intensity training in lowering HbA1c in patients with T2D (Hansen et al. 2009). Therefore, encouraging individuals to increase their total daily incidental (non-exercise) physical activity may yield additional health benefits (Colberg et al. 2016). This approach could initially be beneficial for those who are sedentary/deconditioned and unable/reluctant to participate in more formal exercise.

Flexibility

In addition to aerobic and resistance training, the ADA guidelines also highlight the importance of flexibility training (Colberg et al. 2016). Whilst it does not improve glycaemic control, it does confer other benefits such as improved balance and gait, leading to reduced falls risk in patients with peripheral neuropathy. Importantly, the recommendation is that this is used as an adjunct to aerobic/resistance training, not a replacement (Colberg et al. 2016).

Pre-exercise intervention medical review

Although the risk of cardiovascular events is transiently increased during vigorous-intensity exercise, the overall absolute and relative risks remain low. So the benefits of engaging in regular activity outweigh the modest increase in risk of these adverse events (Riebe et al. 2015; Albert et al. 2000; Whang et al. 2006). The ACSM provide guidelines for pre-participation screening (Riebe et al. 2015) but stress that these should be considered in conjunction with the clinical assessment of each given individual to identify their specific risk, requirements and limitations. Importantly, screening should be appropriate for the intensity of activity prescribed.

Notably, the ADA suggests that necessitating medical clearance for all individuals with T2D may be unnecessary (Colberg et al. 2016). Indeed, initiating any screening protocol beyond usual diabetes care does not necessarily reduce the risk of exercise-induced adverse events in asymptomatic individuals with T2D (Young et al. 2009). However, clinical assessment beyond ongoing diabetes management may be reserved for individuals wishing to engage in activities above the demands of brisk walking or when adverse symptoms are experienced at lower intensities (Colberg et al. 2016). Medical evaluation may include symptom-limited exercise testing at the discretion of the health-care professional whist cardiovascular disease risk should also be considered (Riebe et al. 2015).

It should also be ensured that previously inactive individuals start by performing short sessions of low-intensity exercise before the duration and intensity of exercise are increased progressively, as tolerated, towards desired targets. Sedentary individuals may benefit most from a stepped approach whereby they first aim to reduce sitting time through increasing standing, light ambulation or simple resistance exercises (Henson et al. 2016; Dempsey et al. 2016; McCarthy et al. 2017). If tolerated, light ambulation may then progress to purposeful exercise.

Exercise in the presence of complications

Although exercise is a valuable therapeutic mechanism to improve health and well-being, for the large majority of people with T2D, the presence of T2D complications requires serious consideration. The ADA make a series of recommendations on how to manage exercise in these specific situations (Colberg et al. 2016):

Diabetic retinopathy – In the case of mild retinopathy no alterations are required. However, in moderate to severe retinopathy activities that dramatically increase blood pressure (such as powerlifting) or any activities involving jumping, jarring, head down or breath holding should be avoided. No exercise should be performed for three to six months following a vitreous haemorrhage or laser surgery.

Diabetic kidney disease – In patients with microalbuminuria, exercise transiently increases protein excretion, which can give falsely elevated readings if checked within the subsequent 24-hour period. However, exercise is not thought to worsen the progression to chronic kidney disease and may even prevent it (Johansen 2012). Thus, exercise is safe in all stages of kidney disease, although in end-stage or dialysis-dependent renal disease, exercise should be limited to low intensity, and regular monitoring of renal function is essential.

Peripheral neuropathy – Peripheral neuropathy is exceedingly common in patients with type 2 diabetes and predisposes to ulceration, infection and severe foot deformity. Proper foot care – daily examination, keeping feet dry, use of appropriate footwear with gel/air midsoles – is essential and should be advised to all patients. Patients with active ulcers, amputations or foot deformity should avoid any weight-bearing exercises and opt for arm exercises, swimming or cycling (if possible). Similarly, the presence of autonomic neuropathy may complicate an active lifestyle, so patients should obtain medical approval and discuss symptom-limited exercise testing before commencing formal exercise (Colberg et al. 2016).

Other temporary contraindications include acute systemic infections, severe exacerbations of inflammatory joint disease or musculoskeletal injury, severe hypertension and unstable heart failure.

Exercise in specific situations

Patients on insulin – This was covered in Chapter 11, and similar principles will apply to patients with type 2 diabetes on insulin as for patients with type 1 diabetes.

Pregnancy – Guidance by the American College of Obstetricians and Gynecologists states that aerobic exercise of moderate intensity is safe in pregnancy unless specifically contraindicated (American College of Obstetricians and Gynecologists 2003). Therefore, the ADA recommends that pregnant women with or at risk of diabetes should engage in 20 to 30 minutes of moderate-intensity exercise regularly during pregnancy (Colberg et al. 2016).

Older Adults – Exercise is encouraged in older adults as it carries the additional benefit of reducing the decline in strength and muscle mass observed with advancing age and T2D (Park et al. 2006). Baseline physical strength must be taken into consideration when making decisions about the volume and intensity of the exercise.

Participation in performance sports – Some sports such as motor racing, horse racing, paragliding and boxing carry restrictions. If patients are participating in these sports, they can be referred to the individual sport's regulating body or Diabetes UK for further guidance on these restrictions.

Summary

In summary, exercise practitioners must take an individualised approach to making recommendations for exercise programmes to patients with T2D. Several factors related to the patient's current clinical state will need to be considered when formulating a programme. Both aerobic and resistance training have beneficial effects on glycaemic control as well as other cardiovascular risk factors, and an approach combining both carries the most benefit.

Finally, guidelines promote minimum targets, but patients should be encouraged to engage in as much physical activity and structured exercise as possible. Conversely, in patients for whom 150 minutes per week of moderate exercise may not be achievable, any activity is likely to be of benefit and should therefore be encouraged.

Key points

- T2D is a complex heterogeneous disease that affects around 90% of those individuals with diabetes. The consequences of hyperglycemia are broadly separated into microvascular (nephropathy, neuropathy and retinopathy) and macrovascular complications (coronary artery disease, peripheral arterial disease and stroke).
- Exercise is a valuable therapeutic mechanism to improve health and well-being for the large majority of people with T2D.
- Patients with T2D should be encouraged to adopt a physically active lifestyle that spans the whole continuum of human movement. This includes reducing sedentary behaviours, increasing incidental daily activity and participation in appropriate forms of structured exercise.
- Engagement in exercise will elicit a multitude of acute and chronic benefits via multiple mechanisms. These include (but are not limited to) improved cardiorespiratory fitness, glycaemic control, cardiovascular risk profiles and physical function.

- Given the relative equivalency of metabolic benefits across different modalities, exercise prescription should be guided by individual patient preferences, circumstances and tolerance, in combination with clinical evaluation.
- Some types of exercise and co-existing complications may require additional medical screening and clearance prior to participation.

Case study

AB is a 59-year-old man with type 2 diabetes. He complains of tiredness and daytime sleepiness and is living with obesity, with a body mass index of 40 kg/m^2. He is currently unemployed and spends most of the day sedentary, sitting down watching television. His latest clinical review identified pre-proliferative retinopathy and the presence of calluses. He also has a family history of cardiovascular disease and currently takes a statin and ACE inhibitor for high cholesterol and blood pressure, respectively.

In terms of diabetes medication, he currently takes metformin 500 mg three times a day and gliclazide (sulfonylureas) 80 mg twice a day. His HbA1c remains high at 80 mmol/mol (9.5%). AB has consistently poor glucose control and so requires intensification of his glucose-lowering therapy. The patient does not want to take insulin, so his latest consultation served as a wake-up call.

AB has expressed an interest in exercising again but doesn't know where to start. He has been regularly active in the past and enjoyed walking but has become self-conscious about his appearance and struggles with his mobility. He wants to be able to carry out everyday tasks without feeling out of breath. This includes playing with his grandchildren. He is also concerned about exercise increasing the risk of hypoglycaemia and/or a cardiovascular event.

Case study questions

1. According to the NICE algorithm, what are the potential options regarding medication modification or intensification? Also consider the patient's cardiometabolic profile.
2. Why does the optimisation of glycaemic control carry extra importance for this patient?
3. What are the key things to consider when designing an exercise intervention for this patient?
4. What pre-participation screening would you recommend for this patient, if any?
5. What metabolic adaptations to exercise would contribute to improved glycaemic control and reduced cardiovascular risk factors?

6. Are there any safety considerations for exercise given the patient's current medication regimen?
7. Does the presence of co-morbidities warrant any consideration regarding exercise prescription/management?
8. In the first instance, what would your recommendations be regarding frequency, intensity, time and type?
9. Would there be any contraindications or extra safety considerations to think about if the patient had to start insulin therapy?
10. If a pattern of exercise-related hypoglycaemia becomes apparent, what are some of the options to consider?
11. What behaviour change techniques will you use and why?

TABLE 12.5 At-a-glance summary guide to exercise considerations for people with type 2 diabetes

Condition name	Type 2 diabetes mellitus (T2D)
Pathophysiology summary	T2D is a condition characterised by hyperglycaemia, resulting from defects in insulin secretion, hepatic and peripheral glucose uptake or both. Defects in any of these mechanisms lead to a metabolic imbalance responsible for the development of T2D.
Aims of exercise	To improve glycaemic control (primarily HbA1c), cardiorespiratory fitness, cardiometabolic health profiles, physical function and quality of life and to reduce the risk of micro- and macrovascular complications.
Exercise considerations (including contraindications)	The presence of T2D complications (retinopathy, diabetic kidney disease, peripheral neuropathy) or other contraindications (acute systemic infections, severe exacerbations of inflammatory joint disease or musculoskeletal injury, severe hypertension or unstable heart failure) may require some modifications to exercise regimens.
Frequency	For aerobic activity, aim to not allow more than two days to elapse between exercise sessions. For resistance/flexibility exercises, aim for two to three sessions per week, performed on non-consecutive days.
Intensity	Aim to adopt a physically active lifestyle that spans the whole continuum of human movement. This includes reducing sedentary behaviour and increasing incidental daily physical activity. Moderate to vigorous physical activity is likely to yield the greatest physiological response and therefore benefits.
Time	A minimum of 150 minutes per week for moderate-intensity physical activity or 75 minutes for vigorous-intensity physical activity. Prolonged sitting should be interrupted at least every 30 minutes with either light or moderate physical activity.
Type	Given the relative equivalency of metabolic benefits across different modalities (aerobic and resistance), individual preferences, motivations and circumstances should primarily inform choice and therefore type and mode.
Common medications associated	Biguanides, dipeptidyl peptidase-4 (DPP-4) inhibitors, glucagon-like peptide-1 receptor agonists (GLP-1RAs), sodium-glucose transporter 2 inhibitors (SGLT2i's), sulfonylureas, thiazolidinediones, insulin.

Key safety considerations	Medical clearance for all individuals with T2D may be unnecessary. However, clinical assessment beyond ongoing diabetes management must be reserved for individuals wishing to engage in activities above the demands of brisk walking or when adverse symptoms are experienced at lower intensities. Medical evaluation may include symptom-limited exercise testing at the discretion of the health-care professional.
Effect of exercise on conditions	Both aerobic and resistance training have acute and chronic effects on glycaemic control as well as other cardiovascular risk factors and markers of physical function. This is driven by (amongst other things) beneficial changes in insulin sensitivity through increased skeletal muscle mass, glucose storage, enhanced glucose clearance and improved mitochondrial oxidative capacity.

References

Abate, M., Schiavone, C., Salini, V. And Andia, I., 2013. Management of Limited Joint Mobility in Diabetic Patients. *Diabetes, Metabolic Syndrome and Obesity: Targets and Therapy*, **6**, Pp. 197–207.

Accord Study Group, Accord Eye Study Group, Chew, E.Y., Ambrosius, W.T., Davis, M.D., Danis, R.P., Gangaputra, S., Greven, C.M., Hubbard, L., Esser, B.A., Lovato, J.F., Perdue, L.H., Goff, D.C., Jr, Cushman, W.C., Ginsberg, H.N., Elam, M.B., Genuth, S., Gerstein, H.C., Schubart, U. And Fine, L.J., 2010. Effects of Medical Therapies on Retinopathy Progression in Type 2 Diabetes. *The New England Journal of Medicine*, **363**(3), Pp. 233–244.

Accord Study Group, Cushman, W.C., Evans, G.W., Byington, R.P., Goff, D.C., Jr, Grimm, R.H., Jr, Cutler, J.A., Simons-Morton, D.G., Basile, J.N., Corson, M.A., Probstfield, J.L., Katz, L., Peterson, K.A., Friedewald, W.T., Buse, J.B., Bigger, J.T., Gerstein, H.C. And Ismail-Beigi, F., 2010. Effects of Intensive Blood-Pressure Control in Type 2 Diabetes Mellitus. *The New England Journal of Medicine*, **362**(17), Pp. 1575–1585.

Albert, C.M., Mittleman, M.A., Chae, C.U., Lee, I.M., Hennekens, C.H. And Manson, J.E., 2000. Triggering of Sudden Death from Cardiac Causes by Vigorous Exertion. *The New England Journal of Medicine*, **343**(19), Pp. 1355–1361.

American College of Obstetricians and Gynecologists, 2003. Exercise During Pregnancy and the Postpartum Period. *Clinical Obstetrics and Gynecology*, **46**(2), Pp. 496–499.

Avogaro, A., Albiero, M., Menegazzo, L., De Kreutzenberg, S. And Fadini, G.P., 2011. Endothelial Dysfunction in Diabetes: The Role of Reparatory Mechanisms. *Diabetes Care*, **34**(Suppl 2), Pp. S285–90.

Balducci, S., Zanuso, S., Nicolucci, A., De Feo, P., Cavallo, S., Cardelli, P., Fallucca. S., Alessi, E., Fallucca, F., Pugliese, G. And Italian Diabetes Exercise Study (IDES) Investigators, 2010. Effect of an intensive exercise intervention strategy on modifiable cardiovascular risk factors in subjects with type 2 diabetes mellitus: a randomized controlled trial: the Italian Diabetes and Exercise Study (IDES). *Archives of Internal Medicine*, **170**(20), Pp. 1794–1803. doi: 10.1001/archinternmed.2010.380

Bangalore, S., Fakheri, R., Toklu, B. And Messerli, F.H., 2016. Diabetes Mellitus as a Compelling Indication for Use of Renin Angiotensin System Blockers: Systematic Review and Meta-Analysis of Randomized Trials. *BMJ (Clinical Research Ed.)*, **352**, Pp. I438.

Baron, A.D., Brechtel, G., Wallace, P. And Edelman, S.V., 1988. Rates and Tissue Sites of Non-Insulin- and Insulin-Mediated Glucose Uptake in Humans. *The American Journal of Physiclogy*, **255**(6 Pt 1), Pp. E769–74.

Bianchi, L. And Volpato, S., 2016. Muscle Dysfunction in Type 2 Diabetes: A Major Threat to Patient's Mobility and Independence. *Acta Diabetologica*, **53**(6), Pp. 879–889.

Borg, G.A., 1982. Psychophysical Bases of Perceived Exertion. *Medicine and Science in Sports and Exercise*, **14**(5), Pp. 377–381.

Boule, N.G., Haddad, E., Kenny, G.P., Wells, G.A. And Sigal, R.J., 2001. Effects of Exercise on Glycemic Control and Body Mass in Type 2 Diabetes Mellitus: A Meta-Analysis of Controlled Clinical Trials. *Jama: The Journal of the American Medical Association*, **286**(10), Pp. 1218–1227.

Calmettes, G., John, S.A., Weiss, J.N. And Ribalet, B., 2013. Hexokinase-Mitochondrial Interactions Regulate Glucose Metabolism Differentially in Adult and Neonatal Cardiac Myocytes. *The Journal of General Physiology*, **142**(4), Pp. 425–436.

Cassidy, S., Thoma, C., Hallsworth, K., Parikh, J., Hollingsworth, K.G., Taylor, R., Jakovljevic, D.G. And Trenell, M.I., 2016. High Intensity Intermittent Exercise Improves Cardiac Structure and Function and Reduces Liver Fat in Patients with Type 2 Diabetes: A Randomised Controlled Trial. *Diabetologia*, **59**(1), Pp. 56–66.

Cerf, M.E., 2013. Beta Cell Dysfunction and Insulin Resistance. *Frontiers in Endocrinology*, **4**, P. 37.

Cheung, N., Mitchell, P. And Wong, T.Y., 2010. Diabetic Retinopathy. *Lancet (London, England)*, **376**(9735), Pp. 124–136.

Cholesterol Treatment Trialists' (CTT) Collaboration, Baigent, C., Blackwell, L., Emberson, J., Holland, L.E., Reith, C., Bhala, N., Peto, R., Barnes, E.H., Keech, A., Simes, J. And Collins, R., 2010. Efficacy and Safety of More Intensive Lowering of LDL Cholesterol: A Meta-Analysis of Data from 170,000 Participants in 26 Randomised Trials. *Lancet (London, England)*, **376**(9753), Pp. 1670–1681.

Colberg, S.R., Sigal, R.J., Yardley, J.E., Riddell, M.C., Dunstan, D.W., Dempsey, P.C., Horton, E.S., Castorino, K. And Tate, D.F., 2016. Physical Activity/Exercise and Diabetes: A Position Statement of the American Diabetes Association. *Diabetes Care*, **39**(11), Pp. 2065–2079.

Collamati, A., Marzetti, E., Calvani, R., Tosato, M., D'angelo, E., Sisto, A.N. And Landi, F., 2016. Sarcopenia in Heart Failure: Mechanisms and Therapeutic Strategies. *Journal of Geriatric Cardiology: JGC*, **13**(7), Pp. 615–624.

Davies, M.J., D'alessio, D.A., Fradkin, J., Kernan, W.N., Mathieu, C., Mingrone, G., Rossing, P., Tsapas, A., Wexler, D.J. And Buse, J.B., 2018a. Management of Hyperglycaemia in Type 2 Diabetes, 2018. A Consensus Report by the American Diabetes Association (Ada) and the European Association for the Study of Diabetes (EASD). *Diabetologia*, **61**(12), Pp. 2461–2498.

Davies, M.J., D'alessio, D.A., Fradkin, J., Kernan, W.N., Mathieu, C., Mingrone, G., Rossing, P., Tsapas, A., Wexler, D.J. And Buse, J.B., 2018b. Management of Hyperglycemia in Type 2 Diabetes, 2018. A Consensus Report by the American Diabetes Association (Ada) and the European Association for the Study of Diabetes (EASD). *Diabetes Care*, **41**(12), Pp. 2669–2701.

De Boer, I.H., Bangalore, S., Benetos, A., Davis, A.M., Michos, E.D., Muntner, P., Rossing, P., Zoungas, S. And Bakris, G., 2017. Diabetes and Hypertension: A Position Statement by the American Diabetes Association. *Diabetes Care*, **40**(9), Pp. 1273–1284.

Defronzo, R.A., 2010. Insulin Resistance, Lipotoxicity, Type 2 Diabetes and Atherosclerosis: The Missing Links. The Claude Bernard Lecture 2009. *Diabetologia*, **53**(7), Pp. 1270–1287.

Defronzo, R.A. And Tripathy, D., 2009a. Skeletal Muscle Insulin Resistance is the Primary Defect in Type 2 Diabetes. *Diabetes Care*, **32(**Suppl 2), Pp. S157–163.

Defronzo, R.A. And Tripathy, D., 2009b. Skeletal Muscle Insulin Resistance Is the Primary Defect in Type 2 Diabetes. *Diabetes Care*, **32(**Suppl 2), Pp. S157–163.

Dempsey, P.C., Larsen, R.N., Sethi, P., Sacre, J.W., Straznicky, N.E., Cohen, N.D., Cerin, E., Lambert, G.W., Owen, N., Kingwell, B.A. And Dunstan, D.W., 2016. Benefits for Type 2 Diabetes of Interrupting Prolonged Sitting with Brief Bouts of Light Walking or Simple Resistance Activities. *Diabetes Care*, **39**(6), Pp. 964–972.

Diabetes Control and Complications Trial Research Group, Nathan, D.M., Genuth, S., Lachin, J., Cleary, P., Crofford, O., Davis, M., Rand, L. And Siebert, C., 1993. The Effect of Intensive Treatment of Diabetes on the Development and Progression of Long-Term Complications in Insulin-Dependent Diabetes Mellitus. *The New England Journal of Medicine*, **329**(14), Pp. 977–986.

Dimitriadis, G., Mitrou, P., Lambadiari, V., Maratou, E. And Raptis, S.A., 2011. Insulin Effects in Muscle and Adipose Tissue. *Diabetes Research and Clinical Practice*, **93(**Suppl 1), Pp. S52–59.

Einarson, T.R., Acs, A., Ludwig, C. And Panton, U.H., 2018. Prevalence of Cardiovascular Disease in Type 2 Diabetes: A Systematic Literature Review of Scientific Evidence from Across the World In 2007–2017. *Cardiovascular Diabetology*, **17**(1), Pp. 83-018-0728-6.

Gaede, P., Lund-Andersen, H., Parving, H.H. And Pedersen, O., 2008. Effect of a Multifactorial Intervention on Mortality in Type 2 Diabetes. *The New England Journal of Medicine*, **358**(6), Pp. 580–591.

Garber, C.E., Blissmer, B., Deschenes, M.R., Franklin, B.A., Lamonte, M.J., Lee, I M., Nieman, D.C., Swain, D.P. And American College of Sports Medicine, 2011. American College of Sports Medicine Position Stand. Quantity and Quality of Exercise for Developing and Maintaining Cardiorespiratory, Musculoskeletal, and Neuromotor Fitness in Apparently Healthy Adults: Guidance for Prescribing Exercise. *Medicine and Science in Sports and Exercise*, **43**(7), Pp. 1334–1359.

Gillies, C. L., Abrams, K. R., Lambert, P. C., Cooper, N. J., Sutton, A. J., Hsu, R. T. And Khunti, K., 2007. Pharmacological and lifestyle interventions to prevent or delay type 2 diabetes in people with impaired glucose tolerance: systematic review and meta-analysis. *BMJ*, **334**, Pp. 299. doi:10.1136/bmj.39063.689375.55

Gross, J.L., De Azevedo, M.J., Silveiro, S.P., Canani, L.H., Caramori, M.L. And Zelmanovitz, T., 2005. Diabetic Nephropathy: Diagnosis, Prevention, and Treatment. *Diabetes Care*, **28**(1), Pp. 164–176.

Gu, K., Cowie, C.C. And Harris, M.I., 1998. Mortality in Adults with and Without Diabetes in a National Cohort of the U.S. Population, 1971–1993. *Diabetes Care*, **21**(7), Pp. 1138–1145.

Gulsin, G.S., Henson, J., Brady, E.M., Sargeant, J.A., Wilmot, E.G., Athithan, L., Htike, Z.Z., Marsh, A.M., Biglands, J.D., Kellman, P., Khunti, K., Webb, D., Davies, M.J., Yates, T. And Mccann, G.P., 2020. Cardiovascular Determinants of Aerobic Exercise Capacity in Adults with Type 2 Diabetes. *Diabetes Care*, **43**(9), Pp. 2248–2256.

Gulsin, G.S., Swarbrick, D.J., Athithan, L., Brady, E.M., Henson, J., Baldry, E., Argyridou, S., Jaicim, N.B., Squire, G., Walters, Y., Marsh, A.M., Mcadam, J., Parke, K.S., Biglands, J.D., Yates, T., Khunti, K., Davies, M.J. And Mccann, G.P., 2020. Effects of Low-Energy Diet or Exercise on Cardiovascular Function in Working-Age Adults with Type 2 Diabetes: A Prospective, Randomized, Open-Label, Blinded End Point Trial. *Diabetes Care*, **43**(6), Pp. 1300–1310.

Gupta, S., Rohatgi, A., Ayers, C.R., Willis, B.L., Haskell, W.L., Khera, A., Drazner, M.H., De Lemos, J.A. And Berry, J.D., 2011. Cardiorespiratory Fitness and Classification of Risk of Cardiovascular Disease Mortality. *Circulation*, **123**(13), Pp. 1377–1383.

Hallberg, S.J., Gershuni, V.M., Hazbun, T.L. And Athinarayanan, S.J., 2019. Reversing Type 2 Diabetes: A Narrative Review of the Evidence. *Nutrients*, **11**(4), Pp. 10.3390/Nu11040766.

Hansen, D., Dendale, P., Jonkers, R.A., Beelen, M., Manders, R.J., Corluy, L., Mullens, A., Berger, J., Meeusen, R. And Van Loon, L.J., 2009. Continuous Low- to Moderate-Intensity Exercise Training is as Effective as Moderate- to High-Intensity Exercise Training at Lowering Blood Hba(1c) in Obese Type 2 Diabetes Patients. *Diabetologia*, **52**(9), Pp. 1789–1797.

Harrington, G.N. And Bush, D.R., 2003. The Bifunctional Role of Hexokinase in Metabolism and Glucose Signaling. *The Plant Cell*, **15**(11), Pp. 2493–2496.

Hatting, M., Tavares, C.D.J., Sharabi, K., Rines, A.K. And Puigserver, P., 2018. Insulin Regulation of Gluconeogenesis. *Annals of the New York Academy of Sciences*, **1411**(1), Pp. 21–35.

Heart Outcomes Prevention Evaluation (HOPE) Study Investigators, 2000. Effects of Ramipril on Cardiovascular and Microvascular Outcomes in People with Diabetes Mellitus: Results of the Hope Study and Micro-Hope Substudy. Heart Outcomes Prevention Evaluation Study Investigators. *Lancet (London, England)*, **355**(9200), Pp. 253–259.

Henson, J., Davies, M.J., Bodicoat, D.H., Edwardson, C.L., Gill, J.M., Stensel, D.J., Tolfrey, K., Dunstan, D.W., Khunti, K. And Yates, T., 2016. Breaking up Prolonged Sitting with Standing or Walking Attenuates the Postprandial Metabolic Response in Postmenopausal Women: A Randomized Acute Study. *Diabetes Care*, **39**(1), Pp. 130–138.

Henson, J., Dunstan, D.W., Davies, M.J. And Yates, T., 2016. Sedentary Behaviour as a New Behavioural Target in the Prevention and Treatment of Type 2 Diabetes. *Diabetes/Metabolism Research and Reviews*, **32(**Suppl 1), Pp. 213–220.

Hex, N., Bartlett, C., Wright, D., Taylor, M. And Varley, D., 2012. Estimating the Current and Future Costs of Type 1 and Type 2 Diabetes in the UK, Including Direct Health Costs and Indirect

Societal and Productivity Costs. *Diabetic Medicine: A Journal of the British Diabetic Association*, **29**(7), Pp. 855–862.

Holman, R.R., Paul, S.K., Bethel, M.A., Matthews, D.R. And Neil, H.A., 2008. 10-Year Follow-Up of Intensive Glucose Control in Type 2 Diabetes. *The New England Journal of Medicine*, **359**(15), Pp. 1577–1589.

Howlett, K.F., Andrikopoulos, S., Proietto, J. And Hargreaves, M., 2013. Exercise-Induced Muscle Glucose Uptake in Mice with Graded, Muscle-Specific Glut-4 Deletion. *Physiological Reports*, **1**(3), Pp. E00065.

International Diabetes Federation, 2019, 2019-Last Update, Diabetes Atlas, 9th Edition. Available: Http://Www.Idf.Org/Diabetesatlas [June 2020].

Johansen, K.L. And Painter, P., 2012. Exercise in Individuals with CKD. *American Journal of Kidney Diseases: The Official Journal of the National Kidney Foundation*, **59**(1), Pp. 126–134.

Kalyani, R.R., Metter, E.J., Egan, J., Golden, S.H. And Ferrucci, L., 2015. Hyperglycemia Predicts Persistently Lower Muscle Strength with Aging. *Diabetes Care*, **38**(1), Pp. 82–90.

Kirchhoff, K., Kantartzis, K., Machann, J., Schick, F., Thamer, C., Machicao, F., Fritsche, A., Haring, H.U. And Stefan, N., 2007. Impact of Different Fat Depots on Insulin Sensitivity: Predominant Role of Liver Fat. *Journal of Diabetes Science and Technology*, **1**(5), Pp. 753–759.

Laakso, M., 1999. Hyperglycemia and Cardiovascular Disease in Type 2 Diabetes. *Diabetes*, **48**(5), Pp. 937–942.

Lee, J.H., Lee, R., Hwang, M.H., Hamilton, M.T. And Park, Y., 2018. The Effects of Exercise on Vascular Endothelial Function in Type 2 Diabetes: A Systematic Review and Meta-Analysis. *Diabetology & Metabolic Syndrome*, **10**, Pp. 15-018-0316-7. Ecollection 2018.

Li, G., Zhang, P., Wang, J., An, Y., Gong, Q., Gregg, E.W., Yang, W., Zhang, B., Shuai, Y., Hong, J., Engelgau, M.M., Li, H., Roglic, G., Hu, Y. And Bennett, P.H., 2014. Cardiovascular Mortality, All-Cause Mortality, and Diabetes Incidence After Lifestyle Intervention for People with Impaired Glucose Tolerance in the Da Qing Diabetes Prevention Study: A 23-Year Follow-Up Study. *The Lancet Diabetes & Endocrinology*, **2**(6), Pp. 474–480.

Lindstrom, J., Ilanne-Parikka, P., Peltonen, M., Aunola, S., Eriksson, J.G., Hemio, K., Hamalainen, H., Harkonen, P., Keinanen-Kiukaanniemi, S., Laakso, M., Louheranta, A., Mannelin, M., Paturi, M., Sundvall, J., Valle, T.T., Uusitupa, M., Tuomilehto, J. And Finnish Diabetes Prevention Study Group, 2006. Sustained Reduction in the Incidence of Type 2 Diabetes by Lifestyle Intervention: Follow-Up of the Finnish Diabetes Prevention Study. *Lancet (London, England)*, **368**(9548), Pp. 1673–1679.

Little, J.P., Gillen, J.B., Percival, M.E., Safdar, A., Tarnopolsky, M.A., Punthakee, Z., Jung, M.E. And Gibala, M.J., 2011. Low-Volume High-Intensity Interval Training Reduces Hyperglycemia and Increases Muscle Mitochondrial Capacity in Patients with Type 2 Diabetes. *Journal of Applied Physiology (Bethesda, Md.: 1985)*, **111**(6), Pp. 1554–1560.

Look Ahead Research Group, Wing, R.R., Bolin, P., Brancati, F.L., Bray, G.A., Clark, J.M., Coday, M., Crow, R.S., Curtis, J.M., Egan, C.M., Espeland, M.A., Evans, M., Foreyt, J.P., Ghazarian, S., Gregg, E.W., Harrison, B., Hazuda, H.P., Hill, J.O., Horton, E.S., Hubbard, V.S., Jakicic, J.M., Jeffery, R.W., Johnson, K.C., Kahn, S.E., Kitabchi, A.E., Knowler, W.C., Lewis, C.E., Maschak-Carey, B.J., Montez, M.G., Murillo, A., Nathan, D.M., Patricio, J., Peters, A., Pi-Sunyer, X., Pownall, H., Reboussin, D., Regensteiner, J.G., Rickman, A.D., Ryan, D.H., Safford, M., Wadden, T.A., Wagenknecht, L.E., West, D.S., Williamson, D.F. And Yanovski, S.Z., 2013. Cardiovascular Effects of Intensive Lifestyle Intervention in Type 2 Diabetes. *The New England Journal of Medicine*, **369**(2), Pp. 145–154.

Madsen, S.M., Thorup, A.C., Overgaard, K. And Jeppesen, P.B., 2015. High Intensity Interval Training Improves Glycaemic Control and Pancreatic Beta Cell Function of Type 2 Diabetes Patients. *Plos One*, **10**(8), Pp. E0133286.

Mann, S., Beedie, C. And Jimenez, A., 2014. Differential Effects of Aerobic Exercise, Resistance Training and Combined Exercise Modalities on Cholesterol and the Lipid Profile: Review, Synthesis and Recommendations. *Sports Medicine (Auckland, N.Z.)*, **44**(2), Pp. 211–221.

Mccarthy, M., Edwardson, C.L., Davies, M.J., Henson, J., Rowlands, A., King, J., Bodicoat, D.H., Khunti, K. And Yates, T., 2017. Breaking Up Sedentary Time with Seated Upper Body Activity Can Regulate Metabolic Health in Obese High Risk Adults: A Randomised Crossover Trial. *Diabetes, Obesity & Metabolism*, **19**(12), Pp. 1732–1739.

Mora, S., Cook, N., Buring, J.E., Ridker, P.M. And Lee, I.M., 2007. Physical Activity and Reduced Risk of Cardiovascular Events: Potential Mediating Mechanisms. *Circulation*, **116**(19), Pp. 2110–2118.

Nathan, D.M., Davidson, M.B., Defronzo, R.A., Heine, R.J., Henry, R.R., Pratley, R., Zinman, B. And American Diabetes Association, 2007. Impaired Fasting Glucose and Impaired Glucose Tolerance: Implications for Care. *Diabetes Care*, **30**(3), Pp. 753–759.

National Institute for Health and Care Excellence, 2019a, 2019-Last Update, Type 2 Diabetes in Adults: Management. Available: Https://Www.Nice.Org.Uk/Guidance/Ng28.

National Institute for Health and Care Excellence, 2019b, 2019-Last Update, Diabetic Foot Problems: Prevention and Management. Available: Https://Www.Nice.Org.Uk/Guidance/Ng19.

Park, S.W., Goodpaster, B.H., Strotmeyer, E.S., De Rekeneire, N., Harris, T.B., Schwartz, A.V., Tylavsky, F.A. And Newman, A.B., 2006. Decreased Muscle Strength and Quality in Older Adults with Type 2 Diabetes: The Health, Aging, and Body Composition Study. *Diabetes*, **55**(6), Pp. 1813–1818.

Pesta, D.H., Goncalves, R.L.S., Madiraju, A.K., Strasser, B. And Sparks, L.M., 2017. Resistance Training to Improve Type 2 Diabetes: Working Toward a Prescription for the Future. *Nutrition & Metabolism*, **14**, Pp. 24-017-0173-7. Ecollection 2017.

Richter, E.A. And Hargreaves, M., 2013. Exercise, Glut4, and Skeletal Muscle Glucose Uptake. *Physiological Reviews*, **93**(3), Pp. 993–1017.

Riebe, D., Franklin, B.A., Thompson, P.D., Garber, C.E., Whitfield, G.P., Magal, M. And Pescatello, L.S., 2015. Updating ACSM's Recommendations for Exercise Preparticipation Health Screening. *Medicine and Science in Sports and Exercise*, **47**(11), Pp. 2473–2479.

Rizza, R.A., 2010. Pathogenesis of Fasting and Postprandial Hyperglycemia in Type 2 Diabetes: Implications for Therapy. *Diabetes*, **59**(11), Pp. 2697–2707.

Roberts, C.K., Hevener, A.L. And Barnard, R.J., 2013. Metabolic Syndrome and Insulin Resistance: Underlying Causes and Modification by Exercise Training. *Comprehensive Physiology*, **3**(1), Pp. 1–58.

Robertson, R.P., Harmon, J., Tran, P.O. And Poitout, V., 2004. Beta-Cell Glucose Toxicity, Lipotoxicity, and Chronic Oxidative Stress in Type 2 Diabetes. *Diabetes*, **53(**Suppl 1), Pp. S119–24.

Sarelius, I. And Pohl, U., 2010. Control of Muscle Blood Flow During Exercise: Local Factors and Integrative Mechanisms. *Acta Physiologica (Oxford, England)*, **199**(4), Pp. 349–365

Sears, B. And Perry, M., 2015. The Role of Fatty Acids in Insulin Resistance. *Lipids in Health and Disease*, **14**, Pp. 121-015-0123-1.

Selvin, E., Marinopoulos, S., Berkenblit, G., Rami, T., Brancati, F.L., Powe, N.R. And Golden, S.H., 2004. Meta-Analysis: Glycosylated Hemoglobin and Cardiovascular Disease in Diabetes Mellitus. *Annals of Internal Medicine*, **141**(6), Pp. 421–431.

Shulman, G.I., 2014. Ectopic Fat in Insulin Resistance, Dyslipidemia, and Cardiometabolic Disease. *The New England Journal of Medicine*, **371**(12), Pp. 1131–1141.

Slentz, C.A., Tanner, C.J., Bateman, L.A., Durheim, M.T., Huffman, K.M., Houmard, J.A. And Kraus, W.E., 2009. Effects of Exercise Training Intensity on Pancreatic Beta-Cell Function. *Diabetes Care*, **32**(10), Pp. 1807–1811.

Snowling, N.J. And Hopkins, W.G., 2006. Effects of Different Modes of Exercise Training on Glucose Control and Risk Factors for Complications in Type 2 Diabetic Patients: A Meta-Analysis. *Diabetes Care*, **29**(11), Pp. 2518–2527.

Stratton, I.M., Adler, A.I., Neil, H.A., Matthews, D.R., Manley, S.E., Cull, C.A., Hadden, D., Turner, R.C. And Holman, R.R., 2000. Association of Glycaemia with Macrovascular and Microvascular Complications of Type 2 Diabetes (Ukpds 35): Prospective Observational Study. *BMJ (Clinical Research Ed.)*, **321**(7258), Pp. 405–412.

Umpierre, D., Ribeiro, P.A., Kramer, C.K., Leitao, C.B., Zucatti, A.T., Azevedo, M.J., Gross, J.L., Ribeiro, J.P. And Schaan, B.D., 2011. Physical Activity Advice Only or Structured Exercise Training and Association with Hba1c Levels in Type 2 Diabetes: A Systematic Review and Meta-Analysis. *Jama: The Journal of the American Medical Association*, **305**(17), Pp. 1790–1799.

Whang, W., Manson, J.E., Hu, F.B., Chae, C.U., Rexrode, K.M., Willett, W.C., Stampfer, M.J. And Albert, C.M., 2006. Physical Exertion, Exercise, and Sudden Cardiac Death in Women. *Jama*, **295**(12), Pp. 1399–1403.

Whelton, S.P., Chin, A., Xin, X. And He, J., 2002. Effect of Aerobic Exercise on Blood Pressure: A Meta-Analysis of Randomized, Controlled Trials. *Annals of Internal Medicine*, **136**(7), Pp. 493–503.

Wilcox, G., 2005. Insulin and Insulin Resistance. *The Clinical Biochemist Reviews*, **26**(2), Pp. 19–39.

Wisloff, U., Stoylen, A., Loennechen, J.P., Bruvold, M., Rognmo, O., Haram, P.M., Tjonna, A.E., Helgerud, J., Slordahl, S.A., Lee, S.J., Videm, V., Bye, A., Smith, G.L., Najjar, S.M., Ellingsen, O. And Skjaerpe, T., 2007. Superior Cardiovascular Effect of Aerobic Interval Training Versus Moderate Continuous Training in Heart Failure Patients: A Randomized Study. *Circulation*, **115**(24), Pp. 3086–3094.

Wojtaszewski, J.F., Higaki, Y., Hirshman, M.F., Michael, M.D., Dufresne, S.D., Kahn, C.R. And Goodyear, L.J., 1999. Exercise Modulates Postreceptor Insulin Signaling and Glucose Transport in Muscle-Specific Insulin Receptor Knockout Mice. *The Journal of Clinical Investigation*, **104**(9), Pp. 1257–1264.

Young, L.H., Wackers, F.J., Chyun, D.A., Davey, J.A., Barrett, E.J., Taillefer, R., Heller, G.V., Iskandrian, A.E., Wittlin, S.D., Filipchuk, N., Ratner, R.E., Inzucchi, S.E. And Diad Investigators, 2009. Cardiac Outcomes After Screening for Asymptomatic Coronary Artery Disease in Patients with Type 2 Diabetes: The Diad Study: A Randomized Controlled Trial. *Jama*, **301**(15), Pp. 1547–1555.

Zierath, J.R., Krook, A. And Wallberg-Henriksson, H., 2000. Insulin Action and Insulin Resistance in Human Skeletal Muscle. *Diabetologia*, **43**(7), Pp. 821–835.

13

HYPERTENSION

Alberto Alves, Fernando Ribeiro and Linda Pescatello

Chapter objectives

The aims of this chapter are to:

- Describe the epidemiology, aetiology and pathophysiology of hypertension
- Identify the guidelines for diagnosis and medical management of hypertension
- Explore the effects of different types of exercise training on blood pressure
- Assemble the guidelines for exercise testing and prescription in hypertension
- Discuss safety procedures based on the medication and the response of blood pressure to exercise

Overview of hypertension

Definition

There is a continuous association between higher blood pressure (BP) and increased risk of cardiovascular events (Miura et al., 2001; van den Hoogen et al., 2000). However, different categories based on BP cut-off values have been proposed for assisting clinical decision making. According to the Task Force for the Management of Arterial Hypertension of the European Society of Cardiology (ESC) and the European Society of Hypertension (ESH), hypertension in adults is defined as a resting systolic BP (SBP) in the clinic of ≥ 140 mmHg and/or resting diastolic BP (DBP) ≥ 90 mmHg (Williams et al., 2018). This definition is also followed by the International Society of Hypertension (ISH) (Unger et al., 2020). On the other hand, the American College of Cardiology (ACC)/American Heart Association (AHA) Task Force on Clinical Practice Guidelines (P. K. Whelton et al., 2018) recently proposed a lower threshold for the determination of hypertension (Table 13.1).

The classification of BP for adults is based on the average of the last two out of three or more measurements of seated BP (Unger et al., 2020). Whenever possible, the diagnosis should not be based on a single office visit measurement and should be confirmed with the

DOI: 10.4324/9781315102399-13

TABLE 13.1 Classification of BP levels according to ESC/ESH and ACC/AHA guidelines

	ESC/ESH ★			*ACC/AHA †*		
BP category	*SBP (mmHg)*		*DBP (mmHg)*	*SBP (mmHg)*		*DBP (mmHg)*
Optimal	< 120	and	< 80			
Normal	120–129	and/or	80–84	< 120	and	< 80
High normal★/Elevated†	130–139	and/or	85–89	120–129	and	< 80
Grade 1 hypertension	140–159	and/or	90–99	130–139	or	80–89
Grade 2 hypertension	160–179	and/or	100–109	≥ 140	or	≥ 90
Grade 3 hypertension	≥ 180	and/or	≥ 110			
Isolated Hypertension	≥ 140	and	< 90			

Legend: BP, blood pressure; ESC, European Society of Cardiology; ESH, European Society of Hypertension; DBP, diastolic blood pressure; SBP, systolic blood pressure

Source: Adapted from Whelton et al., 2018; Williams et al., 2018

TABLE 13.2 Definition of hypertension based on office, ambulatory and home BP levels, according to ESC/ESH and ACC/AHA guidelines

	ESC/ESH			*ACC/AHA*		
BP category	*SBP (mmHg)*	*and/or*	*DBP (mmHg)*	*SBP (mmHg)*	*and/or*	*DBP (mmHg)*
Office/Clinic BP	≥ 140		≥ 90	≥ 130		≥ 80
Ambulatory BP						
24-hour mean	≥ 130		≥ 80	≥ 125		≥ 75
Daytime mean	≥ 135		≥ 85	≥ 130		≥ 80
Nighttime mean	≥ 120		≥ 70	≥ 110		≥ 65
Home BP	≥ 135		≥ 85	≥ 130		≥ 80

Legend: ACC/AHA: American College of Cardiology/American Heart Association; BP: blood pressure; DBP: diastolic blood pressure; ESH/ESC: European Society of Hypertension/European Society of Cardiology; SBP: systolic blood pressure

Source: Adapted from Whelton et al., 2018; Williams et al., 2018

use of out-of-office BP measurements such as home BP monitoring (HBPM) or ambulatory BP monitoring (ABPM), when available and feasible (Table 13.2). Out-of-office BP measurement is used in identifying patients with white-coat hypertension or masked hypertension (Williams et al., 2018). White-coat hypertension refers to the untreated patients whose BP is elevated in the office but not during HBPM and ABPM. In contrast, masked hypertension refers to the untreated patients for whom BP is normal in the office but elevated during HBPM and ABPM (Williams et al., 2018). The risk of cardiovascular events is greater among adults with white-coat hypertension than those with true normal BP but lower than those with sustained hypertension (Unger et al., 2020; Williams et al., 2018).

Epidemiology

Hypertension is the most common preventable cause of cardiovascular disease and all-cause mortality in the world (Collaborators, 2018). Worldwide, one in four men and one in five women have raised BP (Collaboration, 2017). The number of adults with raised BP increased from 594 million in 1975 to 1.13 billion in 2015 (Collaboration, 2017) and is estimated to reach 1.56 billion by 2025 (Kearney et al., 2005). This increase at the global level is attributable to population growth and ageing as age-standardised adult mean SBP remained unchanged during the same time period (Collaboration, 2017). The prevalence of hypertension is greater in low- and middle-income countries than in high-income countries and becomes greater with advancing age (Mills et al., 2016). Indeed, hypertension is estimated to affect more than half the population of older adults, which is more than double the affected younger adults (Chow et al., 2013). Moreover, the proportion of US adults with a diagnosis of hypertension has increased from 32.0% (74.1 million) to 45.4% (105.3 million) with the adoption of the 2017 ACC/AHA guidelines. High BP has been consistently responsible for the greatest number of deaths worldwide over the last two decades, overcoming smoking, high fasting plasma glucose, high body mass index, and short gestation for birth weight. It has been estimated that high BP accounted for 10.4 million deaths and 218 million disability-adjusted life-years worldwide in 2017 (Collaborators, 2018).

Aetiology

Hypertension is a complex and heterogenous disorder that originates from the interplay of numerous environmental and genetic factors. In this sense, physical inactivity and high sodium intake are well-established environmental factors that increase the risk of hypertension, stroke and cardiovascular disease (Dempsey et al., 2018; He, Li, & Macgregor, 2013; Strazzullo et al., 2009). Other risk factors, such as obesity, insulin resistance, high alcohol consumption, low potassium intake, low calcium intake, smoking, air and noise pollution and chronic stress, have also been associated with hypertension (Carretero & Oparil, 2000). Family history is also a recognised risk factor of hypertension, as offspring of parents with hypertension show greater predisposition to develop hypertension, even more so if both parents have hypertension (Robert M Carey, 2008). Studies also show a greater correlation of BP values within families than between families, among monozygotic compared with dizygotic twins and in biologic compared to adopted siblings living in the same home (Robert M Carey, 2008). The precise role of common genetic variations in hypertension is complex, as genetic predispositions may influence multiple mechanisms and pathways involved in BP regulation. Multiple common genetic variations have been associated with BP regulation and hypertension, but so far, even their combined genetic scores seem to contribute to a small proportion of the variation in BP that can be explained (Dominiczak, Delles, & Padmanabhan, 2017). Moreover, adherence to a healthy lifestyle, which includes healthy diet, limited alcohol consumption, low urinary sodium excretion, low body mass index and increased physical activity, has been associated with lower BP and lower risk of myocardial infarction, stroke and composite cardiovascular disease regardless of BP genetic risk scores (Pazoki et al., 2018).

Pathology

The regulation of mean arterial pressure is dependent on the balance between cardiac output and total peripheral vascular resistance. While cardiac output depends on numerous factors that regulate heart rate and stroke volume, such as preload, afterload and myocardium contractility, peripheral vascular resistance is mainly determined by changes in diameter of small muscular arteries and arterioles, which, in turn, are primarily influenced by the contractile state of their smooth muscle. Thus, the elevation of mean blood pressure may result from an increase in cardiac output, an increase in total peripheral vascular resistance or a combination of both. Hypertension is usually associated with an increased total peripheral vascular resistance, but changes in cardiac function can also contribute to elevated BP (Mayet & Hughes, 2003).

The pathophysiology of hypertension is extremely complex and multifactorial, depending on the balanced regulation of multiple neural, renal, endocrine and vascular mechanisms (Figure 13.1). The structural and functional changes that occur in the vascular system and are involved in the pathophysiology of hypertension are described elsewhere (Taddei et al., 2018). The small resistance arteries and arterioles play an important role in the regulation of peripheral vascular resistance. The pathogenesis of hypertension involves structural and functional changes in small arteries and microvasculature that seem to contribute to the initiation, maintenance and amplification of elevated BP. These vascular changes comprise remodelling of the small arteries, arterioles and microvasculature, resulting in vascular inflammation, endothelial dysfunction and microvascular rarefaction (Taddei et al., 2018). Moreover, the increase in vascular stiffness and decreased arterial compliance in the large arteries that occur alongside ageing worsen with increasing BP and result in excessive pulsatility in the aorta, which may induce arterial wall barotrauma and damage to small arteries, arterioles and capillaries, due to increased transmission of BP to the microcirculation. These vascular changes are particularly important in low-resistance organs, such as the brain and kidney (Palombo & Kozakova, 2016). The increased pressure load can also lead to several structural changes in the heart in order to normalise myocardial wall stress, ranging from myocardial remodelling to myocardial hypertrophy (increased left ventricular mass). These cardiac changes may impair myocardial relaxation and coronary reserve, leading to the development of diastolic dysfunction, myocardial ischemia and, ultimately, heart failure (Palombo & Kozakova, 2016; Shim, 2011).

Neural mechanisms also seem to play an important role in the pathophysiology of hypertension. Increased sympathetic activation and the consequent the release of neurotransmitters such as noradrenaline promote an increase in heart rate, cardiac contractility and cardiac output as well as enhanced peripheral vasoconstriction and peripheral vascular resistance, which

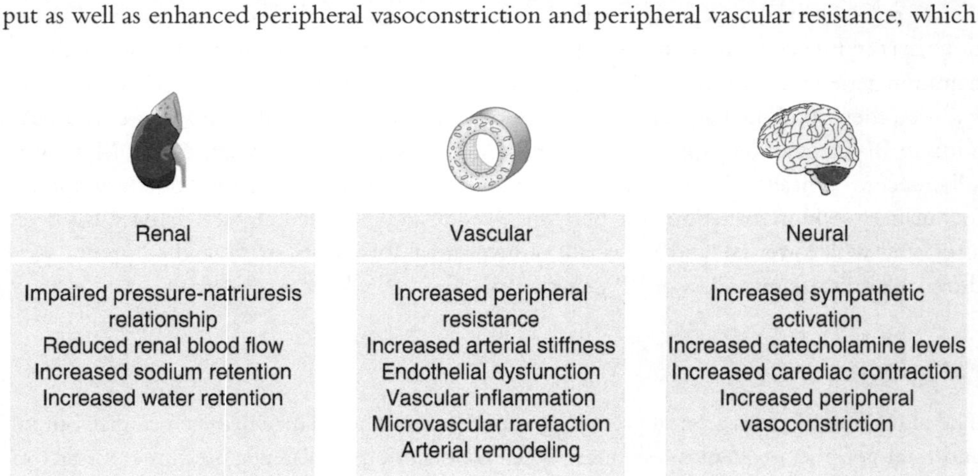

FIGURE 13.1 Complex and multifactorial pathophysiology of hypertension includes neural, renal, endocrine and vascular mechanisms

contribute to sustained increases in BP (Saxena, Ali, & Saxena, 2018). The increased activity of sympathetic nervous system also influences renal sodium and water excretion and is associated with co-morbidities that are known to contribute to the development of hypertension, such as obesity, diabetes, obstructive sleep apnoea and chronic kidney disease (Saxena, Ali, & Saxena, 2018; Taddei et al., 2018).

Renal mechanisms also have an important role in BP homeostasis as impaired renal function is generally associated with hypertension. One important renal-related mechanism is the pressure-natriuresis relationship, in which renal excretion of sodium and water increases when renal arterial pressure increases (Ivy & Bailey, 2014). Sodium equilibrium is essential to extracellular fluid volume and the long-term stabilisation of mean arterial pressure. When working properly, the pressure-natriuresis relationship assures that blood volume and BP return to normal after acute perturbations such as with increased salt intake or peripheral vascular resistance. There is evidence that the pressure-natriuresis relationship is impaired in hypertension, which means that greater levels of arterial pressure are required to promote sodium excretion (Bolivar, 2013). It has been shown that one important cause of this impairment of the pressure-natriuresis relationship is the sustained upregulation of the renin-angiotensin system and consequent chronic elevation in angiotensin II (Taddei et al., 2018). The chronic activation of this powerful vasoactive peptide has been shown to have important effects on renal vasoconstriction, resulting in increased peripheral vascular resistance and reduced renal blood flow and sodium retention, which favour the development of hypertension (Forrester et al., 2018). Angiotensin II also stimulates sodium and water reabsorption in multiple nephron segments and stimulates aldosterone secretion from the adrenal glands to enhance sodium and water retention, raising blood volume and BP (Forrester et al., 2018). In addition, increased intrarenal angiotensin II has important consequences for renal dysfunction induced by high BP, such as increased immune and inflammatory responses, oxidative stress, endothelial dysfunction and interstitial fibrosis (Forrester et al., 2018).

Management and medications

The aim in the treatment, control and management of hypertension is to decrease cardiovascular morbidity and mortality (Brunstrom & Carlberg, 2018; Ettehad et al., 2016). In general, the BP aim in patients with hypertension is to reduce office BP to < 140/90 mmHg (Williams et al., 2018). If treatment is well tolerated, treated BP values should be aimed to 130/80 mmHg or lower in most patients (Williams et al., 2018). Nonetheless, target BP values may vary in older populations and patients with other co-morbid conditions. The ESC/ESH guidelines do not recommend reducing office SBP to < 120 mmHg due to supporting evidence suggesting that SBP values below this threshold may increase the incidence of cardiovascular events and deaths (Williams et al., 2018). It is important to note, though, that there is some disagreement among the professional organisations concerning the BP value to target. For instance, the most recent 2017 AHA/ACC guidelines recommend lowering BP values to < 130/80 mmHg (P. K. Whelton et al., 2018).

Treatment for hypertension includes lifestyle modifications alone or in combination with pharmacological treatment, depending on office BP levels; the presence of other co-morbid conditions such as cardiovascular disease, diabetes and chronic kidney disease; the ten-year cardiovascular disease risk, and the presence of hypertension-mediated organ damage (HMOD). To assess the ten-year cardiovascular disease risk, the AHA/ACC guidelines (P. K. Whelton et al., 2018) use the ASCVD risk calculator, whereas the ESC/ESH guidelines

(Williams et al., 2018) use of the SCORE system coupled with risk modifiers and assessment of HMOD.

A healthy lifestyle is recommended as first line of antihypertensive treatment. The adoption of healthy behaviour is critical in the prevention of hypertension and plays an important role in delaying the progressive increase in BP. In addition, positive changes in lifestyle are believed to enhance the effects of antihypertensive treatment (Williams et al., 2018). These lifestyle changes include salt restriction, healthy diet, moderate consumption of alcohol, weight reduction, smoking cessation and regular physical activity (Table 13.3). Moderate

TABLE 13.3 Lifestyle change recommendations according to ESC/ESH and ACC/AHA guidelines

Lifestyle change	*ESC/ESH recommendations*	*ACC/AHA recommendations*
Salt reduction	Salt restriction to < 5 g per day	Optimal goal is < 1500 mg/d, but aim for at least a 1000 mg/d reduction in most adults
Potassium intake		Aim for 3500–5000 mg/d, preferably by consumption of a diet rich in potassium
Alcohol consumption	Alcohol restriction to less than 14 units per week for men and less than 8 units per week for women	Reduction of alcohol to 2 drinks daily or less in men and 1 drink daily or less in women
Healthy diet	Increased consumption of vegetables, fresh fruits, fish, nuts and unsaturated fats; low consumption of red meat; consumption of low-fat dairy products	Diet rich in fruits, vegetables, whole grains and low-fat dairy products, with reduced content of saturated and total fat
Weight reduction	Weight control to avoid obesity (BMI > 30 kg/m^2; waist circumference > 102 cm in men and > 88 cm in women) and aiming for healthy weight (BMI 20–25 kg/m^2 and waist circumference < 94 cm in men and < 8 cm in women)	Best goal is ideal body weight, but aim for at least a 1 kg reduction in body weight for most adults who are overweight
Regular physical activity	Regular physical activity that includes a minimum of 30 minutes of moderate dynamic aerobic exercise (walking, jogging, cycling or swimming) on five to seven days per week; performance of resistance exercises on two to three days per week is also advisable	Aerobic exercise: 90–150 minutes per week; 65–75% heart rate reserve Dynamic resistance exercise: 90–150 minutes per week; 50–80% of 1-RM; six exercises, three sets per exercise, ten repetitions per set Isometric exercise: four × two minutes (handgrip); one minute rest between exercises; 30–40% maximum voluntary contraction; three sessions per week for eight to ten weeks.
Smoking cessation	Smoking cessation and referral to smoking cessation programs	

Legend: ACC/AHA: American College of Cardiology/American Heart Association; ASCVD: Atherosclerotic Cardiovascular Disease; BMI: body mass index; ESH/ESC: European Society of Hypertension/European Society of Cardiology

Source: Adapted from Whelton et al., 2018; Williams et al., 2018

consumption of coffee and green and black tea, as well as reduced stress and lower exposure to air pollution and cold temperature, have also been recommended as strategies to prevent increases in BP (Unger et al., 2020).

In addition to modifications in lifestyle, drug treatment is recommended for certain classes of patients, although BP thresholds and drug treatment strategies vary among the guidelines of the different professional organisations (Table 13.4) (Bakris, Ali, & Parati, 2019). For the initiation of antihypertensive drug treatment, first-line agents include renin-angiotensin system (RAS) inhibitors, calcium channel blockers (CCB) and thiazide or thiazide-like diuretics. The RAS inhibitors comprise angiotensin-converting enzyme (ACE) inhibitors or angiotensin-II receptor blockers (ARB). European guidelines recommend as initial treatment to most patients a single-pill combination of two drugs of different classes, although in some cases monotherapy is generally considered (Williams et al., 2018). In general, this includes an RAS inhibitor and a calcium channel blocker or a diuretic. A triple-drug combination is recommended to individuals who cannot achieve the target BP with a two-drug combination (Williams et al., 2018). Patients may be considered as having resistant hypertension when BP remains uncontrolled despite the concurrent use of three first-line antihypertensive drugs of different classes. It is fundamental to exclude secondary causes of hypertension and poor adherence to treatment among those with resistant hypertension. The inadequate control of BP must also be confirmed by out-of-office BP monitoring in those patients whose adherence to treatment has been confirmed (Williams et al., 2018). Given the multifactorial aetiology of resistant hypertension, these patients may require a specialist evaluation (R. M. Carey et al., 2018). In patients with resistant hypertension, treatment may comprise the addition of an aldosterone antagonist (spironolactone) or other diuretic, alpha-blocker and beta-blocker. The use of beta-blockers in combination with a drug from the other major classes is recommended in conditions in which there is a specific indication for their use, such as the presence of angina, post-myocardial infarction, heart failure or heart rate control (Williams et al., 2018). There are some differences between the ACC/AHA guidelines and the ESC/

TABLE 13.4 Initiation of drug treatment in patients with hypertension

	ESC/ESH recommendations	*ACC/AHA recommendations*
Indication	High- or very high-risk patients with grade 1 hypertension and with cardiovascular disease, renal disease or HMOD Low moderate–risk patients with grade 1 hypertension and without cardiovascular disease, renal disease or HMOD, after three to six months of lifestyle intervention if BP remains uncontrolled Patients with grade 2 and 3 hypertension In very high-risk patients with high normal BP and cardiovascular disease, drug treatment may also be considered	Adults with stage 1 hypertension with clinical ASCVD or estimated ten-year ASCVD risk ≥ 10% Adults with stage 2 hypertension

Legend: ACC/AHA: American College of Cardiology/American Heart Association; ASCVD: Atherosclerotic Cardiovascular Disease; BP: blood pressure; ESH/ESC: European Society of Hypertension/European Society of Cardiology; HMOD: hypertension-mediated organ damage

Source: Adapted from Whelton et al., 2018; Williams et al., 2018

ESH guidelines (Whelton et al., 2018). For instance, a single-drug treatment is recommended in the initiation of antihypertensive treatment in patients with stage I hypertension. If the BP goal still remains above target, the dosage is increased, and other drug agents are added sequentially to achieve goal BP. The initiation of treatment with two drug agents, either separate or in a fixed-dose combination, is considered in patients with stage II hypertension and an average BP more than 20/10 mmHg above their target BP (Whelton et al., 2018).

Table 13.5 illustrates the effect of front-line antihypertensive medications on the exercise response.

Effects of hypertension on the exercise response

During incremental aerobic exercise, mean BP increases progressively, stemming from an increase in cardiac output and a decrease in peripheral vascular resistance (Powers, 2014). The elevation in mean BP results from an increase in SBP as DBP remains unchanged during incremental aerobic exercise (Powers, 2014). After the exercise session, SBP decreases approximately 6 and 8 mmHg in patients with prehypertension and hypertension, respectively (Carpio-Rivera et al., 2016). The reduction in BP is greater after concurrent exercise (~7 mmHg) followed by aerobic exercise (~6 mmHg) and resistance training exercise (~3 mmHg) (Carpio-Rivera et al., 2016). This blood pressure–lowering effect induced by exercise is known as post-exercise hypotension (PEH). The duration of PEH varies among studies, but there is evidence suggesting that it may persist for 24 hours (Cardoso et al., 2010; Casonatto et al., 2016; Wallace et al., 1999). The mechanisms for PEH have been mostly investigated on aerobic exercise and are not completely understood. Nonetheless, evidence suggests that PEH results, at least in part, from changes in baroreflex control, which lead to a decrease in sympathetic activation to vascular beds, facilitating vasodilation (Brito et al., 2018). Local mechanisms that regulate vasodilation as well as decreased cardiac output due to reduced preload and stroke volume have also been appointed as putative mechanisms of PEH (Brito et al., 2018). Larger reductions in SBP are found when the intensity and duration of the exercise session are higher, the number of sets of resistance exercises is greater and the number of resistance exercises is lower (Carpio-Rivera et al., 2016). It has been shown that the reductions observed immediately after exercise are correlated to those observed following exercise training, which suggests that acute BP responses to exercise may predict the efficacy of long-term chronic training adaptations (Hecksteden, Grutters, & Meyer, 2013; Wegmann et al., 2018). In addition, the acute responses to exercise may help distinguish responders from non-responders to exercise (Lopes et al., 2020) and identify those with hypertensive response to exercise (HRE), even when resting BP levels are controlled (Fletcher et al., 2013). An HRE is associated with increased risk of future hypertension (Matthews et al., 1998), myocardial infarction (Mundal et al., 1996) and stroke (Kurl et al., 2001). Exercise BP response also seems to be a stronger predictor of morbidity and mortality from myocardial infarction than casual BP (Mundal et al., 1996). Men whose BP increases beyond 19.7 mmHg per minute of exercise have a 2.3-fold increased risk of stroke compared to men who increase BP to a level below 16.1 mmHg (Kurl et al., 2001). There is no consensus in the definition of HRE. Some studies have defined HRE as the difference between peak and baseline SBP ≥ 60 mmHg in men and ≥ 50 mmHg in woman during exercise testing, while others suggested an increase in SBP of at least 150 mmHg during light to moderate intensity or SBP at least 210

TABLE 13.5 Medication considerations for exercise for people with hypertension

Class name	*Generic name*	*Brand name*	*Indication*	*Action*	*Side effects*	*Exercise considerations*
Angiotension-converting enzyme (ACE) inhibitors	benzapril captopril enalapril fosinopril lisinopril moexipril perindopril quinapril ramipril trandolapril	Lotensin Lotensin HCT[a] Lotrel[b] Capoten Capozide[a] Epaned Vasotec Vaseretic[a] Lexxel[c] Monopril Monopril HCT[a] Zestril Prinivil Qbrelis Prinzide[a] Zestoretic[a] Univasc Uniretic[a] Aceon Prestalia[b] Accupril Accuretic[a] Altace Mavik Tarka[d]	Hypertension; coronary artery disease; heart failure	Decreases blood pressure by lowering angiotensin-II levels; vasoconstriction; vascular resistance	Dry cough; hypotension; deterioration of renal function; hyperkalaemia; dizziness; fatigue; headaches; insomnia	Lower resting and exercise blood pressure; may predispose to hypotensive response post-exercise; decreased renal function, which is important during exercise-imposed volume depletion

a ACE-I + diuretics (hydrochlorothiazide)
b ACE-I + calcium channel blocker (amlodipine)
c ACE-I + calcium channel blocker (felodipine)
d ACE-I + calcium channel blocker (verapamil)

Class Name	*Generic name*	*Brand name*	*Indication*	*Action*	*Side effects*	*Exercise considerations*
Angiotension-II Receptor Blockers (ARBs)	azilsartan candesartan eprosartan irbesartan losartan olmesartan telmisartan valsartan	Edarbi Edarbyclor[a] Atacand Atacand HCT[b] Teveten Teveten HCT[b] Avapro Avalide[b] Cozaar Hyzaar[b] Benicar Benicar HCT[b] Azor[c] Tribenzor[d] MicardisMiscardis HCT[b] Twynsta[c] Diovan Diovan HCT[b] Exforge[c] Exforge HCT[d]	Hypertension and heart failure	Decreases blood pressure by blocking angiotensin-II receptors	Hypotension; deterioration of renal function; hyperkalemia	Lower resting and exercise blood pressure; may predispose to hypotensive response postexercise and decreased renal function, which is important during exercise-imposed volume depletion

a ARB + diuretic (Chlorthalidone)
b ARB + diuretic (Hydrochlorothiazide)
c ARB + calcium channel blocker
d ARB + diuretic (Hydrochlorothiazide) + calcium channel blocker

(*Continued*)

TABLE 13.5 (Continued)

Class name	*Generic name*	*Brand name*	*Indication*	**Action**	**Side effects**	**Exercise considerations**
Calcium Channel Blockers (CCB)	**dihydropyridines** amlodipine clevidipine felodipine isradipine lercanidipine nicardipine nifedipine nimodipine nisoldipine nitrendipine Nondihydropyridines diltiazem verapamil	Norvasc Cleviprex Plendil DynaCirc DynaCirc CR Zanidip CardeneCardene SR Adalat[a]Procardia XL[a] Procardia[b] Nimotop Nymalize Sular Cardizem Cardizem CD or LA[c] Cartia XT[c] Dilacor XR[c] Tiazac[c] Calan Calan SR[d] Isoptin SR[d] Covera HS[d] Verelan PM[d] Verelan[d] Tarka[e]	Hypertension, angina pectoris, arrhythmia	Decreases blood pressure by preventing calcium from entering the cardiac cells	Bradycardia; tachycardia; headache; dizziness; edema; flushing; asthenia; nausea	Decreases resting and exercise blood pressure; may decrease resting and exercise heart rate; may predispose to hypotensive response postexercise

a Long acting
b Short acting
c Nondihydropyridines (Diltiazem, extended-release)
d Nondihydropyridines (Verapamil, controlled- and extended-release)
e Nondihydropyridines (Verapamil) + angiotension-converting enzyme inhibitors (Trandolapril)

Class name	*Generic name*	*Brand name*	*Indication*	*Action*	*Side effects*	*Exercise considerations*
Diuretics	**Thiazides**	Corzide	Hypertension,	Inhibition	Hyperglycemia;	**Thiazides**
	bendroflumethiazide	Diuril	heart failure	of sodium	glycosuria;	
	chlorothiazide	Hygroton	and edema	reabsorption;	hyperuricemia;	
	chlorthalidone	Microzide Oretic		reduction of	hypochloremic	
	hydrochlorothiazide (HCTZ)	Lozol		extracellular	alkalosis;	
	indapamide	Mykron Zaroxolyn		volume;	hyponatremia;	
	methyclothiazide	Renese		vasodilation	hypokalaemia;	
	metolazone	Bumex			hypomagnesemia;	
	polythiazide	Edecrin			hypercalcemia;	
	Loop diuretics	Lasix			headache; dizziness;	
	bumetanide	Demadex			photosensitivity	
	ethacrynic acid	Midamor Moduretic[a]			reactions; postural	
	furosemide	Hydro-ride[a]			hypotension;	
	forsemide	Dyrenium			paresthesias	
	Potassium-sparing diuretics	Dyazide[b] Maxzide[b]				
	amiloride	Inspra				
	triamterene	Aldactone Aldactazide[c]				
	Aldosterone receptor blockers					
	eplerenone					
	spironolactone					

a Potassium-sparing diuretics (Amiloride) + thiazides (Hydrochlorothiazide)

b Potassium-sparing diuretics (Triamterene) + thiazides (Hydrochlorothiazide)

c Aldosterone-receptor blockers (Spironolactone) + thiazides (Hydrochlorothiazide)

(*Continued*)

TABLE 13.5 (Continued)

Class name	*Generic name*	*Brand name*	*Indication*	*Action*	*Side effects*	*Exercise considerations*
Beta-blockers	acebutolol[a,b] atenolol[b] betaxolol[b] bisoprolol[b] carvedilol[c] esmolol labetalol[c] metoprolol succinate[b] metoprolol tartrate[b] nadolol[c] nebivolol[b] penbutolol[c] pindolol[a,c] propranolol[c] sotalol[c] timolol[c]	Sectral Tenormin Kerlone Zebeta Coreg Brevibloc Trandate Toprol XL Lopressor SR Corgard Bystolic Levatola Viskena Inderal Betapace Blocadren	Hypertension, angina, arrhythmias, acute myocardial infarction, heart failure, migraine headaches, anxiety, hyperthyroidism	Decreases blood pressure and heart rate by preventing binding of epinephrine to its receptors in the heart	Bradycardia; atrioventricular blocks; dizziness; fatigue; nausea; diarrhea; abdominal pain; depression; insomnia; hallucinations; bronchospasm; hypoglycemia; hyperglicemia; hyperkalemia; asthenia; parestesia	Blunts the increase in heart and blood pressure during exercise; may decrease acute aerobic capacity; may affect thermoregulatory regulation

a β-Blockers with intrinsic sympathomimetic activity
b Cardioselective
c Noncardioselective

and 190 mmHg at maximal intensity exercise in men and women, respectively (Kim & Ha, 2016; Sharman et al., 2019). Although not entirely clear, some factors have been suggested as contributing to HRE, including, but not limited to, impaired endothelial vasodilation and enhanced vascular resistance during exercise; increased arterial stiffness, particularly in the older population; and increased activation of the renin-angiotensin system and consequent augmented rise of angiotensin-II during exercise (Kim & Ha, 2016).

In order to prevent an excessive BP response during exercise, it has been suggested to keep SBP ≤ 220 mmHg and/or DBP levels ≤ 105 mmHg (ACSM, 2018). On the other hand, if SBP drops more than 10 mmHg below resting levels, despite an increase in workload, exercise should be stopped (Sharman et al., 2019). In this case, the individual should be advised to visit their physician. It is crucial to educate patients about the immediate reduction of BP after both aerobic and resistance exercise. Promising results suggests that PEH self-monitoring improves exercise adherence among adults with hypertension (Zaleski et al., 2019). It is also important to note that resting SBP ≥ 200 mmHg or DBP ≥ 110 mmHg is a contraindication for exercise (ACSM, 2018). Moreover, in individuals with uncontrolled hypertension (SBP > 160 mmHg), high-intensity exercise is not recommended until BP has been controlled (class III, level of evidence C) (Pelliccia et al., 2020). Valsalva maneuver should also be avoided during resistance training.

The potential effects of antihypertensive medication on the response to exercise should also be considered. Some medications (e.g. alpha-blockers, vasodilators and CCBs) may amplify the BP reductions after the exercise session (ACSM, 2018). For patients on these medications, BP should be monitored after the session, and the cool-down period should be extended as needed. Other antihypertensive medication such as beta-blockers and diuretics may affect thermoregulatory function. Precautions should be taken to avoid heat-related injuries/illnesses for individuals on these medications. Individuals should also be educated about proper fluid intake and symptoms of dehydration. Beta-blockers and diuretics may also increase the predisposition to hypoglycemia in some individuals, particularly patients with diabetes mellitus who take insulin or insulin secretagogues. Precautions should be taken in this situation to avoid adverse hypoglycemic events.

Effects of exercise training

Exercise is universally recommended by all professional societies to lower BP in individuals with hypertension (Table 13.6) because SBP and DBP are reduced on average ~8/~5 mmHg as a result of exercise. These values are clinically meaningful BP reductions based on observed decreases in all-cause (7%), stroke (14%) and coronary heart disease (9%) mortality with a 5 mmHg drop in SBP (Whelton et al., 2002). Furthermore, two recent network meta-analyses showed that exercise interventions are not inferior to antihypertensive medications in reducing blood pressure among individuals with hypertension (Naci et al., 2019; Noone et al., 2020). A network meta-analysis of 391 randomised controlled trials (RCTs) comparing the effects of exercise and medication on SBP concluded that, in individuals with hypertension, the BP reductions induced by exercise are similar to those achieved with antihypertensive medications (e.g. ACE inhibitors, ARB, beta-blockers, CCB and diuretics) (Naci et al., 2019). Noone et al. (2020) reviewed 93 RCTs (n = 32,404) to estimate the comparative efficacy of first-line antihypertensive medications – including ACE inhibitors, ARB, CCB and thiazide-like diuretics – with exercise interventions (including aerobic training and dynamic

TABLE 13.6 Hypertension professional committee recommendations

Professional committee/organisation							
The FITT of the exercise prescription	*ESH/ESC (Williams et al., 2018)*	*ACC/AHA (Whelton et al., 2018)*	*Brazilian Society of Cardiology (Malachias et al., 2016)*	*Exercise and Sport Science Australia (Sharman, Smart, Coombes, & Stowasser, 2019)*	*ACSM (Pescatello, 2019; Pescatello et al., 2019)*	*Canadian Hypertension Education Program (Nerenberg et al., 2018)*	*ISH (Unger et al., 2020)*
Frequency (how often?)	5–7 days/week^{-1}	N/A	5–7 days/week^{-1}	5 days/week^{-1} (moderate) 3 days/week^{-1} (vigorous or HIIT)	Most, preferably all, days of the week	4–7 days/week^{-1} in addition to the routine activities of daily activity	5–7 days/week^{-1}
Intensity (how hard?)	Moderate	Moderate to Vigorous*	Moderate**	Moderate or vigorous or HIIT or a combination of moderate and vigorous***	Low, moderate, or vigorous, with an emphasis on moderate (aerobic: 40 - < 60% of VO_2reserve; resistance: 60–70% 1RM)	Moderate	Moderate or HITT
Time (how long?)	≥ 30 min/day^{-1}	90–150 min/week^{-1}	≥ 30 min/day^{-1} (ideally, 40–50 min/day^{-1})	30 min/day^{-1} (moderate) 20 min/day^{-1} (vigorous) 25 min/day^{-1} (HIIT)	> 20–30 min/day to total > 90–150+ min/week	Accumulation of 30–60 min/day^{-1}	30 min/day^{-1}
Type (what kind?) *Primary*	Aerobic	Aerobic	Aerobic	Aerobic	Aerobic and/or resistance	Aerobic	Aerobic
Evidence rating	Class I level of evidence A	Class I level of evidence A	Grade I level of evidence A	N/A		Grade D‡	N/A

Adjuvant	Dynamic RT 2–3 days/week^{-1}	Dynamic RT, 90–150 min/week^{-1}, 50–80% 1-RM, 3 sets of 10 repetitions, 6 exercises; isometric 4x2 min (handgrip), 1 min rest, 30–40% MVC, 3 sessions·week^{-1} for 8–10 weeks	Dynamic RT 2–3 days/week^{-1}, 1–3 sets, 8–10 exercises for the larger muscle groups (prioritising unilateral exercises), 10–15 repetitions to moderate fatigue, long rest intervals (90–120s)	Dynamic RT ≥ 2 non-consecutive days/week^{-1}, 8–12 repetitions resulting in substantial fatigue, 1 set, 8–10 exercises (multiple sets if time allows); isometric RT 4x2 min (arms/legs), 2–3 min rest, 30% MVC, 3 non-consecutive sessions/week^{-1}	Neuromotor low to moderate intensity, ≥ 2–3 sessions/week of ≥ 20–30 min of multimodal exercise (e.g. yoga, Pilates, tai chi) Flexibility ≥ 2–3 sessions, ≤ 10 min/session, static stretch to the point of slight discomfort for 10–30s with 2–4 reps targeting the major muscle groups	Dynamic or isometric (handgrip) RT	Dynamic RT# 2–3 days/week^{-1}
Evidence rating	N/A	Class I level of evidence A	Grade IIa, level of evidence B	N/A		Grade D‡	N/A

Legend: ACC/AHA: American College of Cardiology/American Heart Association; ACSM: American College of Sports Medicine; ESH/ESC: European Society of Hypertension/European Society of Cardiology; FITT: frequency, intensity, time and type; ISH: International Society of Hypertension; HRR: heart rate reserve; RT, resistance training; VO_2: oxygen uptake

* 65–75% HRR is assumed as the best proven aerobic exercise intensity intervention

** Moderate intensity defined as an intensity that causes noticeable increases in heart rate and breathing (without being breathless); feeling mildly to moderately tired

*** Moderate intensity: 40–59 VO_2reserve or heart rate reserve or 11–13 14–16 Borg rating of perceived exertion 6–20 point scale; vigorous intensity: 60–84 VO_2reserve or heart rate reserve or 14–16 Borg rating of perceived exertion 6–20 point scale

‡ Grade D is the weakest evidence (based on level V evidence: little or no systematic empirical evidence) while Grade A is the strongest evidence (based on Level I evidence or consistent findings from multiple studies of levels II, III or IV); 'higher intensities of exercise are not more effective' was also assigned Grade D

Source: (Malachias et al., 2016, 30–34; Nerenberg et al., 2018, 506–525; Pescatello, 2019a, 849–852; Pescatello, 2019b; Pescatello et al., 2019, 1314–1323; Pescatello et al., 2015, 801–812; Sharman et al., 2019, 837–843; Unger et al., 2020, 1334–1357; Whelton et al., 2018, 1269–1324; Williams et al., 2018, 3021–3104).

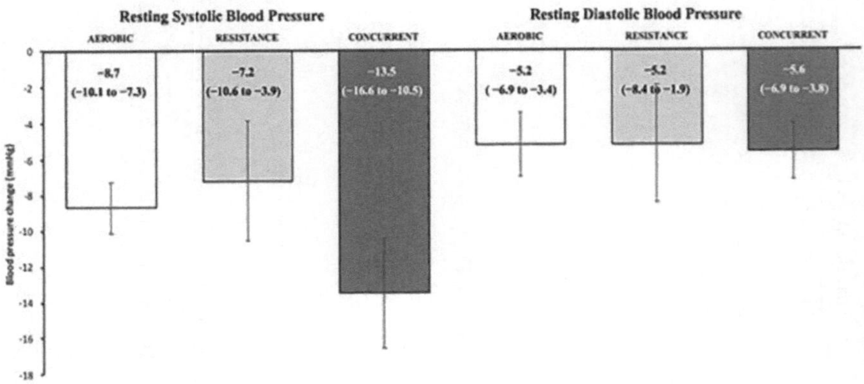

FIGURE 13.2 Blood pressure response to different types of exercise interventions among adults with hypertension. Systolic and diastolic changes (95% CI) as a result of aerobic, resistance and concurrent exercise programs

Source: Adapted from the meta-analysis of Naci et al. (2019) and Cornelissen and Smart (2013), respectively

resistance training) on BP among individuals with hypertension. Despite the bias towards medication trials (81 out of the 93 trials included in the review are related to medications, while only 12 trials are related to exercise), exercise had the second-lowest treatment ranking, just below ARB and CCB. The authors concluded that there was insufficient evidence to suggest that first-line antihypertensive medications significantly reduced BP to a greater extent than did the exercise interventions.

There is also extensive evidence, including several meta-analyses, supporting the antihypertensive effects of different types of exercise (Bersaoui et al., 2020; Borjesson et al., 2016; Boutcher & Boutcher, 2017; Cornelissen & Smart, 2013; Corso et al., 2016; MacDonald et al., 2016; Pescatello et al., 2019; Pescatello, MacDonald, Ash et al., 2015; Pescatello, MacDonald, Lamberti et al., 2015) (Figure 13.2). The following sections provide an overview of the effects of chronic (i.e. long-term effects or training) aerobic (including high-intensity interval training [HIIT]), resistance (dynamic and isometric) and concurrent (aerobic and resistance combined) exercise on BP among individuals with hypertension.

Aerobic exercise

Historically, aerobic exercise has been broadly endorsed by the European and American societies' guidelines and committee statements for prevention, treatment and control of high blood pressure (Table 13.6). Aerobic exercise training has been shown to reduce SBP and DBP by −8 /−5 mmHg among adults with hypertension (Cornelissen & Smart, 2013; Naci et al., 2019; Pescatello et al., 2019). The range of expected reductions with aerobic training vary from −4.9 to −12 mmHg in SBP and −3.4 to −5.8 mmHg in DBP diastolic (Hanssen et al., 2021).

Cornelissen and Smart (2013) performed a comprehensive systematic review and meta-analysis on the antihypertensive effects of aerobic exercise training and reported SBP and DBP reductions of −8.3 (95% CI, −10.7 to −6.0)/−5.2 (95% CI, −6.9 to −3.4) mmHg in

26 study groups with individuals with hypertension. The reductions in BP were greater in individuals with hypertension than in those with prehypertension or normal BP (Cornelissen & Smart, 2013). More recently, Naci et al. (2019) performed a network meta-analysis comparing the effectiveness of different exercise regimens and medications on SBP. They also observed that aerobic exercise reduced SBP by −8.69 mmHg (95% CI: −10.13 to −7.25) among individuals with hypertension (≥ 140 mmHg, n = 3508). The authors did not find a difference between the effects of medications and those of exercise (0.18 mmHg, 95% CI: −1.35 to 1.68) (Naci et al., 2019). It is important to note that the resting BP level is a moderator of the BP response to exercise training. The vast majority of systematic reviews (Cornelissen & Smart, 2013; Fagard & Cornelissen, 2007; Naci et al., 2019; Pescatello et al., 2019) examining the effects of exercise among adults found that the decrease in BP occurred in a dose-response fashion as a function of resting BP, with the greatest reductions observed in those with higher resting BP. For instance, Naci et al. (2019) conducted a sensitivity analysis that showed SBP reductions of 6.84 mmHg (95% CI: −7.90 to −5.76) in trials with individuals with SBP ≥ 130 mmHg at baseline, 8.70 mmHg (95% CI: −10.13 to −7.25) in trials with ≥ 140 mmHg, and 10.74 mmHg (95% CI: −12.70 to −8.77) with ≥ 150 mmHg (Naci et al., 2019). These results suggest that the greatest BP benefits are achieved by those who them need the most: i.e. those with the highest resting BP.

The current exercise recommendations for hypertension are predominantly based on meta-analyses involving European-descendent populations. While high BP affects all segments of the population, African Americans have the highest prevalence of hypertension of any ethnic group in the world, as well as the ethnic disparity in hypertension and hypertension-related outcomes (i.e. uncontrolled BP, target organ damage, end-stage renal disease, stroke) (Carson et al., 2011; Ford, 2011; Howard et al., 2006; Lackland et al., 1995; Rayner & Spence, 2017; Wyatt et al., 2008). The higher rate of hypertension among African Americans and indigenous Africans seems to be related to a greater predispositions to salt sensitivity and suppressed plasma renin: hence, increased susceptibility to sodium retention (Rayner & Spence, 2017). In this regard, in 2002, Whelton and colleagues conducted a meta-analysis with 54 RCTs (2,419 participants) testing the effects of aerobic exercise on BP and reported greater BP reductions among African Americans (−11/−3 mmHg) than among whites (−3/−3 mmHg) and Asians (−6/−7 mmHg) (S. P. Whelton et al., 2002). These results were recently confirmed by a meta-analysis determining the effect of aerobic exercise training on BP in African (4 trials, n = 510) and Asian (22 trials, n = 931) populations (Bersaoui et al., 2020); a reduction in SBP and DBP was found in both ethnic groups – Africans: −12.45 (95% CI: −17.96 to −6.94)/−4.12 (95% CI: −7.18 to −1.05) mmHg; Asians: −7.23 (95% CI: −10.59 to −3.86)/−4.66 (95% CI: −7.08 to −2.23) mmHg – with the reduction in African populations almost doubling the reduction observed in Asian populations (Bersaoui et al., 2020). Despite the low number of studies included in this meta-analysis, particularly in African populations, the benefits of exercise seem to be consistent across different ethnic groups.

Regarding exercise intensity, it should be noted that moderate- (–4.8/–2.3 mmHg) and high-intensity (–3.6/–3.1 mmHg) exercise interventions induced greater reductions in BP than low-intensity exercise (Cornelissen & Smart, 2013), suggesting that the BP response to aerobic exercise is modulated by the intensity of exercise. Nonetheless, even exercise performed at relatively low intensity (e.g. 40–50% VO_2reserve) reduces resting BP (Pescatello et al., 2004). The influence of the exercise intensity has been also investigated on the BP response immediately following exercise (PEH). In this regard, Eicher et al. (2010) observed that the antihypertensive effects of exercise intensity occur in dose-response fashion among adults with pre- to stage 1 hypertension; the largest BP reductions were induced by vigorous-intensity (–11.7–/4.9 mmHg) exercise followed by moderate intensity (–5.4/–2.0 mmHg) and then by low intensity (–2.8/–1.5 mmHg), compared to a non-exercise control session over the course of nine hours after the session.

High-intensity interval training (HIIT)

In recent years, the use of HIIT in clinical populations has become more accepted; in adults with hypertension, HIIT seems to significantly reduce office and ambulatory BP (Boutcher & Boutcher, 2017). HIIT involves alternating periods of short and very high-intensity aerobic exercise (usually at intensities between 85–90% peak heart rate) with periods of recovery or rest (no exercise) of shorter, equal or longer duration. A recent systematic review by Costa et al. comparing the antihypertensive effects of HIIT to moderate-intensity continuous training in adults with pre- to established hypertension supports the benefits of HITT for reducing BP (Costa et al., 2018). The pooled data from the seven studies (164 participants) included in this meta-analysis showed no differences in the reduction of SBP (−0.22 mmHg, 95% CI: −5.36 to 4.92) and DBP (−0.38 mmHg, 95% CI: −3.31 to 2.54) between HIIT (−6.3/−3.8 mmHg) and moderate-intensity continuous training (−5.8/−3.5 mmHg) (Costa et al., 2018). Nevertheless, the seven studies included patients with severe co-morbidities, such chronic heart failure (two trials), coronary heart disease (one trial) and metabolic syndrome (two trials). On the other hand, HIIT typically induces greater increases in aerobic fitness in a shorter period of time and greater benefits in several pathophysiological variables related to the development of hypertension, such as arterial stiffness, endothelial function and insulin resistance (Boutcher & Boutcher, 2017). HIIT could be an alternative exercise strategy when the individual is willing and able to safely go harder than less vigorous continuous training. Regarding safety, no major adverse events were reported in the studies included in the Costa et al. (2018) review; the adverse events reported were related to pain and musculoskeletal injuries. Based on these results, the current exercise prescription recommendations for individuals with hypertension from Exercise and Sport Science Australia include HIIT performed three days per week, 25 minutes per session, four four-minute intervals at 85–95% peak heart rate, separated by three-minute intervals at 50–70% peak heart rate (Sharman et al., 2019).

However, it should be pointed out that a couple of studies in Dahl salt-sensitive rats, an animal model of hypertension, comparing the skeletal muscle (Holloway et al., 2015) and cardiac (Holloway, Bloemberg, da Silva, Simpson et al., 2015) adaptations to four weeks of HIIT versus continuous moderate-intensity aerobic exercise found contrasting results. The authors found that while continuous moderate-intensity exercise resulted in favourable cardiac and skeletal muscle adaptations, HIIT impacted negatively on cardiac function and the overall oxidative capacity of skeletal muscle (Holloway, Bloemberg, da Silva, Quadrilatero et al., 2015; Holloway, Bloemberg, da Silva, Simpson et al., 2015).

In summary, the average reductions in BP (8/5 mmHg) induced by aerobic exercise training seem to be equivalent to the reductions achieved with antihypertensive medication. The exercise-induced BP decrease is greatest in individuals with higher BP. Likewise, the intensity of aerobic exercise seems to be directly related to the BP reductions, with higher intensities inducing the greatest BP reductions. Despite the limited number of studies conducted so far,

HIIT appears to be an alternative with similar antihypertensive effects to continuous exercise; however, the low number of studies and the high burden of co-morbidities in the patients included in HIIT trials to date highlight the need for further large multi-centre prospective studies to confirm the positive multidimensional effects and the safety of HIIT for individuals with hypertension.

Dynamic resistance exercise

Recent evidence suggests that dynamic resistance exercise is as effective as aerobic exercise in reducing BP among individuals with hypertension. MacDonald et al. (2016) analysed 64 controlled studies (71 interventions; n = 2344, of whom 15% were on antihypertensive medication) to determine whether dynamic resistance training alone could lower BP to the level reported with aerobic exercise. On average, the resistance exercise interventions were performed at moderate intensity (65–70% of one repetition maximum), three sessions per week for 14 weeks. Each session was composed, on average, of three sets of 11 repetitions for eight exercises targeting the whole body. A dynamic resistance exercise program reduced SBP and DBP by −5.7 mmHg (95% CI: −9.0 to −2.7 mmHg)/−5.2 mmHg (95%CI: −8.4 to −1.9 mmHg) in adults with hypertension (MacDonald et al., 2016). These results were recently confirmed by Naci et al. (2019), who reported a −7.2 mmHg (95% CI: −10.58 to −3.87) decrease in SBP induced by dynamic resistance exercise in adults with hypertension.

As with aerobic exercise, the BP reductions following dynamic resistance training occur in a dose-response fashion as a function of resting BP. Larger SBP and DBP reductions are observed among those with higher resting BP levels at baseline, with larger reductions reported in individuals with hypertension (−5.7/−5.2 mmHg) than in those with prehypertension (−3.0/−3.3 mmHg), and normal BP (0.0/−1.0 mmHg) (MacDonald et al., 2016).

An interesting moderator of the BP response to dynamic resistance exercise appears to be race/ethnicity. The greatest reductions in BP (−14/−10 mmHg) were observed in studies involving non-white individuals with hypertension (MacDonald et al., 2016). These BP reductions are greater than those reported as a result of aerobic or dynamic resistance exercise among predominantly white populations. If confirmed in future studies that some populations are more likely to respond to dynamic resistance exercise than to aerobic exercise, this type of exercise could become first-line lifestyle treatment for non-white individuals with hypertension.

Presently, most of the recommendations for exercise among individuals with hypertension are to engage in dynamic resistance exercise as a supplement to aerobic exercise (Table 13.6). The latest update of the ACSM exercise recommendations for hypertension acknowledges, for the first time, dynamic resistance exercise as a stand-alone antihypertensive lifestyle therapy (Pescatello, 2019; Pescatello et al., 2019). The general recommendation consists of a moderate-intensity program (i.e. 60–70% of one repetition maximum), comprising 2 to 4 sets of 8 to 12 repetitions for 8 to 10 exercises targeting the major muscle groups on most, preferably all, days of the week (Pescatello, 2019; Pescatello et al., 2019).

In summary, dynamic resistance exercise seems to be as effective as aerobic exercise for reducing BP among individuals with hypertension. The BP reductions are greatest in individuals with higher resting BP. Additionally, the magnitude of the BP reductions appear to be higher in non-white populations, increasing its therapeutic potential – a topic that warrants further investigation.

Concurrent exercise

Interestingly, most of the professional society exercise recommendations for hypertension promote, at least indirectly, the antihypertensive benefits of concurrent exercise training. By recommending aerobic exercise supplemented by dynamic resistance exercise two or three non-consecutive days per week (Table 13.6), it is quite likely that most of the individuals with hypertension would engage in a combination of aerobic and resistance training performed together in a single session or on separate days (that is, concurrent or combined exercise).

A recent network meta-analysis (Naci et al., 2019) comparing the effect of exercise regimens and medications on SBP reported a reduction of −13.5 mmHg (95% CI: −16.6 to −10.5) as a result of a concurrent exercise training program among individuals with hypertension. This reduction is approximately 5 mmHg higher than that induced by aerobic (−8.7 mmHg) or dynamic resistance (−7.2 mmHg) exercise alone among populations with hypertension (Naci et al., 2019). These results are in line with a previous meta-analysis determining the efficacy of concurrent exercise as antihypertensive therapy (Corso et al., 2016). Corso et al. (2016) examined moderate-intensity concurrent aerobic (on average, 55% of VO_2max) and resistance exercise (in general, 60% of one repetition maximum) training performed approximately three days per week, 60 minutes per session, and reported a decrease of −5.3 mmHg (95% CI: −6.4 to −4.2)/−5.6 mmHg (95%CI: −6.9 to −3.8) in SBP and DBP among individuals with hypertension. The authors also found a relationship between the resting levels of BP and the magnitude of the reductions in SBP and DBP, with the greatest reductions observed in those with hypertension (−5.3/−5.6 mmHg), then prehypertension (−2.9/−3.6 mmHg), then normal BP (0.9/−2.5 mmHg). Interestingly, the antihypertensive effects of concurrent exercise were not modulated by the order or proximity (in a single session or on separate days) of the aerobic and resistance exercise components (Corso et al., 2016). Of note, greater BP reductions were reported among individuals with hypertension in studies of higher methodological quality with BP as the primary outcome: −9.2 mmHg (95% CI: −12.0 to −8.0)/−7.7 mmHg (95% CI = −14.0 to −8.0) (Corso et al., 2016).

In summary, combined aerobic and resistance or concurrent exercise training appears to have the potential to elicit the greatest reductions in BP in individuals with hypertension (Figure 13.3). Future studies of high methodological quality with BP as the primary outcome are needed to clearly confirm this potential. Similar to both aerobic and resistance exercise alone, the magnitude of the exercise-induced reduction in BP as a result of a combined exercise training program is dependent on the resting blood pressure levels.

Isometric resistance exercise

The current evidence does not clearly support the benefits of isometric resistance exercise to control BP among populations with hypertension. In contrast to previous reviews, the recent network meta-analysis of Naci et al. (2019) did not find a significant reduction in SBP (−4.92 mmHg, 95% CI: −10.28 to 0.38) as a result of an isometric resistance exercise program in individuals with hypertension. These results contrast with those initially reported in clinical trials and summarised in previous meta-analyses in which isometric exercise was shown to induce significant reductions in BP (Carlson et al., 2014; Cornelissen & Smart, 2013; Inder et al., 2016).

Cornelissen and Smart (2013) pooled four trials to examine the influence of isometric resistance training on BP and found that isometric exercise promoted the largest reductions in SBP (−10.9/−6.2 mmHg) compared to aerobic (−3.5/−2.5 mmHg) and dynamic resistance training (−1.8/−3.2 mmHg) (the results were not significant for DBP), even though the analysis included populations of different BP statuses. In 2016, Inder et al. conducted a meta-analysis of 11 RCTs (six used handgrip and five used leg exercise; n = 302) investigating the effects of isometric resistance training on BP in adults. Only three studies enrolled individuals with hypertension (n = 61). The authors demonstrated an overall decrease in BP of −5.2/−3.9 mmHg; a sub-analysis by BP categories showed a larger mean arterial pressure decrease among individuals with hypertension (−5.9 mmHg [95% CI: −7.9 to −3.9]) than among participants with normal BP (−3.0 mmHg [95% CI: −3.7 to −2.3]), but no significant differences were observed in SBP or DBP between BP categories (Inder et al., 2016). The isometric training protocol typically tested in previous studies consisted of four sets of two minutes of handgrip or leg contractions at 30% of maximal voluntary contraction, separated by one-minute rest periods. Regarding the characteristics of isometric exercise, unilateral (−8.9 vs. −4.6 mmHg) rather than bilateral exercise and arm (−6.9 vs. −4.2 mmHg) rather than leg isometric exercise, respectively, demonstrated a larger reduction in SBP (Inder et al., 2016). These findings led to the incorporation of isometric resistance exercise as an adjunct therapy for managing hypertension by the AHA/ACC (P. K. Whelton et al., 2018) and the Exercise and Sport Science Australia (Sharman et al., 2019) guidelines (Table 13.6).

In summary, isometric resistance exercise may have the potential to produce clinically meaningful reductions in BP; however, due to contrasting reports in the literature, it seems premature to advocate the general use of this form of training to control BP among individuals with hypertension.

Recommendations for exercise testing and exercise programming

Exercise testing

Although the health benefits of exercise are well recognised, there is also an increased risk of cardiovascular disease events associated with the practice of vigorous-intensity exercise (Albert et al., 2000). Individuals with multiple cardiovascular disease risk factors and known or subclinical cardiovascular disease who lead a sedentary lifestyle have a greater likelihood of triggering cardiac events during and after exercise and might benefit the most from risk assessment before their participation in vigorous- or high-intensity exercise programs. The aim of exercise testing is generally to detect the presence of coronary atherosclerotic disease and exercise-induced arrhythmias (Pelliccia et al., 2020). The exercise test may also be useful in the assessment of BP response during exercise and in the determination of the level of cardiorespiratory fitness of the participants, giving additional and valuable information for the development of an exercise prescription (Pelliccia et al., 2020). The assessment of the BP response to exercise is particularly relevant in individuals with hypertension who often have an exaggerated BP response to exercise even if resting BP levels are controlled (Fletcher et al., 2013).

However, hypertension per se is not an indication for routine exercise testing (Fletcher et al., 2013; Riebe et al., 2015). The recommendations for exercise testing for individuals with hypertension will depend on several factors, including, but not limited to, resting BP level, presence of other cardiovascular disease risk factors, target organ damage and presence of cardiovascular, renal or metabolic disease. Clinicians should judge on an individual basis the need for a complete medical examination, exercise test and/or other diagnostic imaging exam. Nonetheless, the following recommendations are suggested for the assessment and interpretation of the BP response to exercise based on the expert opinion and guidelines of several professional organisations, including the AHA and the European Society of Cardiology.

- The exercise test should be postponed if resting SBP exceeds 200 mmHg and/or if DBP exceeds 115 mmHg (Fletcher et al., 2013). The current European Society of Cardiology guidelines on sports cardiology and exercise in patients with cardiovascular disease recommends postponing the maximal exercise test until BP is controlled when SBP is poorly controlled (resting SBP > 160 mmHg) (Pelliccia et al., 2020).
- A resting SBP and/or DBP > 200/110 mmHg is a relative contraindication to exercise testing (Fletcher et al., 2013), while a SBP > 250 mmHg and/or a DBP > 115 mmHg during exercise is an indication for test termination (Fletcher et al., 2013).
- The BP values determining an exaggerated response to exercise are not well established, but it is suggested that SBP ≥ 150 mmHg at light to moderate intensity or SBP ≥ 210/≥ 190 mmHg at maximal-intensity exercise in men or women, respectively, are beyond the upper limits of normal (Sharman et al., 2019).

Exercise programming

The expansion of interest in physical exercise and its application to primary prevention, treatment and control of high BP resulted in an increase in the number of professional societies acknowledging the key importance of exercise in their guidelines for the management of high BP in adults. Table 13.6 summarises the exercise prescription recommendations for individuals with hypertension produced by different organisations, such as the European Society of Hypertension/European Society of Cardiology (Williams et al., 2018), the AHA/ACC (P. K. Whelton et al., 2018), the American College of Sports Medicine (ACSM) (Pescatello, 2019; Pescatello et al., 2019), the Exercise and Sport Science Australia (Sharman et al., 2019), the Brazilian Society of Cardiology (Malachias et al., 2016) and the International Society of Hypertension (Unger et al., 2020). Despite slight variations in terms of frequency (how many sessions per week), intensity (how hard to exercise), time (duration of the exercise session), type (modalities of exercise training), volume (the total amount or dose of exercise) and progression (the rate of increasing the dose of exercise), or the FITT-VP principle), the professional committees/organisations recommend adults with hypertension engage in at least 30 minutes per day^{-1} of moderate to vigorous aerobic exercise five to seven days per week. The recommendation to include dynamic resistant exercise at least as adjuvant is consistent across the different society recommendations (Table 13.6), although the exact FITT prescription to optimally lower BP is not clearly defined.

The latest (2019) update from the ACSM FITT recommendations for hypertension (Pescatello, 2019; Pescatello et al., 2019), based on compelling high-quality contemporary evidence, provides a comprehensive exercise prescription framed by the FITT principle that should result in clinically meaningful reductions in BP among most individuals with hypertension. The exercise training program is recommended to include aerobic exercise or resistance exercise alone combined (concurrent exercise) on most, preferably all, days of the week. Before and after the main component of each exercise session (aerobic and/or resistance), the individuals should perform a period of five to ten minutes warm-up/cool down at an intensity of 10 to 12 on Borg rating of perceived exercise (6–20 point scale); Neuromotor (exercise involving motor skills and/or functional body weight and flexibility exercise such as yoga, Pilates or tai chi) > 20 to 30 minutes per session and flexibility exercise ≤ 10 minutes per session may be offered as adjunct, depending on personal preference. The current ACSM recommendation that integrate flexibility and neuromotor exercise in the program for individuals with hypertension aims to reduce the risk of musculoskeletal injury, increase exercise adherence, improve balance and range of motion and decrease the risk of falls.

The following ACSM FITT-VP exercise prescription recommendations for individuals with hypertension is adapted from (Pescatello, 2019; Pescatello et al., 2019):

Aerobic and/or resistance exercise

- **Frequency:** exercise on most, preferably all, days of the week.
- **Intensity:** low, moderate or vigorous intensity with an emphasis on moderate-intensity exercise. Aerobic: moderate (i.e. 40–59% oxygen uptake reserve or heart rate reserve; rating of perceived exertion 12–13 on a 6–20 scale) to vigorous (i.e. 60–80% oxygen uptake reserve or heart rate reserve; rating of perceived exertion 14–16 on a 6–20 scale) exercise. Resistance: moderate (i.e. 60–70% one repetition maximum; may progress to 80% one repetition maximum).
- **Time:** ≥ 20–30 minutes per day to total ≥ 90 to 150+ minutes per week of continuous or accumulated exercise of any duration. Resistance training should comprise two to four sets of 8 to 12 repetitions of 8 to 10 resistance exercises for each of the major muscle groups per session to total ≥ 20 minutes per session.
- **Type:** Aerobic exercise should emphasise rhythmic activities using large muscle groups such as walking, cycling, jogging, running or swimming. Resistance exercise, also targeting the major muscle groups, may use free weights, resistance bands, functional body weight exercises and/or resistance machines.
- **Volume:** The weekly amount of exercise should total 90 to 150 or more minutes.
- **Progression:** Progression should be offered on an individual basis gradually throughout the program to allow continued adaptation. Include all the FITT components in progression; however, in general, increase only one component of FITT at a time for either aerobic or resistance training. As a suggestion, first increase the duration of exercise by one to five minutes per session until the goal duration has been reached and then increase intensity (5–10% is generally well tolerated) to achieve the recommended volume of weekly exercise. Failure to provide adequate progression may limit the antihypertension benefits of exercise.

It should be noted that exercise prescription for individuals with hypertension should take into account age, co-morbidities, medical history, current BP levels, current level of physical activity, antihypertensive medication use, the presence of other diseases (e.g. cardiovascular, renal and metabolic) (Riebe et al., 2015) and/or target organ damage. These are important factors to consider in the treatment process, and the exercise prescription should be adjusted accordingly.

Summary

Hypertension is a complex and heterogenous disorder that originates from the interplay of numerous environmental and genetic factors. It is defined as the level of blood pressure (office systolic/diastolic ≥ 140 and/or ≥ 90 mmHg), at which the benefits of treatment clearly compensate the risks of treatment, as documented by clinical trials. Regular physical exercise should be encouraged as evidence supports clinically meaningful antihypertensive benefits. Previous clinical trials support clinically meaningful reductions of blood pressure among adults with hypertension as a result of aerobic, resistance and concurrent exercise.

Case study

Medical history

Jane is 58 years old, and she is apparently healthy, with history of hypertension for 14 years. Jane enrolled in the fitness centre to start an exercise program for improving her health and physical fitness. Her weight is 58 kg and BMI 24 kg/m2. Her medications include Exforge (amlodipine + valsartan, 5/80 mg daily) and Aldactazine (spironolactone + Altizide, 25/15 mg daily). Her resting BP is 139/81 mmHg and 24-hour ambulatory BP is 130/75 mmHg. Her LDL-C was 91 $mg.dL^{-1}$, HDL-C was 51 $mg.dL^{-1}$ and total cholesterol was 156 mg/dL. She drinks two glasses of wine at dinner during weekends. She smoked for 10 years but stopped 12 years ago. She also used to run three to four times per week until the age of 30, but currently, her physical activity levels only include walking 20 minutes two days per week (during the weekend) at moderate intensity.

Plan and exercise prescription

Jane's personal trainer encouraged Jane to start an exercise program with 20 minutes of light to moderate intensity (40% V̇O2R or HRR, 11–12 RPE) aerobic exercise on a treadmill, five days per week. Progression initially emphasised increasing exercise duration and then exercise intensity as follows: increase exercise duration gradually by five minutes per week until duration reached 30 minutes per day and exercise intensity by 5% to 10%, progressing from moderate (40–59% V̇O2R or HRR, 12–13 RPE) to vigorous intensity (≥ 60% V̇O2R or HRR, 14–17 RPE), according to her tolerance and preference. Resistance training was added to enhance strength and muscle mass and complement aerobic exercise training (concurrent training) in the management of hypertension. Resistance exercises were incorporated on two days per week, with two days between them. Each resistance exercise session comprised two sets of 10 to 12 repetitions of 8 to 10 resistance exercises for each of the major muscle groups per session at 40% to 50% 1RM and progressing to 60% to 70% 1RM. Flexibility training was incorporated as part of the warm-up and cool down for its general health benefits.

Exercise monitoring and special precautions

To optimise the effects of exercise training, BP was recorded ten minutes before and after each exercise session because self-monitoring of the BP response to exercise has been shown to foster exercise adherence among adults with hypertension. On the other hand, to avoid excessive BP reductions after exercise, given that she is taking calcium channel blockers, the cool down was extended to allow enough time to gradually decrease exercise intensity. Given that Jane was also on diuretics, she was instructed to maintain proper fluid intake during the exercise sessions, especially on hot days, to avoid symptoms of dehydration. In addition, specific instructions to avoid Valsalva maneuver during resistance exercise were given to prevent excessive acute increases in BP.

Key points

- Regular physical exercise – aerobic or resistance or a combination of both (concurrent exercise) – improves blood pressure control and reduces BP levels among individuals with hypertension.
- Adults with hypertension are encouraged to engage in ≥ 20 to 30 minutes per day (totaling ≥ 90 to 150+ minutes per week) of continuous or accumulated exercise of any duration on most days of the week (preferably all).
- The decrease in BP occurs in a dose-response fashion as a function of resting BP, with the greatest antihypertensive effects of exercise observed in individuals with the highest resting BP.

Summary

Short questions

1. What is the definition of hypertension?
2. What is the BP goal in people with hypertension?
3. Indicate the lifestyle changes that are recommended in the treatment of hypertension.
4. State which drugs are considered as first line in the treatment of hypertension.
5. Define post-exercise hypotension.
6. State what activities (exercise type) a person with hypertension should engage in.
7. What is the general recommendation for resistance exercise among individuals with hypertension?
8. How much should the average adult with hypertension exercise per week?
9. Explain how the resting blood pressure levels influence the blood pressure response to exercise.
10. Are the antihypertensive effects of exercise comparable to antihypertensive medication?

TABLE 13.7 At-a-glance summary guide to exercise considerations for people with hypertension

Condition name	*Hypertension*
Pathophysiology summary	Hypertension is a condition diagnosed by persistent high systolic and/or diastolic blood pressure, resulting from renal impairment, endothelial dysfunction and/or impaired autonomic function. Defects in any of these mechanisms lead to increased vascular resistance leading to hypertension.
Aims of exercise	To improve blood pressure control, cardiorespiratory fitness and cardiometabolic health profiles and reduce the risk of micro- and macrovascular complications.
Exercise considerations	The presence of hypertension-related complications (increased risk of stroke or myocardial infarction) require exercise to be limited to moderate intensity to begin with. Interactions between antihypertensive medications and exercise increases the risk of postural/orthostatic hypotension requiring a careful transition between exercises.
Frequency	For aerobic activity, aim for five to seven days per week. For resistance/flexibility exercises, aim for two to three sessions per week performed on non-consecutive days.
Intensity	Aim to adopt a physically active lifestyle, including reducing sedentary behaviour and increasing incidental daily physical activity. Moderate (progressing to vigorous) physical activity is likely to yield the greatest physiological response and therefore benefits. Resistance training 50–80% 1RM.
Time	Accumulation of a minimum of 150 minutes per week for moderate-intensity physical activity (or 75 minutes for vigorous-intensity physical activity). Resistance training: one to three sets of 8–12 repetitions of 6–10 exercises.
Type	The primary exercise mode for modulating blood pressure is aerobic activity, utilising large muscle groups, such as walking, cycling, swimming, dancing or jogging. Isotonic and isometric resistance training exercises are recommended as adjunct exercise therapy.
Common medications	ß-blockers, calcium channel blockers, ACE inhibitors, angiotensin II receptor antagonists and diuretics.
Key safety considerations	Medical referral for individuals with hypertension is useful to indicate other related complications. The referral information is useful to understand the person's medications, particularly multiple antihypertensive medications that increase postural/orthostatic syncope risk with exercise. Take care with exercise transitions and warm up and cool down steadily.
Effect of exercise on conditions	Both aerobic and isometric resistance training have acute and chronic effects on blood pressure control as well as other cardiovascular risk factors associated with elevated blood pressure. These are driven by (amongst other things) enhanced endothelial function, increased capillarisation, improved parasympathetic tone and decreased sympathetic activity, reduced heart rated and cardiac output, enhanced metabolism through increased skeletal muscle mass and improved mitochondrial oxidative capacity.

References

ACSM. (2018). *ACSM's Guidelines for Exercise Testing and Prescription* (10th ed.). Philadelphia: Lippincott Williams & Wilkins.

Albert, C. M., Mittleman, M. A., Chae, C. U., Lee, I. M., Hennekens, C. H., & Manson, J. E. (2000). Triggering of sudden death from cardiac causes by vigorous exertion. *N Engl J Med*, *343*(19), 1355–1361. doi:10.1056/NEJM200011093431902

Bakris, G., Ali, W., & Parati, G. (2019). ACC/AHA versus ESC/ESH on hypertension guidelines: JACC guideline comparison. *J Am Coll Cardiol, 73*(23), 3018–3026. doi:10.1016/j.jacc.2019.03.507

Bersaoui, M., Baldew, S. M., Cornelis, N., Toelsie, J., & Cornelissen, V. A. (2020). The effect of exercise training on blood pressure in African and Asian populations: A systematic review and meta-analysis of randomized controlled trials. *Eur J Prev Cardiol, 27*(5), 457–472. doi:10.1177/2047487319871233

Bolivar, J. J. (2013). Essential hypertension: An approach to its etiology and neurogenic pathophysiology. *Int J Hypertens, 2013*, 547809. doi:10.1155/2013/547809

Borjesson, M., Onerup, A., Lundqvist, S., & Dahlof, B. (2016). Physical activity and exercise lower blood pressure in individuals with hypertension: Narrative review of 27 RCTs. *Br J Sports Med, 50*(6), 356–361. doi:10.1136/bjsports-2015-095786

Boutcher, Y. N., & Boutcher, S. H. (2017). Exercise intensity and hypertension: What's new? *J Hum Hypertens, 31*(3), 157–164. doi:10.1038/jhh.2016.62

Brito, L. C., Fecchio, R. Y., Pecanha, T., Andrade-Lima, A., Halliwill, J. R., & Forjaz, C. L. M. (2018). Postexercise hypotension as a clinical tool: A "single brick" in the wall. *J Am Soc Hypertens, 12*(12), e59–e64. doi:10.1016/j.jash.2018.10.006

Brunstrom, M., & Carlberg, B. (2018). Association of blood pressure lowering with mortality and cardiovascular disease across blood pressure levels: A systematic review and meta-analysis. *JAMA Intern Med, 178*(1), 28–36. doi:10.1001/jamainternmed.2017.6015

Cardoso, C. G., Jr., Gomides, R. S., Queiroz, A. C., Pinto, L. G., da Silveira Lobo, F. Tinucci, T., . . . de Moraes Forjaz, C. L. (2010). Acute and chronic effects of aerobic and resistance exercise on ambulatory blood pressure. *Clinics (Sao Paulo), 65*(3), 317–325. doi:10.1590/S1807-59322010000300013

Carey, R. M. (2008). Pathophysiology of primary hypertension. In *Microcirculation* (pp. 794–895). Amsterdam: Elsevier.

Carey, R. M., Calhoun, D. A., Bakris, G. L., Brook, R. D., Daugherty, S. L., Dennison-Himmelfarb, C. R., . . . Stroke, C. (2018). Resistant hypertension: Detection, evaluation, and management: A scientific statement from the American Heart Association. *Hypertension, 72*(5), e53–e90. doi:10.1161/HYP.0000000000000084

Carlson, D. J., Dieberg, G., Hess, N. C., Millar, P. J., & Smart, N. A. (2014). Isometric exercise training for blood pressure management: A systematic review and meta-analysis. *Mayo Clin Proc, 89*(3), 327–334. doi:10.1016/j.mayocp.2013.10.030

Carpio-Rivera, E., Moncada-Jimenez, J., Salazar-Rojas, W., & Solera-Herrera, A. (2016). Acute effects of exercise on blood pressure: A meta-analytic investigation. *Arq Bras Cardiol, 106*(5), 422–433. doi:10.5935/abc.20160064

Carretero, O. A., & Oparil, S. (2000). Essential hypertension. Part I: Definition and etiology. *Circulation, 101*(3), 329–335. doi:10.1161/01.cir.101.3.329

Carson, A. P., Howard, G., Burke, G. L., Shea, S., Levitan, E. B., & Muntner, P. (2011). Ethnic differences in hypertension incidence among middle-aged and older adults: The multi-ethnic study of atherosclerosis. *Hypertension, 57*(6), 1101–1107. doi:10.1161/HYPERTENSIONAHA.110.168005

Casonatto, J., Goessler, K. F., Cornelissen, V. A., Cardoso, J. R., & Polito, M. D. (2016). The blood pressure-lowering effect of a single bout of resistance exercise: A systematic review and meta-analysis of randomised controlled trials. *Eur J Prev Cardiol, 23*(16), 1700–1714. doi:10.1177/2047487316664147

Chow, C. K., Teo, K. K., Rangarajan, S., Islam, S., Gupta, R., Avezum, A., . . . investigators, P. S. (2013). Prevalence, awareness, treatment, and control of hypertension in rural and urban communities in high-, middle-, and low-income countries. *JAMA, 310*(9), 959–968. doi:10.1001/jama.2013.184182

Collaboration, N. C. D. R. F. (2017). Worldwide trends in blood pressure from 1975 to 2015: A pooled analysis of 1479 population-based measurement studies with 19.1 million participants. *Lancet, 389*(10064), 37–55. doi:10.1016/S0140-6736(16)31919-5

Collaborators, G. B. D. R. F. (2018). Global, regional, and national comparative risk assessment of 84 behavioural, environmental and occupational, and metabolic risks or clusters of risks for 195 countries and territories, 1990–2017: A systematic analysis for the global burden of disease study 2017. *Lancet, 392*(10159), 1923–1994. doi:10.1016/S0140-6736(18)32225-6

Cornelissen, V. A., & Smart, N. A. (2013). Exercise training for blood pressure: A systematic review and meta-analysis. *J Am Heart Assoc, 2*(1), e004473. doi:10.1161/JAHA.112.004473

Corso, L. M., Macdonald, H. V., Johnson, B. T., Farinatti, P., Livingston, J., Zaleski, A. L., . . . Pescatello, L. S. (2016). Is concurrent training efficacious antihypertensive therapy? A meta-analysis. *Med Sci Sports Exerc, 48*(12), 2398–2406. doi:10.1249/MSS.0000000000001056

Costa, E. C., Hay, J. L., Kehler, D. S., Boreskie, K. F., Arora, R. C., Umpierre, D., . . . Duhamel, T. A. (2018). Effects of high-intensity interval training versus moderate-intensity continuous training on blood pressure in adults with pre- to established hypertension: A systematic review and meta-analysis of randomized trials. *Sports Med, 48*(9), 2127–2142. doi:10.1007/s40279-018-0944-y

Dempsey, P. C., Larsen, R. N., Dunstan, D. W., Owen, N., & Kingwell, B. A. (2018). Sitting less and moving more: Implications for hypertension. *Hypertension, 72*(5), 1037–1046. doi:10.1161/HYPERTENSIONAHA.118.11190

Dominiczak, A., Delles, C., & Padmanabhan, S. (2017). Genomics and precision medicine for clinicians and scientists in hypertension. *Hypertension, 69*(4), e10–e13. doi:10.1161/HYPERTENSIONAHA.116.08252

Eicher, J. D., Maresh, C. M., Tsongalis, G. J., Thompson, P. D., & Pescatello, L. S. (2010). The additive blood pressure lowering effects of exercise intensity on post-exercise hypotension. *Am Heart J, 160*(3), 513–520. doi:10.1016/j.ahj.2010.06.005

Ettehad, D., Emdin, C. A., Kiran, A., Anderson, S. G., Callender, T., Emberson, J., . . . Rahimi, K. (2016). Blood pressure lowering for prevention of cardiovascular disease and death: A systematic review and meta-analysis. *Lancet, 387*(10022), 957–967. doi:10.1016/S0140-6736(15)01225-8

Fagard, R. H., & Cornelissen, V. A. (2007). Effect of exercise on blood pressure control in hypertensive patients. *Eur J Cardiovasc Prev Rehabil, 14*(1), 12–17. doi:10.1097/HJR.0b013e3280128bbb

Fletcher, G. F., Ades, P. A., Kligfield, P., Arena, R., Balady, G. J., Bittner, V. A., . . . Prevention. (2013). Exercise standards for testing and training: A scientific statement from the American heart association. *Circulation, 128*(8), 873–934. doi:10.1161/CIR.0b013e31829b5b44

Ford, E. S. (2011). Trends in mortality from all causes and cardiovascular disease among hypertensive and nonhypertensive adults in the United States. *Circulation, 123*(16), 1737–1744. doi:10.1161/CIRCULATIONAHA.110.005645

Forrester, S. J., Booz, G. W., Sigmund, C. D., Coffman, T. M., Kawai, T., Rizzo, V., . . . Eguchi, S. (2018). Angiotensin II signal transduction: An update on mechanisms of physiology and pathophysiology. *Physiol Rev, 98*(3), 1627–1738. doi:10.1152/physrev.00038.2017

Hanssen, H., Boardman, H., Deiseroth, A., Moholdt, T., Simonenko, M., Krankel, N., . . . Leeson, P. (2021). Personalized exercise prescription in the prevention and treatment of arterial hypertension: A consensus document from the European association of preventive cardiology (EAPC) and the ESC council on hypertension. *Eur J Prev Cardiol.* doi:10.1093/eurjpc/zwaa141

He, F. J., Li, J., & Macgregor, G. A. (2013). Effect of longer term modest salt reduction on blood pressure: Cochrane systematic review and meta-analysis of randomised trials. *BMJ, 346*, f1325. doi:10.1136/bmj.f1325

Hecksteden, A., Grutters, T., & Meyer, T. (2013). Association between postexercise hypotension and long-term training-induced blood pressure reduction: A pilot study. *Clin J Sport Med, 23*(1), 58–63. doi:10.1097/JSM.0b013e31825b6974

Holloway, T. M., Bloemberg, D., da Silva, M. L., Quadrilatero, J., & Spriet, L. L. (2015). High-intensity interval and endurance training are associated with divergent skeletal muscle adaptations in a rodent model of hypertension. *Am J Physiol Regul Integr Comp Physiol, 308*(11), R927–934. doi:10.1152/ajpregu.00048.2015

Holloway, T. M., Bloemberg, D., da Silva, M. L., Simpson, J. A., Quadrilatero, J., & Spriet, L. L. (2015). High intensity interval and endurance training have opposing effects on markers of heart failure and cardiac remodeling in hypertensive rats. *PLoS One, 10*(3), e0121138. doi:10.1371/journal.pone.0121138

Howard, G., Prineas, R., Moy, C., Cushman, M., Kellum, M., Temple, E., . . . Howard, V. (2006). Racial and geographic differences in awareness, treatment, and control of hypertension: The reasons for geographic and racial differences in stroke study. *Stroke, 37*(5), 1171–1178. doi:10.1161/01.STR.0000217222.09978.ce

Inder, J. D., Carlson, D. J., Dieberg, G., McFarlane, J. R., Hess, N. C., & Smart, N. A. (2016). Isometric exercise training for blood pressure management: A systematic review and meta-analysis to optimize benefit. *Hypertens Res*, *39*(2), 88–94. doi:10.1038/hr.2015.111

Ivy, J. R., & Bailey, M. A. (2014). Pressure natriuresis and the renal control of arterial blood pressure. *J Physiol*, *592*(18), 3955–3967. doi:10.1113/jphysiol.2014.271676

Kearney, P. M., Whelton, M., Reynolds, K., Muntner, P., Whelton, P. K., & He, J. (2005). Global burden of hypertension: Analysis of worldwide data. *Lancet*, *365*(9455), 217–223. doi:10.1016/S0140-6736(05)17741-1

Kim, D., & Ha, J. W. (2016). Hypertensive response to exercise: Mechanisms and clinical implication. *Clin Hypertens*, *22*, 17. doi:10.1186/s40885-016-0052-y

Kurl, S., Laukkanen, J. A., Rauramaa, R., Lakka, T. A., Sivenius, J., & Salonen, J. T. (2001). Systolic blood pressure response to exercise stress test and risk of stroke. *Stroke*, *32*(9), 2036–2041. doi:10.1161/hs0901.095395

Lackland, D. T., Keil, J. E., Gazes, P. C., Hames, C. G., & Tyroler, H. A. (1995). Outcomes of black and white hypertensive individuals after 30 years of follow-up. *Clin Exp Hypertens*, *17*(7), 1091–1105. doi:10.3109/10641969509033654

Lopes, J., Fonseca, M., Torres-Costoso, A., López-Muñoz, P., Alves, A. J., Magalhães, P., & Ribeiro, F. (2020). Low-and moderate-intensity aerobic exercise acutely reduce blood pressure in adults with high-normal/grade I hypertension. *J Clin Hypertens*.

MacDonald, H. V., Johnson, B. T., Huedo-Medina, T. B., Livingston, J., Forsyth, K. C., Kraemer, W. J., . . . Pescatello, L. S. (2016). Dynamic resistance training as stand-alone antihypertensive lifestyle therapy: A meta-analysis. *J Am Heart Assoc*, *5*(10). doi:10.1161/JAHA.116.003231

Malachias, M. V. B., Franco, R. J., Forjaz, C. L. M., Pierin, A. M. G., Gowdak, M. M., Klein, M., & Matsudo, V. (2016). 7th Brazilian guideline of arterial hypertension: Chapter 6 – non-pharmacological treatment. *Arq Bras Cardiol*, *107*(3 Suppl 3), 30–34. doi:10.5935/abc.20160156

Matthews, C. E., Pate, R. R., Jackson, K. L., Ward, D. S., Macera, C. A., Kohl, H. W., & Blair, S. N. (1998). Exaggerated blood pressure response to dynamic exercise and risk of future hypertension. *J Clin Epidemiol*, *51*(1), 29–35. doi:10.1016/s0895-4356(97)00223-0

Mayet, J., & Hughes, A. (2003). Cardiac and vascular pathophysiology in hypertension. *Heart*, *89*(9), 1104–1109. doi:10.1136/heart.89.9.1104

Mills, K. T., Bundy, J. D., Kelly, T. N., Reed, J. E., Kearney, P. M., Reynolds, K., . . . He, J. (2016). Global disparities of hypertension prevalence and control: A systematic analysis of population-based studies from 90 countries. *Circulation*, *134*(6), 441–450. doi:10.1161/CIRCULATIONAHA.115.018912

Miura, K., Daviglus, M. L., Dyer, A. R., Liu, K., Garside, D. B., Stamler, J., & Greenland, P. (2001). Relationship of blood pressure to 25-year mortality due to coronary heart disease, cardiovascular diseases, and all causes in young adult men: The Chicago heart association detection project in industry. *Arch Intern Med*, *161*(12), 1501–1508. doi:10.1001/archinte.161.12.1501

Mundal, R., Kjeldsen, S. E., Sandvik, L., Erikssen, G., Thaulow, E., & Erikssen, J. (1996). Exercise blood pressure predicts mortality from myocardial infarction. *Hypertension*, *27*(3 Pt 1), 324–329. doi:10.1161/01.hyp.27.3.324

Naci, H., Salcher-Konrad, M., Dias, S., Blum, M. R., Sahoo, S. A., Nunan, D., & Ioannidis, J. P. A. (2019). How does exercise treatment compare with antihypertensive medications? A network meta-analysis of 391 randomised controlled trials assessing exercise and medication effects on systolic blood pressure. *Br J Sports Med*, *53*(14), 859–869. doi:10.1136/bjsports-2018-099921

Noone, C., Leahy, J., Morrissey, E. C., Newell, J., Newell, M., Dwyer, C. P., . . . Molloy, G. J. (2020). Comparative efficacy of exercise and anti-hypertensive pharmacological interventions in reducing blood pressure in people with hypertension: A network meta-analysis. *Eur J Prev Cardiol*, *27*(3), 247–255. doi:10.1177/2047487319879786

Palombo, C., & Kozakova, M. (2016). Arterial stiffness, atherosclerosis and cardiovascular risk: Pathophysiologic mechanisms and emerging clinical indications. *Vascul Pharmacol*, 77, 1–7. doi:10.1016/j.vph.2015.11.083

Pazoki, R., Dehghan, A., Evangelou, E., Warren, H., Gao, H., Caulfield, M., . . . Tzoulaki, I. (2018). Genetic predisposition to high blood pressure and lifestyle factors: Associations with midlife blood pressure levels and cardiovascular events. *Circulation, 137*(7), 653–661. doi:10.1161/CIRCULATIONAHA.117.030898

Pelliccia, A., Sharma, S., Gati, S., Back, M., Borjesson, M., Caselli, S., . . . Group, E. S. C. S. D. (2020). 2020 ESC Guidelines on sports cardiology and exercise in patients with cardiovascular disease. *Eur Heart J.* doi:10.1093/eurheartj/ehaa605

Pescatello, L. S. (2019, June 11). What's new in the ACSM pronouncement on exercise and hypertension? Retrieved from www.acsm.org/home/featured-blogs – homepage/acsm-blog/2019/06/11/new-acsm-pronouncement-exercise-hypertension

Pescatello, L. S., Buchner, D. M., Jakicic, J. M., Powell, K. E., Kraus, W. E., Bloodgood, B., . . . Physical Activity Guidelines Advisory, C. (2019). Physical activity to prevent and treat hypertension: A systematic review. *Med Sci Sports Exerc, 51*(6), 1314–1323. doi:10.1249/MSS.0000000000001943

Pescatello, L. S., Franklin, B. A., Fagard, R., Farquhar, W. B., Kelley, G. A., Ray, C. A., & American College of Sports, M. (2004). American college of sports medicine position stand. Exercise and hypertension. *Med Sci Sports Exerc, 36*(3), 533–553. doi:10.1249/01.mss.0000115224.88514.3a

Pescatello, L. S., MacDonald, H. V., Ash, G. I., Lamberti, L. M., Farquhar, W. B., Arena, R., & Johnson, B. T. (2015). Assessing the existing professional exercise recommendations for hypertension: A review and recommendations for future research priorities. *Mayo Clin Proc, 90*(6), 801–812. doi:10.1016/j.mayocp.2015.04.008

Pescatello, L. S., MacDonald, H. V., Lamberti, L., & Johnson, B. T. (2015). Exercise for hypertension: A prescription update integrating existing recommendations with emerging research. *Curr Hypertens Rep, 17*(11), 87. doi:10.1007/s11906-015-0600-y

Powers, S. (2014). *Exercise Physiology: Theory and Application to Fitness and Performance.* New York: McGraw-Hill Higher Education.

Rayner, B. L., & Spence, J. D. (2017). Hypertension in blacks: Insights from Africa. *J Hypertens, 35*(2), 234–239. doi:10.1097/HJH.0000000000001171

Riebe, D., Franklin, B. A., Thompson, P. D., Garber, C. E., Whitfield, G. P., Magal, M., & Pescatello, L. S. (2015). Updating ACSM's recommendations for exercise preparticipation health screening. *Med Sci Sports Exerc, 47*(11), 2473–2479. doi:10.1249/MSS.0000000000000664

Saxena, T., Ali, A. O., & Saxena, M. (2018). Pathophysiology of essential hypertension: An update. *Expert Rev Cardiovasc Ther, 16*(12), 879–887. doi:10.1080/14779072.2018.1540301

Sharman, J. E., Smart, N. A., Coombes, J. S., & Stowasser, M. (2019). Exercise and sport science Australia position stand update on exercise and hypertension. *J Hum Hypertens, 33*(12), 837–843. doi:10.1038/s41371-019-0266-z

Shim, C. Y. (2011). Arterial-cardiac interaction: The concept and implications. *J Cardiovasc Ultrasound, 19*(2), 62–66. doi:10.4250/jcu.2011.19.2.62

Strazzullo, P., D'Elia, L., Kandala, N. B., & Cappuccio, F. P. (2009). Salt intake, stroke, and cardiovascular disease: Meta-analysis of prospective studies. *BMJ, 339*, b4567. doi:10.1136/bmj.b4567

Taddei, S., Bruno, R. M., Masi, S., & Solini, A. (2018). Epidemiology and pathophysiology of hypertension. In *ESC CardioMed*. Oxford: Oxford University Press.

Unger, T., Borghi, C., Charchar, F., Khan, N. A., Poulter, N. R., Prabhakaran, D., . . . Schutte, A. E. (2020). 2020 International society of hypertension global hypertension practice guidelines. *Hypertension, 75*(6), 1334–1357. doi:10.1161/HYPERTENSIONAHA.120.15026

van den Hoogen, P. C., Feskens, E. J., Nagelkerke, N. J., Menotti, A., Nissinen, A., & Kromhout, D. (2000). The relation between blood pressure and mortality due to coronary heart disease among men in different parts of the world. Seven Countries study research group. *N Engl J Med, 342*(1), 1–8. doi:10.1056/NEJM200001063420101

Wallace, J. P., Bogle, P. G., King, B. A., Krasnoff, J. B., & Jastremski, C. A. (1999). The magnitude and duration of ambulatory blood pressure reduction following acute exercise. *J Hum Hypertens, 13*(6), 361–366. doi:10.1038/sj.jhh.1000797

Wegmann, M., Hecksteden, A., Poppendieck, W., Steffen, A., Kraushaar, J., Morsch, A., & Meyer, T. (2018). Postexercise hypotension as a predictor for long-term training-induced blood pressure reduction: A large-scale randomized controlled trial. *Clin J Sport Med, 28*(6), 509–515. doi:10.1097/JSM.0000000000000475

Whelton, P. K., Carey, R. M., Aronow, W. S., Casey, D. E., Jr., Collins, K. J., Dennison Himmelfarb, C., . . . Wright, J. T., Jr. (2018). 2017 ACC/AHA/AAPA/ABC/ACPM/AGS/APhA/ASH/ASPC/NMA/PCNA Guideline for the prevention, detection, evaluation, and management of high blood pressure in adults: A report of the American college of cardiology/American heart association task force on clinical practice guidelines. *Hypertension, 71*(6), e13–e115. doi:10.1161/HYP.0000000000000065

Whelton, P. K., He, J., Appel, L. J., Cutler, J. A., Havas, S., Kotchen, T. A., . . . National High Blood Pressure Education Program Coordinating, C. (2002). Primary prevention of hypertension: Clinical and public health advisory from the national high blood pressure education program. *JAMA, 288*(15), 1882–1888. doi:10.1001/jama.288.15.1882

Whelton, S. P., Chin, A., Xin, X., & He, J. (2002). Effect of aerobic exercise on blood pressure: A meta-analysis of randomized, controlled trials. *Ann Intern Med, 136*(7), 493–503. doi:10.7326/0003-4819-136-7-200204020-00006

Williams, B., Mancia, G., Spiering, W., Agabiti Rosei, E., Azizi, M., Burnier, M., . . . Group, E. S. C. S. D. (2018). 2018 ESC/ESH guidelines for the management of arterial hypertension. *Eur Heart J, 39*(33), 3021–3104. doi:10.1093/eurheartj/ehy339

Wyatt, S. B., Akylbekova, E. L., Wofford, M. R., Coady, S. A., Walker, E. R., Andrew, M. E., . . . Jones, D. W. (2008). Prevalence, awareness, treatment, and control of hypertension in the Jackson heart study. *Hypertension, 51*(3), 650–656. doi:10.1161/HYPERTENSIONAHA.107.100081

Zaleski, A. L., Taylor, B. A., Park, C. L., Santos, L. P., Panza, G., Kramarz, M. . . . Pescatello, L. S. (2019). Using the immediate blood pressure benefits of exercise to improve exercise adherence among adults with hypertension: A randomized clinical trial. *J Hypertens, 37*(9), 1877–1888. doi:10.1097/HJH.0000000000002115

14

DYSLIPIDAEMIA

Emily Newton and Steven Mann

Chapter Aims

The aims of this chapter are to:

- Define dyslipidaemia and recommended lipid concentrations
- Discuss management of the condition and preventing potential progression
- Explain the benefits and impact of physical activity and exercise
- Present best practice for client-centred exercise prescription using a case study approach

Overview of Dyslipidaemia

Definition

Dyslipidaemia refers to an elevation of both triglycerides (TRI) and total cholesterol (TC) within the blood stream, along with low concentrations of the protective high-density lipoproteins (HDL). TRI are the most common form of fat in the body, storing energy which can be released when needed. Cholesterol is a vital component for several cell functions, such as maintaining a healthy cell membrane and producing a range of steroid hormones. It also aids in digestion through the production of bile. Cholesterol is produced in the liver and is transported via the blood stream. It is not soluble in blood plasma so must be transported via a protein, forming lipoproteins. The three main lipoproteins are low-density lipoprotein (LDL), very low-density lipoprotein (VLDL) and HDL.

LDLs transport most of the body's cholesterol from the liver to the cells that need it. They are commonly known as 'bad' cholesterol as they play a pivotal role in the formation of atherosclerotic plaque in the arteries. VLDLs are also linked to the development of atherosclerosis, transporting TRI from the liver to cells for storage or to be used as fuel. HDL has a vital role, removing excess cholesterol from the arteries so that it can be processed in the liver. High levels of HDL help prevent atherosclerosis, so they are frequently referred to as 'good'

DOI: 10.4324/9781315102399-14

cholesterol. Dyslipidaemia is defined as unhealthy blood lipid concentrations, meaning the 'bad' LDL may be too high or the 'good' HDL could be too low.

TRI and cholesterol are essential for bodily functions; it is only when they rise above the recommended concentrations, as shown in Tables 14.1 and 14.2, that they cause a threat. High concentrations of LDL indicate surplus lipids in the blood that increase the risk of cardiovascular complications. HDL transports lipids back to the liver for recycling and disposal; consequently, high concentrations of HDL are an indicator of a healthy cardiovascular system (Carroll and Lacher, 2012). TRIs in plasma are derived from fats eaten in foods or other energy sources. An excess of TRI in plasma is positively associated with cardiovascular disease (CVD) (da Luz et al., 2008).

Dyslipidaemia is usually symptom free until it progresses to serious conditions such as coronary artery disease (CAD) and peripheral artery disease (PAD). Often, patients will be unaware they have dyslipidaemia until it is diagnosed via a blood test. The most commonly used measure of TC, a measure that includes LDL and HDL, is shown in Table 14.1.

The different effects of LDL and HDL cholesterol on health mean that TC on its own can sometimes be misleading. Exact figures for the components of TC can provide more information and give a clearer indication of risk.

Example: Female client, 65 years, no medical conditions, healthy BMI and blood pressure. Following a routine health check, a concern was raised that her TC was 6.5 mmol/L, classifying as a 'high' reading. When this was broken down, LDL was 3.6 mmol/L, which is borderline high, but HDL was 2.5 mmol/L, which is well above optimal. Whilst the TC indicates risk of CVD, a reason for this could be the exceptional level of HDL. A more sensitive measure could be used here, such as reporting the ratio of total cholesterol against HDL. The lower this figure is the better, with a score of above 6 being considered a high risk factor (Heart UK, 2020). Research indicates that using TC against non-HDL cholesterol could

TABLE 14.1 Normative values for TC, LDL, HDL and TRI concentrations

	mg/dL	*mmol/L*	*Category*
Total Cholesterol	< 200	< 5.2	Desirable
	200–239	5.3–6.2	Borderline high
	> 240	> 6.2	High
Low-Density Lipoprotein Cholesterol	< 100	< 2.6	Desirable
	100–129	2.6–3.34	Near optimal
	130–159	3.36–4.11	Borderline high
	160–189	4.11–4.89	High
	> 190	> 4.9	Very high
High-Density Lipoprotein Cholesterol	> 60	> 1.55	Optimal
	40–60	1.03–1.55	Intermediate
	< 40	< 1.03	Low
Triglycerides	< 150	< 1.7	Optimal
	150–199	1.7–2.3	Borderline high
	200–499	2.3–5.64	High
	> 500	> 5.64	Very high

Source: Adapted from Riebe et al., 2017

TABLE 14.2 Medication considerations for exercise for people with dyslipidaemia

Class name	*Generic name*	*Brand name*	*Indication*	*Action*	*Side effects*	*Exercise considerations*
Statins	atorvastatin simvastatin fluvastati pravastatin rosuvastatin	Lipitor Zocor Lescol Lipostat Crestor	Hypercholesterolemia to lower LDL and TRI levels; may increase HDL	Statins help to manage LDL and TRI levels by inhibiting the enzymes involved in cholesterol synthesis in the liver	Nausea; gastrointestinal upset; headache; dizziness; tiredness; joint and muscle pain, especially in legs	Alternatives and non-weight-bearing exercises may be needed to manage aching in legs
Ezetimibe		Ezetrol	Lowers total cholesterol, LDL and TRI circulating in the blood stream	Helps prevent the body absorbing cholesterol from food in the digestive tract	Gastrointestinal upset; pain; diarrhoea	Avoid exercises that directly work the abdominal muscles, as this may aggravate that area; ensure client is aware of location of nearest toilet
Fibrates	bezafibrate clofibrate fenofibrate gemfibrozil	Bezalip Atromid-S Tricor, Fenobrat Lopid	Elevated TRI; can also reduce LDL and raise HDL	Stimulate enzymes, which can help break down TRI	Gastrointestinal upsets; nausea; stomach pain; can cause kidney stones when used for long periods of time	Avoid exercises that directly work the abdominal muscles, as this may aggravate that area; ensure client remains well hydrated.

Source: Adapted from British Medical Association (2012)

help improve attainment of a healthy concentration as in this ratio, all cholesterol variables are positively associated with CVD (Virani et al., 2012).

Pathology

Dyslipidaemia is associated with many of the risk factors for CVD. Modifiable risk factors include diets high in saturated fat, smoking, physical inactivity, high sedentary behaviour, diabetes and poorly managed blood glucose concentrations, whilst non-modifiable risk factors include ageing, ethnicity and familial hypercholesterolemia. In the UK, 1 in 250 people are estimated to have familial hypercholesterolemia, an inherited condition which causes increased cholesterol concentrations from birth (Heart Matters, 2020). The risk of developing coronary heart disease (CHD) is 13 times higher in people with untreated familial hypercholesterolemia (Nordestgaard et al., 2013). Research indicates that each 0.25 mmol/L (10 mg/dL) increment in non-HDL cholesterol provides an increase in atherosclerotic plaque formation equivalent to one year of ageing (Wiegman et al., 2015), demonstrating the importance of early recognition and lifestyle interventions.

Epidemiology

There is a direct relationship between chronically elevated cholesterol concentrations and CHD (Lloyd-Jones et al., 2004), as reductions in LDL decrease the incidence of heart attacks and ischaemic strokes (Baigent et al., 2010). Individuals with elevated TC concentrations – above 200 mg/dL (5.2 mmol/L) – have approximately twice the risk of CHD as those with optimal concentrations (Roger et al., 2012). The Center for Disease Control and Prevention (CDC, 2011) suggested that this is the case with 71 million US adults, equating to 33.5% of the population. The prevalence of elevated TC is even higher in Europe, where 54% of adults aged 25 and over have total cholesterol levels above the recommended levels (World Health Organisation, 2011).

One-third of all ischaemic heart disease globally is attributed to high cholesterol concentrations (Murray et al., 2003). Whilst age-adjusted prevalence of high cholesterol in the United States lowered from 26.6% (1988–1994) to 25.3% (1994–2004), data from 2013 (Go et al., 2013), suggest that the use of pharmacological cholesterol-lowering substances increased from 11.7% to 40.8% of the adult population during this period. It has long been recognised that reductions in serum cholesterol can reduce CHD risk; for example, reductions of around 0.6 mmol/L can reduce incidence of ischaemic heart disease by 54% at the age of 40 years, reducing to 19% at 80 years (Law, Wald, and Thompson, 1994). Reduction in TC is therefore still considered the 'gold standard' in preventative cardiovascular medicine (Whayne, 2011). This highlights the importance of interventions aimed at reducing serum cholesterol concentrations. Furthermore, the advantages of early intervention have been demonstrated; long-term exposure to 1 mmol/L lower LDL was associated with a 55% reduction in CHD risk while treatment with statin therapy starting in later life required a threefold reduction in LDL to achieve the same magnitude risk reduction (Ference et al., 2012).

Management and Medications

The Health Survey for England (2016) reports lipid-lowering medications are the second-most prescribed medication to adults in England (14%), with antihypertensives being the most widely prescribed (to 15% of the population). Statins are a very common type of lipid-lowering drug which block the action of enzymes involved in manufacturing cholesterol in the liver, resulting in lower cholesterol concentrations in the blood (British Medical Association, 2012). Statins are not only prescribed to people with dyslipidaemia but can also be recommended for anyone at a higher CHD risk, such as diabetics and people with a high incidence of CVD in the family (British Heart Foundation, 2020).

Table 14.2 indicates the effect of the main lipid-lowering medications on acute exercise responses. Side effects will vary between clients and are not limited to those described in the table. Regular blood tests will often be provided to check liver function. It is important to recommend contacting the medical practitioner if a client is experiencing jaundice or rashes, excessive muscle pain or weakness.

Adaptations to exercise sessions may be needed to manage some of the possible side effects of lipid-lowering medications. Anyone with gastrointestinal issues needs to make sure they have access to a toilet in case of faecal urgency, and a change of clothes is recommended. If recommending activity outdoors, such as walking, ensure toilets are available along the route. Avoid any exercises that isolate or put direct pressure on the abdominal muscles as they may be uncomfortable. Clients who are at risk of experiencing dizziness should complete supported exercises such as seated resistance machines. They should remain upright throughout the exercise session and avoid exercises on a potentially unstable surface, such as a Reebok step. If they experience dizziness, they should stop immediately.

If tiredness or weakness is a concern, adapt exercises to ensure they are manageable and alternatives are available on days when the client feels most fatigued. Ensure exercise sessions are varied and interesting to help the client remain engaged and focused. If legs are feeling heavy or achy, vary the mode of exercise and consider switching between upper and lower body as demanded. Ensure long periods of weight-bearing exercise are avoided, and try non-weight bearing-alternatives such as cycling or the rowing machine.

Lifestyle Changes

Reducing or Stopping Smoking

Smoking increases the risk of CVD. and the more cigarettes smoked, the greater the risk. Smoking has a direct impact on TC by raising TRI and lowering the protective HDL. Toxic chemicals in the tobacco prevent the body from repairing damage to the lining of the arteries (endothelium), increasing the likelihood of blood clots (U.S. Department of Health and Human Services, 2010).

Managing Blood Glucose Concentrations

Chronic high circulating blood glucose concentrations can damage the lining of blood vessels, increasing the likelihood of atherosclerosis. Plaque-containing cholesterol and TRI build up inside the arteries over time, hardening and narrowing the arteries. Often people with type 2 diabetes have increased TRI levels, due to increased VLDLs, smaller LDL molecules and low levels of protective HDL, increasing their risk of CVD.

Modifying Diet

A diet high in saturated fats such as processed and fatty meats, butter and cheese, cakes, biscuits and pastries can increase TC. To help reduce cholesterol, clients should try to eat more fresh fruits and vegetables, whole grains, nuts and seeds and oily fish. Clients should be taught how to read food labels to check what type of fat foods contain. They should be advised to focus on home cooking and avoid fast and convenience food which can often be of poor quality.

Effect of Exercise Response

Acute Response to Exercise

It is important to understand the way the body responds to exercise in order to help manage the potential risks. During exercise, cardiac output rises to allow greater circulation of blood. Cardiac output is a combination of stroke volume and heart rate, but stroke volume only increases up to 50% of maximum workload. Above this, increases in cardiac output are solely due to increased heart rate, putting more pressure on the myocardium. Stroke volume rises due to increased preload – that is, the extent to which the ventricles stretch when filling with blood. As heart rate increases, the amount of time the heart is in systole increases, and time in diastole reduces, providing less time for the coronary arteries to receive oxygenated blood. The systolic blood pressure will increase in line with exercise intensity, assisting the boost in blood flow through the vascular system. Increases in systolic pressure can be greater in the upper body than in the lower body, due to the smaller muscle mass and vascular system.

Blood flow changes as the sympathetic nervous system redirects blood from the non-essential areas, such as the digestive system, and redirects it to the working muscles. When exercising, the amount of oxygen extracted from the blood increases, so the amount of oxygen in the venous blood reduces in line with exercise intensity. Changes are also seen in blood plasma as plasma moves from the capillaries into the interstitial fluid space (the fluid-filled area that surrounds a cell). If the temperature of the exercise environment or exercise intensity causes sweating, additional plasma may be lost. Reductions in plasma volume may increase blood viscosity or increase the concentration of substrates being transported in the blood, which is an important consideration when working with clients at risk of CHD.

When working with clients with dyslipidaemia, considerations must be made to ensure heart rate increases steadily and gradually. Increases in heart rate result in a rise in myocardial workload and oxygen demand. Clients with increased lipid levels are at risk of atherosclerosis (plaque build-up in the arteries), and as people age, arteriosclerosis (hardening of the arteries) affects the time needed for the coronary arteries to dilate sufficiently. Arteries with a potentially damaged endothelial lining will require an extended warm up as vasodilation will take longer than in a healthy artery. Exercise sessions should be carefully planned to avoid abrupt changes in body position, which can affect preload, resulting in an increased demand for oxygen to the myocardium. Clients should be encouraged to exercise in an upright position. Supine exercises such as sit-ups reduce blood pooling in the lower limbs, increasing the volume of blood returning to the heart and therefore increasing preload. Quick changes of body position can also cause a drop in blood pressure, resulting in postural hypotension and potential dizziness. During body weight or resistance training, exercise order is important to prevent sudden increases in blood pressure. Exercises should be balanced, alternating muscle groups to prevent overworking smaller upper body muscles. Steady breathing should be encouraged throughout and over gripping avoided to ensure blood pressure remains stable and to avoid the Valsalva manoeuvre (i.e. breath holding).

Managing Exercise Risk

Exercise-associated acute cardiac events generally occur in individuals with structural cardiac disease that has progressed over many years (Thompson et al., 2007). During exercise, raised heart rate and blood pressure can increase in line with intensity, causing stress on artery walls, leading to disruption of plaque. It is important to screen all clients for symptoms of disease; however, clients with dyslipidaemia should be screened particularly thoroughly as this group are already at an increased risk of CVD. Screening processes are needed to manage risk of a cardiac event and ensure the appropriate exercise support and recommendations are provided. As an absolute minimum, a physical activity readiness questionnaire (PARQ) should be used to allow the client to highlight any potential concerns during exercise, such as loss of balance due to dizziness or a bone or joint problem which is worsened by activity. Clients at increased risk of CVD should be asked about potential signs of disease, such as chest pain at rest and breathlessness under low exertion.

Clients with dyslipidaemia should complete a PARQ+, which a more detailed document which asks key questions for each condition. A full medical history, including current activity levels, should be discussed for each client. This will allow any concerns to be highlighted and help provide an indication of functional capacity. All health conditions and physical limitations the client might experience should be considered. A blood pressure reading at rest should be completed as an essential screening tool to highlight potential CVD (see Chapter 13). Always receive a referral from a general practitioner before beginning an exercise programme. In most cases, light-intensity regular walking can be recommended as an appropriate starting point, especially if motivation is high and a delay in beginning exercise would be detrimental. A physically activity lifestyle should be promoted and encouraged at every opportunity. The benefits of physical activity for those with, or at risk of, CHD appear to outweigh the risks (Thompson et al., 2007).

Effects of Exercise Training

Exercise can have a positive effect on the pathogenesis, symptomatology and physical fitness of individuals with dyslipidaemia (Pedersen and Saltin, 2006). Exercise can improve both liver and muscle function, aiding weight loss through increased TRI metabolism. Being with overweight can increase the volume of LDL in the blood, so reducing fat mass will help lower it. Increased physical activity can stimulate enzymes to transport LDL from the blood stream to the liver. Once in the liver cholesterol can be excreted or converted to bile to aid digestion. Exercise can also increase the size of protein particles carrying the cholesterol in the blood stream, which can help increase stability. Regular exercise can increase the muscles' oxidative capacity, leading to increased lipoprotein lipase activity. This appears to enhance the ability of skeletal muscles to utilise lipids as opposed to glycogen, thus reducing plasma lipids (Earnest et al., 2013). Exercise also helps the liver increase HDL concentrations; a mean increase of 4.6% HDL has been reported after examining 50 interventions (Kesaniemi et al., 2001).

It has been suggested that PA which expends between 1,200 and 2,200 kcal per week can elicit favourable changes in HDL concentrations. However, the greatest changes are typically the result of structured and progressive aerobic training (Sassen et al., 2009).

Aerobic Exercise

Aerobic exercise training (AE) is a form of exercise as it is structured and involves an end goal, which is typically to improve fitness. Research indicates that AE can increase HDL concentration, but the impact on LDL and TRI levels has been inconsistent. A review by Leon and Sanchez (2001) revealed at least 12 weeks of moderate- to high-intensity AE provided an average HDL increase of up to 4.6% while TRI levels fell by 3.7% and LDL by 5%. TC remained unchanged, although the HDL:LDL ratio improved considerably. Here, the improvement in HDL is the same as Kesaniemi et al. (2001) demonstrated with increased PA behaviour, but the additional improvements of reduced TRI and LDL may be attributed to the increased intensity during AE compared to PA.

Banz et al. (2003) also demonstrated a positive improvement in HDL concentrations following high-intensity AE. An average increase of 13% HDL was found following a ten-week protocol – training three times a week at 85% HR max for 40 minutes. However, it was reported that HDL was the only component of the lipid profile to improve. Focus needs to be placed on the ratio between TC and HDL, rather than on individual figures.

Nybo et al. (2010) reported that the TC:HDL ratio was the only component of lipid profile significantly improved following a 12-week programme of 150 minutes of exercise a week at 80% HR max in previously untrained participants. This was compared to an intense interval running protocol (five times at two-minute intervals at 95% HR max) for a total time of 40 minutes per week. No improvements in lipid profile were reported following the intense interval programme. When intensity of AE is high during continuous effort, the effects on HDL cholesterol appear to become more consistent.

Dunn et al. (1997) investigated the effects of a six-month AE training programme that progressed from 50% to 85% maximum aerobic power for 20 to 60 minutes three times a week and reported a significant decrease in TC (−0.3 mmol/L) as well as TC:HDL ratio (−0.3). In this case, the intervention period was relatively long, and the intensity was relatively high. In a 16-week study, LeMura et al. (2000) reported significant reductions in plasma TRI (1.4–1.2 mmol/L) and increases in HDL (1.4–1.8 mmol/L) after training three times a week at 70% to 75% HR max for 30 minutes for the first eight weeks, progressing to four times at 85% HR max for 45 minutes thereafter. Data suggests that shorter-term interventions will be effective also if training volume is high enough. Increasing the frequency of training to four times per week may have elicited the additional benefits seen by LeMura et al. in comparison with Banz et al. (three training sessions per week). Further, LeMura et al. observed a 13% reduction in body fat percentage (26.4–22.9%), suggesting the additional volume of training generated an additional metabolic response, a parameter not reported by Banz et al. O'Donovan et al. (2005) controlled training volume to directly assess the impact of training intensity. Sixty-four previously sedentary men were randomly allocated to either a control group, a moderate-intensity exercise group (60% VO_2max) or a high-intensity group (80% VO_2max). Both exercising groups completed three 400-kcal sessions per week for 24 weeks. By setting the session volume in calories, the overall training volume was controlled. Participants were instructed to maintain their dietary habits. It was reported that significant lipid profile improvements occurred only in the high-intensity group, with TOT (6.02–5.48 mmol/L), LDL (4.04–3.52 mmol/L) and non-HDL (4.58–4.04 mmol/L) all decreasing significantly ($p < 0.05$).

Evidence suggests that a moderate-intensity exercise programme will be effective in increasing HDL. To reduce LDL and TRI concentrations, the intensity of aerobic exercise must be increased, something that may not be possible in individuals with limited exercise capacity. Careful consideration needs to be given to the appropriateness of high-intensity continuous aerobic exercise for clients with dyslipidaemia, especially in relation to the increased risk of CVD. Clients who are previously untrained need to begin at a light to moderate intensity, then carefully increase volume, followed by, finally, exercise intensity. Progression needs to be gradual to help prevent overuse injuries. The focus needs to be on long-term lifestyle change, rather than a 12-week intensive programme to reduce lipid concentrations.

Training volume appears to be more important than training intensity for improving lipid profile. There may be a relationship between body fat – which was only lowered in the prolonged group – and cholesterol concentrations, whereby a volume sufficient to elicit changes in fat mass is required to favourably alter lipid profile. The functional capacity, needs and wants of the client need to be carefully considered. A prolonged moderate-intensity aerobic prescription may be much more favoured by clients than a shorter intense programme, but of course, check with the client.

Resistance Training

Resistance training (RT) aims to increase muscular strength and/or endurance utilising external resistance or one's own body (United States Public Health Service, 1996) and may be a more accessible form of exercise for less mobile groups as well as providing an alternative to aerobic training for more mobile individuals (Brooks et al., 2007).

Acute changes in lipid profile following different intensities of RT were examined by Lira et al. (2010). Intensities examined were 50%, 75%, 90% and 110% 1-RM. The final scenario focused on the eccentric phase only, with the lift assisted during the concentric phase. Total training volume was equalised between the groups to ensure that RT intensity was the factor being assessed. TRI clearance was significantly greater following low to moderate intensities at 50% (−14.6 mg/dL) and 75% (−10.7 mg/dL) 1RM compared to higher intensities at 90% (+9.5 mg/dL) and 110% (+12.1 mg/dL). Further, increases in HDL were significantly greater following 50% and 75% 1RM than 110%. The positive impact of low- to moderate-intensity RT may be due to the number of repetitions completed at each intensity, leading to increased activation of total muscle mass. These intensities are a safe starting point for a client new to RT.

Circuit training can also be an appropriate activity for clients with dyslipidaemia. Fett et al. (2009) incorporated RT into circuit training sessions in which no specific weight was designated but in which specific time was allocated to each exercise. Sessions lasted 60 minutes per week and were completed three times a week for one month and four times a week for the second month. Significant reductions were reported in TC (203–186mg/dL) and TRI (122–91mg/dL), further demonstrating that the volume of activity is important, rather than the intensity of the weight lifted. Completing a high number of repetitions when lifting a lower load will ensure the client works within an aerobic capacity, helping the body improve the metabolic capacity of the muscle. Resistance-based exercises can help to encourage fat oxidisation, increase the metabolic capacity of the muscle and help reduce the volume of fat stored in the liver.

Recommendations for Fitness Testing and Exercise Programming

Health and Fitness Testing

Health and fitness testing allows the practitioner to collect important information about the client to establish an appropriate starting point for exercise prescription. This should be completed after a PARQ and discussion of the client's medical history. Tests should be selected which are relatively quick and easy to administer, reliable and inexpensive, to ensure tests can easily be repeated. Tests that could be implemented should first be discussed with the client to ensure they are happy to proceed. Testing frequently happens during the first meeting with a client, so it is important to ensure they are happy to proceed and will not be discouraged by the testing process.

Due to the nature of dyslipidaemia, screening for underlying CVD is essential. At a minimum, resting heart rate and blood pressure should be checked pre-exercise, along with a thorough medical history.

Other tests may be completed depending on the goals and needs of the client, such as anthropometric measures (height, weight, body composition), functional capacity tests (such as (the six-minute walk test, sit-to-stand), and strength or flexibility tests. There are many options here, and this should be tailored to the needs of the client.

Exercise Recommendations

The American College of Sports Medicine (Riebe et al., 2017) has provided recommendations for individuals with dyslipidaemia and without co-morbidities, as shown in Table 14.3. Research indicates that higher-intensity aerobic exercise (O'Donovan et al., 2005) and moderate-intensity resistance training (Lira et al., 2010) can be particularly effective in improving cholesterol concentrations.

The evidence presented for PA highlights a dose-response relationship between activity levels and increases in HDL (Aadahl, Kjaer, and Jørgensen, 2007); therefore, the PA recommendations made are to be considered a minimum. These evidence-based recommendations should aid in the prescription and delivery of interventions to lower cholesterol concentrations.

Key Recommendations for Exercise Programming

- Focus on volume of exercise rather than exercise intensity for clients with low functional capacity.
- In all cases, exercise recommendations must be manageable and maintainable.
- Exercise guidelines should be used as a guide and not a starting point. The prescription must meet the needs of the client as a priority.

TABLE 14.3 Summary of the FITT exercise prescription for people with dyslipidaemia

	Aerobic	*Resistance*	*Flexibility*
Frequency	≥ 5 days per week to maximise calorie expenditure	2–3 days per week	2–3 days per week
Intensity	40–75%VO_2 or HRR	Moderate (50–69% of 1RM) to vigorous (70–85% of 1RM) to improve strength; < 50% 1RM to improve muscular endurance	Stretch to the point of tightness or slight discomfort
Time	30–60 minutes per day; to promote or maintain weight loss, 50–60 minutes or more of daily exercise recommended	2–4 sets, 8–12 repetitions for strength; ≤ 12–20 repetitions for muscular endurance	Hold static stretch for 10–30 seconds; 2–4 repetitions of each exercise
Type	Prolonged, rhythmic activities using large muscle groups (e.g. walking, cycling, swimming)	Resistance machines, free weights and/or body weight	Static, dynamic and/or PNF stretch

Legend: 1RM: one repetition maximum; HRR: heart rate reserve; PNF: proprioceptive neuromuscular facilitation; VO_2R: oxygen uptake reserve
Source: Adapted from Riebe et al., 2017)

TABLE 14.4 Recommendations for varying levels of dyslipidaemia and functional capacity

Cholesterol level maintenance/reduction: Exercise recommendations	
Healthy (Maintaining low LDL & TRI – increasing HDL)	Increase PA to more than 30 minutes a day 5 times a week. Prolonged moderate-intensity AE – 70–80% HR reserve, combined with low-intensity RT – 50% 1RM
Elevated cholesterol/dyslipidaemia (Clearance of LDL & TRI – increasing HDL)	Increase PA to more than 30 minutes a day 5 times a week. Prolonged moderate-intensity AE – 70–80% HR reserve, progressing to 85% HR max (30, 31) combined with moderate-high intensity RT – 75–85% 1RM
Elevated cholesterol/dyslipidaemia – limited mobility (Disabled, elderly populations etc.)	Increase PA as much as is feasible. RT progressing from 50–75% in major muscle groups; can be incorporated into circuit sessions and kept at a moderate intensity

- Be aware of the impact and potential side effects of any medications. Excessive muscle aches, especially in the legs, are a commonly reported side effect and should be referred to the health professional.
- Consider the impact of arteriosclerosis (hardening of the arteries) when working with clients. An extended warm-up will need to be provided to ensure sufficient time for coronary artery dilation.

- When performing resistance-based exercises, ensure that muscle groups are alternated so too much pressure is not placed on the smaller muscle groups of the upper body.
- Take time to educate clients to ensure they understand the importance of exercise and why this is necessary in the management of their condition.
- Some clients may find regular targets and goal setting useful when increasing their activity levels. Take time to speak to the client to establish the most appropriate way to motivate and support.

Case Study

During a routine health check when joining a new medical centre, Mark, an apparently healthy male aged 36 years, received a TC score of 8.2 mmol/L, indicating high risk of CVD. Mark had no previous health concerns and was surprised by this high reading. He was informed that his HDL was moderate at 1.1 mmol/L, but his LDL was very high at 5.2 mmol/L. Mark's resting BP was 134/85 mmHg (suggesting prehypertension) and weight 81 kg with a BMI of 25.6 kg/m^2 (classifying him as overweight). At the time, he had a sedentary and stressful job working in sales. He smoked and consumed on average 12 units of alcohol a week (which is within the UK recommendations). Mark enjoyed physical activity and exercise when he was younger but has struggled to maintain any routine due to high workloads and a young family. He liked walking, dancing and playing football but took part in these activities less than once a week.

Mark chose to focus on immediate lifestyle changes, rather than receiving a prescription for a lipid-lowering medication. He began by reducing saturated fat in his diet, selecting alternatives for animal products such as cheese, butter and whole milk. He became much more aware of the food choices he was making, opting for healthier options and less processed food. At the time of his diagnosis, he also decided to change his career, leaving a sedentary role in sales to become a school caretaker. This dramatically decreased his daily sedentary time and increased low and moderate physical activity behaviour, particularly due to walking more. Alongside an active job, Mark also committed to attend twice-weekly dance classes with his partner once childcare arrangements were in place. However, not all modifiable risk factors were addressed; he continued to consume alcohol and smoke. When the client's blood was tested five months later, his TC had reduced to 5.1 mmol/L (within the desirable range) with an HDL of 1.3 mmol/L and LDL 3.4 mmol/L. Mark's BMI had also reduced slightly to 25.1 kg/m^2. These improvements were very motivating to Mark and supported him to continue to make positive lifestyle choices to further improve his cholesterol profile and finally stop smoking. This highlights the importance of diet modification and regular daily physical activity to positively improve cholesterol concentration.

Summary

Dyslipidaemia is a predominantly asymptomatic condition which can lie undetected, affecting a large segment of the population. It can lead to atherosclerotic CVD and increases the risk of heart attack and stroke. Dyslipidaemia needs to be managed to reduce the risk of a cardiovascular event and ensure optimal concentrations of blood lipids.

Physical activity and exercise can help the management of dyslipidaemia by increasing the 'good' HDL and helping lower the 'bad' LDL and triglyceride. Increasing daily physical activity behaviour can help boost HDL concentration, and higher intensity aerobic exercise has also been shown to have a positive impact on LDL and TRI concentrations. Resistance training at a moderate intensity should be recommended as this has also been shown to be beneficial in cholesterol management. Exercise must be adapted to meet the needs and wants of the client. Changes in lifelong physical activity behaviour should be encouraged, rather than shorter courses of exercise, to support condition management.

Screening must be completed before an exercise programme begins to ensure the client is safe to exercise. This is very important to help establish the exercise intensity and volume most appropriate for the client. Time should be taken to discuss the client's previous medical history and any disease or function limitations, ensuring care is taken to listen to any potential symptoms of cardiovascular disease.

Physical activity and exercise recommendations should focus on enjoyable activities which can be built into the client's weekly routine. Effort should be made to educate about the positive impact activity can have on their condition as well as the wider benefits of living an active lifestyle.

Key Points

- Dyslipidaemia refers to an elevation of both TRI and total cholesterol within the blood stream, along with low concentration of the protective HDL. Total cholesterol over 5.2 mmol/L and HDL below 1 mmol/L indicates dyslipidaemia.
- Lifestyle changes can help manage dyslipidaemia, such as increasing physical activity and reducing sedentary time, making positive dietary choices, managing blood glucose concentrations and stopping or reducing smoking.
- Research indicated that higher-intensity aerobic exercise and moderate-intensity resistance training can have a positive impact on cholesterol concentrations. However, focus should be placed on finding activity that the client enjoys in order to support long-term physical activity behaviour change.

Study Questions

1. What is the definition of dyslipidaemia?
2. How is cholesterol transported around the body?
3. What are the main differences between high- and low-density lipoproteins?
4. What are the recommended total cholesterol and lipoprotein levels for a healthy adult?
5. Why is cholesterol needed by the body?
6. How does dyslipidaemia progress?
7. What medications are used in the treatment of dyslipidaemia?
8. What lifestyle modifications are recommended for people with dyslipidaemia?

TABLE 14.5 At-a-glance summary guide to exercise considerations or people with dyslipidaemia

Condition name	*Dyslipidaemia*
Pathophysiology summary	Dyslipidaemia refers to an elevation of both triglycerides (TRI) and total cholesterol within the blood stream, along with low levels of the protective high-density lipoproteins (HDL).
Aims of exercise	Reduce triglyceride levels and increase high-density lipoproteins.
Exercise considerations (including contraindications)	Consider client's age, medical history and any co-morbidities. It is important to note that dyslipidaemia is asymptomatic; time should be taken to discuss CVD risk factors to establish risk classification. A proper screening should be completed.
Frequency	Aim to exercise 5 days a week, preferably every day if the client is able.
Intensity	Ideally at least moderate intensity, but this will depend on the abilities and co-morbidities of the client.
Time	30–60 minutes of activity.
Type	Aerobic, resistance, flexibility. Most importantly, mode of activity should focus on something the client wants to do.
Common medications associated	Statins, fibrates and ezetimibe can be used to help to lower total cholesterol, LDL and TRI levels as well as to increase HDL.
Key safety considerations	Ensure extended warm-up and cool down provided if the client may have atherosclerosis or arteriosclerosis. The client must be carefully screened to ensure any co-morbidities and medication side effects are known. Offer alternative exercises, especially non–weight bearing. if client is suffering from aching legs. When resistance training, alternate the movement and prime mover to ensure smaller muscle groups are not overworked.
Effect of exercise on condition	Exercise should help increase HDL levels and reduce levels of LDL and TRI circulating in the blood stream.

9. What modes and intensities of activity are recommended for dyslipidaemia?
10. What information should be discussed before a client with dyslipidaemia begins a new physical activity programme?

References

Aadahl M, Kjaer M, Jørgensen T. (2007). Associations between overall physical activity level and cardiovascular risk factors in an adult population. *Eur J Epidemiol.* **22**(6), 369–78.

Baigent C, Blackwell L, Emberson J, Holland LE, Reith C, Bhala N, et al. (2010). Efficacy and safety of more intensive lowering of LDL cholesterol: A meta-analysis of data from 170,000 participants in 26 randomised trials. *Lancet.* **376**(9753), 1670–81.

Banz W, Maher M, Thompson W, Bassett D, Moore W, Ashraf M, et al. (2003). Effects of resistance versus aerobic training on coronary artery disease risk factors. *Exp Biol Med.* **228**(4), 434–40.

British Heart Foundation (2020). Statins [online]. *British Heart Foundation* [Viewed 3 August 2020]. Available from: www.bhf.org.uk/informationsupport/treatments/statins

British Medical Association (2012). *Concise Guide to Medicines and Drugs*. 4th edition. Dorling Kindersley.

Brooks N, Layne JE, Gordon PL, Roubenoff R, Nelson ME, Castaneda-Sceppa C. (2007). Strength training improves muscle quality and insulin sensitivity in Hispanic older adults with type 2 diabetes. *Int J Med Sci.* **4**(1), 19–27.

Carroll MD, Kit BK, Lacher DA. (20120). Total and high-density lipoprotein cholesterol in adults: National health and nutrition examination survey, 2009–2010. *NCHS Data Brief.* **92**, 1–8.

Centre for Disease Control (2011). Vital signs: Prevalence, treatment, and control of high levels of low-density lipoprotein cholesterol. *United States, 1999–2002 and 2005–2008*. **60**(4), 109–14.

da Luz P, Favarato D, Faria-Neto JJ, Lemos P, Chagas A. (2008). High ratio of triglycerides to HDL-cholesterol predicts extensive coronary disease. *Clinics*. **63**(4), 427–32.

Dunn A, Marcus B, Kampert J, Garcia M, Kohl Hr, Blair S. (1997). Reduction in cardiovascular disease risk factors: 6-month results from project active. *Prev Med*. **26**(6), 883–92.

Earnest CP, Artero EG, Sui X, Lee DC, Church TS, Blair SN. (2013). Maximal estimated cardiorespiratory fitness, cardiometabolic risk factors, and metabolic syndrome in the aerobics center longitudinal study. *Mayo Clin Proc*. **88**(3), 259–70.

Ference BA, Yoo W, Alesh I, Mahajan N, Mirowska KK, Mewada A, et al. (2012) Effect of long-term exposure to lower low-density lipoprotein cholesterol beginning early in life on the risk of coronary heart disease: A mendelian randomization analysis. *J Am Coll Cardiol*. **60**(25), 2631–9.

Fett C, Fett W, Marchini J. (2009). Circuit weight training vs jogging in metabolic risk factors of overweight/obese women. *Arq Bras Cardiol*. **93**(5), 519–25.

Go AS, Mozaffarian D, Roger VL, Benjamin EJ, Berry JD, Borden WB, et al. (2013). Heart disease and stroke statistics – 2013 update: A report from the American Heart Association. *Circulation*. **127**(1), 6–245.

Health Survey for England (2016). Prescribed medications [online]. *Health Survey for England* [Viewed 3 August 2020]. Available from: http://healthsurvey.hscic.gov.uk/media/63790/HSE2016-pres-med.pdf

Heart Matters (2020). Focus on familial hypercholesterolemia [online]. *British Heart Foundation* [Viewed 3 August 2020]. Available from: www.bhf.org.uk/informationsupport/heart-matters-magazine/medical/familial-hypercholesterolaemia

Heart UK. (2020). Getting a cholesterol test [online]. *Heart UK* [Viewed 3 August 2020]. Available from: www.heartuk.org.uk/cholesterol/getting-a-cholesterol-test

Kesaniemi Y, Danforth EJ, Jensen M, Kopelman P, Lefèbvre P, Reeder B. (2001). Dose-response issues concerning physical activity and health: An evidence-based symposium. *Med Sci Sports Exerc*. **33**(6), 351–8.

Law MR, Wald NJ, Thompson SG. (1994). By how much and how quickly does reduction in serum cholesterol concentration lower risk of ischaemic heart disease? *BMJ*. **308**(6925), 367–72.

LeMura L, von Duvillard S, Andreacci J, Klebez J, Chelland S, Russo J. (2000). Lipid and lipoprotein profiles, cardiovascular fitness, body composition, and diet during and after resistance, aerobic and combination training in young women. *Eur J Appl Physiol*. **82**(5–6), 451–8.

Leon A, Sanchez O. (2001). Response of blood lipids to exercise training alone or combined with dietary intervention. *Med Sci Sports Exerc*. **33**(6), 502–15.

Lira F, Yamashita A, Uchida M, Zanchi N, Gualano B, Martins EJ, et al. (2010). Low and moderate, rather than high intensity strength exercise induces benefit regarding plasma lipid profile. *Diabetol Metab Syndr*. **2**, 31.

Lloyd-Jones DM, Wilson PW, Larson MG, Beiser A, Leip EP, D'Agostino RB, et al. (2004). Framingham risk score and prediction of lifetime risk for coronary heart disease. *Am J Cardiol*. **94**(1), 20–4.

Murray CJ, Lauer JA, Hutubessy RC, Niessen L, Tomijima N, Rodgers A, et al. (2003). Effectiveness and costs of interventions to lower systolic blood pressure and cholesterol: A global and regional analysis on reduction of cardiovascular-disease risk. *Lancet*. **361**(9359), 717–25.

Nordestgaard BG, Chapman MJ, Humphries SE, Ginsberg HN, Masana L, Descamps O. (2013). A European atherosclerosis society consensus panel. Familial hypercholesterolaemia is underdiagnosed and undertreated in the general population: Guidance for clinicians to prevent coronary heart disease: Consensus statement of the European atherosclerosis society. *Eur Heart J*. **34**(45), 3478–90.

Nybo L, Sundstrup E, Jakobsen M, Mohr M, Hornstrup T, Simonsen L, et al. (2010). High-intensity training versus traditional exercise interventions for promoting health. *Med Sci Sports Exerc*. **42**(10), 1951–8.

O'Donovan G, Owen A, Bird S, Kearney E, Nevill A, Jones D, et al. (2005). Changes in cardiorespiratory fitness and coronary heart disease risk factors following 24 wk of moderate- or high-intensity exercise of equal energy cost. *J Appl Physiol*. **98**(5), 1619–25.

Pedersen B, Saltin B. (2006). Evidence for prescribing exercise as therapy in chronic disease. *Scand J Med Sci Sports*. **16**(1), 3–63.

Riebe D, Ehrman J, Liguori G, Magal M. (2017). *American College of Sports Medicine Guidelines for Exercise Testing and Prescription*. 10th edition. Wolters Kluwer.

Roger VL, Go AS, Lloyd-Jones DM, Benjamin EJ, Berry JD, Borden WB, et al. (2012). Heart disease and stroke statistics – 2012 update: A report from the American heart association. *Circulation*. **125**(1), 2–220.

Sassen B, Cornelissen VA, Kiers H, Wittink H, Kok G, Vanhees L. (2009). Physical fitness matters more than physical activity in controlling cardiovascular disease risk factors. *Eur J Cardiovasc Prev Rehabil*. **16**(6), 677–83.

Thompson PD, Franklin BA, Balady GJ, Blair SN, Corrado D, Estes M. (2007). Exercise and acute cardiovascular events. *Circulation*. **115**, 2358–68.

United States Public Health Service (1996). *Office of the Surgeon General, Centers for Disease Control, Prevention, President's Council on Physical Fitness, & Sports. Physical Activity and Health: A Report of the Surgeon General*. Jones & Bartlett Learning.

U.S. Department of Health and Human Services (2010). *A Report of the Surgeon General. How Tobacco Smoke Causes Disease: What It Means to You. Centers for Disease Control and Prevention, National Center for Chronic Disease Prevention and Health Promotion*. Office on Smoking and Health.

Virani SS, Wang D, Woodard LD, Chitwood SS, Landrum CR, Zieve FJ, et al. (2012). Non-high-density lipoprotein cholesterol reporting and goal attainment in primary care. *J Clin Lipidol*. **6**(6), 545–52.

Whayne TF. (2011). Atherosclerosis: Current status of prevention and treatment. *Int J Angiol*. **20**(4), 213–22.

Wiegman A, Gidding SS, Watts GF, Chapman MJ, Ginsberg HN, Cuchel M, et al. (2015). European atherosclerosis society consensus panel. Familial hypercholesterolaemia in children and adolescents: Gaining decades of life by optimizing detection and treatment. *Eur Heart J*. **36**(36), 2425–37.

World Health Organisation (2011). *Global Status Report on Noncommunicable Diseases 2010: Description of the Global Burden of NCDs, Their Risk Factors and Determinants*. World Health Organisation.

15

ASTHMA

John Dickinson and Suraj Rajput

Chapter aims

The aims of this chapter are to:

- Briefly introduce asthma and discuss pharmacological and non-pharmacological therapy
- Demonstrate that although exercise is a trigger for asthma, it can also be used as an effective therapy for the management of the disease
- Discuss how to assess fitness and monitor changes over time in asthma patients
- Discuss types of exercise that are appropriate for individuals with mild, moderate and severe asthma

Introduction to asthma

Asthma is an obstructive airway disease in which individuals will intermittently experience a reduction in expiratory airflow. Asthma airway obstruction is a result of smooth muscle contraction, inflammation and remodelling in the lower airways that can be reversed and controlled with suitable therapy. Asthma can manifest itself in a variety of ways, and symptoms include wheezing, coughing, excess mucus production and breathlessness. These symptoms can vary among individuals, especially when individuals are exposed to triggers such as cold air, exercise, viral upper airway respiratory infection, cigarette smoke, pollution and respiratory allergens.

Records of asthma prevalence suggest that since the 1960s, asthma has been increasing. For example, between 1978 and 1988, asthma prevalence in school children living in Wales increased 5% (Burr et al., 1989), and in Scotland, the chance of children developing lifetime asthma increased from 10% in 1989 to 20% in 1994 (Omran and Russel, 1996). Similar increases in adult asthma were reported by Brogger et al. (2003), showing that the risk of asthma in adults aged less than 40 years living in Norway had tripled between 1972 and 1999. Asthma prevalence over this period increased from 3.6% to 7.6% in males and from 3.2% to 10.7% in females. However, over the past 20 years, asthma prevalence in UK seems to be

DOI: 10.4324/9781315102399-15

plateauing, with the prevalence of adults with asthma between approximately 9% and 12% (Asthma UK, 2019; British Lung Foundation, 2019).

Asthma pathophysiology

In healthy airways, the smooth muscle surrounding the bronchioles and bronchi are relaxed, and the bronchial epithelium is not inflamed, which allows an individual to ventilate their lungs with relative ease when at rest or exercising. During an asthma 'attack', the airways display inflammation, smooth muscle contraction and mucosal gland hyper-secretion (Fireman, 2003). The triggers and mechanisms underlying asthma are multi-factorial. A brief description of the series of events that lead to the development of asthma is presented in Box 15.1.

BOX 15.1 DEVELOPMENT OF ASTHMA FOLLOWING ACUTE EXPOSURE TO A TRIGGER

- Exposure of lower airways to a specific asthma trigger (e.g. pollen, pollution, dust, dry air).
- Rapid activation of airway mast cells and macrophages.
- Mast cells and macrophages release pro-inflammatory mediators such as histamine, eicosanoids, leukotrienes, prostaglandin and reactive oxygen species, which induce contraction of the airway smooth muscle, mucus secretion and vasodilatation.
- The pro-inflammatory mediators induce vascular leakage, which contains plasma protein that induces thickening of the airway wall (airway remodelling).
- The combined result is a narrowing of the airway lumen, resulting in reduced expiratory airflow.

The bronchial epithelium cells are in a key position where gene-environment and environment-environment interactions can occur. The bronchial epithelium acts as a barrier between the internal environment of the body and the external environment, and it is continuously exposed to gaseous and particulate components of the external environment. Thus, the bronchial epithelium is involved in many of the reactions that lead to asthma.

When exposed to inhaled pollutants, infectious agents and other particulate matter (i.e. asthma triggers), the bronchial epithelium acts as a protective barrier. When the epithelium is exposed to these irritants, it releases pro-inflammatory mediators that help protect the lungs. Salvi et al. (2000) demonstrated that diesel exhaust particles cause epithelial activation with increased expression of interleukin-8 (IL-8), which was consistent with the observed increase in neutrophils in bronchial biopsies and lavage fluid following exposure. Following exposure to asthma triggers, a healthy bronchial epithelium is able to repair itself rapidly. This enables the down regulation of the inflammatory response caused by acute exposure to potential asthma triggers. When an asthmatic bronchial epithelium is exposed to potential asthma triggers, it has an increased susceptibility to inflammation due to an increase in the production of remodelling growth factors and mucus production as well as an inability to repair rapidly

(Holgate, 2002). This inadequate repair response and epithelial damage may lead to heightened airway responsiveness, a failure to metabolise agonists, the destruction of the diffusion barrier altering permeability of airway mucosa, the depletion of epithelial-derived relaxant factors and loss of enzymes responsible for degrading pro-inflammatory neuropeptides. The implications of this are an increase in asthma symptoms, exacerbation frequency and severity.

Decreased baseline airway calibre and exaggerated airway narrowing result in restricted expiratory airflow that is typified by a reduced forced expiratory volume in one second (FEV_1) (Table 15.1). In a 15-year follow-up study, Lange et al. (1998) conducted measurements of FEV_1 in asthmatics and non-asthmatics. The study was conducted between 1976 and 1994 and included 17,506 participants, of whom 1,095 had asthma. Among women and men, and among smokers and non-smokers, the decline in FEV_1 over time was greater in participants with asthma. The average drop in FEV_1 for a non-asthmatic was 22 ml per year and 38 ml per year for an asthmatic. It is normal to expect a reduction in lung function over time (years) in non-asthmatics, but the reduction in lung function seems to be accelerated in individuals with asthma. There is limited evidence to demonstrate that effective management of asthma utilising preventative inhaler therapy (e.g. inhaled corticosteroids) can prevent the decline in pulmonary function. However, it is likely that inhaled corticosteroids will, at least partially, prevent pulmonary function decline in people with asthma (O'Byrne et al., 2019).

Diagnosis of asthma

The diagnosis of asthma should involve a patient history accompanied by objective airway assessments, including spirometry (NICE, 2017). Objective evidence includes measurement of pulmonary function via a maximal flow-volume loop (Miller et al., 2005). Objective evidence should also include either evidence of airway bronchodilation (e.g. FEV_1 improves 12% following inhalation of up to 400 μg of salbutamol) and/or evidence of bronchoconstriction following either a direct (methacholine) or indirect (e.g. exercise) airway challenge (see Box 15.1). The severity of asthma can be defined as mild, moderate and severe, using the patient's baseline forced expiratory volume in one second (FEV_1) (Table 15.1).

Despite the adoption of spirometry as the main objective measurement for asthma diagnosis, the procedure does involve patients producing good technique and maximal effort. It has previously been demonstrated that the quality of spirometry can be variable between patients and only provides a snapshot of airway function (Gannon et al., 1999). In addition to maximal

TABLE 15.1 Severity of asthma defined by baseline FEV_1

Severity	*Definition*
Mild	FEV_1 greater than 80% of predicted value. Mild intermittent asthma is defined as having symptoms less than twice a week, and mild persistent asthma is defined as having symptoms more often than twice a week.
Moderate	FEV_1 of between 60% and 80% of predicted value. They may use rescue medication (e.g. inhaled salbutamol) relatively frequently and have some limitations to daily activities.
Severe	FEV_1 of less than 60% of predicted value with extreme limitation in normal activity. Severe asthmatics are likely to use rescue medication several times a day.

flow-volume loops, pulmonary function and health can also be measured using assessments that require less patient compliance with technique.

Airway resistance measured via impulse oscillometry (IOS) can be recorded during steady rested breathing and does not require maximal effort from patients. IOS provides specific detail regarding an individual's airway mechanics and is more sensitive to changes in airway resistance than FEV_1 (Larsen et al., 2009). The fraction of exhaled nitric oxide (FeNO) has been shown to be representative of airway eosinophilic inflammation, which can be a marker for a number of various asthma phenotypes (Price et al., 2019; Dweik et al., 2011). It has been shown to be useful as an additional diagnostic tool for asthma (Schneider et al., 2013). Incorporating additional measures of respiratory function such as IOS and FeNO may improve accuracy of asthma diagnosis and reduce occurrence of under and over diagnosis of asthma (Kavanagh et al., 2019).

Using objective assessments (e.g. spirometry, airway challenges) to support asthma diagnosis can improve accuracy and reduce costs associated with misdiagnosis (Pakhale et al., 2011). However, many medical practitioner diagnoses of asthma do not incorporate complete objective assessments. It has previously been reported that 33% of physician-diagnosed asthma are inappropriate (Aaron et al., 2017). In a Canadian study, the lifetime costs for asthma misdiagnosed was $4,000 per patient for the medications alone (Pakhale et al., 2011). It is therefore imperative that a secure diagnosis of asthma is made using objective assessments and that these objective assessments are also used to monitor the management of asthma.

Medical management of asthma

No therapy exists to eliminate asthma; therefore, current therapy is targeted at managing the condition, symptoms and episodes of 'attacks'. In particular, asthma therapy attempts to reduce airway inflammation and protect against and reverse bronchoconstriction. Ultimately, the aim of asthma therapy is to allow an individual with asthma to take part in any activity they wish symptom-free. There are a range of pharmacological and non-pharmacological therapies available that have been shown to reduce asthma severity and symptoms (Table 15.2).

Inhaler therapy

Inhaler therapy in the form of inhaled β_2-agonists (e.g. salbutamol) and inhaled corticosteroids (e.g. beclomethasone) are the recommended forms of therapy for mild to moderate asthma

TABLE 15.2 Current therapy available for asthma

Pharmacologic	*Non-pharmacologic*
Inhaled short-acting β_2-agonists (e.g. salbutamol)	Exercise training
Inhaled long-acting β_2-agonists (e.g. salmeterol)	High-intensity warm-up prior to exercise
Inhaled corticosteroids (e.g. beclomethasone)	Change of environment
Oral eukotriene receptor antagonists	Breathing exercises
Inhaled sodium chromoglycate	Low-salt diet
Oral corticosteroids	Poly-unsaturated fatty acids (e.g. fish oils)
Oral β_2-agonists	Anti-oxidants (vitamin C and E)

(NICE, 2017). These two forms of therapy provide complementary protective effects to prevent asthma, with inhaled β_2-agonists, protecting against and reversing airway smooth muscle constriction and inhaled corticosteroids acting against the inflammatory process related to the development of asthma.

Use of inhaled β_2-agonists in isolation is not recommended as a therapy for asthma if the patient is using them more than three times a week (NICE, 2017). Daily sole use of inhaled β_2-agonists may lead to 1) development of tolerance and reduction in the duration of their protective effect, 2) increase in asthma severity and 3) prolonged recovery of lung function after an asthma attack (Anderson and Brannan, 2004). These responses are believed to be due to desensitisation of the β_2-receptors on mast cells leading to greater mediator release.

Inhaled corticosteroids are seen as the protective form of asthma therapy as they control inflammatory processes and reduce the occurrence of symptoms. A number of studies have demonstrated that treatment with inhaled corticosteroids reduces the number of airway inflammatory cells, including mast cells, eosinophils and lymphocytes (Ward et al., 2002). Most studies conducted on inhaled corticosteroids suggest that these effects are usually seen after two weeks of treatment (Chanez et al., 2004); however, therapy must be maintained in order to continue to benefit from the therapy. Several studies have demonstrated asthmatics using inhaled corticosteroids have an improved airway epithelium (Lundgren et al., 1988; Laitinen, Laitinen and Haahtela, 1992; Heino et al., 1988). However, no single study has demonstrated that inhaled corticosteroids are able to fully restore normality to the airway epithelium layer (Lundgren et al., 1988).

Despite corticosteroids controlling airway inflammation and remodelling, they do not provide full attenuation to acute airway hyperresponsiveness in all individuals with asthma. For example, it has been demonstrated that treatment with inhaled corticosteroids attenuated acute airway hyperresponsiveness in over 50% of people with exercise-induced asthma (Henriksen and Dahl, 1983; Henriksen, 1985; Vathenen et al., 1991; Farrero et al., 1995). In contrast, studies have shown benefits from regular use of inhaled steroids in patients with mild asthma, even in those whose forced expiratory volume in one second (FEV_1) is > 90% predicted (Pauwels et al., 2003).

There are numerous non-pharmacological strategies (see Table 15.2) that can be utilised to support the treatment of asthma (Dickinson, Amirav and Hostrup, 2018). There are promising findings that utilising these non-pharmacological strategies can reduce asthma symptoms and severity and improve asthma control; however, the evidence requires larger-scale studies, and future studies are encouraged before any recommendations are implemented. There is currently insufficient evidence to support the use of any non-pharmacological asthma therapy in the absence of regular pharmaceutical asthma therapy. Exercise practitioners should therefore ensure that pharmacological interventions are to hand at all times.

How do we know if asthma is controlled?

Following diagnosis and the patient being prescribed therapy, a follow-up appointment should be arranged where lung function assessments are repeated. It can also be beneficial to ask the patient to complete an asthma control questionnaire (Juniper et al., 2006), which will address the symptoms the patient is experiencing and the number of times they are using emergency therapy (e.g. inhaled salbutamol). Regular (6 to 12 months) follow-up appointments are helpful for asthmatics to gauge how well they are responding to treatment and for

TABLE 15.3 Gold-standard criteria for asthma control using the asthma control questionnaire

2 or more per week of	(a) Fewer than 2 days with symptom score greater than 1
	(b) Rescue β2-agonist use on fewer than 2 days and on no more than 4 occasions
	(c) Peak expiratory flow greater than 80% predicted every day
All of	• No night-time awakenings
	• No exacerbations (need for oral corticosteroids)
	• No emergency department visits/hospitalisations
	• No treatment-related adverse events enforcing a change in asthma therapy

Source: Adapted from Juniper et al. (2006, 616–621).

practitioners to ensure the patient is remaining compliant with their asthma management plan and using inhalers and other therapy appropriately. The gold-standard criteria for patients having asthma control are presented in Table 15.3.

Exercise as a therapy for asthma

Exercise is estimated to be a trigger for between 80% and 90% of people with asthma. However, physical activity is important in the rehabilitation of patients with asthma (Carlsen and Carlsen, 2002) since physical fitness can be poor in asthmatics (Garfinkel et al., 1992; Malkia and Impivaara, 1998). Despite this, elite athletes are also more susceptible to asthma-related conditions than the general population (Dickinson et al., 2005).

A typical barrier is that people with asthma may be put off exercising as it triggers their asthma, and they can experience significant symptoms. However, people with asthma can learn to control their asthma appropriately to prevent/reduce exercise-induced respiratory symptoms and benefit from the positive health effects of exercise. In fact, there is clear evidence that individuals with asthma can perform as elite athletes and win Olympic gold medals (Fitch, 2012).

Acute response to exercise in people with asthma

One of the preventative steps a person with asthma can take to control their asthma is to avoid environments (e.g. high pollution, pollen) and activities that trigger their asthma. So why exercise if exercise is a trigger for the majority of individuals with asthma? This is a challenging topic, and it is clear some health professionals may become protective about how much exercise (if any) should be recommended. There may be a fear among people with asthma about what exercise is safe and possible. For these reasons, it has been previously reported that children with asthma are likely to be less active than their non-asthmatic peers and that people with asthma have a lower aerobic fitness level than their non-asthmatic peers (Williams et al., 2010). This is a concern and may put people with asthma who do not engage with an active lifestyle at an increased risk of developing cardiovascular and metabolic conditions.

Evidence suggests that when individuals with asthma engage in a regular exercise programme, they will experience a reduction in respiratory symptoms, improved asthma control, reduction in use of an emergency inhaler (e.g. salbutamol), reduction in hospitalisations due to asthma, reduction in airway inflammation, improvement in fitness, improved mood and reductions in body fat (Eichenberger et al., 2013). Furthermore, in a meta-analysis, Carsen

TABLE 15.4 Medication considerations for exercise for people with asthma

Class name	*Generic name*	*Brand name*	*Indication*	*Action*	*Side effects*	*Exercise considerations*
Inhaled short-acting β_2-agonists	salbutamol	Ventolin	Inhale 200–400 µg prior to physical activity or when patient feels symptomatic	Bronchodilator	Arrhythmias; dizziness; headache; hypokalaemia (with high doses); nausea; palpitations; tremor	Patient's heart rate may be raised slightly after inhalation of salbutamol; patient should inhale 200–400 µg 20 minutes prior to moderate- or high- intensity activity that is likely to initiate asthma symptoms Monitor use during session; if patient regularly needs inhaled salbutamol again during the session, this may be a sign that their asthma is not optimally managed, or they have a co-existing respiratory condition that needs resolving
Inhaled long-acting β_2-agonists	salmeterol	Serevent	Inhale 50 µg twice daily; dose may be increased to 100 micrograms twice daily in more severe airway obstruction	Bronchodilator	Arrhythmias; dizziness; headache; hypokalaemia (with high doses); nausea; palpitations; tremor	Patient should inhale dose of salmeterol at least one hour prior to physical activity, ideally with corticosteroid and inhaling doses morning and evening Should not be used as a rescue inhaler during exercise; use salbutamol
Inhaled corticosteroids	fluticosone	Flixotide	Initially 100–500 µg twice daily; dose may be increased according to severity of asthma; doses above 500 µg twice daily initiated by a specialist	Anti-inflammatory	Headache; oral candidiasis; altered taste; voice alteration	Monitor salbutamol use during exercise; if patient regularly needs inhaled salbutamol again during the session, this may be a sign that their asthma is not optimally managed and corticosteroid dose needs to be adjusted, or they have a co-existing respiratory condition that needs resolving

Oral leukotriene receptor antagonists	montelukast	Singulair	10 mg once daily; dose to be taken in the evening	Anti-inflammatory	Diarrhoea; fever; gastrointestinal discomfort; headache; nausea; skin reactions; upper respiratory tract infection; vomiting	Monitor salbutamol use during exercise; if patient regularly needs inhaled salbutamol again during the session, this may be a sign that their asthma is not optimally managed and corticosteroid dose needs to be adjusted, or they have a co-existing respiratory condition that needs resolving
Inhaled sodium chromoglycate	cromolyn	Intal	Inhale 10 mg four times a day; additional dose may also be taken before exercise; increase to 10 mg six to eight times a day if necessary; maintenance 5 mg four times a day (5 mg is equivalent to one puff)	Anti-inflammatory	Cough; headache; pneumonia eosinophilic; rhinitis; throat irritation	Monitor use during session. If patient regularly needs inhaler during the session, this may be a sign that their asthma is not optimally managed, or they have a co-existing respiratory condition that needs resolving
Oral corticosteroids	prenisolone	Prelone	40–50 mg daily for 5–14 days	Anti-inflammatory	Anxiety; abnormal behaviour; cataract subcapsular; cognitive impairment; Cushing's syndrome; electrolyte imbalance; fatigue; fluid retention; gastrointestinal discomfort; headache; impaired healing; hirsutism; hypertension; increased risk of infection; menstrual cycle irregularities; altered mood; nausea; osteoporosis; peptic ulcer; psychotic disorder; skin reactions; sleep disorders; weight increase	Patients using oral corticosteroids are likely to be recovering from severe asthma exacerbation; it is not recommended that patients using this therapy engage in planned exercise until advised to do so by the medical practitioner managing their care

et al. (2013) demonstrated that across 21 studies including 772 people with asthma, physical training was well tolerated with no adverse events reported. Physical training showed marked improvement in aerobic fitness. These studies provide clear evidence that people with controlled asthma should be encouraged to participate in regular exercise training without fear of symptom exacerbation.

It is clear that exercise is a powerful tool in the management of asthma; however, practitioners working with people with asthma should consider what types of exercises are appropriate and whether the exercise should be conducted within an exercise referral setting or independently. Otherwise, the chronic effects of exercise training for people with asthma are the same as for the general population.

Exercise programmes for people with asthma

Exercise is one of the most effective treatments for patients with asthma. Exercise engagement is critical to the management and treatment of asthma patients. Exercise programmes can take place in a variety of environments including a gym class, a gym setting within local communities or home exercise programmes.

The American Thoracic Society (Spruit et al., 2015) listed two main key objectives of rehabilitation:

1. To control and relieve symptoms and physiological complications of the respiratory disease
2. To provide an educational component in order to ensure patients are able to manage and achieve optimal care for their respiratory condition

Patients with asthma who are looking for support to engage in exercise may benefit from working with a multidisciplinary team, which could consist of a physiotherapist, exercise practitioners, respiratory physiologists, nurses, consultants etc., depending on the location of the programme and the resources available to patients.

Patients who have respiratory conditions and have limited exercise ability, persistent symptoms, poor quality of life due to reduced activity etc. should all be considered for structured exercise rehabilitation programmes regardless of their age, gender or lung function results (physiological impairment).

The following are possible stages of enrolment onto a rehabilitation programme for patients with asthma, but it is important to note this will vary depending on the resources and professionals involved and the differences in locations.

Choosing the patient for an exercise rehabilitation programme

Precautions and contraindications to exercise:

Most patients are able to exercise to varying degrees and intensity; however, it is important to ensure that patients who have considerable risk during exercise are stabilised prior to commencing the programme (British Thoracic Society, 2013, 2016).

- Precautions to enrolling a patient onto a rehabilitation programme include significant orthopaedic impairments (e.g. severe osteoarthritis) and neurological impairments (e.g.

debilitating stroke, severe Parkinson's). This comprises a group of conditions that will not benefit patient outcomes and could worsen their existing conditions.

Contraindications include:

- Aortic aneurysm greater than 5.5 cm
- Unstable cardiac disease
- Severe pulmonary hypertension > 40 mmHg

It is important to note that patients must have a stable heart condition and appropriate pre-screening done prior to starting an exercise programme.

Asthma patient assessment prior to exercise engagement

The patient assessment should normally be undertaken by either a health-care professional or exercise practitioner. It involves taking a comprehensive history from the patient to ensure they are suitable for rehabilitation/exercise. The patient's goals and concerns are outlined and enable the programme coordinator to set specific exercises to achieve these (ideally SMART) goals.

A medical and physical examination should be undertaken in an acute or community setting, which should include lung function (for diagnostic tests to determine severity of asthma), musculoskeletal assessment and strength tests, review of medication and general observations (e.g. heart rate, blood pressure, saturation of oxygen).

If these are unavailable, exercise practitioners in a gym setting should ensure that the patient has a stable heart condition and can also use tools such as the Asthma Quality of Life Questionnaire (AQLQ) (Box 15.2) to analyse their activities and how asthma affects activities of daily living, especially for those with moderate to severe asthma.

BOX 15.2 ASTHMA QUALITY OF LIFE QUESTIONNAIRE

- Asthma Quality of Life Questionnaire (AQLQ) measures functional impairment.

www.qoltech.co.uk/aqlq.html

Some of the key reasons for a person with asthma being referred for exercise are dyspnoea and fatigue. In view of this, the rating of perceived exertion (RPE) scale or modified dyspnoea scale based on the Borg scale can be used to monitor aerobic and resistance exercise intensity by the person or the exercise practitioner (Figure 15.1).

Fitness assessments

Once it is established that the patient is suitable and stable for exercise, it is important to measure their exercise limits and abilities in order to derive a specific individualised exercise programme.

Shortness of Breath Modified Borg Dyspnea Scale	
0	Nothing at all
0.5	Extremely Slight (just noticeable)
1	Very Slight
2	Slight
3	Moderate
4	Somewhat Severe
5	Severe
6	
7	Very Severe
8	
9	Extremely Severe (almost maximal)
10	Maximal

FIGURE 15.1 Modified dyspnoea scale

For services that have the appropriate resources, a cardiopulmonary exercise test (CPET) will give a true reading of the patient's abilities and will measure their lung function, flow volume loops, peak oxygen consumption (VO_2max), anaerobic threshold, heart performance during exercise and exercise 12 lead ECG.

However, due to a lack of recourses and funding in some areas, CPET is not always possible. Therefore, in most areas with limited resources and set-up, the common ways to assess patients are the six-minute walk test (6MWT) and the incremental shuttle walk test (ISWT).

The six-minute walk test (6MWT)

This is a submaximal exercise test that entails measurement of distance walked over a span of six minutes.

- The patients are required to walk around two cones 30 metres apart as fast and as long as they can in six minutes.
- Participants are allowed to slow down if they are breathless and can stop and have a rest if their breathlessness is extreme. They are encouraged to carry on walking once they are able to do so.
- Their pre and post heart rate, saturation of oxygen and dyspnea are measured.
- Numerous outcome measures can be derived from a six-minute walk test: percentage of predicted six-minute walk distance, miles per hour, METs and target heart rate.
- Refer to the ATS clinical guidance (ATS, 2002) as a reference for conducting the 6MWT.

For exercise practitioners, it is important to understand the normative values for the 6MWT in order to evaluate the patient's ability and fitness. According to Camarri et al. (2006), the average six-minute walk distance (6MWD) was 659 ± 62 m (range 484–820 m) for individuals who did not have respiratory concerns. Males typically walked 59 ± 13 m farther than females. This is important for the exercise practitioner to take into consideration when assessing male and female patients.

Incremental shuttle walk test

This was developed to simulate a cardiopulmonary exercise test using a field-walking test (Holland, Spruit and Singh, 2015).

- The patient is required to walk around two cones set nine metres apart (so the final track is ten metres) in time to a set of auditory beeps played on a CD.
- Initially, the walking speed is very slow, but each minute, the required walking speed progressively increases.
- The patient walks for as long as they can until they are either too breathless or can no longer keep up with the beeps, at which time the test ends.
- The number of shuttles is recorded. Each shuttle represents a distance of ten metres (i.e. each time the patient reaches a cone is one shuttle).
- The results of the ISWT can be used to prescribe the intensity of walking training based on maximal heart rate. See Table 15.4 for normative ISWT average distance covered.
- Refer to clinical guidance as a reference for conducting the ISWT (Holland, Spruit and Singh, 2015).

Developing an exercise programme for people with asthma

Exercises will vary depending on the nature, setting and structure of the rehabilitation centre or gym. The American College of Sports Medicine (ACSM, 2018) suggest walking and utilising large muscle groups three to five days per week, and the ATS advises individuals to exercise at 60% to 75% of maximal work rate for 20 to 30 minutes two to five times a week.

For a rehabilitation programme (with an exercise practitioner), it is recommended that patients attend at least one or two supervised sessions a week and carry on a home exercise programme in addition to this (one or two days), with most programmes running for 12 weeks.

It is important to note that with asthma patients, the environment plays an integral part in their symptoms; therefore all care should be taken to ensure that the surroundings are adequate to exercise: for example, having optimum, controlled temperature in a gym setting

TABLE 15.5 Normative values for the distance covered during an incremental shuttle walk test

Age (years)	*Average Distance (m)*
17–40	897
40–49	824
50–59	788
60–69	699
≥ 70	633

Source: Harrison et al., 2013)

(well-ventilated rooms, humidified warm air). If patients are exercising outdoors, factors such as dry air, allergens and air pollution can trigger their symptoms. In instances like these, participants are advised to have appropriate exercise attire (such as a snood/scarf to cover their nose and mouth to warm the air they breathe in).

Prior to any exercise, asthma patients should engage in a pre-exercise warm-up. A well-coordinated warm-up has the following benefits:

- Raises body temperature and increases blood flow to the muscles, hence preventing muscle injuries
- Helps stimulate the nervous system and enables the body to anticipate increase physical activity behaviour
- Helps muscles, joints and tendons to be ready for the forces they will be put under while exercising
- Helps increase the respiratory rate and facilitate a coordinated breathing effort to prevent acute shortness of breath and panic.

A comprehensive warm-up programme should be no more than 15 minutes and aim to increase the heart rate and respiratory rate gradually. It should include general aerobic exercise and static and dynamic stretching. An example of a warm-up is shown in Box 15.3:

BOX 15.3 EXAMPLE OF A PRE-EXERCISE WARM-UP FOR PATIENTS WITH ASTHMA

- Walking or cycling for five to ten minutes, gradually increasing the intensity (measured by either heart rate or dyspnoea scale)
- Jumping jacks (ten reps)
- Lunges (ten reps)
- Squats (ten reps)
- Thoracic and hip rotations
- Static stretching of the larger muscle groups (hamstrings, quadriceps, calves)

NOTE: Participants can use reliever medication (e.g. Ventolin) if needed prior to starting exercise to optimise their output.

Exercises for people with mild asthma

People with mild asthma generally have an FEV_1 greater than 80% of predicted value. Mild intermittent asthma is defined as having symptoms less than twice a week, and mild persistent asthma is defined as having symptoms more than twice a week.

As long as the symptoms are well controlled (see Table 15.3), people with asthma should be able to complete most forms of exercise within the capabilities of their current fitness status. There is clear evidence that individuals with mild asthma who engage in exercise can expect to experience a reduction in symptoms and improvements in general well-being. Emtner, Herala and Stalenheim (1996) tested 26 adults who underwent a ten-week supervised rehabilitation programme. Following a six-minute submaximal cycle ergometer test and 12-minute walk test, patients exercised at a target intensity of 80% to 90% of their predicted maximal heart rate. In the first two weeks of the programme, patients exercised daily in an indoor swimming pool, and for the next eight weeks, patients underwent 45-minute sessions twice a week. After the programme, the cycle ergometer test showed an average decrease in heart rate of 12 beats per minute and average increase of 111 metres during the 12-minute walk.

For patients with mild asthma, it is well known that prescribing exercise intensity to > 80% maximal heart rate produces results that show significant improvements in quality of life, management of symptoms, increased physical activity behaviour and improvement in VO_2peak following exercises as shown by the studies mentioned earlier and as evidenced by a systematic review carried out by Ram, Robinson and Black (2000).

There are no specific exercise regimes for mild asthma, but they should include at least 30 minutes of cardiovascular exercises working at intensity > 80% maximal heart rate. It is also recommended that participants work at this intensity at least three times a week.

Exercise prescription for moderate to severe asthma

To be able to set up a programme of exercise for moderate to severe asthma patients, it is important to understand the differences in severity. Moderate asthma patients have an FEV_1 of between 60% and 80% of their predicted value. They may use rescue medication (e.g. inhaled salbutamol) relatively frequently and have some limitations to daily activities. Severe asthma patients, on the other hand, have a FEV_1 of less than 60% of the predicted value with extreme limitation in normal activity. Severe asthmatics are likely to use rescue medication several times a day.

The significance of the severity of asthma as described here will determine the exercise prescription regime. Severe asthmatic patients will need regular or longer rest periods during exercise. They will have reduced endurance and higher Borg scores and may use their rescue medication more frequently than the moderate asthmatic patients. Hence, severe asthma patients' exercise regimes will need to be tailored to accommodate their symptoms and ability.

The exercise intensity for the moderate and severe asthma patients will be lower than that of the mild patients. This will generally be set at 50% or 80% of their maximal heart rate and will vary depending on each individual's stage and any other co-morbidity such as cardiac conditions (pulmonary hypertension, heart failure), diabetes, osteoarthritis, obesity, recurrent chest infections etc.

Case studies demonstrate the impact of exercise prescription for people with moderate and severe asthma.

Certain evaluation tools can be used to determine how effective the exercises prescribed are.

Examples of some tools (not extensive) used in analysis of the patient's mental state and how their activities of daily living are affected are shown next:

- Patient health questionnaire (PHQ-9) – reviews depression signs

  www.cqaimh.org/pdf/tool_phq9.pdf

- General anxiety disorder questionnaire (GAD-7) – assesses the patient's anxiety levels
- St George's Respiratory Questionnaire (SGRQ) – measures health status and quality of life

A reduction of 4 units suggests a clinically significant difference for SGRQ.

CASE STUDIES OF A MODERATE AND SEVERE PATIENT, BOTH ENGAGING IN EXERCISE PROGRAMMES

Moderate patient:

Patient X: 56-year-old female with a FEV_1 of 69%

Outcome measures tested for Patient X are as follows:

Outcome measure	*Pre-assessment*	*Post-assessment*
SGRQ	66.77	58.66
PHQ-9	10	2
GAD-7	4	0
Six-minute walk test (metres)	310	476
One rep max (bicep curl)	2.8	3.7
Grip strength (KG)	5	16
MRC	3	3
Borg	2	0

Severe patient:

Patient Y has severe asthma with an FEV1 of 53%

Outcome measures tested for Patient Y are as follows:

Outcome measure	*Pre-assessment*	*Post-assessment*
SGRQ	71.78	51.16
PHQ-9	16	4
GAD-7	6	2
Six-minute walk test (metres)	200	450
One rep max (bicep curl)	6.4	8
Grip strength (KG)	28	34
MRC	4	2
Borg	3	0

The programme:

Both patients were in the same cohort.

Warm-up exercises were conducted in gym hall (20 metres length) with controlled temperature:

The warm-up exercises included:

Five minutes of walking, getting up to 50–60% of maximal heart rate.

Thoracic and hip rotations, knee bends and calf raises. These were followed by another five minutes of walking.

After the warm-up, both patients started with 30 minutes of cardiovascular exercises as follows:

- 20 minutes of walking (length of 20 metres a lap).

Patient X had to walk 43 laps (860 metres) to achieve 70% HR_{6peak}.
Patient Y had to walk 20 laps (400 metres) to achieve 60% HR_{6peak}.

- 5 minutes of cycling at the same intensity.
- This was followed by 5 minutes doing step-ups.

Upon conclusion of the cardiovascular exercise, patients then proceeded to perform strength training. This was done at 60% of their one rep maximum (bicep curl).

- Three sets of ten reps of bicep curls, upright row and chest press.
- Three sets of ten reps of sit-to-stand.

NOTE: For patients who are able to perform compound exercises such as deadlifts, overhead presses, lunges, squats etc., a programme of three sets of ten reps would be beneficial in building muscle bulk. This is progressed by increasing the repetitions or resistance. However, consideration must be taken in view of the patients Borg scores to minimise dyspnoea.

Cool down:

- Five minutes of gentle relaxed walking to bring the heart rate back to its resting state.
- Cervical and thoracic stretches.
- Hamstring and quadriceps stretching.
- Calf stretches.

Each patient's exercise intensity was increased after two to three weeks by increasing their walk times, increasing resistance of the weights and working at higher intensity of their HR_{6peak} to allow progression of exercise and improve fitness. Patients exercised for an average of 45 to 60 minutes. This was followed by an education talk that included topics such as managing breathlessness, managing anxiety and depression, inhaled medications, benefits of exercise etc.

Patients attend two supervised sessions a week and are encouraged to continue with a home exercise program for at least another two days a week.

In conclusion, the case studies show a significant improvement in patient outcomes.

Patient X had a clinically significant change of 8.11 in the SGRQ scores, improved by 166 metres on the walk test and showed a reduction in resting Borg scores.

Patient Y had a highly significant change in SGRQ (20.62), along with an increased walking distance of 250 metres. These tools are viable options for exercise practitioners/instructors to use to measure the impact of exercise training for asthma patients.

A further key point in the patient's journey is to monitor the exercise training programme and adapt this to the individual's needs. Monitoring can be simple in view of using the Borg and MRC scores to assess the effectiveness of the exercise programme and to help assess the context of aerobic exercise intensity. The practitioner should adapt the programme and challenge the patient constantly in order to gain maximum output within the patient's abilities. If possible, the practitioner should monitor the patient's heart rate and oxygen levels and ensure these are within the set parameters (e.g. 70% HR_{6peak}). This monitoring process allows a quantitative approach to training periodisation, and the rate of perceived exertion can also be useful in allowing the patient to maximise their training load.

Helping a person with asthma become an independent exerciser

Following a comprehensive rehabilitation programme or exercise regime, many local councils and gym settings offer an exercise referral scheme (ERS). Health-care professionals can refer individuals for exercise sessions at the gym for a 12-week period for free or at a subsidised fee. An exercise programme similar to the one shown earlier is formulated for the individual and reviewed by the exercise practitioner. Following completion of this programme, individuals are offered a subsidised membership to join the local gym. If an individual is reluctant to enter a gym setting, local councils have outdoor walking or cycling programmes which could be an alternative to a gym-based exercised programme.

Summary

There is a vast amount of evidence to support the inclusion of exercise in the care of people with mild to severe asthma. Exercise can encourage the development of endurance and physical capacity. With the appropriate guidance, most individuals can learn to control symptoms and continue to improve their physical and mental functionality.

Study tasks

1. What type of airway disease is asthma, and what are the main symptoms an asthmatic may report?
2. What is the underlying cause of asthma development?
3. What are the potential problems that an asthma patient may face if they use inhaled β_2-agonists in isolation of any other therapy?
4. What are the potential benefits of engaging in exercise for people with asthma?
5. What precautions should be taken to ensure the environment is suitable for patients with asthma to exercise?
6. What intensity and frequency of aerobic exercise should people with mild asthma be encouraged to engage in?

7. In what ways may a severe asthma patient need to modify an exercise programme, compare to a moderate asthma patient?
8. What assessments can be used to diagnose asthma?
9. What assessments of cardiopulmonary fitness could be used prior to an asthma patient engaging in an exercise programme?
10. What are the criteria to define whether asthma is well controlled?

TABLE 15.6 At-a-glance summary guide to exercise considerations for people with asthma

Condition name	*Asthma*
Pathophysiology summary	Obstructive airway disease. Airway obstruction is driven by airway inflammation and smooth muscle contraction resulting in reduced airflow on expiration.
Aims of exercise	Improve control of breathing, reduce airway inflammation, improve control of respiratory symptoms during exercise. Improve quality of life and comorbidities associated with asthma.
Exercise considerations (include contraindications)	Uncontrolled asthma is a contraindication. Be aware of triggers for asthma, such as cold, animals, allergens, to avoid around exercise. Use a long acting inhaler if required and ensure participant exercises with their rescue inhaler. Include a progressive warm-up to reduce the risk of exercise-induced asthma.
Frequency	3–4 times per week
Intensity	Mild asthma >80% HR_{max} Moderate asthma 70–80% HR_{max} Severe asthma 60–70% HR_{max}
Time	30–60 minutes
Type	Variety of cardiovascular and strength.
Common medications associated.	Inhaled β2-Agonists (e.g. salbutamol) Inhaled corticosteroids (e.g. beclomethasone).
Key safety considerations	Ensure participants have rescue inhalers available when engaging in exercise. Ensure participants asthma is under control prior to engaging in exercise.
Effect of exercise on conditions	Reduce respiratory symptoms during exercise Improved health status Improved quality of life Reduced use of rescue inhalers Reduced hospitalisations

References

Aaron, S., Vandemheen, K., FitzGerald, J., Ainslie, M., Gupta, S., Lemière, C., Field, S., McIvor, R., Hernandez, P., Mayers, I., Mulpuru, S., Alvarez, G., Pakhale, S., Mallick, R. & Boulet, L. (2017). 'Reevaluation of Diagnosis in Adults with Physician-Diagnosed Asthma'. *Journal of the American Medical Association*, vol. 317(3), pp. 269–279.

American College of Sports Medicine. (2018) *Guidelines for Exercise Testing and Prescription*. Tenth Edition. www.acsm.org/docs/default-source/publications-files/acsm-guidelines-download-10th-edabf32a97415a400e9b3be594a6cd7fbf.pdf?sfvrsn=aaa6d2b2_0. Accessed 21st January 2020.

American Thoracic Society. (2002). 'ATS Statement: Guidelines for the Six-Minute Walk Test'. *American Journal of Respiratory and Critical Care Medicine*, vol. 166, pp. 111–117.

Anderson, S. & Brannan, J. (2004). 'Long Acting β_2-Adrenoceptor Agonists and Exercise Induced Asthma'. *Pediatric Drugs*, vol. 6, pp. 1–15.

Asthma UK. (2019). *Asthma Facts and Statistics*. www.asthma.org.uk/about/media/facts-and-statistics/. Accessed 5th June 2019.

British Lung Foundation. (2019). *Asthma Statistics*. https://statistics.blf.org.uk/asthma. Accessed 5th June 2019.

British Thoracic Society. (2013) 'BTS Guidelines on Pulmonary Rehabilitation in Adults Thorax'. *An International Journal of Respiratory Medicine*, vol. 68, supplement 2.

British Thoracic Society. (2016). *SIGN 153, British Guidelines on the Management of Asthma: A National Clinical Guideline Revised 2016*. https://www.brit-thoracic.org.uk/quality-improvement/guidelines/asthma/.

Brogger, J., Bakke, P., Eide, G., Johansen, B., Andersen, A. & Gulsvik, A. (2003). 'Long-Term Changes in Adult Asthma Prevalence'. *European Respiratory Journal*, vol. 21, pp. 468–472.

Burr, M., Butland, B., King, S. & Vaughan-Williams, E. (1989). 'Changes in Asthma Prevalence: Two Surveys 15 Years Apart'. *Archives of Disease in Children*, vol. 64, pp. 1452–1456.

Camarri, B., Eastwood, P., Cecins, N., Thompson, P. & Jenkins, S. (2006). 'Six Minute Walk Distance in Healthy Subjects Aged 55–75 Years'. *Respiratory Medicine*, vol. 100, pp. 658–665.

Carlsen, K.H. & Carlsen, K.C. (2002). 'Exercise Induced Asthma'. *Paediatric Respiratory Reviews*, vol. 3, p. 154.

Carson, K.V., Chandratilleke, M.G., Picot, J., Brinn, M.P., Esterman, A.J. & Smith, B.J. (2013). 'Physical Training for Asthma'. *The Cochrane Database of Systematic Review*, vol. 9, pp. CD001116.

Chanez, P., Bourdin, A., Vachier, I., Godard, P., Bousquet, J. & Vignola, A. (2004). 'Effects of Inhaled Corticosteroids on Pathology in Asthma and Chronic Obstructive Pulmonary Disease'. *Proceeding of the American Thoracic Society*, vol. 1, pp. 184–190.

Dickinson, J., Amirav, I. & Hostrup, M. (2018). 'Nonpharmacologic Strategies to Manage Exercise-Induced Bronchoconstriction'. *Immunology and Allergy Clinics of North America*, vol. 38, pp. 245–258.

Dickinson, J., Whyte, G., McConnell, A. & Harries, M. (2005). 'Impact of Changes in the IOC-MC Asthma Criteria: A British Perspective'. *Thorax*, vol. 60, pp. 629–632.

Dweik, R., Boggs, P., Erzurum, S., Irvin, C., Leigh, M., Lundberg, J., Olin, A., Plummer, A. & Taylor, D. (2011). 'American Thoracic Society Committee on Interpretation of Exhaled Nitric Oxide Levels (FENO) for Clinical Applications: An Official ATS Clinical Practice Guideline: Interpretation of Exhaled Nitric Oxide Levels (FENO) for Clinical Applications'. *American Journal of Respiratory and Critical Care Medicine*, vol. 184(5), pp. 602–615.

Eichenberger, P., Diener, S., Kofmehl, R. & Spengler, C. (2013). 'Effects of Exercise Training on Airway Hyperreactivity in Asthma: A Systematic Review and Meta-Analysis'. *Sports Medicine*, vol. 43, pp. 1157–1170.

Emtner, M., Herala, M. & Stalenheim, G. (1996). 'High-Intensity Physical Training in Adults with Asthma: A 10-Week Rehabilitation Program'. *Chest*, vol. 109(2), pp. 323–330.

Farrero, E., Llunell, A., Canete, C., Rodriguez, B., Manresa, F. & Romero, P. (1995). 'Inhaled Steroids Treatment and Withdrawal in Asthmatic Children'. *Allergologia et Immunopathologia*, vol. 23, pp. 182–188.

Fireman, P. (2003). 'Understanding Asthma Pathophysiology'. *Allergy and Asthma Proceedings*, vol. 24, pp. 79–83.

Fitch, K. (2012). 'An Overview of Asthma and Airway Hyper-Responsiveness in Olympic Athletes'. *British Journal of Sports Medicine*, vol. 46, pp. 413–416.

Gannon, P., Belcher, J., Pantin, C. & Burge, P. (1999). 'The Effect of Patient Technique and Training on the Accuracy of Self-Recorded Peak Expiratory Flow'. *European Respiratory Journal*, vol. 14(1), pp. 28–31.

Garfinkel, S.K., Kesten, S., Chapman, K.R. & Rebuck A.S. (1992). 'Physiologic and Non-Physiologic Determinants of Aerobic Fitness in Mild to Moderate Asthma'. *The American Review of Respiratory Disease*, vol. 145, pp. 741–745.

Harrison, S., Greening, N., Houchen-Wolloff, L., Bankart, J., Morgan, M., Steiner, M. & Singh, S. (2013). 'Age-Specific Normal Values for the Incremental Shuttle Walk Test in a Healthy British Population'. *Journal of Cardio Pulmonary Rehabilitation and Prevention*, vol. 33(5), pp. 309–313.

Heino, M., Karjalainen, J., Ylikoski, J., Laitinen, A. & Laitinen, L. (1988). 'Bronchial Ciliogenesis and Oral Steroid Treatment in Patients with Asthma'. *British Journal of Diseases of the Chest*, vol. 82, pp. 175–178.

Henriksen, J. (1985). 'Effect of Inhalation of Corticosteroids on Exercise Induced Asthma: Randomised Double Blind Crossover Study of Budesonide in Asthmatic Children'. *British Medical Journal*, vol. 291, pp. 248–249.

Henriksen, J. & Dahl, R. (1983). 'Effects of Inhaled Budesonide Alone and in Combination with Low-Dose Terbutaline in Children with Exercise-Induced Asthma'. *American Review of Respiratory Diseases*, vol. 128, pp. 993–997.

Holgate, S. (2002). 'Asthma: More Than an Inflammatory Disease'. *Current Opinion in Allergy and Clinical Immunology*, vol. 2, pp. 27–29.

Holland, A., Spruit, H. & Singh, S. (2015). 'How to Carry Out a Field Walking Test in Chronic Respiratory Disease'. *Breathe*, vol. 11(2), pp. 128–139.

Juniper, E.F., Bousquet, J., Abetz, L. & Bateman, E.D. (2006). 'Identifying 'Well-Controlled' and 'Not Well-Controlled' Asthma Using the Asthma Control Questionnaire'. *Respiratory Medicine*, vol. 100, pp. 616–621.

Kavanagh, J., Jackson, D. & Kent, B. (2019). 'Over- and Under-Diagnosis in Asthma'. *Breathe*, vol. 15(1), pp. e20–e27.

Laitinen, L., Laitinen, A. & Haahtela, T. (1992). 'A Comparative Study of the Effects of an Inhaled Corticosteroid, Budesonide, and a Beta 2-Agonist, Terbutaline, on Airway Inflammation in Newly Diagnosed Asthma: A Randomized, Double-Blind, Parallel-Group Controlled Trial'. *Journal of Allergy and Clinical Immunology*, vol. 90, pp. 32–42.

Lange, P., Parner, J., Vestibo, J., Schnohr, P. & Jensen, G. (1998). 'A 15 Year Follow Up Study of Ventilatory Function in Adults with Asthma'. *New England Journal of Medicine*, vol. 339, pp. 1194–1200.

Larsen, G., Morgan, W., Heldt, G., Mauger, D., Boehmer, S., Chinchilli, V., Lemanske, R. Jr., Martinez, F., Strunk, R., Szefler, S., Zeiger, R., Taussig, L., Bacharier, L., Guilbert, T., Radford, S., Sorkness, C. & Childhood Asthma Research and Education Network of the National Heart, Lung, and Blood Institute. (2009). 'Impulse Oscillometry Versus Spirometry in a Long-Term Study of Controller Therapy for Pediatric Asthma'. *The Journal of Allergy and Clinical Immunology*, vol. 123(4), pp. 861–867.

Lundgren, R., Soderberg, M., Horstedt, P. & Stenling, R. (1988). 'Morphological Studies of Bronchial Mucosal Biopsies from Asthmatics Before and After Ten Years of Treatment with Inhaled Steroids'. *European Respiratory Journal*, vol. 1, pp. 883–389.

Malkia, E. & Impivaara, O. (1998). 'Intensity of Physical Activity and Respiratory Function in Subjects with and Without Bronchial Asthma'. *Scandinavian Journal of Medicine & Science in Sports*, vol. 8, pp. 27–32.

Miller, M., Hankinson, J., Brusasco, V., Burgos, F., Casaburi, R., Coates, A., Crapo, R., Enright, P., van der Grinten, C.P.M., Gustafsson, P., Jensen, R., Johnson, D.C., MacIntyre, N., McKay, R., Navajas, D., Pedersen, O.F., Pellegrino, R., Viegi, G. & Wanger, J. (2005). 'Standardisation of Spirometry'. *European Respiratory Journal*, vol. 26, pp. 319–338.

National Institute for Health and Care Excellence. (2017). *Asthma: Diagnosis, Monitoring and Chronic Asthma Management*. NICE Guideline, 29th November. www.nice.org.uk/guidance/ng80. Accessed 27th December 2019.

O'Byrne, P., Fabbri, L.M., Pavord, I.D. et al. (2019). 'Asthma Progression and Mortality: The Role of Inhaled Corticosteroids'. *European Respiratory Journal*, vol. 54. doi:10.1183/13993003.00491-2019.

Omran, M. & Russell, G. (1996). 'Continuing Increase in Respiratory Symptoms and Atopy in Aberdeen Schoolchildren'. *British Medical Journal*, vol. 312, p. 34.

Pakhale, S., Sumner, A., Coyle, D., Vandemheen, K. & Aaron, S. (2011). '(Correcting) Misdiagnoses of Asthma: A Cost Effectiveness Analysis'. *BMC Pulmonary Medicine*, vol. 11, p. 27. doi:10.1186/1471-2466-11-27.

Pauwels, R., Sears, M., Campbell, M., Villasante, C., Huang, S., Lindh, A., Petermann, W., Aubier, M., Schwabe, G. & Bengtsson, T. (2003). 'Formoterol as Relief Medication in Asthma: A World-wide Safety and Effectiveness Trial'. *European Respiratory Journal*, vol. 22, pp. 787–794.

Price, D., Bosnic-Anticevich, S,. Pavord, I., Roche, N., Halpin, D., Bjermer, L., Usmani, O., Brusselle, G., Ming, S. & Rastogi, S. (2019). 'Association of Elevated Fractional Exhaled Nitric Oxide Concentration and Blood Eosinophil Count with Severe Asthma Exacerbations'. *Clinical and Translational Allergy*, vol. 9, p. 41. doi:10.1186/s13601-019-0282-7.

Ram, F., Robinson, S. & Black, P. (2000). 'Effects of Physical Training in Asthma: A Systematic Review'. *British Journal of Sports Medicine*, vol. 34(3), pp. 162–167.

Salvi, S., Nordenhall, C., Blomberg, A., Rudell, B., Pourazar, J., Kelly, F., Wilson, S., Sandstrom, T., Holgate, S. & Frew, A. (2000). 'Diesel Exhaust Induces Expression of IL-8 and GRO in Bronchial Epithelium in Human Airways'. *American Journal of Respiratory Critical Care Medicine*, vol. 161, pp. 550–557.

Schneider, A., Schwarzbach, J., Faderl, B., Welker, L., Karsch-Völk, M. & Jörres, R. (2013). 'FENO Measurement and Sputum Analysis for Diagnosing Asthma in Clinical Practice'. *Respiratory Medicine*, vol. 107(2), pp. 209–216.

Spruit, M.A., Pitta, F., McAuley, E., ZuWallack, R.L. & Nici, L. (2015). 'Pulmonary Rehabilitation and Physical Activity in Patients with Chronic Obstructive Pulmonary Disease'. *American Journal of Respiratory and Critical Care Medicine*, vol. 192(8), pp. 924–933.

Vathenen, A., Knox, A., Wisniewski, A. & Tattersfield, A. (1991). 'Effect of Inhaled Budesonide on Bronchial Reactivity to Histamine, Exercise, and Eucapnic Dry Air Hyperventilation in Patients with Asthma'. *Thorax*, vol. 46, pp. 811–816.

Ward, C., Pais, M., Bish, R., Reid, D., Feltis, B., Johns, D. & Walters, E. (2002). 'Airway Inflammation, Basement Membrane Thickening and Bronchial Hyperresponsiveness in Asthma'. *Thorax*, vol. 57, pp. 309–316.

Williams, B., Hoskins, G., Pow, J., Neville, R., Mukhopadhyay, S. & Coyle, J. (2010). 'Low Exercise Among Children with Asthma: A Culture of Over Protection?'. *British Journal of General Practice*, vol. 60, pp. e319–e326.

16

LOW BACK PAIN

James Fisher, Hopin Lee and Paul Hendrick

Chapter Aims

The aims of this chapter are to:

1. Describe lumbar and trunk anatomy and the role these musculoskeletal structures play in low back pain (LBP) and exercise prescription
2. Describe the pathology of LBP and appreciate current medications and medical management for persons living with LBP
3. Identify appropriate assessment strategy prior to implementation of an exercise programme for a person with LBP
4. Understand the acute responses to a bout of exercise and chronic adaptations to an exercise intervention for a person with LBP
5. Describe the deconditioning hypothesis
6. Explain the boom-or-bust phenomenon relating LBP and recovery
7. Support the reader to feel confident in prescribing exercise to a person with LBP

Introduction

The following chapter will outline lumbar and trunk anatomy and the pathology of non-specific low back pain (NSLBP). It will then discuss current medical management and contemporary evidence in the use and prescription of exercise for the management of NSLBP. The chapter is divided into several sections, and whilst the pathology section will help an exercise practitioner consider potential causes, and the medication section will help with understanding of medical management, it is important to remember that LBP is a symptom, not a diagnosis (Bono, 2004). In that sense, and since weakness of the lumbar muscles appears related to LBP (Mayer et al., 1999; Risch et al., 1993), an emphasis is placed on the benefits of muscle-strengthening exercise. However, additional exercise treatments are discussed, and a multimodal, client-centric approach is encouraged for management of this condition.

DOI: 10.4324/9781315102399-16

16.1 Lumbar Anatomy

To fully understand LBP, the consequences for a person, and the potential exercise-based remedies, a thorough and detailed anatomical knowledge is essential. The lumbar spine consists of five vertebrae situated above the fused vertebrae of the sacrum (Figure 16.1). The sacroiliac joint is of significance when considering lumbar problems and connects the spine to the pelvis. The lumbar vertebrae increase in size as you descend anatomically from lumbar vertebrae one (L1) to lumbar vertebrae five (L5). The fifth lumbar vertebra articulates with the sacroiliac joint. The vertebrae are separated by intervertebral discs and connected through multiple ligaments and muscles.

The primary muscles of the lumbar spine include:

- The **quadratus lumborum** (Figure 16.2), which originates on the posterior iliac crest and iliolumbar ligament and inserts on the transverse process of L1–L4 and inferior border of the 12th rib

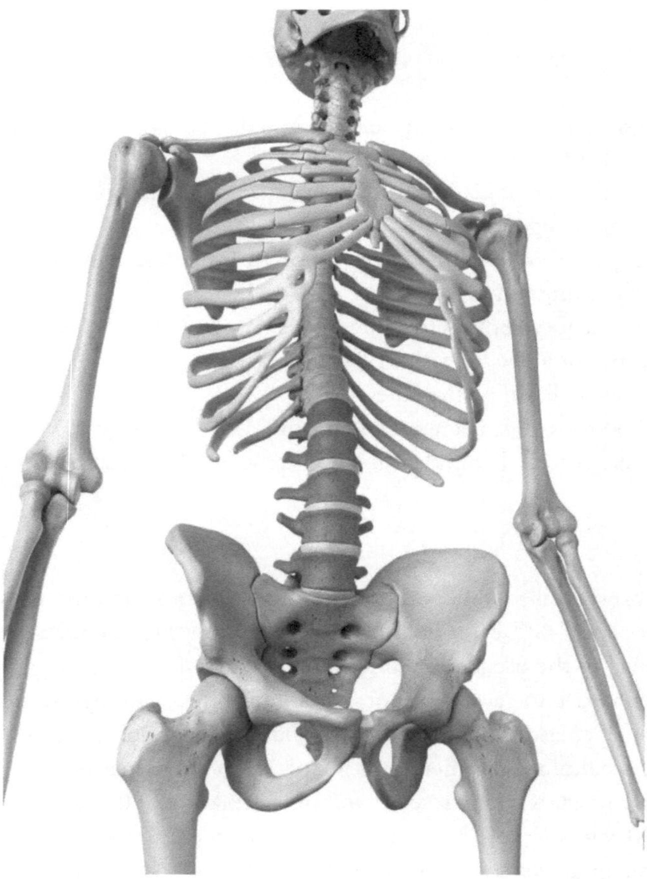

FIGURE 16.1 Lumbar Spine

Source: Shutterstock ID: 296153237

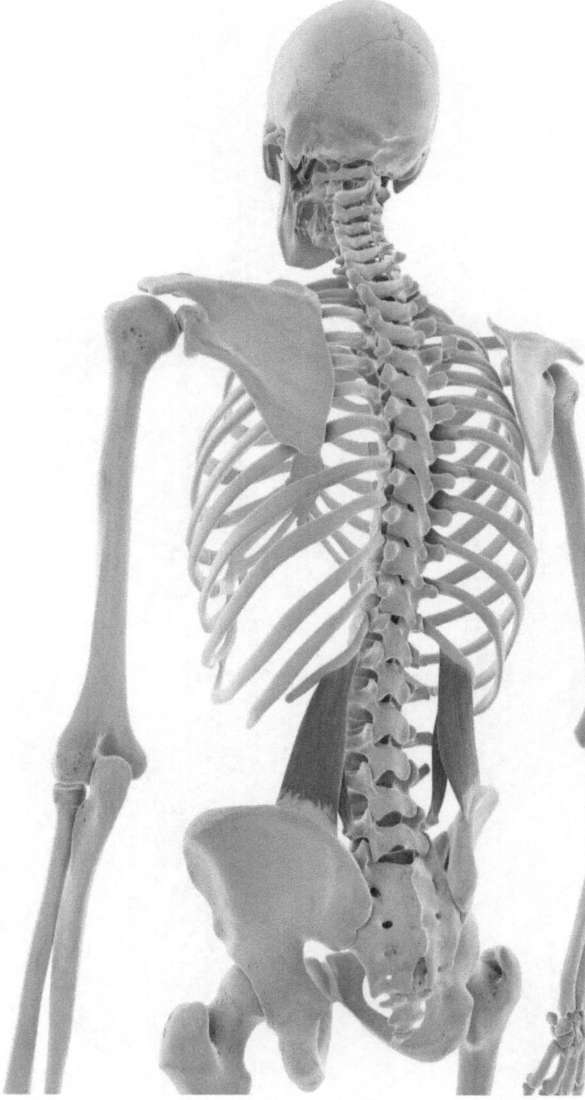

FIGURE 16.2 Quadratus Lumborum

Source: Shutterstock ID: 1544639363

- The **multifidus** (Figure 16.3), which originates on the posterior sacrum, posterior iliac spine and processes of L5-cervical (C)4 and inserts on to the spinous process two to four vertebrae above the origin
- The **iliocostalis** (Figure 16.4), which originates on the medial iliac crest, thoracolumbar aponeurosis and posterior surface of ribs 3 through 12 and inserts on the posterior surface of ribs 1–12 and transverse processes of C4–C7
- The **longissimus** (Figure 16.5), which originates on the thoracolumbar aponeurosis, transverse processes of L5-thoracic (T)1 and articular processes of C4-C7 and inserts

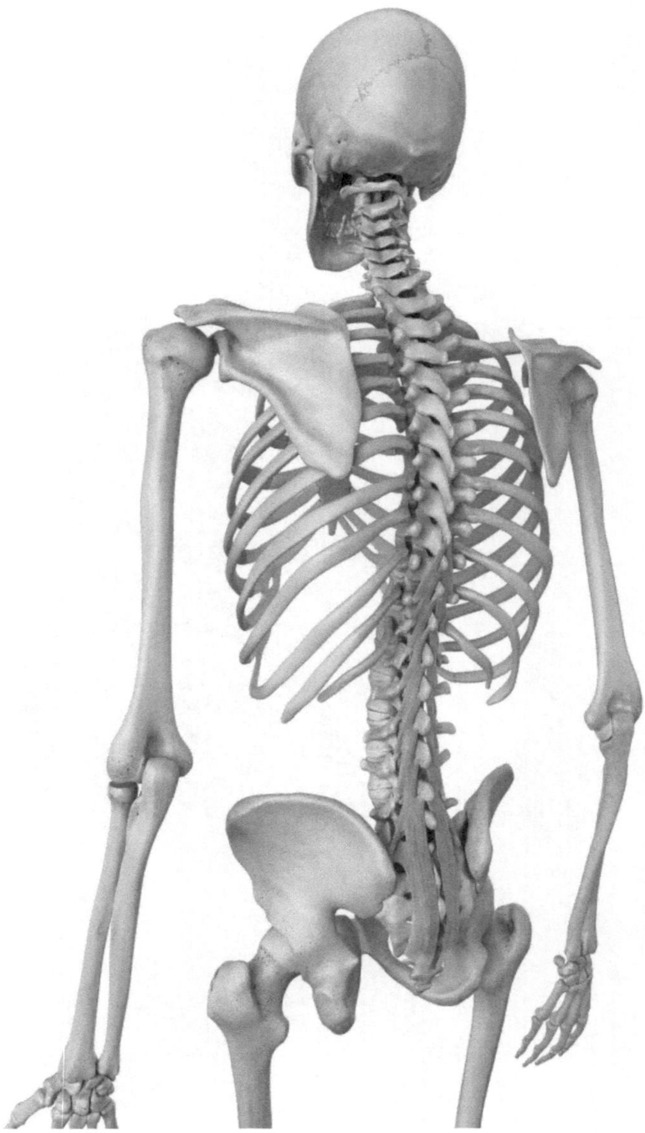

FIGURE 16.3 Multifidus

Source: Shutterstock ID: 293549282

on the transverse processes of T1–T12 and C2–C6, posterior surface of ribs 3–12 and mastoid process of the temporal bone

- The **spinalis** (Figure 16.6), which originates on the spinous processes of L2–T11 and T2–C7 and ligament nuchae and inserts on the spinous processes of T1–T8 and C2–C4 and between the superior and inferior nuchal lines of the occiput

When these muscles contract bilaterally, they act to produce extension of the spine; however, when contracted unilaterally, these muscles work to produce lateral flexion.

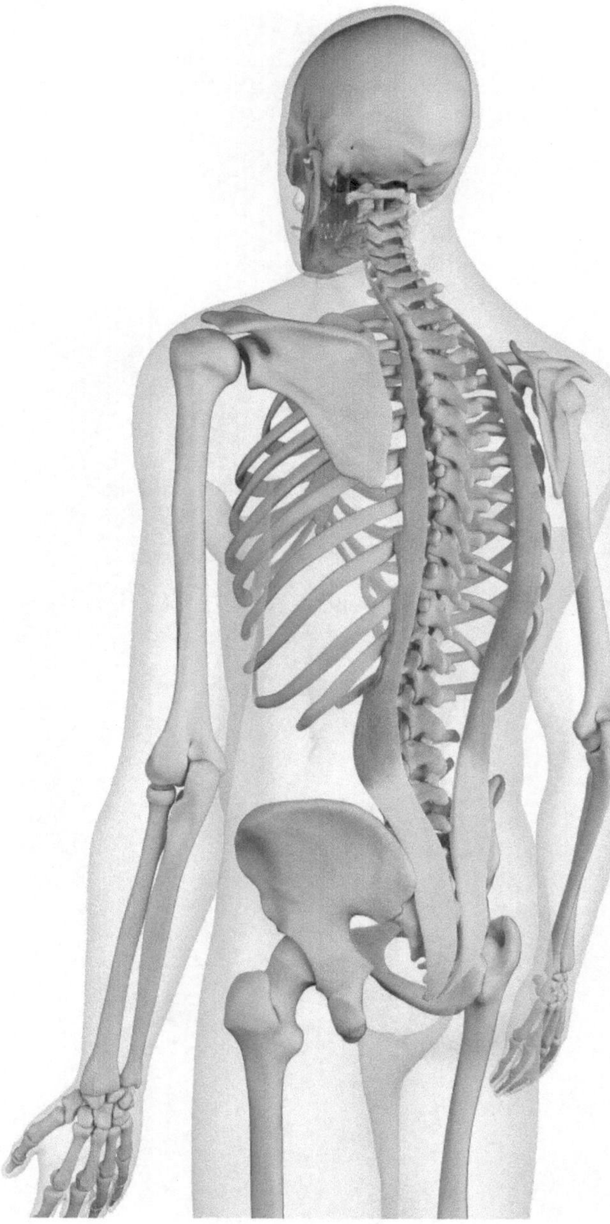

FIGURE 16.4 Iliocostalis

Source: Shutterstock ID: 303077270

The primary muscles of the trunk are also of interest; these include:

- The **transverse abdominus** (Figure 16.7), which originates on the internal surfaces of ribs 7–12 and inserts on the abdominal aponeurosis
- The **diaphragm** (Figure 16.8), which originates on ribs 7–12, inner surfaces of costal cartilages, xiphoid processes of sternum and bodies of L1-L2

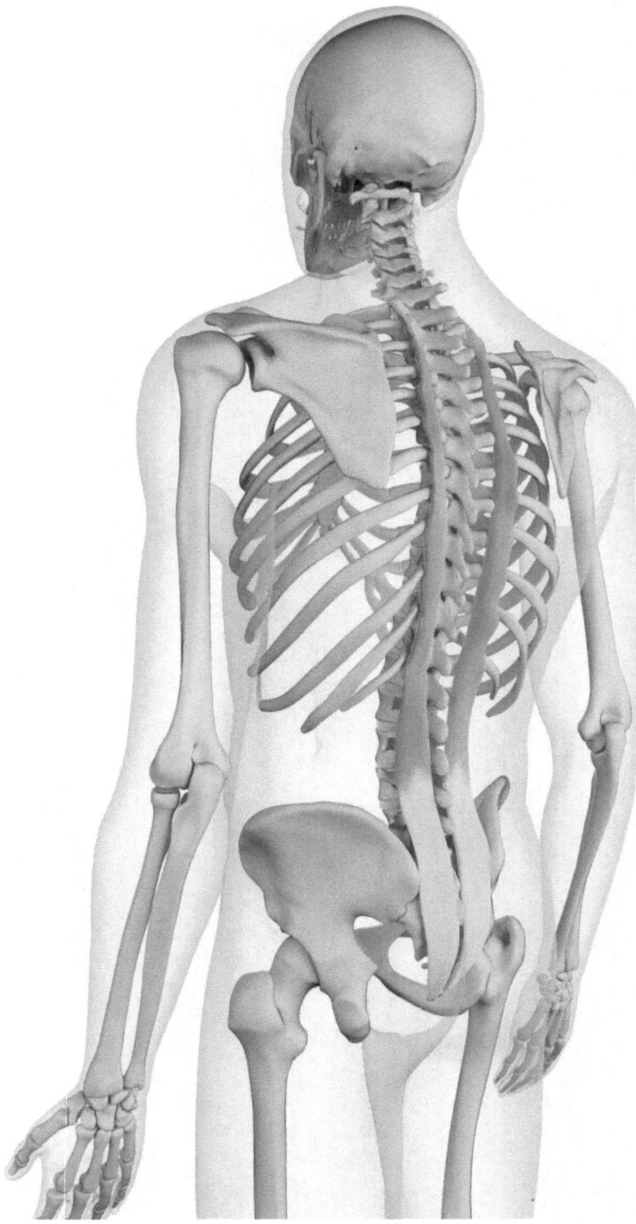

FIGURE 16.5 Longissimus

Source: Shutterstock ID: 303071012

- The **external oblique** (Figure 16.9), which originates on the external surfaces of ribs 5–12 and inserts on the anterior crest of ilium, pubic tubercle and abdominal aponeurosis
- The **internal oblique** (Figure 16.10), which originates on the thoracolumbar aponeurosis, iliac crest and lateral inguinal ligament and inserts on the internal surfaces of ribs 10–12 and abdominal aponeurosis.

These muscles act to provide spinal stabilisation. The internal and external oblique also produce rotation of the spine in ipsilateral and contralateral directions, respectively.

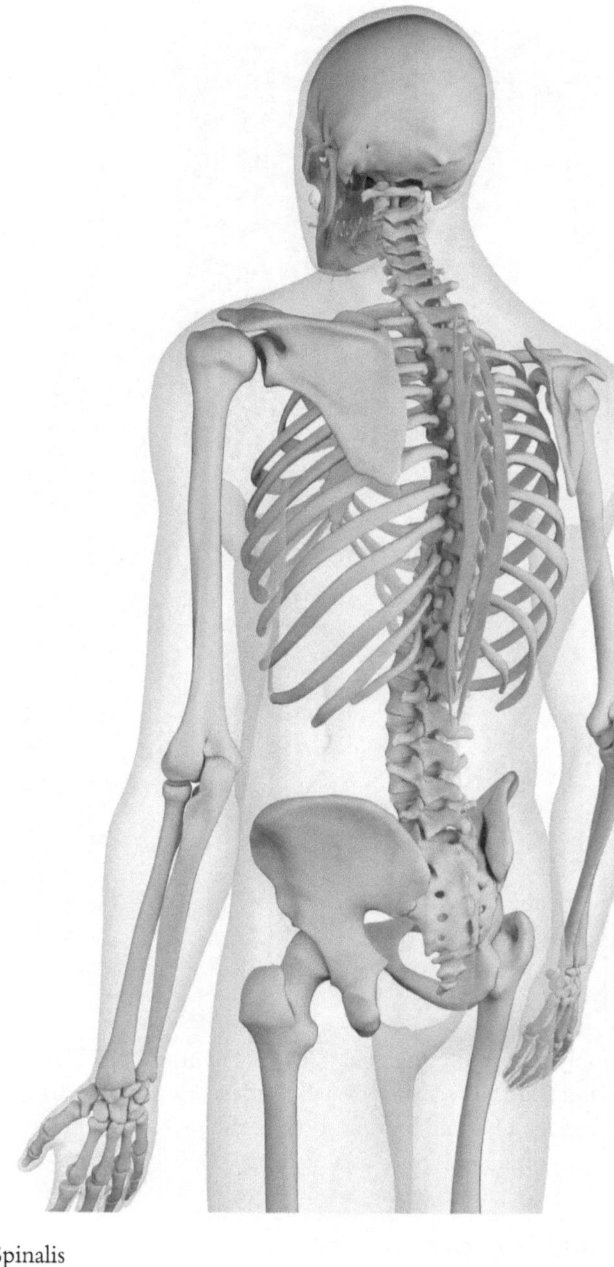

FIGURE 16.6 Spinalis

Source: Shutterstock ID: 303066767

16.2 Overview of Pathology

Occurrence and Socioeconomic Cost

LBP is one of the most endemic musculoskeletal problems in Western society, and lifetime prevalence rates are estimated to be at around 80% to 90% (Hoy et al., 2010). Consequently, it is one of the most common reasons for health-care consultation (Jöud, Petersson, & Englund, 2012) and has significant cost and societal impact with time off work and inability to return to

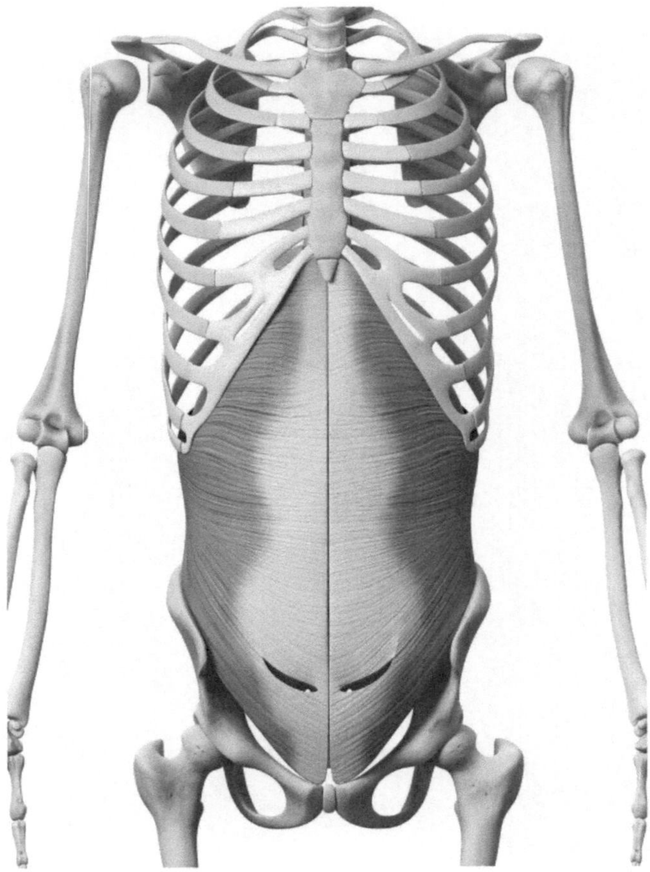

FIGURE 16.7 Transverse Abdominus

Source: Shutterstock ID: 223318138

usual function commonly reported (Hoy et al., 2014). The impact of LBP is ranked highest in terms of disability and sixth in terms of overall burden (Hoy et al., 2014), and therefore, effective strategies to manage LBP and prevent some of the myriad of effects of pain chronicity are highlighted as key considerations (Costa et al., 2013).

Characterisation and Chronicity

LBP is a condition characterised by pain located in the lower lumbar region and buttocks, with potential referral into the legs, particularly the posterior thigh and calf. The most common criterion definitions in the literature suggests that chronic LBP be categorised as continuous pain for a period equal to or greater than three months (Meucci, Fassa, & Faria, 2015). The percentage of people who live with LBP who go on to develop chronicity has been estimated to be as high as 70% (Itz, Geurts, Van Kleef, & Nelemans, 2013), and it is this group of people who pose significant cost and disability issues, with a significant proportion reporting ongoing issues following an episode of LBP (Costa et al., 2012).

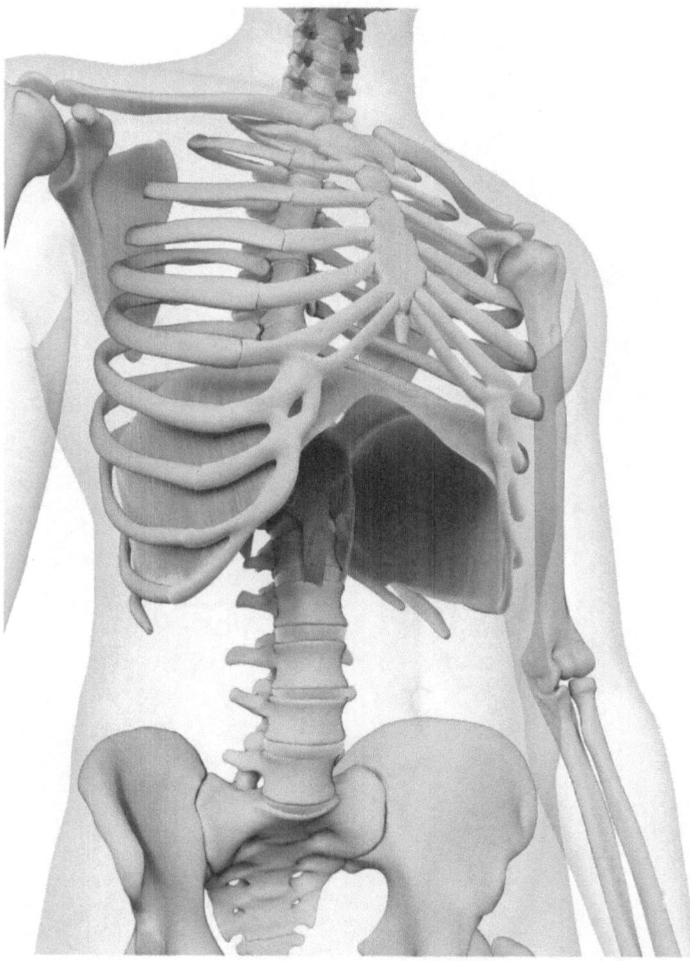

FIGURE 16.8 Diaphragm

Source: Shutterstock ID: 303082082

A proportion report having recurrent flare-ups and remissions whilst for others, the condition will become more long-standing and chronic (Dunn, Jordan, & Croft, 2006). Issues of recurrence and chronicity for people with LBP are critical to understand in the management of this condition, as is the unique 'lived experience' (Bunzli, Watkins, Smith, Schutze, & O'Sullivan, 2013) as the effects are different for each individual. It is therefore clear that this chronic condition has multiple effects on an individual and that their experiences of the condition and the way they cope with it are important to understand in management. This mode of assessment and management also aligns with a bio-psycho-social approach to the assessment, management and classification (McCarthy, Arnall, Strimpakos, Freemont, & Oldham, 2004). Such an approach looks at factors which contribute to the ongoing pain as well as facilitators and forms part of a comprehensive assessment and management approach for this condition (Waddell & Burton, 2005). The treatment for a person with LBP first requires consideration of the potential etiology and pathologies underlying the condition.

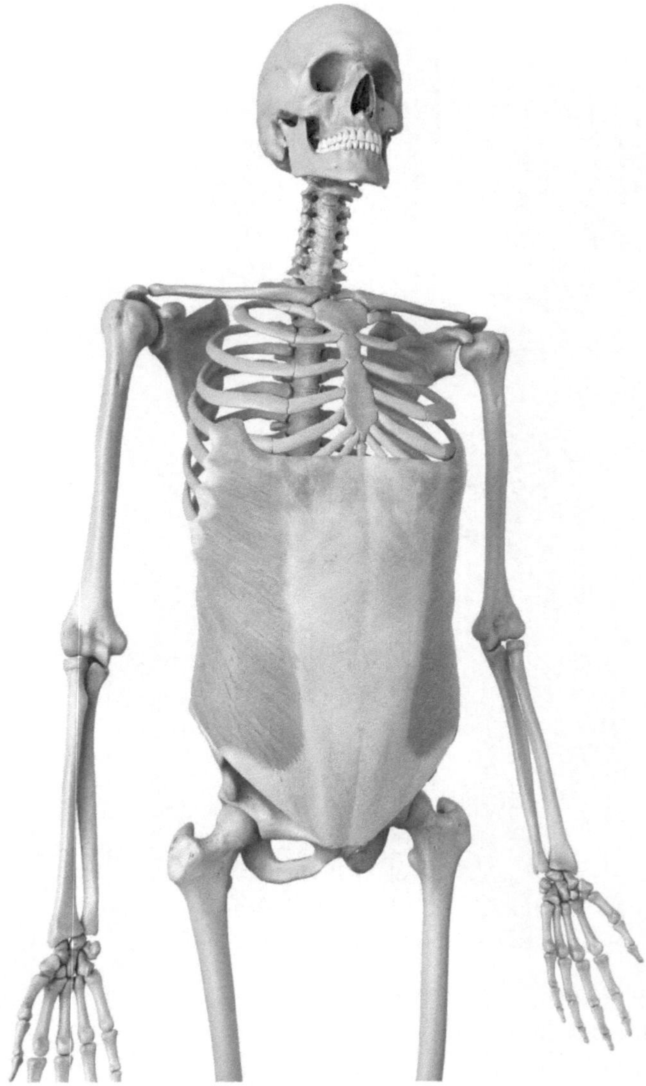

FIGURE 16.9 External Oblique

Source: Shutterstock ID: 293559047

Specific LBP

It is important to recognise those people who do not fit the criteria for non-specific LBP. These people represent a relatively smaller percentage of people presenting with chronic symptoms, estimated at 10% to 15% (Slade, Patel, Underwood, & Keating, 2015). These people may present with so called 'red flags' which represent non-benign spinal symptoms and include potential fracture, infection, inflammation, vascular insult, cauda equina and systemic illnesses, all of which can masquerade as spinal pain (Monie, Fazey, & Singer, 2016; Verhagen, Downie, Popal, Maher, & Koes, 2016). Differential diagnosis of this group is based on a

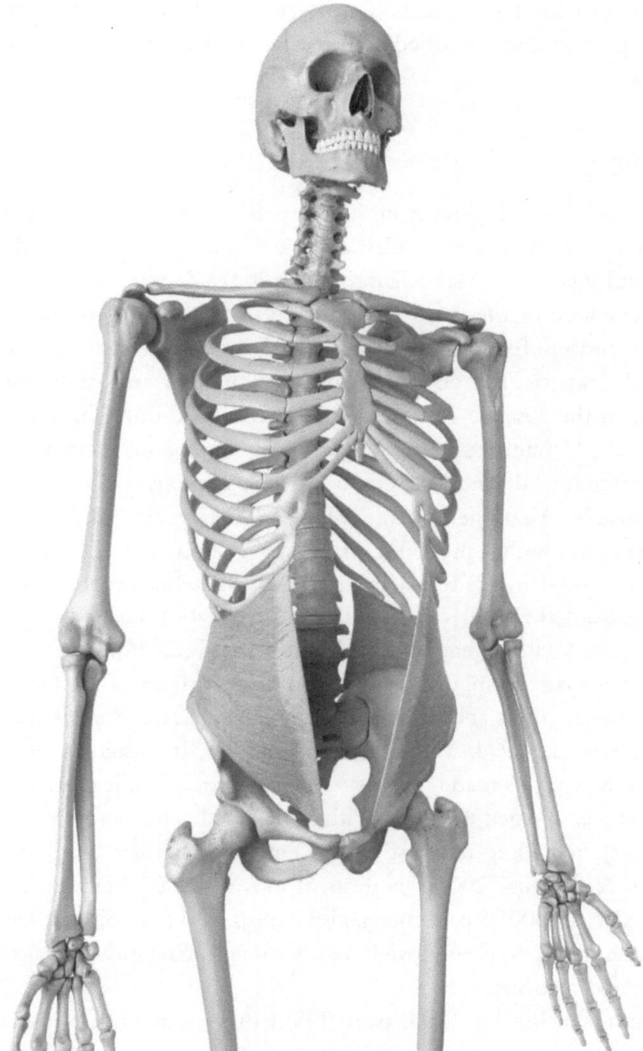

FIGURE 16.10 Internal Oblique

Source: Shutterstock ID: 293554241

thorough history and assessment, including pain history and behaviours, associated signs and symptoms, relevant medical history and family history, general overall health and consideration of the age of the person and other co-morbidities, including cardiovascular, respiratory, orthopedic and rheumatological conditions (Monie et al., 2016).

Also, within the group are those people who present with conditions for which there is a clear pathoanatomical diagnosis, including spinal stenosis (identified as a narrowing of the spaces within the spine, putting pressure on the nerves travelling through the spine), ankylosing spondylitis (an inflammatory condition which can cause vertebrae to fuse), discitis (inflammation in the intervertebral disc, usually resulting from infection) and radiculopathy (pinched nerve) with neurological signs (Deyo, Jarvik, & Chou, 2014). It is important that these people are 'flagged' and identified and that targeted specific management is instigated where appropriate.

Non-specific LBP

The development of pain can arise from any structure that possesses a nerve supply. Key structures that have been implicated in LBP include the disc, facet joints and sacroiliac joints, nerves, muscles and ligaments (Manchikanti et al., 2001; Zhang, Guo, Guo, & Wu, 2009). However, it is recognised that for most people with LBP, it is not possible to provide a clear pathoanatomical diagnosis. Indeed, radiological and diagnostic classification within this group is often equivocal, and findings do not correlate with signs and/or symptoms (Pillastrini et al., 2012) and, in the absence of serious underlying conditions, do not improve clinical outcomes (Chou, Fu, Carrino, & Deyo, 2009). This group has been classified as non-specific in that 'specific' differential diagnosis based on a tissue pathology module of pain is not always feasible and or possible (Airaksinen et al., 2006). Key diagnostic classifications have focused on three main structures within the spine: 1) the disc (Ogon et al., 2015), 2) the facet joints (Manchikanti et al., 2004) and 3) the sacroiliac joints (Manchikanti et al., 2001). Discogenic pain (pain arising from the disc) can include disc herniation and prolapse as well as disc degeneration associated with an ageing spine (Fardon et al., 2014). Furthermore, facet joint sprains, strains and arthritic changes within the articular surfaces of the facet joint, as well as changes in the sacroiliac joints and supporting ligaments, have also been attributed to causes of LBP (Schwarzer et al., 1994; Van Kleef et al., 2010). It should be acknowledged that differential diagnosis is problematic, and several diagnostic classification systems have been investigated. These classify people living with LBP based on a number of diagnostic variables (Riddle, 1998), including response to movement (Machado, De Souza, Marcelo Von Sperling, Ferreira, & Ferreira, 2006), patterns of movement (O'Sullivan, 2005), prognostic indicators (Jellema et al., 2005), pain mechanisms (Nijs et al., 2015) and beliefs (O'Sullivan, 2005). The assessment process is employed in each case to help guide management and facilitate rehabilitation and recovery.

People with non-specific low back pain (NSLBP) present with a myriad of signs and symptoms, and much of this is potentially linked to the process of pain central sensitisation (Sanzarello et al., 2016). As a result of this process, there are changes in the way that sensory information is processed within the peripheral and central nervous systems (CNS), resulting in changes in the way that people perceive and react to painful and non-painful stimuli, including tissue loading and movement (O'Neill, Manniche, Graven-Nielsen, & Arendt-Nielsen, 2007; Roussel et al., 2013). These are important considerations when assessing people with chronic pain and when considering whether the chronic pain is more strongly linked to mechanical and nociceptive elements with a more direct link to tissue loading and/or to changes in the pain processing pathways within the CNS.

It is therefore important for medical professionals to triage, through assessment, any person presenting with LBP to rule out more serious and/or potentially sinister causes of LBP if suspected. Once this has been done, referral can occur, and diagnosis should focus around management decisions and how contributory factors might influence a person's response to exercise and physical activity (Deyo, 2002).

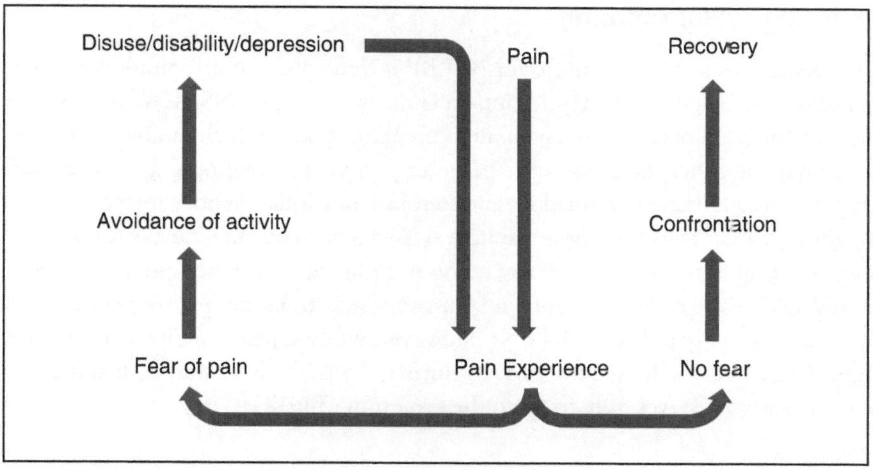

FIGURE 16.11 Fear-avoidance Model

16.3 Medication and Medical Management for People with LBP

In the UK, the National Institute for Health and Care Excellence (NICE) guidelines provide a process for the assessment and management of persons living with LBP. These should be a primary consideration in the prescription of exercise to ensure an interdisciplinary approach is adopted, placing the client at the centre of any interventional strategies. In most cases, a stratified management approach will be adopted, considering both need and intensity of support. Wherever the client places along the spectrum, exercise guidance/prescription is essential, unless contraindicated. As a result of specific diagnoses, exercise is an important part of both maintaining normal daily function and managing recovery from LBP. It is important that, where feasible, acute LBP is resolved swiftly since evidence supports that fear avoidance only intensifies as LBP continues from acute to chronic (Grotle, Vøllestad, Veierød, & Brox, 2004). As Figure 16.11 identifies, fear of pain and the concurrent avoidance of activity can result in escalating negative physiological and psychosocial experiences. The effects of common pharmacological treatments on the exercise response are the same as for osteoarthritis, presented in Table 18.1.

Active and Passive Treatment Strategies

Less intensive strategies for people with LBP might include recommendations to remain active/continue with normal daily activities as well as providing guidance on self-management. More complex strategies should outline specific exercise programmes with or without manual therapy and/or the use of psychological support, potentially in the form of cognitive behavioural therapy (CBT). Irrespective of the degree of intensity it is unlikely that exercise should be avoided, and indeed, physical inactivity is associated with higher degrees of LBP and disability (Teichtahl et al., 2015). Manual therapies in the form of manipulation, mobilisation or soft tissue treatment should only be considered as an adjunct to exercise strategies. And indeed, massage and pharmacological interventions are considered passive treatments that serve only to remedy the resultant symptoms (e.g. pain), not the cause of NSLBP (Shipton, 2018).

Pharmacological Intervention

Typical pharmacological interventions for NSLBP include use of non-opioid painkillers (e.g. paracetamol or codeine); non-steroid anti-inflammatory drugs (NSAIDs) (e.g. ibuprofen, naproxen, diclofenac); opioid-based painkillers on prescription, which inhibit neurotransmission of impulses at either the presynaptic nerve or postsynaptic neuron (e.g. dihydrocodeine, amitriptyline, gabapentin and tramadol); and steroidal anti-inflammatory injections (e.g. cortisone). Since many medications have resultant side effects such as fatigue, muscle stiffness and dizziness, it is important to consider any medication being used when prescribing exercise. Specifically, in the case of steroidal anti-inflammatory injections, people are generally advised to avoid strenuous activity for several days. However, whilst a pharmacological approach can reduce pain and thus might allow return to normal daily activity/exercise, it still exists as a passive treatment that serves only to abate the symptom of LBP.

Cognitive Behavioural Therapy and Cognitive Functional Therapy

An additional treatment strategy in conjunction with exercise is that of psychological intervention, normally in the form of CBT. The psychology of pain, fear avoidance and exercise form a complex relationship. Typically, CBT/cognitive functional therapy (CFT) intends to help a person with LBP by altering the way they think about their pain, as well as affecting behaviours. Interventions are often aimed at helping individuals 'make sense of their pain' through positive beliefs such as reduced fear, increased awareness, enhanced understanding and control of pain, adaptive coping, enhanced self-efficacy, confidence etc. (Khodadad, Letafatkar, Hadadnezhad, & Shojaedin, 2020). A systematic review from 1999 supports the use of CBT in producing positive changes for domains of pain experience, cognitive coping and reduced behavioural expression of pain (Morley, Eccleston, & Williams, 1999). It is also noteworthy that individualised treatment might produce more favourable outcomes than group-based strategies. A recent multi-centre randomised controlled trial (RCT) reported that one-to-one CFT, including interview, physical assessment by a physiotherapist. and resultant intervention. including: 1) 'making sense of pain', 2) Exposure with 'control' and 3) lifestyle change, was more efficacious in the reduction of disability at 6 and 12 months than a group-based exercise and education intervention (O'Keeffe, O'Sullivan, Purtill, Bargary, & O'Sullivan, 2020). However, whilst CBT appears to support multiple positive improvements, the efficacy of CBT in pain science education, graded exposure and multimodal interventions appears most effective for behaviour modification and compliance with exercise (Barbari, Storari, Ciuro, & Testa, 2020).

16.4 Risk Factors, Screening and Assessment

Risk Factors

A number of risk factors exist which predispose a person to NSLBP. Epidemiological research has reported risk factors to include jobs requiring repetitive heavy lifting, use of jackhammers or other similar tools/machinery (e.g. those with whole-body vibration) and prolonged operation of motor vehicles (Frymoyer et al., 1983). Furthermore, a higher prevalence of NSLBP exists in older adults, and specifically males compared to females, as well as those who have a low level of job satisfaction or poor working conditions (Valat, Goupille, &

Vedere, 1997). In addition, persons with LBP were more likely to be cigarette smokers with greater tobacco consumption (measured by the number of cigarettes per day and the number of years of exposure) equating to more severe LBP (Frymoyer et al., 1983). Finally, there is evidence suggesting that living with overweight and/or obesity might be linked to LBP (Valat et al., 1997). Based on this information, exercise practitioners should identify modifiable risk factors such as tobacco consumption and begin to address physical inactivity and obesity where possible within the capabilities of anyone living with LBP. Of course, epidemiological research does not identify causal relationships; however, whilst these factors might not individually be direct causes of LBP, they might do so in combination or lead to chronicity following prolonged exposure.

Screening for Contraindications

As an exercise practitioner working in an exercise referral scheme (ERS), it is important that you impress upon the client the need for them first to obtain medical referral prior to your provision of any exercise prescription. This step is important medically and legally in knowing that any exercise is not going to negatively impact medical diagnosis (for example, in a person with a posterior protrusion of the intervertebral disc, lumbar flexion exercises would be contraindicated). People with LBP should then undergo a thorough exercise risk assessment before exercise prescription (Shephard, 1988). As well as helping determine current physical activity behaviour (e.g. through the use of the international physical activity questionnaire [IPAQ]) (Lee, Macfarlane, Lam, & Stewart, 2011), this step provides an important part of identifying any additional conditions, injuries, or contraindications that might otherwise interfere with exercise prescription, examples of which might include pregnancy, osteoporosis, hypertension etc. There are few contraindications to low back exercise (Hancock, 2014); however, practitioners should treat each person individually and assess each exercise based on a risk-reward strategy.

Pain and Functional Assessment

The process of LBP treatment should result from both the assessment methods and a decision-making process to ensure both the safety of the person and the mediation of their dedication to exercise prescription. LBP assessment can often use quantifiable methods such as the Oswestry Disability Index (ODI), in which a person answers questions with numerical values about how any pain impacts their daily function (Fairbank & Pynsent, 2000), or a visual analogue scale (VAS), whereby a person simply places a vertical line intersecting a horizontal line to denote their current pain (Aoki et al., 2012). Alternatively, functional measures might be used to demonstrate the outcome of the experience of pain: e.g. strength (Bruce-Low et al., 2012), trunk range of motion (Tousignant, Poulin, Marchand, Viau, & Place, 2005), isolated lumbar range of motion (Graves et al., 1990a), balance and coordination (Behennah, Conway, Fisher, Osborne, & Steele, 2018) and muscular endurance (Conway, Behennah, Fisher, Osborne, & Steele, 2016). Since adherence to and compliance with exercise prescription for LBP are typically low (Middleton, 2004), an objective assessment of LBP and/or its functional impacts can be an important part of the initial exercise uptake. The exercise intervention, in turn, can lead to a greater reduction in pain as well as improvement in function. Any assessment and decision-making process is shown to be preferable and promote greater participation when it includes the person living with LBP (Slade, Patel, Underwood, & Keating,

2014). Furthermore, education on exercise and self-management can help those living with LBP better manage their condition (Cooper, Smith, & Hancock, 2009).

Any form of fitness testing is identifiable as exercise and therefore should not contravene medical referral, there should be no pre-existing contraindications identified from a health assessment, and the testing should link to the client goals and should be distinguishable in the informed consent documentation. Pre-testing based around the variables identified in a goal-setting session can be an important part of helping a person identify objective measures of functionality. Objective functional capacity tests include the six-minute walk test and the five-minute stair-climbing task (Smeets, Hijdra, Kester, Hitters, & Knottnerus, 2006). Trunk muscular endurance can be assessed using both the Biering-Sorensen test (Latimer, Maher, Refshauge, & Colaco, 1999), which requires the client to lie prone with arms folded across the chest and maintain the body in the unsupported position, and the prone straight-leg-raise test (Massoud Arab, Salavati, Ebrahimi, & Ebrahim Mousavi, 2007). However, the Biering-Sorensen test has shown inconsistent results with regard to reproducibility (Alaranta, Hurri, Heliövaara, Soukka, & Harju, 1994; Latimer, Maher, Refshauge, & Colaco, 1999). This is likely a result of multi-joint trunk extension, rather than isolated lumbar extension, evidenced by the fatigue of the hip extensors during the Biering-Sorensen test (Kankaanpää, Laaksonen, Taimela, Hänninen, & Airaksinen, 1998).

The gold standard for low-back strength assessment is the isolated lumbar extension machine (MedX, Ocala, FL). This is due to the range of pelvic restraints (Figure 16.12), ensuring that all movement is restricted to the lumbar region, rather than trunk extension through pelvic rotation (Graves et al., 1994; Smith, Bissell, Bruce-Low, & Wakefield, 2011; Steele, Bruce-Low, & Smith, 2015). Using this device, the range of motion of the lumbar spine can be objectively assessed, and isometric torque can be quantifiably measured

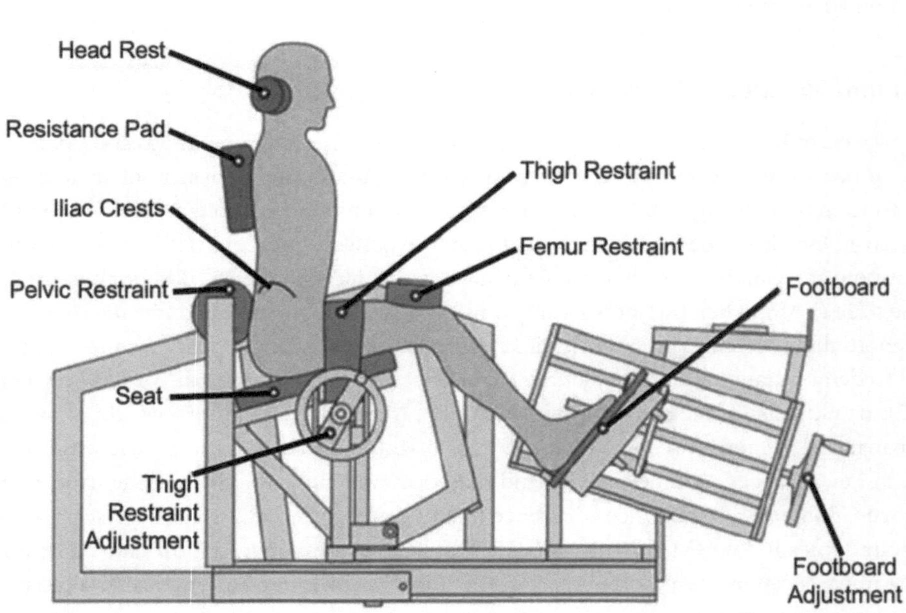

FIGURE 16.12 MedX Isolated Lumbar Extension Machine Pelvic Restraint System

anywhere within that range of motion (Graves et al., 1990a). Finally, measures of balance (Ruhe, Fejer, & Walker, 2011), which has been shown to be altered in LBP populations, might be utilised; the star excursion balance test (Behennah et al., 2018) requires a person to maintain a single-leg stance with their dominant leg while reaching with the contralateral leg as far along eight specified directions as possible. The client then returns to the centre of the grid on both feet while maintaining balance. Re-testing of these methods can reinforce positive physiological responses to exercise, as well as producing encouraging psychological emotions towards exercise. Knowing a timescale for re-assessment/testing can help a client with their mental approach to exercise over the short term, enhancing adherence and compliance. Notably, a person should have some contribution to the exercise prescription, perhaps in frequency and, ideally, type of exercise, to reinforce participation and identify and overcome potential barriers.

16.5 Acute Response to Exercise

Psychology of Exercise

Chronic pain is also associated with psychological distress and changes in the processing, perceptions and behavioural adaptations to pain (Waddell, Main, Morris, Di, & Gray, 1984). Such changes include increased fear avoidance behaviours, reduced pain self-efficacy and catastrophising around movement, exercise and activity (Kent & Keating, 2008; Wertli et al., 2014). People with these beliefs and behaviours have poorer prognosis with less tolerance for physical activity and exercise as a result of these behavioural adaptations to the pain (Crombez, Eccleston, Van Damme, Vlaeyen, & Karoly, 2012; Wideman et al., 2013). As a result, the management of these people employing exercise and physical activity also needs to take these psychological factors into consideration.

An important factor in the exercise treatment of LBP is being adaptable enough to consider different exercise philosophies and ensure not solely treating the ailment but rather, treating the person. In this sense, education and involvement in exercise methodologies will enhance adherence and compliance (Cooper et al., 2009; Slade et al., 2014), producing a more positive response. Furthermore, it maybe that for some people, exercise and physical activity do not reduce pain substantially but do improve quality of life and mobility. This issue also highlights the importance of recognising the bio-psycho-social nature of chronic pain (Gatchel, 2013) and, even more, the unique lived experience of LBP, as well as individual expectations around management and factors which influence its course. The multi-dimensional nature of pain also emphasises the fact that multiple outcomes should be considered when looking at the effects of an exercise or physical activity intervention for people with chronic pain (Dagenais, Tricco, & Haldeman, 2010). These outcomes include pain, disability, self-efficacy, fear avoidance, psychological distress, mood, sleep quality and fatigue levels, as well as biomechanical factors such as muscular strength and endurance (Searle, Spink, Ho, & Chuter, 2015; Van Middelkoop et al., 2011).

Exercise and physical activity interventions have demonstrated improvements in overall mental health, mood and the reduction of psychological distress (Hoffman & Hoffman, 2007; Penedo & Dahn, 2005) and depression in adult populations (Krogh, Nordentoft, Sterne, & Lawlor, 2011). Such mechanisms are potentially due to alterations in the way people think and feel about exercise and pain and alterations in the processing of pain (De Moor, Beem,

Stubbe, Boomsma, & De Geus, 2006; Peluso & Andrade, 2005). These offer potential mechanisms for improved function and pain reductions through exercise prescription. However, a key part of adherence and compliance is returning for repeated exercise therapy for the duration of an intervention. An exercise practitioner must recognise that the acute responses to exercise might not be immediately conducive to encouraging return (for example, a person might feel muscular soreness resulting from a bout of exercise) and work with a person presenting with LBP to acknowledge these acute responses.

Pain

Whilst massage therapy exists as a passive treatment to LBP, its popularity is likely a product of the immediate reductions in pain, disability and anxiety, as well as increases in pain pressure threshold (Buttagat, Eungpinichpong, Chatchawan, & Kharmwan, 2011). However, studies have suggested that exercise itself can act as an analgesic through a phenomenon termed exercise-induced hypoalgesia (Naugle, Fillingim, & Riley, 2012). It has been hypothesised that the endogenous opioid system is triggered by exercise-induced activation of arterial baroreceptors following increases in heart rate and blood pressure (Koltyn & Umeda, 2006; Nijs, Kosek, Van Oosterwijck, & Meeus, 2012). In support, moderate aerobic exercise (25 minutes at 70% peak aerobic uptake on a cycle ergometer) is shown to produce immediate reductions in LBP lasting up to 30 minutes post-exercise cessation (Hoffman, Shepanski, MacKenzie, & Clifford, 2005). Furthermore, a plethora of studies have supported isometric contractions of direct and indirect limbs reducing pain perception in asymptomatic persons (Naugle et al., 2012). Likewise, dynamic muscle actions using a typical resistance training protocol (e.g. bench press, leg press, pull-downs, and overhead press/arm extensions, for three sets of ten repetitions at 75% one-repetition maximum) can also reduce pain perception in asymptomatic persons (Focht & Koltyn, 2009; Koltyn & Arbogast, 1998). Research considering symptomatic persons is more limited, has predominantly considered persons living with fibromyalgia syndrome and has used isometric muscle actions. However, the evidence suggests that pain perception is also reduced (Naugle et al., 2012). To date, it appears that no published research has considered the acute effects of direct and indirect exercise on pain perception in people living with LBP. However, evidence suggests that exercise protocols which are painful might offer a small but significant benefit over pain-free exercise (Smith et al., 2017). Consequently, persons undertaking specific exercise to strengthen the lumbar extensors and improve spinal stabilisation ought to be advised that muscular pain during a bout of exercise should not be considered a barrier to a successful outcome.

Fatigue and Discomfort

At present, there are limited studies considering acute fatigue following specific lumbar/trunk exercise. However, a recent study of specific isolated lumbar extension exercise reported greater fatigue following a lighter load (50% maximal voluntary contraction) than a heavier load (80% maximal voluntary contraction) exercise condition (Stuart, Steele, Gentil, Giessing, & Fisher, 2018). Whilst this might not be surprising due to the greater number of repetitions performed and the longer time under load for the lighter-load condition, it is of notable importance for the functionality of persons with LBP. Furthermore, studies have suggested that lighter-load exercise infers greater degrees of discomfort than heavier loads when exercise is performed to a high degree of effort (Fisher, Stuart, Steele, Gentil, & Giessing, 2018; Stuart et al., 2018). This is also true of other muscles (Farrow, Steele, Behm, Skivington, & Fisher, 2020) and is of importance since medical professionals and exercise practitioners are often cautious and, as a result, prescribe lighter loads for exercise to people symptomatic of LBP. Based on this research, exercise prescription for people with LBP should consider more moderate loads to avoid unnecessarily long-exercise duration as well as needless high fatigue and discomfort.

A final study considering fatigue response reported significant reductions in force as a result of performing the kettlebell swing exercise (Edinborough, Fisher, & Steele, 2016). Whilst fatigue was less statistically significantly than with the isolated lumbar extension exercise, this is supported by a forthcoming discussion pertaining to muscle activation and kettlebell swings as a potentially efficacious and low-tech method of strengthening the lumbar extensors and reducing LBP. This exercise has been anecdotally advocated for the reduction in LBP as a result of the bracing contraction at the top of the movement.

Muscle Activation

A key method of assessing the effectiveness of an exercise is through the use of surface electromyography (sEMG). In brief, sEMG can measure the electrical activity across a muscle and provide a proxy measure for the degree to which muscle fibers are being recruited; a higher EMG amplitude represents a greater recruitment of muscle fibers and thus a more forceful contraction. However, assessing the acute response through muscle activation is not necessarily indicative of chronic adaptations in strength or hypertrophy. Practitioners reading research are encouraged to be cautious over the interpretation of sEMG data, specifically of the multifidus and lumbar muscles, where crosstalk (readings from synergist muscles) can impact outcome data (De Luca, 1997; Stokes, Henry, & Single, 2003). Furthermore, sEMG measurements can provide no data on low-back pain symptoms and functionality. However, a number of studies have considered sEMG and electrical amplitude across the lumbar extensors, from which we are able to identify the potential efficacy of an exercise by appreciating whether it appropriately contracts the desired musculature. We have summarised the current body of research herein.

Multiple studies have compared the performance of isolated lumbar extension exercise to that of trunk extension exercise through the use of pelvic restraints, some of which report that single-joint lumbar extension (Figure 16.12) in which the pelvis is restricted produces greater activation of the muscles of the lumbar spine (Da Silva, Larivière, Arsenault, Nadeau, & Plamondon, 2009; Lee, 2015; San Juan et al., 2005), while others report no differences between single-joint lumbar- and multi-joint trunk-extension exercises (Udermann et al., 1999; Walsworth, 2004). However, the issue of sEMG in these studies is compounded by variance in load. The studies suggesting greater activation of the lumbar musculature all used relatively light loads (40–50% one-repetition maximum) (Da Silva et al., 2009; Lee, 2015; San Juan et al., 2005), whereas the studies reporting no differences between isolated lumbar extension and trunk extension used heavier loads (~80% one-repetition maximum) (Udermann et al., 1999; Walsworth, 2004). Load is well established as a factor for consideration when using sEMG; a heavier load will produce greater sEMG readings because a greater number of motor units and corresponding muscle fibers are required to contract synchronously to overcome that load. However, whilst the use of a lighter load will produce lower sEMG amplitude values, with each successive repetition, there is dropout and subsequent sequential recruitment of additional motor units to continue performing repetitions (Fisher, Steele, & Smith, 2017).

Studies considering sEMG and trunk extension exercise using a Roman chair have shown significant activation of the lumbar extensors (Larivière et al., 2011; Mayer, Verna, Manini, Mooney, & Graves, 2002). However, data suggests lower activation of the muscles of the lower back compared to the hip extensor muscles (Larivière et al., 2011). Interestingly, analysis of kinematics in this study showed a progressive decrease (11°) in the lumbar range of motion and a concurrent increase in hip (2°) and thoracic (7°) range of motion during the exercise (Larivière et al., 2011). This might support the efficacy of this exercise for initial repetitions, but as repetitions are continued, fatigue of the lumbar extensors causes a shift in the mechanics of the exercise. A further study highlighted that, where pelvic rotation is restricted in the Roman chair exercise, the lumbar extensor activation can be increased (Mayer et al., 2002), and furthermore, where the angle of the Roman chair is altered from 45° to horizontal, the lumbar muscle activation increases further (Mayer et al., 1999). Notably, lumbar activation is also increased when the pelvic rotation is restricted in floor-based exercises such as the prone trunk extension (dorsal raise) and other co-contraction spinal stabilisation exercises (Shirado, Ito, Kaneda, & Strax, 1995). Exercises such as abdominal hollowing (Vezina & Hubley-Kozey, 2000), single leg lift and single left coupled with contralateral arm extension (bird-dog) from four-point kneeling (Stevens et al., 2007) have also shown muscle activation of the erector spinae group and multifidus specifically, although these were notably lower than other trunk muscles (external oblique and rectus abdominus) in asymptomatic persons.

Other studies have considered sEMG and reported notable amplitude along the lumbar extensors during hip extension exercises (see Figure 16.13) such as the Romanian (Chulvi-Medrano et al., 2010), sumo and conventional deadlift variations (Escamilla, Francisco, Kayes, Speer, & Moorman, 2002). Evidently, the lumbar muscles are activated in performance of hip extension exercise; however, this is to maintain a neutral spine rather than produce lumbar extension. Finally, a case study has reported around 50% maximal voluntary contraction of the lumbar extensors during a kettlebell swing (hip extension) exercise using only 16 kg (McGill & Marshall, 2012). The authors also reported that by the nature of the abdominal bracing and abdominal muscular pulses, the kettlebell swing can provide a unique loading pattern to the lumbar and trunk muscles, which might support restoration and enhancement of low back health (McGill & Marshall, 2012). Chronic adaptations to exercise types will be discussed in the next section. However, whilst sEMG data can suggest exercise efficacy based on muscle activation, we should remain cautious that sEMG is not necessarily indicative of chronic adaptations to exercise.

Motor Control

People living with LBP often present with trunk muscle motor control deficiencies. For example, in persons with LBP, activity of the multifidus is often delayed (MacDonald, Moseley, & Hodges, 2009) and reduced (Danneels et al., 2002; Sihvonen, Lindgren, Airaksinen, & Manninen, 1997), and concurrent activity of the superficial trunk muscles is increased compared to asymptomatic persons (Arendt-Nielsen, Graven-Nielsen, Svarrer, & Svensson, 1996; Hodges & Moseley, 2003a; Radebold, Cholewicki, Polzhofer, & Greene, 2001). This change in motor control appears to impact spinal loading and movement biomechanics and likely

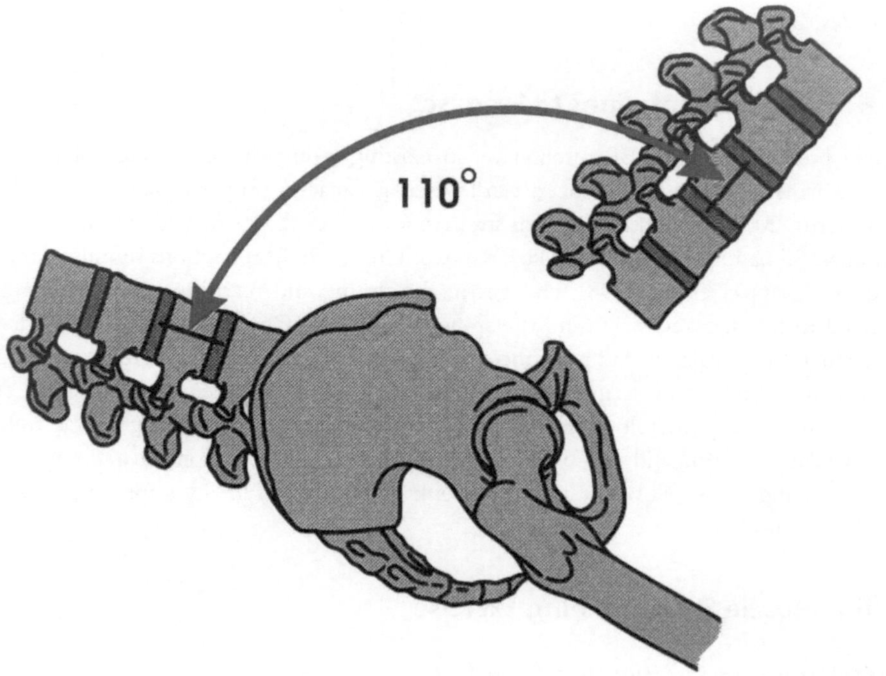

FIGURE 16.13 Hip Extension Using Solely Pelvic Rotation

increases the recurrence of LBP (Hodges & Moseley, 2003b). Repeated voluntary contraction of specific muscles has been shown to be more effective than co-contraction training of the trunk muscles for immediate improvements in motor control in people with LBP (Hall, Tsao, MacDonald, Coppieters, & Hodges, 2009). Furthermore, whilst specific motor training of the paraspinal muscles and trunk extension tasks appear equally efficacious in improving motor control timing of the lumbar multifidus during rapid-arm tasks, only the motor training exercise produced increases in muscle activation of the multifidus during slow trunk movements (Tsao, Druitt, Schollum, & Hodges, 2010). Consequently, prescription of exercises might best focus on specific and deliberate contraction of muscles rather than compound movements for both acute responses and chronic training adaptations.

Boom or Bust

Behavioural adaptions to pain also include people who develop a boom-or-bust relationship with their pain (Birkholtz, Aylwin, & Harman, 2004). People living with LBP will often overdo physical activity when the pain is feeling better and then, as a result, have an exacerbation of their pain and consequently reduce their physical activity. Such behaviours are commonly reported (Cane, Nielson, McCarthy, & Mazmanian, 2013) and act as a potential barrier to effective management of pain through activity and exercise (Andrews, Strong, & Meredith, 2015). Pain education and the use of various exercise programmes including graded physical activity use conditioning to encourage healthy behaviours by engaging in activities with tolerable pain to achieve functional goals (Macedo, Smeets, Maher, Latimer, & McAuley, 2010).

16.6 Chronic Adaptations to Exercise

People presenting with LBP often have co-existing reductions in a range of physiological impairments, including reduced cardiovascular capacity (Smeets, Wittink, Hidding, & Knottnerus, 2006), diminished lumbar strength (Graves et al., 1990), reduced spinal mobility (Thomas, Silman, Papageorgiou, Macfarlane, & Croft, 1998), reductions in muscular endurance (Kankaanpää et al., 1998), changes in the timing and recruitment of muscle groups involved in moving and stabilising the spine (van Dieën, Cholewicki, & Radebold, 2003) and reductions in balance and proprioception (Behennah et al., 2018; Verbunt et al., 2003). In providing exercise prescription for a person with LBP, an exercise professional should acknowledge these physiological deficiencies with respect to the client goals, as well as to improve daily function and quality of life. Specific exercise prescription can attempt to resolve the underlying cause of LBP or at the least enhance quality of life by improving these functional measures.

16.6.1 Muscle Strengthening Exercise

The Deconditioning Hypothesis

A well-established theory is that of the deconditioning hypothesis, whereby a reduction in muscular size and strength of the lumbar extensors (possibly due to gluteal and hamstring dominance for trunk extension movement) is a causal factor in LBP, which, in turn, results in disuse of these muscles, leading to further deconditioning (Steele, Bruce-Low, & Smith, 2014). This is not necessarily a product of typical muscular deconditioning with age but is exaggerated as a result of the specific disuse of the lumbar muscles. It was earlier stated that occupations that require repetitive heavy lifting can be a risk factor for LBP. This is likely a result of the dominance of the leg and hip extensor muscles through lifting and subsequent adaptations in strength whilst the lumbar extensors are challenged through this movement but do not receive adequate stimulus to adapt.

In addition, physical inactivity can be a risk factor. In some population groups, people who performed poorly in markers of physical function were strongly associated with inactivity and LBP (Tagliaferri et al., 2020). Supporting this, atrophy of the lumbar muscles (Wallwork, Stanton, Freke, & Hides, 2009) and altered recruitment patterns seem to support recurrence and continuance of LBP, potentially resulting from disuse and inactivity (Danneels et al., 2000; MacDonald, Moseley, & Hodges, 2009). Conclusively, physical activity and exercise seem to be integral to maintaining and improving quality of life and physical function in people with LBP, and physical activity of sufficient intensity of effort to improve physical fitness (e.g. muscular strength and endurance and aerobic capacity) shows reductions in LBP (Heneweer, Picavet, Staes, Kiers, & Vanhees, 2012). Exercise is further recommended since, based on the deconditioning hypothesis, it treats the cause of the pain. In contrast, passive approaches to LBP, such as most types of medication, as well as massage and acupuncture, only serve to treat the symptoms of LBP. Based on the deconditioning hypothesis, exercising the lumbar extensors and spinal stabilisers at an intensity of effort high enough to improve muscular strength and function can serve to reduce the severity and recurrence of LBP (Carpenter & Nelson, 1999; Risch et al., 1993; Steele, Bruce-Low, & Smith, 2015).

Approaches to Exercise Prescription

Exercise interventions include targeting a range of outcome measures, typically strength, flexibility, neuro-muscular motor control, aerobic fitness and stability (Hayden, Van Tulder, & Tomlinson, 2005). Of course, these should be selected based on client goals and assessment. Current evidence shows pain reduction and functional improvements are greater where components of an exercise programme include targeting strength increases of key trunk and pelvic muscles and coordination/stabilisation exercises. However, the evidence for aerobic exercises is less clear (Searle et al., 2015). Indeed, the largest effect size of all the exercise groupings was noted in the strength/resistance trials that concentrated on whole-body and trunk muscles. The results of subgroup analysis show preliminary support for exercises that target multiple muscle groups (Searle et al., 2015). However, exercise dosage, including duration, load and method of training, are still unclear in relation to how they affect LBP, so these variables should be managed in consultation with each individual. The following sections will discuss different approaches to exercise focused on strengthening the muscles of the lumbar spine, trunk and pelvis.

Different Types of Back Extension

A key concept herein is the difference between single-joint isolated lumbar extension and multi-joint trunk extension. The former is movement of only the lumbar vertebrae through flexion and extension and is normally accomplished through restraining movement of the pelvis in some way, whereas the latter includes pelvic rotation through shortening of the gluteal and hamstring muscles. This is often referred to as lumbo-pelvic rhythm. Figures 16.13 through 16.15 (reproduced with permission) demonstrate that back extension movement can be achieved in three separate ways (Jones, 1993).

Hip extension can be performed solely by rotation of the pelvis (Figure 16.13). The lumbar vertebrae effectively remain unmoved (although musculature supporting the vertebrae will contract isometrically to stabilise and retain a natural lumbar curve). However, the hip-extension movement comes from the gluteal and hamstring muscles rotating the pelvis. Examples of this movement are typically Romanian deadlift, kettlebell swing, and squat exercises.

Trunk extension can be performed as a compound movement of pelvic rotation and lumbar extension (Figure 16.14). As in Figure 16.13, pelvic rotation has been performed by contracting the gluteal and hamstring muscles; however, in addition, the lumbar extensor muscles have contracted to perform extension/hyperextension of the lumbar spine. Examples of this movement are typically Roman chair and dorsal raise exercises, which notably do not show the same degree of pelvic rotation shown in Figure 16.14 but which do produce significant activation of the hip-extension musculature.

Isolated lumbar extension is shown in Figure 16.15. This is normally achieved through a restraint system preventing pelvic rotation (e.g. thigh restraint and/or seatbelt and/or footboard) on an exercise machine. This might also be achieved to some extent when using a

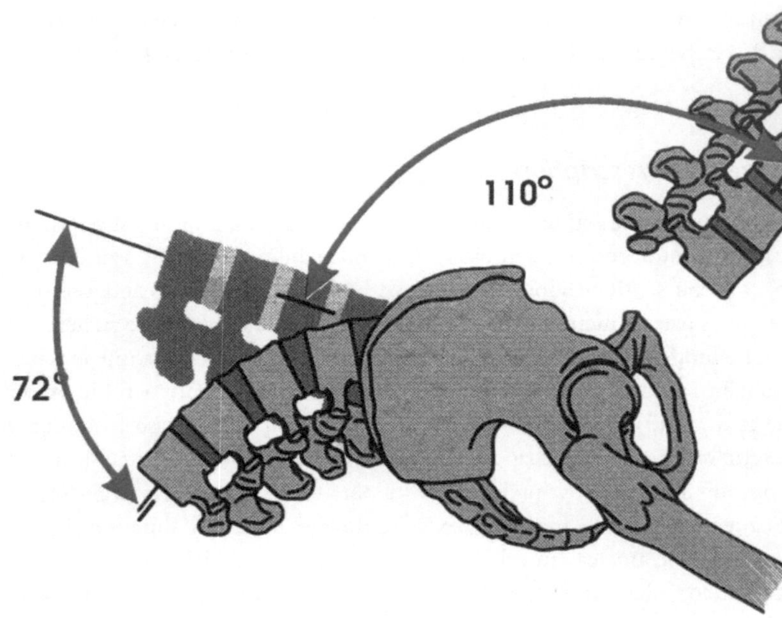

FIGURE 16.14 Trunk Extension Using Combined Pelvic Rotation and Lumbar Extension

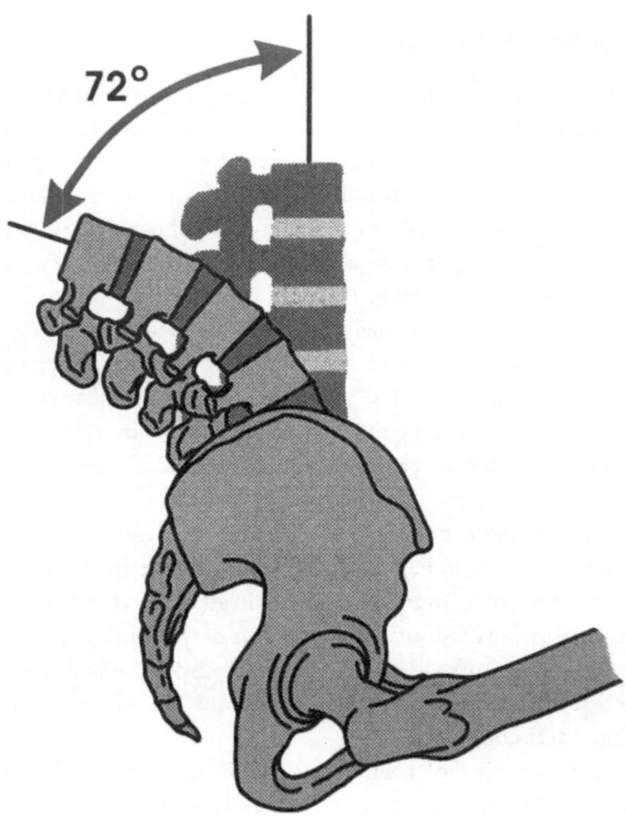

FIGURE 16.15 Isolated Lumbar Extension

Roman chair in such a way that the pelvis is positioned against the pad, preventing hip rotation (Mayer et al., 2002).

Isolated Lumbar Extension Exercise

As stated, the lumbar extensors can be effectively isolated through a series of pelvic restraints (e.g. Figure. 16.12) preventing the hip extensor (gluteal and hamstring) muscles from assisting in lumbar extension exercise. A large body of research has supported the use of isolated lumbar extension exercise in producing significant increases in lumbar strength (Fisher, Bruce-Low, & Smith, 2013; Fisher et al., 2018) and concurrent reductions in LBP (Bruce-Low et al., 2012; Carpenter & Nelson, 1999; Risch et al., 1993; Steele et al., 2015) and disability (Steele et al., 2019) – although variability in response should be expected (Steele et al., 2017). Furthermore, this training modality has been proven efficacious using low volume (e.g. single set) and low frequency (e.g. once a week and even once every two weeks) protocols (Bruce-Low et al., 2012; Fisher et al., 2013; Graves et al., 1990b; Steele, Fitzpatrick, Bruce-Low, & Fisher, 2015). Notably, this low-volume, low-frequency approach has also produced significant hypertrophy in lumbar muscles (Foster et al., 1993), as well as increases in the bone-mineral density of the lumbar vertebrae in older adults as a result of a six-month intervention (Pollock et al., 1992). The efficacy of this approach is so well documented that it has been suggested to be the best option for treating LBP (Mayer, Mooney, & Dagenais, 2008). Notably, other research has considered alternative lumbar extension machines that do not fixate the pelvis and therefore do not isolate the lumbar extensors; however, these have failed to demonstrate increases in strength of the lumbar muscles when tested in isolation (Graves et al., 1994).

In one of the largest RCTs considering LBP, the MedX isolated lumbar extension machine (Figure 16.12) was used to treat 627 people with LBP (Nelson, Miller, Hogan, Wegner, & Kelly, 1995). The study included males and females aged between 14 and 65 years and having experienced LBP for an average of 26 months prior to treatment. Participants completed one hour of supervised exercise twice per week, during which time they completed isolated lumbar extension exercise, as well as aerobic exercise and strength training of other muscles (hamstrings, glutei and abdominals). Participants completed an average of 18 sessions (range 4–35) prior to discharge, when they were (nearly) pain-free and were no longer making objective increases in spinal function. Clients also received education where they watched videos, learned body mechanics and read specific literature.

At discharge, 76% of participants were graded by their response to exercise as excellent (46%) or good (30%) denoting substantial pain relief and improvement in strength. A further 14% were graded poor, showing strength increases but little or no reduction in LBP. All participants were then provided with a home exercise device to continue progressive resistance exercise of the trunk muscles. At an average of 13 months post discharge, participants (n = 495) completed a survey of their current lumbar status; of those attaining good or excellent results at discharge, 94% reported continued or maintained improvement. Whilst this study clearly supports the efficacy of isolated lumbar extension exercise, it also demonstrates the importance of education and continuous adherence to exercise for the lumbar and trunk muscles. Furthermore, whilst isolated lumbar extension exercise appears the gold standard for specifically training the lumbar extensors, an obvious limitation is the cost and potential inaccessibility of equipment which might properly stabilise the pelvis, preventing rotation and isolating the lumbar spine. Consequently, more low-tech methodologies have been investigated.

Trunk Extension Exercise

Trunk extension exercise is typically a back-extension movement in which pelvic rotation is permitted, allowing activation of the hip extensor muscles (Figure 16.14). For the purposes of this chapter, this refers to Roman chair and dorsal raise exercises and back-extension resistance machines without pelvic restraint. The 45° Roman chair exercise (discussed previously in the context of acute responses in muscle activation) has been shown to increase trunk extension endurance (as measured by the Biering-Sorenson test) by 42% in asymptomatic persons following an eight-week training intervention (Verna et al., 2002). However, even after a 12-week progressive resistance training intervention, participants failed to show any increases in isolated lumbar extension strength, suggesting that there had been no training adaptation to the lumbar extensor muscles specifically (Mayer, Udermann, Graves, & Ploutz-Snyder, 2003; Verna et al., 2002). Prone dorsal raise and leg lift when stabilised at the pelvis and combined with other spinal stabilisation exercises can produce increases in the cross-sectional area of the multifidus when a five-second pause is maintained in the maximally contracted position (Danneels et al., 2001). Finally, trunk extension and flexion exercises performed on Nautilus resistance machines showed increases in both flexion and extension strength as well as the lumbar extensor cross-sectional area (Parkkola, Kujala, & Rytökoski, 1992). However, it is not clear to what extent the pelvis might have been restrained or how these responses might compare to other exercises.

Hip Extension

Hip extension exercise is defined herein as an exercise in which the lumbar spine remains neutral in position, and movement occurs through rotation of the pelvis (Figure 16.13). Whilst it is likely that the lumbar extensors play a key role in stabilising the spine to prevent unwanted spinal flexion, they are not considered the prime movers in these exercises. However, intervention studies have reported favourable outcomes from the use of kettlebell swing exercises in people with LBP, including a reduction in low back pain (Jay et al., 2011) and improvements in postural coordination (Jay et al., 2013). As mentioned previously, this exercise has been hypothesised to be beneficial in reducing LBP as a result of the bracing spinal stabilisation in the final/finishing position of the exercise, rather than as a result of the hip extension element. Notably, the participants, whilst symptomatic, were relatively low in LBP (they rated their pain 2.8 out of 10, reducing to 1.4 following an eight-week intervention) (Jay et al., 2011, 2013). However, this exercise might not be suitable for those experiencing higher degrees of LBP.

Other studies have reported that hip extension exercises such as the Romanian deadlift (Fisher et al., 2013), back squat and hip thrust (Hammond et al., 2019) provide no training effect to the lumbar extensors when tested for isolated isometric strength increases in asymptomatic persons. To date, there are no published studies considering the efficacy of these exercises in reduction of pain in people with LBP.

Spinal Stabilisation

Alternate theories have proposed that no single muscle is key to achieving lumbar spine stability, and thus recommendations have focused on rehabilitation programmes to involve the entire spinal and trunk musculature. The evidence suggests that spinal stabilisation exercises focused on trunk stability (facilitation of deep muscles of the spine) can be more effective than manual therapy or education alone (Goldby, Moore, Doust, & Trew, 2006), as well as reducing recurrence of LBP at one and three years (305 and 35%, respectively) (Hides, Jull, & Richardson, 2001). Other studies have suggested that spinal stabilisation is equally effective as other forms of general exercise in the management of LBP (Slade & Keating, 2006; Smith, Littlewood, & May, 2014). Strengthening exercises for the lumbar spine follow basic principles (Akuthota, Ferreiro, Moore, & Fredericson, 2008) whereby muscle strength and endurance are first assessed using muscle endurance tests such as the Biering-Sorenson test, pelvic side bridge/plank endurance test (quadratus lumborum endurance strength, leg-lowering test for lower abdominal strength), modified Trendelenburg test or single-leg squat test. Following this, co-contraction exercises such as the front bridge/plank, side bridge/plank and bird-dog, which require maintenance of a neutral lumbar curve, are performed (McGill, 2015).

In addition, lateral flexion exercises to stimulate coactivation of the extensors and flexors (Konrad, Schmitz, & Denner, 2001) and hollowing and bracing exercises (e.g. the cat-camel) have also been evidenced for the training of the transverse abdominus and internal oblique (Barnett & Gilleard, 2005) in people with LBP. However, contradictory evidence exists. Following three months of rehabilitation, including single-leg lift and single-leg lift coupled with contralateral arm extension (bird-dog) from four-point kneeling, prone bilateral hip extension and other exercises intended to co-contract the spinal stabilisers, there were no increases in spinal flexion or extension strength or muscle activation of the rectus abdominus, external oblique and multifidus (Arokoski, Valta, Kankaanpää, & Airaksinen, 2004).

Nevertheless, spinal stabilisation exercises have been shown to improve balance, reduce pain and increase the lumbar multifidus cross-sectional area in people with NSLBP (Chung, Lee, & Yoon, 2013). Furthermore, other research has reported that spinal stabilisation exercises such as hip extension from four-point kneeling (in combination with other trunk extension exercises) can produce meaningful increases in the multifidus cross-sectional area only when there is an isometric pause (five seconds) at the maximally contracted position (Danneels et al., 2001). Based on the literature underpinning the use of isolated lumbar extension exercise, it appears that multiple modalities of training the lumbar extensors and spinal stabilising muscles can be used; however, an emphasis should be placed on the quality and intensity of the contraction to ensure sufficient stimulus for strength increases, muscle hypertrophy and reduction in LBP.

16.6.2 Aerobic Exercise

It would be remiss not to discuss the potential benefits of aerobic exercise on LBP. Multiple studies have supported pain improvement (measured by pain pressure threshold, visual analogue scale and pain questionnaires) over interventions lasting between 6 and 12 weeks through the use of aerobic exercise on LBP (Chan, Mok, & Yeung, 2011; Chatzitheodorou, Kabitsis, Malliou, & Mougios, 2007; Chatzitheodorou, Mavromoustakos, & Milioti, 2008; Shnayderman & Katz-Leurer, 2013). However, the studies using lower intensities, walking at 50% heart rate reserve (HRR) (Shnayderman & Katz-Leurer, 2013) and increasing intensity weekly from 40% HRR up to 85% HRR throughout the intervention (Chan et al., 2011) showed increases comparable to traditional physiotherapeutic approaches including passive treatments and spinal stabilisation exercises. In studies with higher intensities (85% HRR) across 12-week interventions, participants showed similar decreases in pain (Chatzitheodorou et al., 2007; Chatzitheodorou et al., 2008) to those in the studies using lower intensities (Chan et al., 2011; Shnayderman & Katz-Leurer, 2013). In review, it has been suggested that aerobic exercise at 40% to 60% HRR should be promoted for NSLBP rehabilitation (Gordon & Bloxham, 2016).

16.6.3 Flexibility Training

Lastly, some studies have supported the inclusion of specific flexibility training in exercise prescription to decrease LBP (measured by VAS). In an RCT of 40 women with NSLBP, a group performing non-weight-bearing exercise, including mobility and stability exercises for the lumbo-pelvic spine, improved lumbar flexion and extension and decreased pain after a four-week intervention (Masharawi & Nadaf, 2013). In other research, six weeks of Pilates classes (one hour once a week) have improved hamstring and lower-back flexibility and reduced NSLBP (Gladwell, Head, Haggar, & Beneke, 2006), and a systematic review reported reductions in LBP for persons undertaking yoga (Cramer, Lauche, Haller, & Dobos, 2013). In addition to specific flexibility training, isolated lumbar extension resistance exercise has been shown to increase range of motion assessed using both isolated lumbar flexion/extension tests and functional tests such as the Shober's flexion test (Bruce-Low et al., 2012).

16.7 Exercise Prescription to Improve the Condition

This section will summarise these findings from acute and chronic responses to exercise for the management of NSLBP. It is important to remember that these processes should follow referral from a medical professional to confirm the nonexistence of any medical conditions that are contraindicative of the assessment and exercise prescription outlined.

Prior to exercise prescription, objective assessments of pain and function should be performed in accordance with each person's goals and experiences. Ultimately, these assessments will guide any exercise treatment. The body of research suggests that exercise for the management of LBP should be aligned with an education programme to support the individual and include a focus on the isolation of specific lumbar exercises. This is encouraged to help train the neuromuscular system to be better able to recruit these muscles, as well as improve strength and function and reduce mechanisms underpinning LBP. Evidence suggests this is done best using pelvic restraints preventing pelvic rotation where possible. Where this is not possible, and in addition, these exercises should be supplemented with spinal stabilisation exercises to improve trunk function, as well as additional muscle-strengthening exercises for the whole body, unless contraindicated. Exercise supervision is encouraged, and a controlled repetition duration with a pause at maximally contracted positions ensures the full activation of the desired muscles. A comprehensive whole-body muscle strengthening programme should serve to reduce pain through exercise-induced hypoalgesia as well as convey the multitude of additional physiological and psychological benefits of muscle-strengthening exercise (Fisher, Steele, Gentil, Giessing, & Westcott, 2017). All exercise should be performed to a high level of effort, using a moderate but manageable load, sufficient to catalyze adaptations in muscular strength and function. Particularly light weights might be avoided due to the high discomfort associated with the prolonged time under load. Intensity of effort appears more important than volume (number of sets performed) as well as frequency of exercise. Finally, for a holistic multi-modal approach, moderate-intensity aerobic exercise (40–60% HRR) and flexibility training for the lumbo-pelvic complex might also be included to both improve function and decrease pain. Whilst painful exercise should be avoided where possible to optimise adherence and compliance, people should be advised that muscular pain during a bout of exercise is not a barrier to successful outcome. Exercise practitioners are advised to make to clients aware of the potential boom-or-bust scenario and encourage them to use graded activity in their daily life.

Based on the research, whilst exercise prescription should be specific to an individual, centred around their goals, pain and function, exercise prescription should include

- Exercise to target the lumbar muscles specifically (e.g. isolated lumbar extension, Roman chair, dorsal raise etc., potentially with pelvic restraint where possible)
- Spinal stabilisation exercises to provide co-contraction to the other musculature of the trunk (e.g. front plank, side plank, bird-dog etc.)
- Additional muscle strengthening exercises (e.g. overhead press, chest press/press-up variant, seated row/pull-down exercise, seated knee extension and leg curl exercises and other supplementary exercises for smaller muscles (e.g. biceps and triceps) where appropriate/possible
- Moderate-intensity aerobic exercise (40–60% HRR)
- Flexibility exercises for the lumbo-pelvic complex

16.8 Case Study

Vijay is a 38-year-old male who presented with a five-year history of non-specific chronic low back pain. On multiple occasions, Vijay had been prescribed painkillers and other non-steroidal anti-inflammatory medication; however, he expressed reluctance to use pharmaceutical remedies over a prolonged period. He had also sought massage and acupuncture, but these treatments failed to deliver anything more than temporary symptomatic relief. Vijay has a young daughter and is encouraged by her efforts to exercise, so he sought exercise guidance to improve his own health and fitness and perhaps improve his management of LBP.

The exercise practitioner reviewed a medical referral confirming no contraindications to muscle-strengthening exercise and performed a pre-exercise medical assessment and client lifestyle questionnaire confirming client motivation and goals. Under consultation, Vijay signed informed consent acknowledging understanding of the assessment and exercise programming.

Vijay completed a revised Oswestry low back pain and disability index, as well as a star excursion balance test, range of motion test and isometric strength test for his lumbar muscles using an isolated lumbar extension machine. His results confirmed considerable and regular pain as well as poor balance and coordination in posterior movements, limited range of motion into flexion and weakness in his lumbar muscles.

It was agreed between Vijay and the exercise practitioner to undertake once-weekly isolated lumbar extension strength training and, concurrently, complete a whole-body muscle strengthening programme consisting of eight to ten additional exercises. Notably, this programme also included spinal stabilisation exercises, including the front bridge/plank and side bridge/side plank. Whilst once a week appears a low frequency, this fitted with Vijay's schedule, and he adopted a minimal dose approach to avoid disengagement and allowed frequency to be increased if necessary/appropriate. Furthermore, Vijay was engaging in aerobic exercise in the form of walking for around 30 minutes, two or three times week on his own time. Vijay's enthusiasm throughout the first ten weeks was positive, and at reassessment, there was a clear reduction in pain and improvement in balance, strength, and range of motion. Based on this positive response, Vijay requested an increase in frequency of strength training sessions up to twice a week. Following a further ten weeks, Vijay continued to increase his functionality, although he showed lesser reductions in his LBP. Upon consultation, Vijay acknowledged that he had returned to playing cricket and gardening, hobbies he often enjoyed for many hours at a time, and that often resulted in increases in LBP for the subsequent 24 to 48 hours. The exercise practitioner addressed that these activities might be exacerbating his LBP and, whilst not discouraging participation, suggested that the time they were undertaken for should be managed. An education session was completed to assist Vijay in his understanding of LBP and graded exercise treatment.

At the time of Vijay's discharge, he had full range of motion and greater-than-normal low-back strength when tested using an isolated lumbar extension machine. His balance had also shown improvements, and objective assessment confirmed considerable reduction in low-back pain. Vijay was provided education as to how to complete a whole-body strength training program at his local gym, which included use of a low-back extension machine and the performance of spinal stabilisation exercises. Vijay was also enjoying attending a yoga class and other circuit-based fitness classes, which he felt improved his health and fitness as well as helping manage his low-back pain.

16.9 Summary/Key Points

- LBP is one of the most endemic musculoskeletal problems in Western society, and lifetime prevalence rates are estimated to be at around 80% to 90%.
- The percentage of people who suffer from LBP who go onto to develop chronicity has been estimated to be as high as 70%.
- Massage, acupuncture and pharmacological interventions are considered passive treatments that serve only to remedy the resultant symptoms, not the cause of LBP.
- People with LBP often have a range of physiological impairments, including diminished lumbar strength, reduced spinal mobility and reductions in balance and proprioception.
- Exercise is integral to improving quality of life and physical function in people with LBP, and, based on the deconditioning hypothesis, exercise treats the cause of the pain.
- Muscle-strengthening exercise of sufficient intensity of effort to improve physical fitness shows reductions in LBP.

- Exercises for LBP can be divided based on multi-joint hip and trunk extension and single-joint lumbar extension.

Study Tasks

1. Briefly explain the anatomy and function of the lumbar spine.
2. Describe the impact of LBP on Western society.
3. Define the prevalence and transition from acute to chronic low back pain.
4. Explain your understanding of the fear-avoidance model.
5. Massage, acupuncture and pharmaceutical treatments for LBP might not present a long-term remedy; please explain why.
6. People presenting with LBP often have what other co-existing physiological conditions?
7. Describe the deconditioning hypothesis.
8. Describe the three types of back-extension exercise and the differentiators, providing example exercises.
9. Describe the biomechanics of spinal stabilisation exercises.
10. Explain your understanding of a boom-or-bust relationship with LBP.

TABLE 16.1 At-a-Glance Summary Guide to Exercise Considerations for People with Low Back Pain

Pathophysiology Summary	NSLBP is characterised by pain located in the lower lumbar region and buttocks with potential referral into the legs, particularly the posterior thigh and calf. Key diagnostic classifications have focused on three main structures within the spine: the disc (e.g. disc herniation and prolapse as well as disc degeneration), facet joints (e.g. sprains, strains and arthritic changes within the articular surfaces of the facet joint) and changes in the sacroiliac joints and supporting ligaments.
Aims of Exercise	1. Alleviate pain symptoms through exercise-induced hypoalgesia. 2. Strengthen the muscles of the lumbar spine and trunk. 3. Reduce low back pain prevalence and severity.
Exercise Considerations (Including Contraindications)	Prescription should include muscle-strengthening exercise, spinal stabilisation exercise, aerobic exercise and flexibility training. Specific attention should be given to each person since pain presents as a lived experience and is not the same between any two people. Contraindications to low back muscle-strengthening exercise are limited but include any medically identified red flags and osteoporosis. Contraindications can also include hypertension and pregnancy, though exercise can normally be managed with restrictions in these groups.
Frequency	One to seven times a week, depending upon other variables.
Intensity of Effort	Muscle-strengthening exercise should be performed to a high degree of effort. Aerobic exercise can be more moderate (40–60% HRR).
Intensity of Load	Muscle strengthening should be completing using a load permitting 8 to 12 repetitions.
Time	For muscle strengthening, time under load should be ~60 to 90 seconds per exercise set. For aerobic exercise, bouts of ≥ 25 minutes are encouraged.
Type	Muscle-strengthening exercise and aerobic exercise.

(Continued)

TABLE 16.1 (Continued)

Common Medications Associated	Non-steroid anti-inflammatory drugs (NSAIDs) (e.g. ibuprofen, naproxen, diclofenac). Opioid-based painkillers (e.g. dihydrocodeine, amitriptyline, gabapentin and tramadol). Steroidal anti-inflammatory injections (e.g. cortisone).
Key Safety Considerations	Typical medications can have resultant side effects such as fatigue, muscle stiffness and dizziness, which should be considered. Other safety considerations include limited range of motion in lumbar flexion and extension and soreness during exercise.
Effect of Exercise on Conditions	Acutely, specific exercise might incur delayed onset muscle soreness or even soreness during the exercise, although this is noted not to negatively impact positive chronic adaptations. Patients are likely to experience acute reductions in pain as a result of exercise-induced hypoalgesia. Chronic adaptations to resistance exercise are the strengthening of the lumbar muscles and, ultimately, the reduction in prevalence and severity of low back pain.

References

Airaksinen, O., Brox, J. I., Cedraschi, C., Hildebrandt, J., Klaber-Moffett, J., Kovacs, F., et al. (2006). European guidelines for the management of chronic nonspecific low back pain. *European Spine Journal, 15*(Suppl 2), s192.

Akuthota, V., Ferreiro, A., Moore, T., & Fredericson, M. (2008). Core stability exercise principles. *Current Sports Medicine Reports*, 7(1), 39–44.

Alaranta, H., Hurri, H., Heliövaara, M., Soukka, A., & Harju, R. (1994). Non-dynamometric trunk performance tests: Reliability and normative data. *Scandinavian Journal of Rehabilitation Medicine, 26*(4), 211–215.

Andrews, N. E., Strong, J., & Meredith, P. J. (2015). Avoidance or incapacitation: A discussion on definition and validity of objective measures of avoidance, persistence, and overactivity. *The Clinical Journal of Pain, 31*(7), 670–672.

Aoki, Y., Sugiura, S., Nakagawa, K., Nakajima, A., Takahashi, H., Ohtori, S., et al. (2012). Evaluation of nonspecific low back pain using a new detailed visual analogue scale for patients in motion, standing, and sitting: Characterizing nonspecific low back pain in elderly patients. *Pain Research and Treatment*. doi: 10.1155/2012/680496.

Arendt-Nielsen, L., Graven-Nielsen, T., Svarrer, H., & Svensson, P. (1996). The influence of low back pain on muscle activity and coordination during gait: A clinical and experimental study. *Pain, 64*(2), 231–240.

Arokoski, J. P., Valta, T., Kankaanpää, M., & Airaksinen, O. (2004). Activation of lumbar paraspinal and abdominal muscles during therapeutic exercises in chronic low back pain patients. *Archives of Physical Medicine and Rehabilitation, 85*(5), 823–832.

Barbari, V., Storari, L., Ciuro, A., & Testa, M. (2020). Effectiveness of communicative and educative strategies in chronic low back pain patients: A systematic review. *Patient Education and Counseling, 103*(5), 908–929.

Barnett, F., & Gilleard, W. (2005). The use of lumbar spinal stabilization techniques during the performance of abdominal strengthening exercise variations. *The Journal of Sports Medicine and Physical Fitness, 45*(1), 38–43.

Behennah, J., Conway, R., Fisher, J., Osborne, N., & Steele, J. (2018). The relationship between balance performance, lumbar extension strength, trunk extension endurance, and pain in participants with chronic low back pain, and those without. *Clinical Biomechanics, 53*, 22–30.

Birkholtz, M., Aylwin, L., & Harman, R. M. (2004). Activity pacing in chronic pain management: One aim, but which method? part one: Introduction and literature review. *British Journal of Occupational Therapy, 67*(10), 447–452.

Bono, C. M. (2004). Low-back pain in athletes. *Journal of Bone and Joint Surgery, 86*(2), 382–396.

Bruce-Low, S., Smith, D., Burnet, S., Fisher, J., Bissell, G., & Webster, L. (2012). One lumbar extension training session per week is sufficient for strength gains and reductions in pain in patients with chronic low back pain ergonomics. *Ergonomics, 55*(4), 500–507.

Bunzli, S., Watkins, R., Smith, A., Schutze, R., & O'Sullivan, P. (2013). Lives on hold: A qualitative synthesis exploring the experience of chronic low-back pain. *The Clinical Journal of Pain, 29*(10), 907–916.

Buttagat, V., Eungpinichpong, W., Chatchawan, U., & Kharmwan, S. (2011). The immediate effects of traditional Thai massage on heart rate variability and stress-related parameters in patients with back pain associated with myofascial trigger points. *Journal of Bodywork and Movement Therapies, 15*(1), 15–23.

Cane, D., Nielson, W. R., McCarthy, M., & Mazmanian, D. (2013). Pain-related activity patterns: Measurement, interrelationships, and associations with psychosocial functioning *The Clinical Journal of Pain, 29*(5), 435–442.

Carpenter, D. M., & Nelson, B. W. (1999). Low back strengthening for the prevention and treatment of low back pain. *Medicine and Science in Sports and Exercise, 31*, 18–24.

Chan, C. W., Mok, N. W., & Yeung, E. W. (2011). Aerobic exercise training in addition to conventional physiotherapy for chronic low back pain: A randomized controlled trial. *Archives of Physical Medicine and Rehabilitation, 92*(10), 1681–1685.

Chatzitheodorou, D., Kabitsis, C., Malliou, P., & Mougios, V. (2007). A pilot study of the effects of high-intensity aerobic exercise versus passive interventions on pain, disability, psychological strain, and serum cortisol concentrations in people with chronic low back pain. *Physical Therapy, 87*(3), 304–312.

Chatzitheodorou, D., Mavromoustakos, S., & Milioti, S. (2008). The effect of exercise on adrenocortical responsiveness of patients with chronic low back pain, controlled for psychological strain. *Clinical Rehabilitation, 22*(4), 319–328.

Chou, R., Fu, R., Carrino, J. A., & Deyo, R. A. (2009). Imaging strategies for low-back pain: Systematic review and meta-analysis. *The Lancet, 373*(9662), 463–472.

Chulvi-Medrano, I., García-Massó, X., Colado, J. C., Pablos, C., de Moraes, J. A , & Fuster, M. A. (2010). Deadlift muscle force and activation under stable and unstable conditions. *The Journal of Strength & Conditioning Research, 24*(10), 2723–2730.

Chung, S., Lee, J., & Yoon, J. (2013). Effects of stabilization exercise using a ball on mutifidus cross-sectional area in patients with chronic low back pain. *Journal of Sports Science & Medicine, 12*(3), 533.

Conway, R., Behennah, J., Fisher, J., Osborne, N., & Steele, J. (2016). Associations between trunk extension endurance and isolated lumbar extension strength in both asymptomatic participants and those with chronic low back pain. *Paper Presented at the Healthcare, 4*(3), 70.

Cooper, K., Smith, B. H., & Hancock, E. (2009). Patients' perceptions of self-management of chronic low back pain: Evidence for enhancing patient education and support. *Physiotherapy, 95*(1), 43–50.

Costa, L. D. C. M., Maher, C. G., Hancock, M. J., McAuley, J. H., Herbert, R. D., & Costa, L. O. (2012). The prognosis of acute and persistent low-back pain: A meta-analysis. *Canadian Medical Association Journal, 184*(11), e613–e624.

Costa, L. D. C. M., Koes, B. W., Pransky, G., Borkan, J., Maher, C. G., & Smeets, R. J. (2013). Primary care research priorities in low back pain: An update. *Spine, 38*(2), 148–156.

Cramer, H., Lauche, R., Haller, H., & Dobos, G. (2013). A systematic review and meta-analysis of yoga for low back pain. *The Clinical Journal of Pain, 29*(5), 450–460.

Crombez, G., Eccleston, C., Van Damme, S., Vlaeyen, J. W., & Karoly, P. (2012). Fear-avoidance model of chronic pain: The next generation. *The Clinical Journal of Pain, 28*(6), 475–483.

Dagenais, S., Tricco, A. C., & Haldeman, S. (2010). Synthesis of recommendations for the assessment and management of low back pain from recent clinical practice guidelines. *The Spine Journal, 10*(6), 514–529.

Danneels, L. A., Coorevits, P., Cools, A., Vanderstraeten, G., Cambier, D., Witvrouw E., et al. (2002). Differences in electromyographic activity in the multifidus muscle and the iliocostalis lumborum between healthy subjects and patients with sub-acute and chronic low back pain. *European Spine Journal, 11*(1), 13–19.

Danneels, L. A., Vanderstraeten, G. G., Cambier, D. C., Witvrouw, E. E., Bourgois, J., Dankaerts, W., et al. (2001). Effects of three different training modalities on the cross sectional area of the lumbar multifidus muscle in patients with chronic low back pain. *British Journal of Sports Medicine, 35*(3), 186–191.

Danneels, L. A., Vanderstraeten, G. G., Cambier, D. C., Witvrouw, E. E., De Cuyper, H. J., & Danneels, L. (2000). CT imaging of trunk muscles in chronic low back pain patients and healthy control subjects. *European Spine Journal, 9*(4), 266–272.

Da Silva, R., Larivière, C., Arsenault, A. B., Nadeau, S., & Plamondon, A. (2009). Pelvic stabilization and semisitting position increase the specificity of back exercises. *Medicine Science in Sports Exercise, 41*(2), 435.

De Luca, C. J. (1997). The use of surface electromyography in biomechanics. *Journal of Applied Biomechanics, 13*(2), 135–163.

De Moor, M. H., Beem, A. L., Stubbe, J. H., Boomsma, D. I., & De Geus, E. J. (2006). Regular exercise, anxiety, depression and personality: A population-based study. *Preventive Medicine, 42*(4), 273–279.

Deyo, R. A. (2002). Diagnostic evaluation of LBP: Reaching a specific diagnosis is often impossible. *Archives of Internal Medicine, 162*(13), 1444–1447.

Deyo, R. A., Jarvik, J. G., & Chou, R. (2014). Low back pain in primary care. *British Medical Journal, 349*, g4266.

Dunn, K. M., Jordan, K., & Croft, P. R. (2006). Characterizing the course of low back pain: A latent class analysis. *American Journal of Epidemiology, 163*(8), 754–761.

Edinborough, L., Fisher, J. P., & Steele, J. (2016). A comparison of the effect of kettlebell swings and isolated lumbar extension training on acute torque production of the lumbar extensors. *The Journal of Strength & Conditioning Research, 30*(5), 1189–1195.

Escamilla, R. F., Francisco, A. C., Kayes, A. V., Speer, K. P., & Moorman, C. T. (2002). An electromyographic analysis of sumo and conventional style deadlifts. *Medicine and Science in Sports and Exercise, 34*(4), 682–688.

Fairbank, J. C., & Pynsent, P. B. (2000). The Oswestry disability index. *Spine, 25*(22), 2940–2953.

Fardon, D. F., Williams, A. L., Dohring, E. J., Murtagh, F. R., Rothman, S. L. G., & Sze, G. K. (2014). Lumbar disc nomenclature: Version 2.0: Recommendations of the combined task forces of the North American spine society, the American society of spine radiology and the American society of neuroradiology. *The Spine Journal, 14*(11), 2525–2545.

Farrow, J., Steele, J., Behm, D. G., Skivington, M., & Fisher, J. P. (2020). Lighter-load exercise produces greater acute-and prolonged-fatigue in exercised and non-exercised limbs. *Research Quarterly for Exercise and Sport*, 1–11.

Fisher, J. P., Bruce-Low, S., & Smith, D. (2013). A randomized trial to consider the effect of Romanian deadlift exercise on the development of lumbar extension strength. *Physical Therapy in Sport, 14*(3), 139–145.

Fisher, J. P., Steele, J., Gentil, P., Giessing, J., & Westcott, W. L. (2017). A minimal dose approach to resistance training for the older adult; the prophylactic for aging. *Experimental Gerontology, 99*, 80–86.

Fisher, J. P., Steele, J., & Smith, D. (2017). High-and low-load resistance training: Interpretation and practical application of current research findings. *Sports Medicine, 47*(3), 393–400.

Fisher, J. P., Stuart, C., Steele, J., Gentil, P., & Giessing, J. (2018). Heavier-and lighter-load isolated lumbar extension resistance training produce similar strength increases, but different perceptual responses, in healthy males and females. *PeerJ, 6*, e6001.

Focht, B. C., & Koltyn, K. F. (2009). Alterations in pain perception after resistance exercise performed in the morning and evening. *The Journal of Strength & Conditioning Research, 23*(3), 891–897.

Foster, D., Avillar, M., Pollock, M., Graves, J., Dudley, G., Woodard, D., et al. (1993). Adaptations in strength and cross-sectional area of the lumbar extensor muscles following resistance training. *Medicine & Science in Sports & Exercise, 25*(5), S47.

Frymoyer, J. W., Pope, M. H., Clements, J. H., Wilder, D. G., MacPherson, B., & Ashikaga, T. (1983). Risk factors in low-back pain. an epidemiological survey. *Journal of Bone and Joint Surgery, 65*(2), 213–218.

Gatchel, R. J. (2013). The biopsychosocial model of chronic pain. *Clinical Insights: Chronic Pain, 5*, 5–17.

Gladwell, V., Head, S., Haggar, M., & Beneke, R. (2006). Does a program of Pilates improve chronic non-specific low back pain? *Journal of Sport Rehabilitation, 15*(4), 338–350.

Goldby, L. J., Moore, A. P., Doust, J., & Trew, M. E. (2006). A randomized controlled trial investigating the efficiency of musculoskeletal physiotherapy on chronic low back disorder. *Spine, 31*(10), 1083–1093.

Gordon, R., & Bloxham, S. (2016). A systematic review of the effects of exercise and physical activity on non-specific chronic low back pain. *Paper Presented at the Healthcare, 4*(2), 22.

Graves, J. E., Pollock, M. L., Carpenter, D. M., Leggett, S. H., Jones, A., MacMillan, M., et al. (1990a). Quantitative assessment of full range-of-motion isometric lumbar extension strength. *Spine, 15*(4), 289–294.

Graves, J. E., Pollock, M. L., Foster, D., Leggett, S. H., Carpenter, D. M., Vuoso, R., et al. (1990b). Effect of training frequency and specificity on isometric lumbar extension strength. *Spine, 15*(6), 504.

Graves, J. E., Webb, D. C., Pollock, M. L., Matkozich, J., Leggett, S. H., Carpenter, D. M., et al. (1994). Pelvic stabilization during resistance training: Its effect on the development of lumbar extension strength. *Archives of Physical Medicine and Rehabilitation, 75*(2), 210–215.

Grotle, M., Vøllestad, N. K., Veierød, M. B., & Brox, J. I. (2004). Fear-avoidance beliefs and distress in relation to disability in acute and chronic low back pain. *Pain, 112*(3), 343–352.

Hall, L., Tsao, H., MacDonald, D., Coppieters, M., & Hodges, P. W. (2009). Immediate effects of co-contraction training on motor control of the trunk muscles in people with recurrent low back pain. *Journal of Electromyography and Kinesiology, 19*(5), 763–773.

Hammond, A., Perrin, C., Steele, J., Giessing, J., Gentil, P., & Fisher, J. P. (2019). The effects of a 4-week mesocycle of barbell back squat or barbell hip thrust strength training upon isolated lumbar extension strength. *PeerJ, 7*, e7337.

Hancock, M. (2014). Approach to low back pain-physiotherapy. *Australian Family Physician, 43*(3), 117.

Hayden, J. A., Van Tulder, M. W., & Tomlinson, G. (2005). Systematic review: Strategies for using exercise therapy to improve outcomes in chronic low back pain. *Annals of Internal Medicine, 142*(9), 776–785.

Heneweer, H., Picavet, H. S. J., Staes, F., Kiers, H., & Vanhees, L. (2012). Physical fitness, rather than self-reported physical activities, is more strongly associated with low back pain: Evidence from a working population. *European Spine Journal, 21*(7), 1265–1272.

Hides, J. A., Jull, G. A., & Richardson, C. A. (2001). Long-term effects of specific stabilizing exercises for first-episode low back pain. *Spine, 26*(11), e243–e248.

Hodges, P. W., & Moseley, G. L. (2003a). Pain and motor control of the lumbopelvic region: Effect and possible mechanisms. *Journal of Electromyography and Kinesiology, 13*(4), 361–370.

Hodges, P. W., & Moseley, G. L. (2003b). Pain and motor control of the lumbopelvic region: Effect and possible mechanisms. *Journal of Electromyography and Kinesiology, 13*(4), 361–370.

Hoffman, M. D., & Hoffman, D. R. (2007). Does aerobic exercise improve pain perception and mood? A review of the evidence related to healthy and chronic pain subjects. *Current Pain and Headache Reports, 11*(2), 93–97.

Hoffman, M. D., Shepanski, M. A., MacKenzie, S. P., & Clifford, P. S. (2005). Experimentally induced pain perception is acutely reduced by aerobic exercise in people with chronic low back pain. *Journal of Rehabilitation Research & Development, 42*(2).

Hoy, D., March, L., Brooks, P., Blyth, F., Woolf, A., Bain, C., et al. (2014). The global burden of low back pain: Estimates from the global burden of disease 2010 study. *Annals of the Rheumatic Diseases, 73*(6), 968–974.

Hoy, D., March, L., Brooks, P., Woolf, A., Blyth, F., Vos, T., et al. (2010). Measuring the global burden of low back pain. *Best Practice & Research Clinical Rheumatology, 24*(2), 155–165.

Itz, C. J., Geurts, J. W., Van Kleef, M., & Nelemans, P. (2013). Clinical course of non-specific low back pain: A systematic review of prospective cohort studies set in primary care. *European Journal of Pain, 17*(1), 5–15.

Jay, K., Frisch, D., Hansen, K., Zebis, M. K., Andersen, C. H., Mortensen, O. S., et al. (2011). Kettlebell training for musculoskeletal and cardiovascular health: A randomized controlled trial. *Scandinavian Journal of Work, Environment & Health*, 196–203.

Jay, K., Jakobsen, M. D., Sundstrup, E., Skotte, J. H., Jørgensen, M. B., Andersen, C. H., et al. (2013). Effects of kettlebell training on postural coordination and jump performance: A randomized controlled trial. *The Journal of Strength & Conditioning Research*, *27*(5), 1202–1209.

Jellema, P., Van Der Windt, Daniëlle AWM, Van Der Horst, Henriëtte E, Twisk, J. W., Stalman, W. A., & Bouter, L. M. (2005). Should treatment of (sub) acute low back pain be aimed at psychosocial prognostic factors? Cluster randomised clinical trial in general practice. *British Medical Journal*, *331*(7508), 84.

Jones, A. (1993). *The lumbar spine, the cervical spine and the knee*. Ocala, FL: MedX Corporation.

Jöud, A., Petersson, I. F., & Englund, M. (2012). Low back pain: Epidemiology of consultations. *Arthritis Care & Research*, *64*(7), 1084–1088.

Kankaanpää, M., Laaksonen, D., Taimela, S., Kokko, S., Airaksinen, O., & Hänninen, O. (1998). Age, sex, and body mass index as determinants of back and hip extensor fatigue in the isometric Sørensen back endurance test. *Archives of Physical Medicine and Rehabilitation*, *79*(9), 1069–1075.

Kent, P. M., & Keating, J. L. (2008). Can we predict poor recovery from recent-onset nonspecific low back pain? A systematic review. *Manual Therapy*, *13*(1), 12–28.

Khodadad, B., Letafatkar, A., Hadadnezhad, M., & Shojaedin, S. (2020). Comparing the effectiveness of cognitive functional treatment and lumbar stabilization treatment on pain and movement control in patients with low back pain. *Sports Health*, *12*(3), 289–295.

Koltyn, K. F., & Arbogast, R. W. (1998). Perception of pain after resistance exercise. *British Journal of Sports Medicine*, *32*(1), 20–24.

Koltyn, K. F., & Umeda, M. (2006). Exercise, hypoalgesia and blood pressure. *Sports Medicine*, *36*(3), 207–214.

Konrad, P., Schmitz, K., & Denner, A. (2001). Neuromuscular evaluation of trunk-training exercises. *Journal of Athletic Training*, *36*(2), 109.

Krogh, J., Nordentoft, M., Sterne, J. A., & Lawlor, D. A. (2011). *The effect of exercise in clinically depressed adults: Systematic review and meta-analysis of randomized controlled trials*. Database of Abstracts of Reviews of Effects (DARE): Quality-Assessed Reviews [Internet]. London: Centre for Reviews and Dissemination.

Larivière, C., Da Silva, R. A., Arsenault, A. B., Nadeau, S., Plamondon, A., & Vadeboncoeur, R. (2011). Specificity of a back muscle roman chair exercise in healthy and back pain subjects. *Medicine and Science in Sports and Exercise*, *43*(1), 157.

Latimer, J., Maher, C. G., Refshauge, K., & Colaco, I. (1999). The reliability and validity of the Biering – Sorensen test in asymptomatic subjects and subjects reporting current or previous nonspecific low back pain. *Spine*, *24*(20), 2085.

Lee, P. H. (2015). Enhanced muscle activity during lumbar extension exercise with pelvic stabilization. *Journal of Exercise Rehabilitation*, *11*(6), 372.

Lee, P. H., Macfarlane, D. J., Lam, T. H., & Stewart, S. M. (2011). Validity of the international physical activity questionnaire short form (IPAQ-SF): A systematic review. *International Journal of Behavioral Nutrition and Physical Activity*, *8*(1), 115.

MacDonald, D., Moseley, G. L., & Hodges, P. W. (2009). Why do some patients keep hurting their back? evidence of ongoing back muscle dysfunction during remission from recurrent back pain. *Pain®*, *142*(3), 183–188.

Macedo, L. G., Smeets, R. J., Maher, C. G., Latimer, J., & McAuley, J. H. (2010). Graded activity and graded exposure for persistent nonspecific low back pain: A systematic review. *Physical Therapy*, *90*(6), 860–879.

Machado, L. A. C., De Souza, Marcelo Von Sperling, Ferreira, P. H., & Ferreira, M. L. (2006). The McKenzie method for low back pain: A systematic review of the literature with a meta-analysis approach. *Spine*, *31*(9), e254–e262.

Manchikanti, L., Boswell, M. V., Singh, V., Pampati, V., Damron, K. S., & Beyer, C. D. (2004). Prevalence of facet joint pain in chronic spinal pain of cervical, thoracic, and lumbar regions. *BMC Musculoskeletal Disorders*, *5*(1), 15.

Manchikanti, L., Singh, V., Pampati, V., Damron, K. S., Barnhill, R. C., Beyer, C., et al. (2001). Evaluation of the relative contributions of various structures in chronic low back pain. *Pain Physician, 4*(4), 308–316.

Masharawi, Y., & Nadaf, N. (2013). The effect of non-weight bearing group-exercising on females with non-specific chronic low back pain: A randomized single blind controlled pilot study. *Journal of Back and Musculoskeletal Rehabilitation, 26*(4), 353–359.

Massoud Arab, A., Salavati, M., Ebrahimi, I., & Ebrahim Mousavi, M. (2007). Sensitivity, specificity and predictive value of the clinical trunk muscle endurance tests in low back pain. *Clinical Rehabilitation, 21*(7), 640–647.

Mayer, J. M., Graves, J. E., Robertson, V. L., Pierra, E. A., Verna, J. L., & Ploutz-Snyder, L. L. (1999). Electromyographic activity of the lumbar extensor muscles: Effect of angle and hand position during roman chair exercise. *Archives of Physical Medicine and Rehabilitation, 80*(7), 751–755.

Mayer, J. M., Mooney, V., & Dagenais, S. (2008). Evidence-informed management of chronic low back pain with lumbar extensor strengthening exercises. *The Spine Journal, 8*(1), 96–113.

Mayer, J. M., Udermann, B. E., Graves, J. E., & Ploutz-Snyder, L. L. (2003). Effect of roman chair exercise training on the development of lumbar extension strength. *Journal of Strength and Conditioning Research, 17*(2), 356–361.

Mayer, J. M., Verna, J. L., Manini, T. M., Mooney, V., & Graves, J. E. (2002). Electromyographic activity of the trunk extensor muscles: Effect of varying hip position and lumbar posture during roman chair exercise. *Archives of Physical Medicine and Rehabilitation, 83*(11), 1543–1546.

McCarthy, C. J., Arnall, F. A., Strimpakos, N., Freemont, A., & Oldham, J. A. (2004). The biopsychosocial classification of non-specific low back pain: A systematic review. *Physical Therapy Reviews, 9*(1), 17–30.

McGill, S. M. (2015). *Low back disorders: Evidence-based prevention and rehabilitation*. Champaign, IL: Human Kinetics.

McGill, S. M., & Marshall, L. W. (2012). Kettlebell swing, snatch, and bottoms-up carry: Back and hip muscle activation, motion, and low back loads. *The Journal of Strength & Conditioning Research, 26*(1), 16–27.

Meucci, R. D., Fassa, A. G., & Faria, N. M. X. (2015). Prevalence of chronic low back pain: Systematic review. *Revista De Saude Publica, 49*, 73.

Middleton, A. (2004). Chronic low back pain: Patient compliance with physiotherapy advice and exercise, perceived barriers and motivation. *Physical Therapy Reviews, 9*(3), 153–160.

Monie, A. P., Fazey, P. J., & Singer, K. P. (2016). Low back pain misdiagnosis or missed diagnosis: Core principles. *Manual Therapy, 22*, 68–71.

Morley, S., Eccleston, C., & Williams, A. (1999). Systematic review and meta-analysis of randomized controlled trials of cognitive behaviour therapy and behaviour therapy for chronic pain in adults, excluding headache. *Pain, 80*(1–2), 1–13.

Naugle, K. M., Fillingim, R. B., & Riley, J. L. (2012). A meta-analytic review of the hypoalgesic effects of exercise. *The Journal of Pain, 13*(12), 1139–1150.

Nelson, B. W., Miller, M., Hogan, M., Wegner, J. A., & Kelly, C. (1995). The clinical effects of intensive, specific exercise on chronic low back pain: A controlled study of 895 consecutive patients with 1-year follow up. *Orthopedics, 18*(10), 971–981.

Nijs, J., Apeldoorn, A., Hallegraeff, H., Clark, J., Smeets, R., Malfliet, A., et al. (2015). Low back pain: Guidelines for the clinical classification of predominant neuropathic, nociceptive, or central sensitization pain. *Pain Physician, 18*.

Nijs, J., Kosek, E., Van Oosterwijck, J., & Meeus, M. (2012). Dysfunctional endogenous analgesia during exercise in patients with chronic pain: To exercise or not to exercise? *Pain Physician, 15*(3S), eS205–eS213.

Ogon, I., Takebayashi, T., Takashima, H., Tanimoto, K., Ida, K., Yoshimoto, M., et al (2015). Analysis of chronic low back pain with magnetic resonance imaging T2 mapping of lumbar intervertebral disc. *Journal of Orthopaedic Science, 20*(2), 295–301.

O'Keeffe, M., O'Sullivan, P., Purtill, H., Bargary, N., & O'Sullivan, K. (2020). Cognitive functional therapy compared with a group-based exercise and education intervention for chronic low back pain: A multicentre randomised controlled trial (RCT). *British Journal of Sports Medicine, 54*(13), 782–789.

O'Neill, S., Manniche, C., Graven-Nielsen, T., & Arendt-Nielsen, L. (2007). Generalized deep-tissue hyperalgesia in patients with chronic low-back pain. *European Journal of Pain, 11*(4), 415–420.

O'Sullivan, P. (2005). Diagnosis and classification of chronic low back pain disorders: Maladaptive movement and motor control impairments as underlying mechanism. *Manual Therapy, 10*(4), 242–255.

Parkkola, R., Kujala, U., & Rytökoski, U. (1992). Response of the trunk muscles to training assessed by magnetic resonance imaging and muscle strength. *European Journal of Applied Physiology and Occupational Physiology, 65*(5), 383–387.

Peluso, M. A. M., & Andrade, L. H. S. G. D. (2005). Physical activity and mental health: The association between exercise and mood. *Clinics, 60*(1), 61–70.

Penedo, F. J., & Dahn, J. R. (2005). Exercise and well-being: A review of mental and physical health benefits associated with physical activity. *Current Opinion in Psychiatry, 18*(2), 189–193.

Pillastrini, P., Gardenghi, I., Bonetti, F., Capra, F., Guccione, A., Mugnai, R., et al. (2012). An updated overview of clinical guidelines for chronic low back pain management in primary care. *Joint Bone Spine, 79*(2), 176–185.

Pollock, M. L., Garzarella, L., Graves, J. E., Carpenter, D. M., Leggett, S. H., Lowenthal, D., et al. (1992). Effects of isolated lumbar extension resistance training on bone mineral density of the elderly. *Medicine & Science in Sports & Exercise, 24*(5), S66.

Radebold, A., Cholewicki, J., Polzhofer, G. K., & Greene, H. S. (2001). Impaired postural control of the lumbar spine is associated with delayed muscle response times in patients with chronic idiopathic low back pain. *Spine, 26*(7), 724–730.

Riddle, D. L. (1998). Classification and low back pain: A review of the literature and critical analysis of selected systems. *Physical Therapy, 78*(7), 708–737.

Risch, S. V., Norvell, N. K., Pollock, M. L., Risch, E. D., Langer, H., Fulton, M., et al. (1993). Lumbar strengthening in chronic low back pain patients. physiologic and psychological benefits. *Spine, 18*(2), 232–238.

Roussel, N. A., Nijs, J., Meeus, M., Mylius, V., Fayt, C., & Oostendorp, R. (2013). Central sensitization and altered central pain processing in chronic low back pain: Fact or myth? *The Clinical Journal of Pain, 29*(7), 625–638.

Ruhe, A., Fejer, R., & Walker, B. (2011). Center of pressure excursion as a measure of balance performance in patients with non-specific low back pain compared to healthy controls: A systematic review of the literature. *European Spine Journal, 20*(3), 358–368.

San Juan, J. G., Yaggie, J. A., Levy, S. S., Mooney, V., Udermann, B. E., & Mayer, J. M. (2005). Effects of pelvic stabilization on lumbar muscle activity during dynamic exercise. *The Journal of Strength & Conditioning Research, 19*(4), 903–907.

Sanzarello, I., Merlini, L., Rosa, M. A., Perrone, M., Frugiuele, J., Borghi, R., et al. (2016). Central sensitization in chronic low back pain: A narrative review. *Journal of Back and Musculoskeletal Rehabilitation, 29*(4), 625–633.

Schwarzer, A., Aprill, C., Derby, R., Fortin, J., Kine, G., & Bogduk, N. (1994). The relative contributions of the disc and zygapophyseal joint in chronic low back pain. *Spine, 19*(7), 801–806. Retrieved from https://journals.lww.com/spinejournal/Abstract/1994/04000/The_Relative_Contributions_of_the_Disc_and.13.aspx.

Searle, A., Spink, M., Ho, A., & Chuter, V. (2015). Exercise interventions for the treatment of chronic low back pain: A systematic review and meta-analysis of randomised controlled trials. *Clinical Rehabilitation, 29*(12), 1155–1167.

Shephard, R. J. (1988). PAR-Q, Canadian home fitness test and exercise screening alternatives. *Sports Medicine, 5*(3), 185–195.

Shipton, E. A. (2018). Physical therapy approaches in the treatment of low back pain. *Pain and Therapy, 7*(2), 127–137.

Shirado, O., Ito, T., Kaneda, K., & Strax, T. E. (1995). Electromyographic analysis of four techniques for isometric trunk muscle exercises. *Archives of Physical Medicine and Rehabilitation, 76*(3), 225–229.

Shnayderman, I., & Katz-Leurer, M. (2013). An aerobic walking programme versus muscle strengthening programme for chronic low back pain: A randomized controlled trial. *Clinical Rehabilitation, 27*(3), 207–214.

Sihvonen, T., Lindgren, K., Airaksinen, O., & Manninen, H. (1997). Movement disturbances of the lumbar spine and abnormal back muscle electromyographic findings in recurrent low back pain. *Spine, 22*(3), 289–295.

Slade, S. C., & Keating, J. L. (2006). Trunk-strengthening exercises for chronic low back pain: A systematic review. *Journal of Manipulative and Physiological Therapeutics, 29*(2), 163–173.

Slade, S. C., Patel, S., Underwood, M., & Keating, J. L. (2014). What are patient beliefs and perceptions about exercise for nonspecific chronic low back pain?: A systematic review of qualitative studies. *The Clinical Journal of Pain, 30*(11), 995–1005.

Slade, S. C., Patel, S., Underwood, M., & Keating, J. (2015). What are patient beliefs and perceptions about exercise for non-specific chronic low back pain: A systematic review of qualitative research. *Physiotherapy, 101*, e1407.

Smeets, R. J., Hijdra, H. J., Kester, A. D., Hitters, M. W., & Knottnerus, J. A. (2006). The usability of six physical performance tasks in a rehabilitation population with chronic low back pain. *Clinical Rehabilitation, 20*(11), 989–997.

Smeets, R. J., Wittink, H., Hidding, A., & Knottnerus, J. A. (2006). Do patients with chronic low back pain have a lower level of aerobic fitness than healthy controls?: Are pain, disability, fear of injury, working status, or level of leisure time activity associated with the difference in aerobic fitness level? *Spine, 31*(1), 90–97.

Smith, B. E., Hendrick, P., Smith, T. O., Bateman, M., Moffatt, F., Rathleff, M. S., et al. (2017). Should exercises be painful in the management of chronic musculoskeletal pain? A systematic review and meta-analysis. *British Journal of Sports Medicine, 51*(23), 1679–1687.

Smith, B. E., Littlewood, C., & May, S. (2014). An update of stabilisation exercises for low back pain: A systematic review with meta-analysis. *BMC Musculoskeletal Disorders, 15*(1), 416.

Smith, D., Bissell, G., Bruce-Low, S., & Wakefield, C. (2011). The effect of lumbar extension training with and without pelvic stabilization on lumbar strength and low back pain 1. *Journal of Back and Musculoskeletal Rehabilitation, 24*(4), 241–249.

Steele, J., Bruce-Low, S., & Smith, D. (2014). A reappraisal of the deconditioning hypothesis in low back pain: Review of evidence from a triumvirate of research methods on specific lumbar extensor deconditioning. *Current Medical Research and Opinion, 30*(5), 865–911.

Steele, J., Bruce-Low, S., & Smith, D. (2015). A review of the specificity of exercises designed for conditioning the lumbar extensors. *British Journal of Sports Medicine, 49*(5), 291–297.

Steele, J., Fisher, J., Bruce-Low, S., Smith, D., Osborne, N., & Newell, D. (2017). Variability in strength, pain, and disability changes in response to an isolated lumbar extension resistance training intervention in participants with chronic low back pain. *Paper Presented at the Healthcare, 5*(4), 75.

Steele, J., Fisher, J., Perrin, C., Conway, R., Bruce-Low, S., & Smith, D. (2019). Does change in isolated lumbar extensor muscle function correlate with good clinical outcome? A secondary analysis of data on change in isolated lumbar extension strength, pain, and disability in chronic low back pain. *Disability and Rehabilitation, 41*(11), 1287–1295.

Steele, J., Fitzpatrick, A., Bruce-Low, S., & Fisher, J. (2015). The effects of set volume during isolated lumbar extension resistance training in recreationally trained males. *PeerJ, 3*, e878.

Stevens, V. K., Vleeming, A., Bouche, K. G., Mahieu, N. N., Vanderstraeten, G. G., & Danneels, L. A. (2007). Electromyographic activity of trunk and hip muscles during stabilization exercises in four-point kneeling in healthy volunteers. *European Spine Journal, 16*(5), 711–718.

Stokes, I. A., Henry, S. M., & Single, R. M. (2003). Surface EMG electrodes do not accurately record from lumbar multifidus muscles. *Clinical Biomechanics, 18*(1), 9–13.

Stuart, C., Steele, J., Gentil, P., Giessing, J., & Fisher, J. P. (2018). Fatigue and perceptual responses of heavier-and lighter-load isolated lumbar extension resistance exercise in males and females. *PeerJ, 6*, e4523.

Tagliaferri, S. D., Armbrecht, G., Miller, C. T., Owen, P. J., Mundell, N. L., Felsenberg, D., et al. (2020). Testing the deconditioning hypothesis of low back pain: A study in 1182 older women. *European Journal of Sport Science, 20*(1), 17–23.

Teichtahl, A. J., Urquhart, D. M., Wang, Y., Wluka, A. E., Oâ€™Sullivan, R., Jones, G., et al. (2015). Physical inactivity is associated with narrower lumbar intervertebral discs, high fat content of paraspinal muscles and low back pain and disability. *Arthritis Research & Therapy, 17*(1), 114.

Thomas, E., Silman, A. J., Papageorgiou, A. C., Macfarlane, G. J., & Croft, P. R. (1998). Association between measures of spinal mobility and low back pain: An analysis of new attenders in primary care. *Spine, 23*(3), 343–347.

Tousignant, M., Poulin, L., Marchand, S., Viau, A., & Place, C. (2005). The Modified – Modified Schober test for range of motion assessment of lumbar flexion in patients with low back pain: A study of criterion validity, intra-and inter-rater reliability and minimum metrically detectable change. *Disability and Rehabilitation, 27*(10), 553–559.

Tsao, H., Druitt, T. R., Schollum, T. M., & Hodges, P. W. (2010). Motor training of the lumbar paraspinal muscles induces immediate changes in motor coordination in patients with recurrent low back pain. *The Journal of Pain, 11*(11), 1120–1128.

Udermann, B. E., Graves, J. E., Donelson, R. G., Ploutz-Snyder, L., Boucher, J. P., & Iriso, J. H. (1999). Pelvic restraint effect on lumbar gluteal and hamstring muscle electromyographic activation. *Archives of Physical Medicine and Rehabilitation, 80*(4), 428–431.

Valat, J., Goupille, P., & Vedere, V. (1997). Low back pain: Risk factors for chronicity. *Occupational Health and Industrial Medicine, 2*(37), 77.

van Dieën, J. H., Cholewicki, J., & Radebold, A. (2003). Trunk muscle recruitment patterns in patients with low back pain enhance the stability of the lumbar spine. *Spine, 28*(8), 834–841.

Van Kleef, M., Vanelderen, P., Cohen, S. P., Lataster, A., Van Zundert, J., & Mekhail, N. (2010). 12 pain originating from the lumbar facet joints. *Pain Practice, 10*(5), 459–469.

Van Middelkoop, M., Rubinstein, S. M., Kuijpers, T., Verhagen, A. P., Ostelo, R., Koes, B. W., et al. (2011). A systematic review on the effectiveness of physical and rehabilitation interventions for chronic non-specific low back pain. *European Spine Journal, 20*(1), 19–39.

Verbunt, J. A., Seelen, H. A., Vlaeyen, J. W., van de Heijden, Geert J, Heuts, P. H., Pons, K., et al. (2003). Disuse and deconditioning in chronic low back pain: Concepts and hypotheses on contributing mechanisms. *European Journal of Pain, 7*(1), 9–21.

Verhagen, A. P., Downie, A., Popal, N., Maher, C., & Koes, B. W. (2016). Red flags presented in current low back pain guidelines: A review. *European Spine Journal, 25*(9), 2788–2802.

Verna, J. L., Mayer, J. M., Mooney, V., Pierra, E. A., Robertson, V. L., & Graves, J. E. (2002). Back extension endurance and strength: The effect of variable-angle roman chair exercise training. *Spine, 27*(16), 1772–1777.

Vezina, M. J., & Hubley-Kozey, C. L. (2000). Muscle activation in therapeutic exercises to improve trunk stability. *Archives of Physical Medicine and Rehabilitation, 81*(10), 1370–1379.

Waddell, G., & Burton, A. K. (2005). Concepts of rehabilitation for the management of low back pain. *Best Practice & Research Clinical Rheumatology, 19*(4), 655–670.

Waddell, G., Main, C. J., Morris, E. W., Di, M. P., & Gray, I. C. (1984). Chronic low-back pain, psychologic distress, and illness behavior. *Spine, 9*(2), 209–213.

Wallwork, T. L., Stanton, W. R., Freke, M., & Hides, J. A. (2009). The effect of chronic low back pain on size and contraction of the lumbar multifidus muscle. *Manual Therapy, 14*(5), 496–500.

Walsworth, M. (2004). Lumbar paraspinal electromyographic activity during trunk extension exercises on two types of exercise machines. *Electromyography and Clinical Neurophysiology, 44*(4), 201–207.

Wertli, M. M., Eugster, R., Held, U., Steurer, J., Kofmehl, R., & Weiser, S. (2014). Catastrophizing – a prognostic factor for outcome in patients with low back pain: A systematic review. *The Spine Journal, 14*(11), 2639–2657.

Wideman, T. H., Asmundson, G. G., Smeets, R. J. M., Zautra, A. J., Simmonds, M. J., Sullivan, M. J., et al. (2013). Re-thinking the fear avoidance model: Toward a multi-dimensional framework of pain-related disability. *Pain, 154*(11), 2262.

Zhang, Y., Guo, T., Guo, X., & Wu, S. (2009). Clinical diagnosis for discogenic low back pain. *International Journal of Biological Sciences, 5*(7), 647.

APPENDICES

Appendix A: Biering-Sorensen Trunk Endurance Test

This is a timed measure used to assess the endurance of the trunk extensor muscles. The goal of the Biering-Sorensen test is to maintain a horizontal position by isometrically contracting the trunk extensors for as long as possible.

The patient lies prone on an examining table/massage couch with the upper edge of the iliac crests in alignment with the edge of the table/couch.

The lower body is fixed to the table by three straps around the pelvis, knees and ankles. With the arms folded across the chest, the patient isometrically maintains the upper body in a horizontal position while time is recorded.

If a person experiences no difficulty in holding the position for greater than 240 seconds, then the test is stopped.

Assessment is generally performed between time points to gauge improvements.

Appendix B: Star Excursion Balance Test (SEBT)

This is a dynamic test that is a measure of balance requiring strength, flexibility and proprioception. The goal of the SEBT is to maintain single-leg stance on one leg while reaching as far as possible with the contralateral leg.

To set up the test, cut four strips of tape to a length of six to eight feet each. Two pieces will be used to form a '+', with the other two being placed over top to form an 'x' so that a star shape is formed. It is important that all lines are separated from each other by a 45° angle.

The person performing the test must maintain their balance on one foot while using the other foot to reach as far as possible in the eight different directions. The person (standing on their left foot, for example) must reach once in each of the following directions: anterior, anteromedial, medial, posteromedial, posterior, posterolateral, lateral and anterolateral.

Assessment might consider differences in distance reached in specific directions, differences between left and right limbs to identify imbalances or differences between time points to identify improvements in balance and coordination.

Appendix C: Prone Straight-Leg Raise (SLR) Test

This can be used as a timed muscular endurance test or an assessment of range of motion.

To perform the prone SLR test, start by finding a suitable place to lie down that is free from obstructions.

Lie face down (prone) on the floor. Gently tighten your core muscles by keeping your abdominal muscles engaged. You should still be able to breathe while doing this.

Keeping your abdominals engaged and your knees straight, slowly lift one leg up backwards. You should keep your knee straight as your thigh lifts from the floor. Be sure you do not rotate your back or your pelvis while lifting your leg.

Assessment is often performed between left and right limbs to identify imbalances or between time points to identify improvements in endurance and/or range of motion.

17

RHEUMATOID ARTHRITIS

George Metsios and Antonis Stavropoulos-Kalinoglou

Chapter aims

The aims of this chapter are to develop a clear understanding of:

- The epidemiology, pathophysiology, and mechanisms of rheumatoid arthritis
- The effects of exercise (acute and chronic) on rheumatoid arthritis synptoms and systemic manifestations
- How to develop effective and individualised exercise prescription in people living with rheumatoid arthritis

1. Rheumatoid arthritis: general concepts

1.1 Definition and clinical manifestations

Rheumatoid arthritis (RA) was first described in the 1800s as a new form of gout under the designation 'primary asthenic gout'. Several distinctive characteristics of the disease, including predominance in women, a chronic course, involvement of many joints from the onset and a decline in general health, were identified (Landre-Beauvais, 2001). The term RA was later introduced to characterise this disease. Rheumatoid (from Greek: ρεύμα [*rhevma*], meaning the flow, and the suffix *-oid* meaning similar to, alike) signifies the chronic cyclic nature of the disease, which is characterised by periods of increased activity (flares) and others of remission. Arthritis (from Greek: άρθρωση [*arthrosi*], meaning joint, and suffix *-it is*, meaning inflammation) is literally the inflammation of the joints (Onions et al., 1996).

Thus, RA is a systemic chronic inflammatory disorder of cyclic nature that affects mainly synovial joints (Hunder, 2005). More specifically, it affects any joint where cartilage overlies bone and with a joint cavity lined by a synovial membrane that contains synovial fluid. The changes to the synovium (i.e. oedema, increased vascularity and hyperplasia), the primary site of inflammation in RA, are important to the course of the disease (Buch and Emery, 2002).

DOI: 10.4324/9781315102399-17

TABLE 17.1 Functional capacity classification of rheumatoid arthritis

Class	*Description*
I	No limitations.
II	Function is adequate for normal activities despite joint discomfort or limitation of motion.
III	Function is inadequate for most self-care and vocational activities.
IV	Patient is largely or wholly unable to manage self-care and may be restricted to a wheelchair or bed.

Source: Adapted from Steinbrocker et al. (1949)

Most common symptoms include joint pain, swelling and stiffness – especially following prolonged periods of inactivity (e.g. morning stiffness following sleep). Also, other characteristics signs of inflammation – redness and warmth – are often present in the affected joints (Hunder, 2005). Symptoms usually initiate over a period of several weeks to months; however, in almost a third of all RA patients, disease onset is rapid, occurring over a few days or weeks. At the initial stages of the disease, the majority of patients present with oligoarthritis (i.e. fewer than six joints affected), often asymmetric; monoarthritis is very rare. Stiffness following prolonged periods of rest (e.g. sleep) is also noted as are signs of fatigue (Hunder, 2005). As the disease progresses, the majority of patients develop polyarthritis and experience unexplained flares and remissions. Even though the course of the disease differs among individuals, most RA patients develop destructive arthritis, which can be disabling (Scott et al., 2000).

Among patients with long-standing disease (i.e. > 10 years), only 17% are free from any disability while 16% are completely disabled (Sherrer et al., 1986). As early as 1949 (Steinbrocker et al., 1949), this difference in disease outcomes was known, and a classification of the functional limitations of the disease was proposed (Table 17.1). This classification is important in the planning of future health needs and treatment, including exercise prescription.

1.2 Epidemiology

RA is the most common inflammatory arthritis. Despite some variation among different populations, in Northern Europe and North America a prevalence of 0.5% to 1%, with an annual incidence of 20 to 50 new cases per 100.000 inhabitants, is usually reported (Alamanos and Drosos, 2005). These values are slightly lower than some older reports (Doran et al., 2002); however, it is not clear whether this is a true reduction in RA prevalence or merely a reflection of different methods used to identify RA patients. Similarly, current guidelines to diagnose RA (Aletaha et al., 2010) have improved accuracy of diagnosis (Radner et al., 2014) and are able to identify sufferers early (Humphreys et al., 2012), which could affect prevalence figures in the future. While RA may affect anyone at any age, women have a two- to threefold higher rate of it, and symptoms most commonly occur during or after the fifth decade of life (Alamanos and Drosos, 2005).

Among RA patients, disability, often manifesting as premature work cessation, is a common feature. In the first three years following diagnosis, almost a quarter of patients may stop working. This figure increases to more than a third by 10 years and more than half by 25 years after diagnosis, with most of these cases attributed directly to arthritis (Allaire et al., 2008). However, when the disease is better controlled, almost a third of these patients may return to work but could need further support (Allaire et al., 2008).

RA has also been shown to reduce life expectancy by three to ten years, depending on the severity of the disease and age at onset (Erhardt et al., 1989). The increases in life expectancy recorded in the general population over the past decades are not reflected in RA patients (Glennas et al., 2000; Buch and Emery, 2002). The causes of death do not differ significantly between RA patients and the general population, but they occur at a younger age. The main cause of death in RA is cardiovascular disease (CVD), which is both more prevalent and more likely to lead to death in these patients than in the general population (Kitas and Erb, 2003). Novel therapies may be effective in reducing inflammation and should also limit the development of CVD; however, this is not reflected in the incidence of CVD events among RA patients (Crowson et al., 2013).

1.3 Aetiology and pathophysiology

The aetiology of RA is not clear. It is believed that RA is triggered when an immunogenetically susceptible host is exposed to an antigen. In this manner, an acute inflammatory reaction is initiated. In contrast to the normal course of inflammation, when the antigen has been repelled, this reaction is not terminated. Instead, it recognises some of the tissues in the joints as foreign and attacks them (autoimmune reaction). It is this chronic, uncontrolled phase of the inflammation that ultimately destroys the joints. The antigen(s) that trigger the initial inflammation have not been positively recognised; however, several potential risk factors have been identified. Among them, the most consistent include genetic susceptibility, female gender, a family history of RA, exposure to tobacco (Deane et al., 2017), previous infection – especially by the Epstein-Barr virus (Kumar et al., 2015) and obesity (George and Baker, 2016; Stavropoulos-Kalinoglou et al., 2011a).

It has been proposed that a genetic component is involved in the pathogenesis of RA. Among various genes investigated, the human leukocyte antigen (HLA) alleles show the strongest links with RA. HLA is a part of the major histocompatibility complex (MHC) of genes, located in chromosome six. It is responsible for the encoding Class I and II molecules, which present T-cells with antigens. Most of RA patients (65–80%) have the HLA-DR4 or DR1 allele or both. These alleles share a common region of four amino acids located in the antigen-binding cleft of the DR molecule adjacent to the T-cell receptor. This is referred to as 'the shared' or 'the rheumatoid epitope' and is presumably the specific binding site of the antigen that initiates the inflammation of the joints (Kumar et al., 2015).

MHC Class II molecules, carrying the antigen, cause naive T-cells to divide and differentiate. Activated T-cells release a number of bioactive molecules called cytokines. Angiogenic cytokines, such as vascular endothelial growth factor, induce angiogenesis and increase vascular permeability (Marrelli et al., 2011). The adhesion of leukocytes (i.e. T-cells, mainly CD4 + helper T-cells; B-cells; macrophages) to the endothelium is initially controlled by E-selectin, an adhesion molecule that forms low-affinity bonds with the leukocytes and causes them to slow down and roll along the blood vessel wall (Ospelt and Gay, 2008). Migration of these cells to the site of inflammation is then facilitated by other adhesion molecules, such as intercellular adhesion molecules and vascular cell adhesion molecules (Malik and Lo, 1996). Cytokines, such as TNFα, IL-1, IL-6 and IL-8, are again implicated in this process by inducing the expression of adhesion molecules on endothelial cells and leukocytes (Mojcik and Shevach, 1997; Nassonov et al., 2000). The main noticeable structural changes are oedema, increased vascularity and hyperplasia of the synovium, which manifest clinically as joint swelling and pain (Buch and Emery, 2002).

These manifestations progress with advancing disease; synovial hyperplasia is enhanced until the synovium becomes invasive at the site of the joint where the synovium attaches to the bone or cartilage. This causes the formation of a distinctive tissue, called 'pannus', in which a large concentration of matrix metalloproteinases is observed (Ospelt and Gay, 2008). Pannus causes destruction of extracellular matrix, leading to the characteristic joint erosions observed in RA (Ospelt and Gay, 2008; Buch and Emery, 2002).

Cytokines, especially tumour necrosis factor alpha (TNFα), and interleukins 1 (IL-1) and 6 (IL-6) are involved in each step of the process. They are produced de novo in response to an immune stimulus by a wide variety of cells and can have autocrine, paracrine and endocrine effects. TNFα is responsible to a greater extent for the proliferative and inflammatory aspects of the disease, whereas IL-1 is for its destructive aspects. IL-6 seems to be implicated more in the systemic effects of RA (Buch and Emery, 2002). Central to these processes are the effects of cytokines on transcription factors, especially the nuclear factor kappa beta (NF-κB) and the activator protein one (AP-1) pathways (Okamoto et al., 2008). Cytokines are also largely responsible for the systemic effects of RA and its extra articular manifestations (Choy, 2012). These include, amongst others, cardiovascular aspects, muscle mass loss, neuropathy and pulmonary and ocular conditions.

1.4 Diagnosis and treatment

While the exercise practitioner is not involved in any way in the diagnosis or pharmaceutical treatment of the conditions, it is imperative to develop a good understanding of the processes involved in both and especially to understand the potential interactions of medication with exercise prescription.

One of the great challenges facing medical professionals is the correct and early identification of a patient with RA. While there is not a definitive test that would diagnose the condition, an algorithm has been proposed. The key aim of this algorithm is to distinguish, 'among patients with undifferentiated inflammatory synovitis, factors that best discriminate between those who are at great risk for persistent or erosive disease' (Aletaha et al., 2010). Based on this algorithm, for a patient to be diagnosed with definitive RA, they need to have confirmed synovitis in at least one joint, and no alternative diagnosis should better explain the synovitis. If this is true, the patients are assessed in four domains: 1) number and site of involved joints, 2) serologic abnormality, 3) elevated acute-phase response and 4) symptom duration. These are scored to a maximum total of ten; for a patient to be diagnosed with RA, they need to score ≥ 6/10 (Aletaha et al., 2010).

RA patients are often taking several different drugs at the same time (Treharne et al., 2007). It is thus difficult to include them all in the same chapter; however, when working with any RA patient, it is imperative for the exercise practitioner to receive a full list of medications that the patient is on and investigate the potential interaction with exercise prescription.

To date, there is no known cure for RA. However, several different pharmaceutical approaches to manage the condition are available. Their main aims are to relieve symptoms (e.g. joint pain, swelling and stiffness) or to decelerate the progression of joint damage. The choice of medication depends on the severity of the disease and its symptoms, as well as the response of the patient to them. The most commonly used approaches are described next.

Analgesics: More commonly known as painkillers, they aim at pain relief rather than reduction of inflammation. The most commonly prescribed analgesic is paracetamol. Codeine is another analgesic, which is sometimes prescribed as a combined medicine with paracetamol.

Non-steroidal anti-inflammatory drugs (NSAIDs): Several different types of NSAIDs exist. Ibuprofen and aspirin are those most commonly used. Diclofenac, fenoprofen, flurbiprofen and cyclooxigenase-2 (COX-2) inhibitors are also frequently prescribed in RA. Like analgesics, NSAIDs help relieve pain while they can also reduce stiffness and inflammation. However, they do not affect disease progression. They act by blocking the action of the enzyme cyclooxygenase. This enzyme, especially its second form (i.e. COX-2), produces prostaglandins which are involved in the inflammatory cascade of RA (Crofford, 2000). When taken in high doses or over a long period of time, NSAIDs can cause complications, such as digestive problems, stomach bleeding, kidney and liver damage, tinnitus (ringing in the ears) and high blood pressure (Joint Formulary Committee, 2017). COX-2 inhibitors are generally less harmful to the stomach; however, they might increase CVD risk (Funk and Fitzgerald, 2007).

Corticosteroids: These are effective in reducing pain and inflammation and might also limit joint damage. They are most often prescribed on a short-term basis, during a disease flare. Relief is rapid, and the effects can last from a few weeks to several months, depending on the severity of the disease. Such drugs act directly on the immune system and lower its response to the antigen (Vane and Botting, 1996). However, this may lower the immune response of the body against harmful agents (Franchimont, 2004). Other side effects of corticosteroids include weight gain, osteoporosis, easy bruising, muscle weakness and thinning of the skin (Joint Formulary Committee, 2017). They can also worsen diabetes and glaucoma and increase risk for CVD (Panoulas et al., 2008).

Disease-modifying anti-rheumatic drugs (DMARDs): DMARDs aim to reduce the destructive effect of inflammation on the joints. However, their effects may take months before they are noticeable; thus, early and aggressive intervention is now a major target of RA management. Methotrexate, sulfasalazine, hydroxychloroquine and leflunomide can be prescribed either alone or in combination with each other; older drugs, such as gold injections and penicillamine, are now rarely used. Each drug has a different mechanism of action, but all aim to reduce joint damage by limiting inflammation in the joints and surrounding tissues (Joshi and Dhaneshwar, 2014).

Biologics: This groups of DMARDs includes tumour necrosis factor alpha (TNFα) inhibitors, therapies against interleukin-1 and -6 receptor as well as CD 20, T-cell costimulatory modulators, as well as targeted DMARDs (Janus Kinase inhibitors – Jak). These are some of the most effective drugs for RA as the may reduce symptoms rapidly and decelerate or even halt disease progression. Their mechanisms of action vary significantly, but the main advancement compared to conventional DMARDs is that they target a specific cytokine. This has significantly improved clinical efficacy and joint destruction while showing an enhanced safety profile (Tugwell et al., 2011).

The effects of common pharmacological treatments on the exercise response in people with rheumatoid arthritis are summarised in Table 17.2.

Surgery: While surgery is reserved for the more severe cases of RA, a large proportion of patients might undergo such a procedure (Fevang et al., 2007). The rates, however, have

TABLE 17.2 Medication considerations for exercise for people with rheumatoid arthritis

Class name	*Generic name*	*Brand name*	*Indication*	*Action*	*Side effects*	*Exercise considerations*
Analgesics	paracetamol	Panadol OA	Mild to moderate pain	Inhibition of prostagladin synthesis; activation of serotonergic pathways	Rare: acute generalised exanthematous pustulosis; malaise; skin reactions; Stevens-Johnson syndrome; toxic epidermal necrolysis Frequency not known: blood disorders; leucopenia; neutropenia; thrombocytopenia	None specific
Non-steroidal anti-inflammatory drugs (NSAIDs)	ibuprofen		Pain and inflammation in rheumatic disease	Non-selective inhibition of cyclooxygenase (COX); COX is essential for prostaglandin synthesis via the arachidonic acid pathway	With systemic use: Rare: alveolitis; aseptic meningitis (patients with connective-tissue disorders such as systemic lupus erythematosus may be especially susceptible); hepatic damage; interstitial fibrosis associated with NSAIDs can lead to renal failure; pancreatitis; papillary necrosis associated with NSAIDs can lead to renal failure; pulmonary eosinophilia; Stevens-Johnson syndrome; toxic epidermal necrolysis; visual disturbances Frequency unknown: angioedema; blood disorders; bronchospasm; colitis (induction or exacerbation of); Crohn's disease (induction or exacerbation of); depression; diarrhoea; dizziness; drowsiness; fluid retention (rarely precipitating congestive heart failure); gastro-intestinal bleeding; gastro-intestinal discomfort; gastro-intestinal disturbances; gastro-intestinal ulceration; haematuria; headache; hearing disturbances; hypersensitivity reactions; insomnia; nausea; nervousness; photosensitivity; raised blood pressure; rashes; renal failure (especially in patients with pre-existing renal impairment); tinnitus; vertigo	None specific, but watch for side effects such as diziness and high blood pressure and treat accordingly

(*Continued*)

TABLE 17.2 (Continued)

Class name	*Generic name*	*Brand name*	*Indication*	*Action*	*Side effects*	*Exercise considerations*
Disease-modifying anti-rheumatic drugs (DMARDs)	methotrexate		Moderate to severe active RA	Inhibition of dihydrofolate reductase, which is central in purines and pyrimidines synthesis	Abdominal discomfort; acne; alopecia; anaphylactic reactions; anorexia; arthralgia; blood disorders; changes in nail pigmentation; changes in skin pigmentation; chills; chronic pulmonary fibrosis; confusion; conjunctivitis; cystitis; diarrhoea; dizziness; drowsiness; dyspepsia; dysuria; ecchymosis; fever; furuncolosis; gastro-intestinal bleeding; gastro-intestinal ulceration; haematuria; headache; hepatotoxicity; hypotension; impotence; injection-site reactions; insomnia; interstitial pneumonitis; malaise; menstrual disturbances; mood changes; mucositis; myalgia; myelosuppresion; nausea; neurotoxicity; osteoporosis; paraesthesia; pericardial tamponade; pericarditis; photosensitivity; pleuritic pain; precipitation of diabetes; pruritus; pulmonary fibrosis; pulmonary oedema; rash; reduced libido; renal failure; Stevens-Johnson syndrome; telangiectasia; thrombosis; toxic epidermal necrolysis; toxic megacolon; urticaria; vaginitis; vasculitis; visual disturbance; vomiting	None specific, however any infections or other side effects need to be reported
Biologics	Anti-TNFa inhibitor	Etanercept	Moderate to severe active rheumatoid arthritis (alone or in combination with methotrexate) when the response to other disease-modifying antirheumatic drugs is inadequate; severe, active and progressive rheumatoid arthritis not previously treated with methotrexate	Soluble TNF receptor that binds specifically to circulating TNF and reduces its bioavailabilty and thus its action on its target cells	Uncommon: interstitial lung disease; new onset or worsening psoriasis; rash; skin cancer; uveitis Rare: demyelinating disorders; lymphoma; seizures; Stevens-Johnson syndrome; vasculitis Very rare: toxic epidermal necrolysis Frequency not known: abdominal pain; anaemia; antibody formation; aplastic anaemia; appendicitis; blood disorders; cutaneous ulcer; depression; diabetes mellitus; fever; gastritis; headache; hypersensitivity reactions; inflammatory bowel disease; injection-site reactions; leucopenia; leukaemia; lupus erythematosus-like syndrome; macrophage activation syndrome; malignancy; nausea; oesophagitis; pancytopenia; pruritus; solid tumours; thrombocytopenia; vomiting; worsening heart failure	None known, however some side effects may impact the ability of the patient to exercise

This is only an indicative list of medications that RA patients might be on

Source: Information for this table was extracted from the relevant sections of the BNF (Joint Formulary Committee, 2017)

reduced significantly over the past decades, mainly as a result of more effective treatment options (Fevang et al., 2007; Louie and Ward, 2009). Yet arthroplasty (reconstruction or replacement of the affected joint) or osteotomy (shortening or lengthening of the bone) is often performed on RA patients. Their prognosis is usually good, and the patient should regain full function following rehabilitation.

Considerations for exercise prescription: All the aforementioned drugs have side effects, some of which are common or serious. Each patient needs to be reviewed on an individual basis, and exercise prescription should be decided following consideration of any specific side effects the patient is presenting with. Some of the drugs may exacerbate arrhythmias or even lead to heart disease; it is not clear, however, if exercise may actually improve such effects. Further, due to their mechanisms of action, some drugs, especially biological agents, may reduce the immune response, making patients susceptible to infections; maintaining a hygienic environment and limiting contact with potential sources of infection while exercising (e.g. other users of the exercise facility who may have an infection) may be required. It is also important to remember that RA patients very often present with other conditions needing pharmacological treatment (e.g. high blood pressure, dyslipidaemia). Thus, having a complete list of the medications they are using is imperative.

1.5 The multidisciplinary team and communication with the referring medical practitioner

For most patients suffering from chronic conditions, their general practitioner (GP) is central to the multidisciplinary team (MDT). Moreover, the relevant medical team have a significant input in the management of the condition. To date, there are very few facilities that offer specialised exercise referral schemes (ERS) for RA patients, but it has been shown that even in existing cardiac rehabilitation facilities, such patients can exercise and experience significant benefits (Stavropoulos-Kalinoglou et al., 2013; Metsios et al., 2014).

From an exercise practitioner perspective, it is important to develop a clear understanding of the specific needs and abilities of each patient. A full medical record, including diagnosis and sites of inflammation and joint damage, as well as a complete list of medication, needs to be shared between the medical team and the exercise practitioner. It is usually beneficial if this is accompanied by a letter summarising the main medical considerations of the patient, including any co-morbidities. Based on these, the exercise practitioner will be able to develop a clear fitness testing strategy in order to assess the exercise capacity and any movement limitations of the patient and then provide an individualised exercise prescription. The benefits of exercise on RA and the ways it can be integrated into the management of the condition are detailed next.

2. Effects of physical activity on disease-related symptoms and systemic manifestations in RA

Evidence accumulated over the last few years has demonstrated that physical activity and/or exercise results in beneficial effects on the health of RA patients. These beneficial effects can be distinguished into two main categories: disease-related symptoms and systemic manifestations.

2.1 Effects of physical activity on disease-related symptoms

The main disease-related symptoms of RA include functional disability, inflammation, fatigue and pain. Robust evidence, in the form of systematic reviews and meta-analyses, clearly demonstrates now that involvement in physical activity and/or exercise results in improvements that beneficially impact the main disease-related symptoms of RA. The most recent systematic review and meta-analysis is from the Cochrane Collaboration, published in 2009. It highlights that engaging RA patients in exercise results in significant improvements in aerobic capacity and strength, which, in turn, can reduce pain and improve physical function within 12 weeks of exercising (Hurkmans et al., 2009). Exercise causes beneficial adaptations in cardiac, pulmonary and vascular function and structure (Joyner and Green, 2009; Gielen et al., 2010; McCarthy et al., 2015), which are the main reasons for the observed significant improvements in cardiorespiratory fitness in response to exercise. Importantly, the largest randomised controlled trial (RCT) on exercise in RA revealed that functional ability significantly improves in exercising RA patients versus RA controls, a phenomenon thought to be related to the concomitant improvements in aerobic capacity of the exercising patients (De Jong et al., 2003). This trial also investigated, for the first time, radiographic damage (i.e. damage in articular structures identified via X-ray); although it was initially concluded that patients should avoid exercising joints with extensive radiographic damage, a subsequent 18-month follow-up study demonstrated that exercise is safe for both small and large joints as well as those with extensive damage (De Jong et al., 2009). It is worth noting that, although these results are very promising, radiographic damage was a secondary outcome in this study that was not adequately powered, and thus, these results should be treated with caution. More studies are required in this field to replicate these findings.

Inflammation is considered the hallmark of RA and contributes to the main symptomatology of the disease, particularly pain, fatigue and functional disability. Evidence now exists to show that involvement in exercise has a major dose-dependent anti-inflammatory effect. In RA, joints that have been affected by the disease are characterised by initially local and then circulating overexpression of IL-6, IL-1 and TNFa. The cross-talk of these cytokines results in a vicious cycle in which overexpression of one causes overexpression of these other key inflammatory molecules, thereby enhancing the autoimmune inflammatory response. However, during exercise, the kinetics of these pro-inflammatory cytokines are different from sepsis/inflammation, which is the reason it has been suggested that exercise has an anti-inflammatory effect. In specific, exercise-induced mRNA, overexpression of IL-6 does not coincide with relevant increases in IL-1 and TNFa, but with enhanced stimulation of anti-inflammatory cytokines: namely, interleukin 10, soluble tumour necrosis factor receptor and interleukin 1 receptor antagonist (Benatti and Pedersen, 2015). This may suggest that an acute session of exercise promotes an anti-inflammatory phenotype. In line with this, macrophage (inflammation-induced) induction of IL-6 depends on the upstream and downstream signalling of IL-6, induced by the activation of NF-kB and necessitates the presence of TNFα (Pedersen and Febbraio, 2008). In contrast, intramuscular (exercise-induced) induction of IL-6 is produced without an a priori overexpression of TNFα or NF-kB activation and is regulated by an interaction between the nuclear factor of activated T-cells and glycogen-p38 mitogen-activated protein kinase pathways (Munoz-Canoves et al., 2013). Therefore, it has been suggested that acutely (during a bout of exercise), exercise-induced IL-6 production is intensity dependent and non-inflammatory as it acts as a trigger for hepatic glycogenolysis and lipolysis (Benatti and Pedersen, 2015) to enable energy deriving to the exercising muscles. In the long term, the anti-inflammatory effects of exercise are thought to be the result of the reduction in the size of adipocytes. Specifically, obesity (i.e. hypertrophy and hyperplasia of adipose cells) results in an excess of macronutrients in adipose tissue cells, causing them to stimulate inflammatory mediators (IL-6, IL-1 and TNFa) and increases in adiponectin, thus promoting the predisposition of inflammatory states and oxidative stress (Saltiel and Olefsky, 2017). The inciting aetiology for these observations has been proposed to be hypoxia, which, is turn, promotes the necrosis and infiltration of macrophages into adipose tissue, promoting the inflammatory states seen in adiposity. In contrast, the most recent systematic review and meta-analysis on the effects of exercise versus hypocaloric diets on adiposity revealed that exercise can result in a greater loss of visceral fat even in the absence of weight loss (Verheggen et al., 2016). Consequently, exercise can potentially reduce inflammation via the observed reductions in the size of adipocytes. It is worth mentioning that although the long-term anti-inflammatory responses have not been studied per se in RA (i.e. investigation of acute phase reactants or pro-inflammatory cytokines as primary outcomes), research in diabetes, a low-grade inflammatory condition, reveals that exercise can significantly reduce acute inflammatory load (i.e. C-reactive protein) (Hayashino et al., 2014).

Fatigue is a very prevalent symptom of RA, with approximately 40% of RA patients reporting severe fatigue levels similar to those seen in patients with chronic fatigue syndrome (Repping-Wuts et al., 2007). The exact mechanisms of fatigue are currently unknown in RA; however, risk factors thought to exacerbate fatigue in RA are psychological factors, pain and physical inactivity but not inflammation (Hewlett et al., 2011). A meta-analysis of five RCTs with low risk of bias revealed that aerobic exercise is an effective intervention to reduce fatigue levels in RA; however the effects were small (Rongen-van Dartel et al., 2015). More research is required in this area to determine the exact effects of exercise on fatigue in RA; however, the current preliminary findings are promising.

2.2 Effects of physical activity on systemic manifestations

RA has significant systemic involvement: namely, skin, ocular, oral, gastrointestinal, pulmonary, renal, neurological and haematological manifestations that vary according to disease severity. Research studies investigating the effects of exercise on the aforementioned manifestations are currently lacking.

Perhaps the most prevalent systemic manifestation of RA is the development of cardiovascular disease (CVD) (Kitas and Gabriel, 2011). Moreover, patients with RA experience a condition termed 'rheumatoid cachexia', which is characterised by reduced muscle mass at the presence of unchanged or slightly increased total body mass that further deteriorates their functional ability. For both these systemic manifestations, research studies collectively have shown that physical activity and/or exercise can help reverse the phenomena that predispose patients to either increase their CVD risk or experience rheumatoid cachexia.

Exercise and cardiovascular disease risk in RA

Based on the evidence that has accumulated over the last few decades, exercise is now considered a cornerstone in the management of cardiovascular disease. Cochrane Collaboration meta-analyses highlight that exercise-based cardiac rehabilitation is an effective means of reducing cardiovascular mortality (but not overall mortality) and risk of hospitalisation, as well as patient-important outcomes, such as quality of life (Anderson et al., 2016). Cardiac rehabilitation is also cost-effective; however, more research is required to determine the most cost-effective exercise dosage (Shields et al., 2018).

Relevant studies in RA have started emerging during the last few years. In terms of cost, there is preliminary evidence demonstrating associations between reduced physical activity with an increased number of hospital admissions as well as days of hospitalisation of RA patients (Metsios et al., 2011). Moreover, with regards to CVD risk and exercise, there is evidence in RA revealing that increasing physical activity and/or cardiorespiratory fitness is associated with an improved cardiovascular profile, including a reduced ten-year CVD risk, blood pressure, lipid profile and insulin resistance (Metsios et al., 2015a, 2009b). However, the effects of physical activity and/or exercise on hard clinical CVD outcomes, such as cardiovascular mortality or myocardial infarction in RA, are currently lacking.

The CVD risk of RA patients has been evaluated indirectly in clinical trials and systematic reviews via the use of cardiorespiratory fitness as a primary outcome (De Jong et al., 2003; Rouse et al., 2014; Stavropoulos-Kalinoglou et al., 2013; Metsios et al., 2008b), given its strong association with multiple different CVD outcomes (Metsios et al., 2015a). In these studies, cardiorespiratory fitness significantly increases as a result of exercise in RA, which is also in line with an earlier 2009 RA and exercise meta-analysis (Hurkmans et al., 2009). Multiple CVD outcomes have been investigated in response to exercise in a controlled trial, in which RA patients were matched for their age, gender and body mass index and allocated into two groups: combined aerobic and resistance training versus usual care controls who only received general information about the benefits of exercise at baseline. The combined results of this trial revealed that a six-month exercise programme can significantly improve blood pressure, lipid profile and micro- and macro-vascular function and reduce oxidative stress, percent body fat and ten-year CVD probability (Metsios et al., 2014; Stavropoulos-Kalinoglou et al., 2013, Wadley et al., 2014). These results, however, must be treated with caution as appropriately designed RCTs with specific CVD outcomes are currently required to confirm these findings.

Exercise and rheumatoid cachexia

Rheumatoid cachexia is a syndrome that accompanies RA. This is a syndrome first described by Roubenoff and colleagues (Roubenoff et al., 1994) and is thought to be driven by pro-inflammatory cytokines with the predominance of TNFa (a similar pathway with cancer cachexia) (Gould et al., 2013) and results in significant alterations in energy metabolism, favouring increased fat deposition and reduced muscle mass (Metsios et al., 2008a; Walsmith and Roubenoff, 2002). As a result of this, patients with RA retain their body mass; however, their body composition characteristics are significantly different to age- and weight-matched adults; the resulting body composition phenotype that is characterised by increased adiposity or reduced muscle mass may further promote CVD risk (Metsios et al., 2009a; Summers et al., 2010; Stavropoulos-Kalinoglou et al., 2011b), as well as deteriorated functional disability (Metsios and Lemmey, 2015; Walsmith and Roubenoff, 2002). As a result of these observations, it has been suggested that the BMI cut-off points for RA patients should change from 25 to 23 kg/m^2 for living with overweight and from 30 to 28 kg/m^2 for living with obesity (Stavropoulos-Kalinoglou et al., 2007). Unfortunately, despite the increasing research interest that this specific area of investigation has attracted, at present, there is a lack of uniform criteria for defining rheumatoid cachexia, As a result of this, the prevalence of this syndrome ranges from 8% to 67% in this population (Summers et al., 2010); thus, its associations with disease-related and systemic manifestations can vary.

Given the initial hypothesis that rheumatoid cachexia is a TNFa-driven syndrome, it was hypothesised that blocking TNFa via anti-TNFa medication could potentially reverse this. However, studies in early and long-standing RA patients revealed that anti-TNFa medication up to six months does not favourably alter the body composition of RA patients (Marcora et al., 2006; Metsios et al., 2007). However, extensive research work from Lemmey and colleagues demonstrates that progressive resistance training is safe and has significant beneficial effects on increasing muscle mass and reducing adiposity in RA, with additional improvements in functional ability parameters (Lemmey et al., 2009b; Marcora et al., 2005). These findings are particularly important since even the new treat-to-target approaches fail to successfully normalise body composition in RA (Lemmey et al., 2009b). The recommended public health guidelines, therefore, for performing resistance exercise training twice per week may hold great promise for improving different adverse effects of RA in this patient population.

3. Development of effective and individualised exercise prescription in rheumatoid arthritis

For many years, rheumatology health-care professionals were advising patients with RA to rest, mainly due to fear of exacerbating disease symptoms. However, based on the accumulated knowledge from research, physical activity and/or exercise is evidently a safe and effective intervention for improving the management of disease-related symptoms and systemic manifestations in RA (Hurkmans et al., 2009; Metsios and Lemmey, 2015; Rongen-Van Dartel et al., 2015). Therefore, it would be expected that exercise and/or physical activity would be more actively promoted for the management of RA. Unfortunately, this is not the case.

There are several different reasons for the lack of exercise implementation in both clinical practise and the community for the management of RA.

Lack of provision for health-care practitioners: It has previously been shown that there is a lack of provision of specific guidelines on how to develop safe and effective exercise programmes in RA or how to promote brief exercise and/or physical activity within RA clinical practise (Metsios and Lahart, 2015). It can be assumed, therefore, that the existence of such guidelines, particularly if they were tailored to clinical practise (i.e. brief advise) could potentially make a positive impact in increasing physical activity levels. Specifically, in other non-communicable diseases such as hypertension, which is a highly prevalent co-morbidity in RA (Panoulas et al., 2007, 2008), recent RCTs revealed that simple physician-led physical activity advice to increase steps per day, followed up in subsequent routine visits, has major beneficial effects in improving disease-related outcomes with very good sustainability (Dasgupta et al., 2017; Maruthur et al., 2009). Moreover, recommendations have started to emerge recently to make physical activity a priority in clinical practise as well as to suggest how this can be done in a time-efficient manner (Berra et al., 2015). Specifically, the recommendations suggest to briefly educate patients about the beneficial effects of physical activity, physically write a prescription working up to 30 minutes of physical activity per day (with the potential use of a pedometer), and following up on these targets in subsequent visits (Berra et al., 2015). This approach needs to be appropriately evaluated in relevant RCTs; however, it holds good promise as it builds on the well-known doctor-patient relationship, which is a key stimulus for beneficial changes in patient behaviours and patient satisfaction (Doyle et al., 2013).

The contribution of exercise professionals to the overall management of RA is also important. The exercise professional should be able to individualise exercise prescription according to patients' needs, functional ability and preferences, to enable long-term adherence. Guidelines on how to assess the RA patient, individualise exercise prescription, monitor progress and progressively increase intensities to achieve maximum health benefits for RA patients do exist (Metsios et al., 2015b).

Patient barriers: Lack of time and cost of exercise are amongst the main barriers reported by RA patients, which is similar to what is seen in the healthy population (Veldhuijzen Van Zanten et al., 2015). However, a systematic review revealed that the most frequent barriers stopping RA patients engaging with physical activity and/or exercise are relevant to their disease symptoms: specifically, fatigue, pain and functional disability (Veldhuijzen Van Zanten et al., 2015). Moreover, fear of aggravating the damage in the joints as well as lack of knowledge about the benefits of physical activity and the absence of RA-specific physical activity programmes were also reported as main barriers. Therefore, it can be argued that the absence of relevant provision and patient empowerment around these matters has significantly limited the engagement of RA patients in physical activity. This is in line with findings from the last two decades, which consistently demonstrate that physical activity levels and cardiorespiratory fitness in RA remain significantly lower than in the healthy population (Metsios et al., 2015a). Sokka et al. (2008) suggest that despite the recent research advances in RA and physical activity research/knowledge, little has changed.

Research studies suggest that this overall lack of provision and support for physical activity in healthcare is recognised by RA patients (Wilcox et al., 2006), while in contrast, information about physical activity from rheumatology health-care practitioners can, in fact, increase physical activity behaviour in people living with RA (Terpstra et al., 1992). However, in the absence of RA-specific physical activity programmes, it is unlikely that ERS will be effective in increasing the uptake of and adherence to a physically active lifestyle by RA patients as this barrier is also a recognised key factor for the low physical activity behaviour seen in people living with RA. In support of this, patients with CVD who attend cardiac rehabilitation experience high dropout rates and, importantly, return to sedentary behaviours post cardiac rehabilitation due to the lack of relevant support (Dalal et al., 2015). Consequently, the sustainability and, as a result of this, the effectiveness and cost effectiveness of physical activity interventions suffer significantly. It is paramount that any ERS for RA patients provide long-term support to participants and, more importantly, link into their standard care in a way that the MDT is aware of their engagement and progress in exercise.

3.1. Embedding exercise referral in clinical practise

While exercise referral is a well-established avenue for various conditions, there are very few schemes that accommodate RA patients specifically. As mentioned previously, a reluctance by medical practitioners to promote exercise and the lack of expertise among exercise practitioners are the key drivers behind this. However, there are some steps that could reverse this and increase exercise participation among RA patients. Given the significant and constant involvement of the medical practitioners in RA management and their central role in ERS, a small part of the following section discusses the steps they could follow in order to facilitate exercise referral. However, the main focus is on the steps exercise professionals should follow to ensure the development and application of an effective exercise programme for RA patients.

Step 1: Capacity building of frontline health-care practitioners

The lack of physical activity implementation in clinical practice may have several different reasons. One of the predominant factors is that medical school curricula do not incorporate physical activity modules; nor is physical activity within the continuous personal development of health-care professionals. As a result, specific knowledge of how physical activity and/or exercise can impact disease-related and systemic outcomes in RA is lacking. Relevant initiatives with great potential are available at national level (Gates et al., 2017). It must be noted herein that the capacity building of health-care professionals to ameliorate the significant individual and societal burden of non-communicable disease is a primary target of the World Health Organization and the National Institute of Health and Care Excellence (NICE, 2014; WHO, 2015). The exact methods by which this can be achieved are still under development. However, informing medical professionals of the benefits of exercise is paramount. Informed specialists will be able to guide the development of appropriate referral schemes and direct their patients to them.

Step 2: Patient empowerment

Informed practitioners may also better relay relevant information to patients. As with any lifestyle change, it is imperative that the patient understands the importance of the change and commits to it. Patient education programmes in RA (Zangi et al., 2015) and other conditions (Lopez-Vargas et al., 2016) have shown promising results; however, there is very little information on patient education and exercise in RA.

Patients with RA are currently treated via treat to target, an approach that aims to achieve remission or lower disease activity. Irrespective of the disease activity of the RA patient, physical activity advice should be relayed to the patient as early as possible following diagnosis. If the disease activity of the patient is uncontrolled at the time, the importance of future engagement in physical activity should be mentioned; also, patients should be advised to engage in as much physical activity as possible, even if that is limited to daily tasks around the house. If the patient is in remission/has low disease activity, physical activity should be briefly discussed and promoted, and they should be referred to a trained exercise specialist. Medical professionals should be involved in the process of monitoring the engagement of their patients in exercise programmes by discussing it in subsequent routine consultations. The aforementioned capacity building of health-care practitioners could significantly facilitate this process.

A schematic representation of how to implement physical activity advice in routine clinical settings is presented in Figure 17.1.

Step 3: Incorporating exercise referral into the management of rheumatoid arthritis

As with many chronic conditions, the ability of a patient with RA to exercise is defined by the severity of the condition. Thus, the first step in successful ERS is symptom control

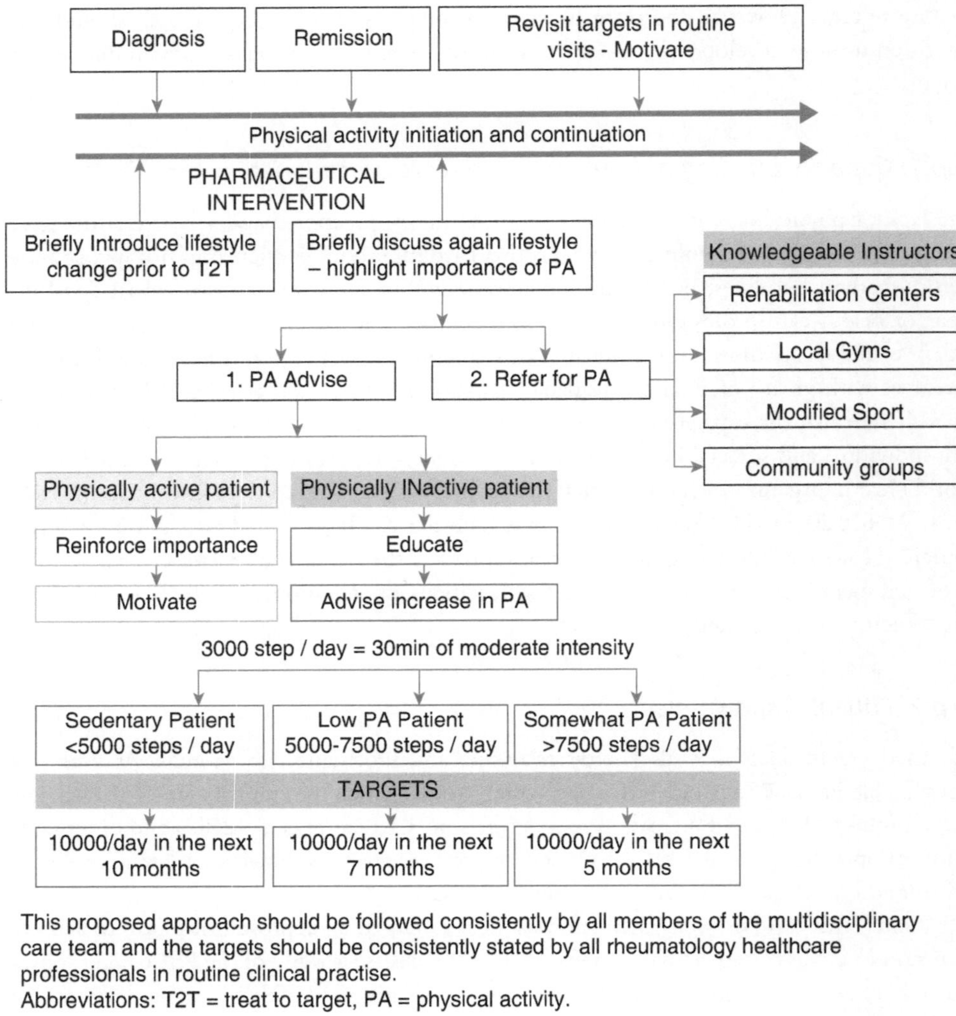

FIGURE 17.1 Process of increasing physical activity and exercise participation among people with rheumatoid arthritis in clinical practice

(Metsios et al., 2015b). However, irrespective of disease activity, all RA patients should be encouraged to do as much exercise as they can. Given that exercise is a long-term intervention, its importance should be highlighted constantly by all parties involved in patient management.

The importance of exercise in the management of RA has been highlighted in various parts of this chapter, and ERS needs to become an integral part of patient management. Inclusion of RA patients in existing ERS is beneficial to and safe for them (Stavropoulos-Kalinoglou et al., 2013). Such programmes are, in most cases, suitable for RA patients, and staff can be trained to accommodate the specific needs of RA patients.

Special considerations for exercising patients with rheumatoid arthritis

The key consideration related to the RA population is that of movement limitation due to structural changes in joints or joint pain. RA patients often have limited or altered range of motion in some of their joints. This may limit their ability to perform specific exercises or even use the affected joints effectively. If this is the case, the exercise practitioner will need to adapt any such exercises. Similarly, it is often difficult for RA patients to sit on the floor and then stand back up. Floor exercises should be avoided, at least in the early stages of exercise referral, and replaced with seated or standing alternatives. In the case of structural changes to the joint, such exercise adaptations may be permanent. However, if movement limitations are due to joint pain, it is not uncommon for these limitations to be reduced with exercise. In such cases, re-evaluating movement ability of the patient in frequent intervals – e.g. every four to six weeks – is essential.

A common manifestation of RA is disease flares (Landre-Beauvais, 2001). These are periods of high disease activity that will acutely affect a patient's ability to exercise. They cause significant pain and general malaise; during flares, patients find it very difficult to perform even their daily activities, let alone exercise. During such periods, patients should be advised to try and move as much as possible, but in most cases, attending exercise sessions will be impossible. Following a flare, depending on its severity and duration, patients may have experienced a significant decline in their fitness levels and possible movement capacity. It is essential that their functional ability and fitness is re-evaluated upon re-entry into the programme. Re-entry into exercise interventions following a flare has not been studied specifically. However, anecdotal evidence suggests that regular communication with patients while they are away may facilitate re-entry and increase participation to the programme after that.

Also, even though exercise is beneficial for RA and does not cause any further damage to the joints – if anything, it protects them – several RA patients report acute joint pain following an exercise session. This pain usually goes away within a few hours. However, it is the duty of the exercise professional to discuss this with the patients and reassure them about it. If the pain persists for more than 12 hours (i.e. into the following morning), then part of the exercise prescription might need to be re-evaluated. Usually, lowering the intensity and reducing the repetitions will address this.

Finally, RA is often accompanied by several co-morbidities, most commonly CVD. A full CPET will often reveal previously undiagnosed cardiac issues. If any such issues are known or identified during the pre-exercise testing process, RA patients should be referred to the relevant medical specialist. Exercise prescription should be primarily for this condition, considering the special considerations of RA.

3.2 Development of exercise programmes for patients with rheumatoid arthritis

Several studies have looked at the potential benefits of exercise in RA (Metsios et al., 2015b; Metsios and Lemmey, 2015; Cooney et al., 2011). Evidence overwhelmingly suggests that exercise is safe and effective for this group of patients. In general, RA patients are able to perform any type of exercise that has been studied and certainly the type of exercise usually associated with ERS – i.e. gym-based circuit training (Metsios et al., 2008b; Stavropoulos-Kalinoglou et al., 2013). However, for an exercise programme to be effective, there are some key criteria that need to be met. These are discussed in detail next.

Patient engagement and the role of the motivational interview

As with any exercise programme, the exercise referral process should start with a face-to-face interview between the exercise practitioner and the patient. The ultimate aim of this interview is to help the patient appreciate the benefits and importance of exercise so that they engage with the programme (Morgan, 2005). Moreover, this interview provides the exercise practitioner with the chance to extract relevant information from the patients that may have been omitted from previous discussions with other members of the team. Such information could include disease characteristics, current and historic severity of symptoms, previous experience of exercise and current physical activity behaviour and likes and dislikes relevant to exercise, as well as any other health issues the patient may experience. The information gathered is useful for the design of the programme. Also, the interview process helps build rapport between the parties involved (Mechanic and Schlesinger, 1996). The interview should conclude with an agreement on the goals that the patient aspires to achieve by following the exercise programme, as well as the monitoring tools that will be used. Common goals include attendance and adherence to sessions, physiological outcomes such as improvement in fitness (e.g. distance covered during a six-minute walk test) or reduction in weight and physical activity goals such as an increase in step count.

Pre-participation screening

Patients with RA have a high prevalence of CVD. Worryingly, in many cases, CVD remains undiagnosed until an episode occurs. Thus, pre-participation screening in RA patients is essential. Using existing questionnaires, such as that of the ACSM (Riebe et al., 2015), is the absolute minimum. It is strongly recommended that blood pressure also be tested as hypertension is often undiagnosed in RA patients (Panoulas et al., 2008). For optimum risk evaluation and exercise prescription, full cardiopulmonary exercise testing (CPET) should be pursued.

Exercise capacity testing in rheumatoid arthritis

At the basis of an individualised exercise prescription lies a suitable testing battery. This needs to be developed and adjusted according to the available equipment and expertise as well as the needs of each patient. In this section, a general approach to exercise testing will be presented. Specific tests can be found in relevant textbooks (e.g. ACSM guidelines for exercise testing and prescription).

Aerobic capacity: As mentioned previously, for safety reasons and also for optimum exercise prescription, a full CPET should be pursued. Several studies have performed CPET with RA patients, and they seem to be able to complete such tests as safely and effectively as other populations (Liff et al., 2019; Stavropoulos-Kalinoglou et al., 2013). Caution should be applied when selecting the mode of exercise as some patients might have movement limitations in a specific joint. For example, a patient might not be able to bend their knees fully; thus, cycling might not be suitable. Is it also important to remember that RA patients often have very low aerobic capacity; thus, initial intensity and intensity increments need to be relatively small. Following warm-up at very low intensity, cycling protocols usually start at 0–25w with a rate of increase of no more than 15–20w per minute while treadmill protocols could start at 2kph with an increment of 0.5kph every minute (Stavropoulos-Kalinoglou et al., 2013). The equation of Hansen et al. (1984) is also suitable for cycling protocols. In the absence of CPET equipment and expertise, a simple test such as the sis-minute walk test (De Santana et al., 2014) can produce useful results for aerobic capacity.

Strength: Muscle wasting is a common feature of RA, and incorporating resistance exercises in the prescription is very important. Evaluation of strength is key in optimising resistance exercise prescription. Most studies that have used resistance exercise have performed various types of repetition maximum testing (RM). While 1RM protocols are generally considered highly valid and reliable in the general population (Seo et al., 2012) and have been used in RA (Lemmey et al., 2009a), they are challenging for the patients to perform. Alternatively, submaximal RM protocols ranging from 3–8RM can be used (Flint-Wagner et al., 2009; Baillet et al., 2011). Importantly, most studies have shown that exercise prescription based on these protocols elicits significant benefits for the patients.

Flexibility: In general, flexibility testing and prescription in RA has been overlooked. Most studies evaluating range of motion have focused on joint movement, and there is very little information on exercise per se. However, some of the common flexibility tests can be adapted for RA patients. The test most commonly used in RA is the sit-and-reach test (De Santana et al., 2014). It often needs to be adapted in such a way that the patients don't need to sit on the floor; a chair sit-and-reach option can be used instead (Jones et al., 1998).

Exercise prescription in rheumatoid arthritis

As mentioned earlier, there is no type of exercise that RA patients can't or shouldn't do collectively. However, given the large variation in symptoms, affected joints and disease severity, RA is one of the conditions that warrants individualised exercise prescription (Metsios et al., 2015b; Stavropoulos-Kalinoglou et al., 2013). This should be based on the key information on patient movement ability, disease characteristics and exercise preferences collected during the initial interview; the results of exercise capacity testing; and the available facilities and expertise.

General principles for exercise prescription in RA: Even though, currently, there are not specific guidelines for exercise prescription in RA, some general principles should be adhered to by all programmes. It is important to understand that these patients may have very low levels of fitness, significant movement limitations and minimal experience of exercise. Also, many patients are likely to be older adults. Consequently, any exercise programme should be easy initially and become progressively harder. The first few sessions should serve as familiarisation with the equipment and the requirements of the programme. It is important for patients to feel safe before they try to achieve their exercise targets. In previous programmes, up to four supervised sessions (two weeks) have been used for familiarisation (Stavropoulos-Kalinoglou et al., 2013).

Intensity and duration of the exercises should be reviewed every four to six weeks or when the patient or the exercise practitioner feels that it is needed. It is often difficult to formally re-evaluate the patient; however, monitoring intensity and effort (discussed later in this chapter) during sessions may provide some useful feedback.

Aerobic Exercise: This should form the bulk of the exercise prescription. Initial frequency should be two or three days per week, with a gradual progression to up to five days per week. More frequent exercise should be viewed with caution so that the joints are given sufficient time to recover. However, in patients with good levels of fitness and controlled disease, higher frequency should be considered.

The minimum aim would be to accumulate the widely recommended 150 minutes of moderate-intensity physical activity or 75 minutes of vigorous physical activity (or any combination of the two) per week, as identified by many nations' physical activity guidelines. Commonly, exercise intensities of 60% to 80% of maximal aerobic capacity have been shown to elicit the greatest benefits and be well tolerated by RA patients. Higher-intensity exercise (> 90% of maximal aerobic capacity) has been tried and proven safe and effective in RA (Sandstad et al., 2015); such approaches could be used but should be reserved for patients who are progressing well with their exercise programme.

The type of exercise is usually the greatest challenge for the exercise practitioner. The exercise programme should be adapted to the abilities of each patient. Commonly, a circuit type of session incorporating different types of exercise (e.g. 2–4 minutes on treadmill, bike, cross-trainer with a brief 1–2 minute rest period in between) will work well for RA patients; this approach places adequate stress on the cardiovascular and pulmonary systems while the joints are used in different ranges of motion that follow different loading patterns.

Resistance exercise: This should be introduced gradually, usually after the first month. Fixed weights and machines are usually easier for patients to use than free weights and may prevent injuries due to poor technique.

In the first instance, an entire session would be used to introduce the patient to the exercises and familiarise them with the function of the equipment and the movement. Is it not uncommon for patients to need several sessions before they are able to be fully independent in using weight-lifting equipment while having the appropriate technique. Until this has been achieved, frequency should be limited to one or two sessions per week.

However, most commonly, resistance exercises would follow the aerobic component of the exercise programme and again be performed in a circuit-training fashion in every session (Stavropoulos-Kalinoglou et al., 2013). Caution is needed with this approach if the person is attending three or more sessions per week. It is advisable not to exercise the same muscle group more than twice per week (Ralston et al., 2018).

Intensity should be very low in the first few sessions. Their aim is familiarisation and not inducing any physiological responses. However, as the patient becomes more confident, a target of 40% to 60% of estimated 1RM should be achieved. Higher intensities could be explored with well-accustomed patients in the later stages of the referral programme.

The greatest challenge is restrictions to range of motion. While RA patients will generally be able to perform most exercises, some limitations in range of movement may prevent them from doing a specific exercise or using some equipment. A common example is the pectoral machine; many patients have limited shoulder movement, and they find it hard to get into position to use this machine. Adjusting the starting position, if the machine allows, or using an alternative exercise (e.g. dumbbell exercises) may be needed. The same problem (i.e. limitations in shoulder mobility) may prevent them from performing a lateral pull-down. Again, adjusting the starting position or using an alternative exercise may be needed. These are only some examples of the challenges facing the exercise professional; good knowledge of exercise adaptations and access to relevant recourses are essential.

Flexibility: As indicated earlier, there is very limited information on flexibility training for RA. Most relevant studies have looked at range of motion and functional capacity. However, most utilise methods of physiotherapy rather than a formal exercise programme. However, physiotherapy can improve mobility and partly restore range of motion in the affected joints without aggravating the disease (Bergstra et al., 2014). Also, a common finding of exercise trials is an improvement in the functional capacity of these patients (Rahnama and Mazloum, 2012).

In practice, flexibility exercises should aim to improve range of movement of the affected joints and also increase the person's overall mobility. They are often included in the warm-up and cool down of the sessions. The effectiveness of this approach has not been formally evaluated.

Exercise type: Some studies have evaluated the benefits of tai-chi and yoga; however, to date, the evidence is too limited and weak to be able to safely conclude their utility (Akyuz and Kenis-Coskun, 2018). Despite the limited evidence, both types of exercise show promising results and, as with all other forms of exercise, seem safe for RA patients. Tai-chi has been shown to reduce swelling and pain while improving overall quality of life (Shin et al., 2015; Uhlig et al., 2010; Wang, 2008). However, these findings are not consistent (Uhlig et al., 2010). Yoga seems to positively affect indices of disease activity (Telles et al., 2011; Singh et al., 2011), pain and quality of life (Bosch et al., 2009; Moonaz et al., 2015).

Hydrotherapy and aquatic exercise are often suggested for RA as the buoyancy of water minimises the forces applied on the joints. Indeed, some studies have evaluated the potential benefits of such exercises. Hydrotherapy programmes have been shown to improve mood states and patient satisfaction, reduce pain and joint tenderness and increase grip strength. While again, these are positive effects, the evidence is not strong enough to reach definitive conclusions (Al-Qubaeissy et al., 2013).

In ERS, exercises such as the ones discussed here can be useful. They could provide an alternative to the routine of the standard gym-based sessions and enhance enjoyment for the patient. However, their effectiveness needs to be further evaluated.

Compliance monitoring

Making sure that the patients are doing what they need to be doing is essential for the success of any exercise programme. Various tools can be used to evaluate compliance in an exercise programme.

Attendance: The first part of compliance is attendance. A monitoring system which records when the patients visit the exercising facility needs to be in place. It is advised that this system is known to the patients so that they understand the facility is keeping a record of their attendance.

Adherence: There is no common definition of adherence to exercise sessions (Bailey et al., 2018). However, one approach that has been effectively used is adherence to exercise prescription in terms of completing the prescribed exercises and achieving intensity targets (Stavropoulos-Kalinoglou et al., 2013). This can be achieved in different ways in a pragmatic setting.

Perceived Effort: A common and easy method to assess exercise intensity is the rate of perceived exertion, often referred to as the Borg scale (Scherr et al., 2013). This is a useful tool to estimate intensity, in the absence of any other equipment, in patients with heart rate (HR) limitations (e.g. chronotropic incompetence) or taking medication that may affect HR (e.g. beta blockers). Also, it is very useful for resistance exercise (Day et al., 2004). Commonly, at the start of the programme a target of 11 to 13 RPE should be set, gradually progressing to 13 to 15 RPE. Higher intensities can be introduced later in the programme in the form of high-intensity interval training or shorter bouts of exercise (Sandstad et al., 2015).

Target heart rate: In most cases, any individualised exercise prescription will provide the patients with a target heart rate (tHR). This is a narrow range of HR that the patient should aim to achieve during each exercise. HR can be easily monitored throughout a session with a suitable device and the values fed back to the supervisor. Also, most modern equipment has a built-in function for HR monitoring.

Case study task

A 54-year-old lady is referred to you for her exercise presciption. She was diagnosed with RA six years ago. Since then, she has been on various NSAIDs and DMARDs, which were effective in reducing symptoms but did little in limiting disease progression. Her main areas of concern are her hips. She is able to walk but only at a slow pace. She often complains about lasting pain in the knees following walks to the shops, and she associates any form of physical activity with increased pain.

Currently, she is on an anti-TNFa agent (etanercept, weekly injection) while also taking methotrexate (15 mg/week). Other than her RA, she is in good health; however, she is hypertensive and has been on an ACE inhibitor for the past three years.

The main aims of your first discussion are to identify her attitude towards exercise and her willingness to include regular exercise in her lifestyle and also to investigate what type of exercise and in what setting she would prefer to perform. The next step will be to develop a fitness-testing battery before prescribing her exercise programme.

Your initial discussions reveal that she has not exercised in years. Even before the diagnosis of RA, she led a sedentary lifestyle. She has never been to the gym, and she very rarely walks or does any outdoor activities. She seems apprehensive about exercising on her own and prefers to attend a supervised facility, at least for the first few months. You describe how your exercise referral scheme works and that there are instruction and supervision available. She agrees to start exercising there and seems keen to try different exercises.

You now need to decide on exercise type and intensity. Think about available equipment, what is possible and what is meaningful to assess. You can use her heart rate reserve to calculate intensity for this exercise (use a resting HR of 82), but consider using more accurate assessments in real life. Based on this, come up with an exercise prescription that will increase her HR to 40% to 60% of her HRR for the first few sessions. Then progress towards 70% based on her responsivness. Also, taking into account her movement limiations, identify a few resistance exercises that she should be able to perform safely and in a controlled maner.

Summary/Key points

- RA is a chronic, inflammatory condition that affects the joints; however, it has several extra-articular manifestations which significantly affect the patient.
- Exercise is safe and has several benefits for RA patients.
- Exercise prescription needs to be individualised.
- Individaulisation should be based on:
    - Medically relevant information from the managing physician (including diagnosis and sites affected by RA, medication, co-morbidities).
    - Fitness testing.

Study tasks

1. What are the main symptoms of rheumatoid arthritis?
2. How common is aheumatoid arthritis, and who is more likely to be affected by it?
3. Which cytokines and transcription factors are central in the development and progression of RA?
4. Which are the main drug classes used in the treatment of RA?
5. What information needs to be communicated from the physicians to the exercise professional prior to the start of an exercise referral programme?
6. What are the benefits of exercise for RA disease symptoms?
7. What are the effects of exercise on cardiovascular risk?
8. What are the effects of exercise on rheumatoid cachexia?
9. What are the main barriers to exercise among RA patients?
10. What are the main considerations for exercise testing in RA?
11. What are the key consideration for exercise prescription in RA?

TABLE 17.3 At-a-glance summary guide to exercise considerations for people with rheumatoid arthritis

Condition name	*Rheumatoid arthritis*
Pathophysiology summary	The cause of RA is unknown. However, it is thought that when a genetically susceptible person is exposed to an environmental stimulus, RA develops. It usually has a rapid onset, causing significant pain and swelling to the joints, eventualy leading to movement limitation and damage. Cytokines (especially TNFa, IL-1 and IL-6) as well as some transcription pathways (NF-κβ) and (AP-1) are central to the developemnt and progression of RA.
Aims of exercise	The main aim of exercise, in the post-rehabilitation phase, is to: • improve overall fitness • maintain or even improve functional capacity • reduce co-morbidity, especially cardiovascular disease and rheumatoid cachexia • reduce disability and increase independance
Exercise considerations	RA patients often have significant movement limitations. These should be taken into account when designing an exercise programme. However, there is no evidence to suggest that any patient, even those with excesive joint damage, should refrain from exercise.

(*Continued*)

TABLE 17.3 (Continued)

Condition name	*Rheumatoid arthritis*
	During flares, patients might not be able to exercise at all. However, they should be advised to do as much as possible. Even some indicative exercises could be provided. Following return to normal function and depending on length of absence, they may need to be re-introduced to their exercise programme gradually. Changes in medication may cause fluctuations in disease activity. These are usually short term and should not affect the patient for more than a few days. However, training might need to be adapted. Co-morbidities are common among RA patients, and these should be evaluated seperately and dealt with accordingly.
Frequency	First weeks: Introduction with low frequency (2–3 days/week) with one resistance session. Thereafter: Three to five days with two resistance sessions (can be combined with the aerobic session). Possible progression to higher frequency based on the patient's abilities and wishes.
Intensity	Starting at a low intensity of 40% to 60% HRR or RPE and progressively increasing to 70%. Higher-intensity exercise can be used and could improve effectiveness and adherence.
Time	An accumulation of 150 minutes per week of moderate exercise, 75 minutes per week of high-intensity exercise or any combination of the two is advised.
Type	Any type of exercise that is tolerated by the patient and achieves the targets set by the exercise professional can be used. A combination of aerobic and resistance exercises should be pursued.
Common medications associated	RA patients may take several different types of medication. Those aimed at managing the disease are classed as analgesics, NSAIDs, corticosteroids, DMARDs and biologics. Medication for co-morbidities is often prescribed.
Key safety considerations	Unfamiliarity with exercise: Some patients will not have exercised for decades. They need to be introduced gradually to their prescription. Movement limitations: Most will have some movement limitations; these need to be taken into account when designing the intervention. Disease flares: During a flare, movement might be limited. They will need to take time off their exercise programme to recover and then be reintroduced to it. Co-morbidities: Many will have co-morbidities with implications for exercise prescription more important that RA itself. These need to be identified. Medication: RA patients are on several different drugs, and some may change often. A detailed list and frequent follow-up are needed.
Effect of exercise on conditions	Improved function, reduced fatigue and pain, improved overall health – including cardiovascular risk profile – possible reduction in disease activity.

References

Akyuz, G. & Kenis-Coskun, O. 2018. The efficacy of Tai Chi and Yoga in rheumatoid arthritis and spondyloarthropathies: A narrative biomedical review. *Rheumatol Int*, 38, 321–330.

Alamanos, Y. & Drosos, A. A. 2005. Epidemiology of adult rheumatoid arthritis. *Autoimmun Rev*, 4, 130–136.

Aletaha, D., Neogi, T., Silman, A. J., Funovits, J., Felson, D. T., Bingham, C. O., Birnbaum, N. S., Burmester, G. R., Bykerk, V. P., Cohen, M. D., Combe, B., Costenbader, K. H., Dougados, M., Emery, P., Ferraccioli, G., Hazes, J. M., Hobbs, K., Huizinga, T. W., Kavanaugh, A., Kay, J., Kvien, T. K., Laing, T., Mease, P., Menard, H. A., Moreland, L. W., Naden, R. L., Pincus, T., Smolen, J. S., Stanislawska-Biernat, E., Symmons, D., Tak, P. P., Upchurch, K. S., Vencovsky, J., Wolfe, F. & Hawker, G. 2010. 2010 rheumatoid arthritis classification criteria: An American college of rheumatology/European league against rheumatism collaborative initiative. *Ann Rheum Dis*, 69, 1580–1588.

Allaire, S., Wolfe, F., Niu, J. & Lavalley, M. P. 2008. Contemporary prevalence and incidence of work disability associated with rheumatoid arthritis in the US. *Arthritis Care Res*, 59, 474–480.

Al-Qubaeissy, K. Y., Fatoye, F. A., Goodwin, P. C. & Yohannes, A. M. 2013. The effectiveness of hydrotherapy in the management of rheumatoid arthritis: A systematic review. *Musculoskelet Care*, 11, 3–18.

Anderson, L., Thompson, D. R., Oldridge, N., Zwisler, A. D., Rees, K., Martin N. & Taylor, R. S. 2016. Exercise-based cardiac rehabilitation for coronary heart disease. *Cochrane Database Syst Rev*, CD001800.

Bailey, D. L., Holden, M. A., Foster, N. E., Quicke, J. G., Haywood, K. L. & Bishop, A. 2018. Defining adherence to therapeutic exercise for musculoskeletal pain: A systematic review. *BJS*, 098742.

Baillet, A., Vaillant, M., Guinot, M., Gaudin, P. & Juvin, R. 2011. Efficacy of resistance exercises in rheumatoid arthritis: Meta-analysis of randomized controlled trials. *Rheumatology*, 51, 519–527.

Benatti, F. B. & Pedersen, B. K. 2015. Exercise as an anti-inflammatory therapy for rheumatic diseases-myokine regulation. *Nat Rev Rheumatol*, 11, 86–97.

Bergstra, S. A., Murgia, A., Te Velde, A. F. & Caljouw, S. R. 2014. A systematic review into the effectiveness of hand exercise therapy in the treatment of rheumatoid arthritis. *Clin Rheumatol*, 33, 1539–1548.

Berra, K., Rippe, J. & Manson, J. E. 2015. Making physical activity counseling a priority in clinical practice: The time for action is now. *JAMA*, 314, 2617–2618.

Bosch, P. R., Traustadottir, T., Howard, P. & Matt, K. S. 2009. Functional and physiological effects of yoga in women with rheumatoid arthritis: A pilot study. *Altern Ther Health Med* 15, 24–31.

Buch, M. & Emery, P. 2002. The aetiology and pathogenesis of rheumatoid arthritis. *Hospital Pharmacist*, 9, 5–10.

Choy, E. 2012. Understanding the dynamics: Pathways involved in the pathogenesis of rheumatoid arthritis. *Rheumatology*, 51, v3–v11.

Cooney, J. K., Law, R. J., Matschke, V., Lemmey, A. B., Moore, J. P., Ahmad, Y., Jones, J. G., Maddison, P. & Thom, J. M. 2011. Benefits of exercise in rheumatoid arthritis. *J Aging Res*, 2011, 681640–681640.

Crofford, L. J. 2000. The role of COX-2 in rheumatoid arthritis synovial tissues. *Arthritis Research*, 1, S30–S30.

Crowson, C. S., Liao, K. P., Davis, J. M., Solomon, D. H., Matteson, E. L., Knutson, K. L., Hlatky, M. A. & Gabriel, S. E. 2013. Rheumatoid arthritis and cardiovascular disease. *Am Heart J*, 166, 622–628, e1.

Dalal, H. M., Doherty, P. & Taylor, R. S. 2015. Cardiac rehabilitation. *BMJ*, 351, h5000.

Dasgupta, K., Rosenberg, E., Joseph, L., Cooke, A. B., Trudeau, L., Bacon, S. L., Chan, D., Sherman, M., Rabasa-Lhoret, R. & Daskalopoulou, S. S. 2017. Physician step prescription and monitoring to improve ARTERial health (SMARTER): A randomized controlled trial in type 2 diabetes and hypertension. *Diabetes Obes Metab*, 17.

Day, M. L., Mcguigan, M. R., Brice, G. & Foster, C. 2004. Monitoring exercise intensity during resistance training using the session RPE scale. *J Strength Cond Res*, 18, 353–58.

Deane, K. D., Demoruelle, M. K., Kelmenson, L. B., Kuhn, K. A., Norris, J. M. & Holers, V. M. 2017. Genetic and environmental risk factors for rheumatoid arthritis. *Best Pract Res Clin Rheumatol*, 31, 3–18.

De Jong, Z., Munneke, M., Kroon, H. M., Van Schaardenburg, D., Dijkmans, B. A., Hazes, J. M. & Vliet Vlieland, T. P. 2009. Long-term follow-up of a high-intensity exercise program in patients with rheumatoid arthritis. *Clin Rheumatol*, 28, 663–671.

De Jong, Z., Munneke, M., Zwinderman, A. H., Kroon, H. M., Jansen, A., Ronday, K. H., Van Schaardenburg, D., Dijkmans, B. A., Van Den Ende, C. H., Breedveld, F. C., Vliet Vlieland, T. P. & Hazes, J. M. 2003. Is a long-term high-intensity exercise program effective and safe in patients with rheumatoid arthritis? Results of a randomized controlled trial. *Arthritis Rheum*, 48, 2415–2424.

De Santana, F. S., Da Cunha Nascimento, D., De Freitas, J. P. M., Miranda, R. F., Muniz, L. F., Santos Neto, L., Da Mota, L. M. H. & Balsamo, S. 2014. Assessment of functional capacity in patients with rheumatoid arthritis: implications for recommending exercise. *Revista Brasileira de Reumatologia (English Edition)*, 54, 378–385.

Doran, M. F., Pond, G. R., Crowson, C. S., O'fallon, W. M. & Gabriel, S. E. 2002. Trends in incidence and mortality in rheumatoid arthritis in Rochester, Minnesota, over a forty-year period. *Arthritis Rheum*, 46, 625–631.

Doyle, C., Lennox, L. & Bell, D. 2013. A systematic review of evidence on the links between patient experience and clinical safety and effectiveness. *BMJ Open*, 3.

Erhardt, C. C., Mumford, P. A., Venables, P. J. & Maini, R. N. 1989. Factors predicting a poor life prognosis in rheumatoid arthritis: An eight-year prospective study. *Ann Rheum Dis*, 48, 7–13.

Fevang, B. T., Lie, S. A., Havelin, L. I., Engesaeter, L. B. & Furnes, O. 2007. Reduction in orthopedic surgery among patients with chronic inflammatory joint disease in Norway, 1994–2004. *Arthritis Rheum*, 57, 529–532.

Flint-Wagner, H. G., Lisse, J., Lohman, T. G., Going, S. B., Guido, T., Cussler, E., Gates, D. & Yocum, D. E. 2009. Assessment of a sixteen-week training program on strength, pain, and function in rheumatoid arthritis patients. *J Clin Rheumatol*, 15, 165–171.

Franchimont, D. 2004. Overview of the actions of glucocorticoids on the immune response: A good model to characterize new pathways of immunosuppression for new treatment strategies. *Annals of the New York Academy of Sciences*, 1024, 124–137.

Funk, C. D. & Fitzgerald, G. A. 2007. COX-2 inhibitors and cardiovascular risk. *J Cardiovasc Pharmacol*, 50, 470–479.

Gates, A. B., Kerry, R., Moffatt, F., Ritchie, I. K., Meakins, A., Thornton, J. S., Rosenbaum, S. & Taylor, A. 2017. Movement for movement: exercise as everybody's business? *Br J Sports Med*, 51, 767–768.

George, M. D. & Baker, J. F. 2016. The obesity epidemic and consequences for rheumatoid arthritis care. *Curr Rheumatol Rep*, 18, 6.

Gielen, S., Schuler, G. & Adams, V. 2010. Cardiovascular effects of exercise training: molecular mechanisms. *Circulation*, 122, 1221–1238.

Glennas, A., Kvien, T. K., Andrup, O., Karstensen, B. & Munthe, E. 2000. Recent onset arthritis in the elderly: A 5 year longitudinal observational study. *J Rheumatol*, 27, 101–108.

Gould, D. W., Lahart, I., Carmichael, A. R., Koutedakis, Y. & Metsios, G. S. 2013. Cancer cachexia prevention via physical exercise: Molecular mechanisms. *J Cachexia Sarcopenia Muscle*, 4, 111–124.

Hansen, J. E., Sue, D. Y. & Wasserman, K. 1984. Predicted values for clinical exercise testing. *Am Rev Respir Dis*, 129, S49–S55.

Hayashino, Y., Jackson, J. L., Hirata, T., Fukumori, N., Nakamura, F., Fukuhara, S., Tsujii, S. & Ishii, H. 2014. Effects of exercise on C-reactive protein, inflammatory cytokine and adipokine in patients with type 2 diabetes: A meta-analysis of randomized controlled trials. *Metabolism*, 63, 431–440.

Hewlett, S., Chalder, T., Choy, E., Cramp, F., Davis, B., Dures, E., Nicholls, C. & Kirwan, J. 2011. Fatigue in rheumatoid arthritis: Time for a conceptual model. *Rheumatol (Oxford)*, 50, 1004–1006.

Humphreys, J. H., Verstappen, S. M. M., Hyrich, K. L., Chipping, J. R., Marshall, T. & Symmons, D. P. M. 2012. The incidence of rheumatoid arthritis in the UK: Comparisons using the 2010 ACR/EULAR classification criteria and the 1987 ACR classification criteria. Results from the Norfolk Arthritis register. *Ann Rheum Dis*, 72.

Hunder, G. G. 2005. *Atlas of rheumatology*, Philadelphia: Current Medicine.

Hurkmans, E., Van Der Giesen, F. J., Vliet Vlieland, T. P., Schoones, J. & Van Den Ende, E. C. 2009. Dynamic exercise programs (aerobic capacity and/or muscle strength training) in patients with rheumatoid arthritis. *Cochrane Database Syst Rev*, CD006853.

Joint Formulary Committee. 2017. *British National Formulary*, London: BMJ Group and Pharmaceutical Press.

Jones, C. J., Rikli, R. E., Max, J. & Noffal, G. 1998. The reliability and validity of a chair sit-and-reach test as a measure of hamstring flexibility in older adults. *Res Q Exerc Sport*, 69, 338–343.

Joshi, P. & Dhaneshwar, S. S. 2014. An update on disease modifying antirheumatic drugs. *Inflamm Allergy Drug Targets*, 13, 249–261.

Joyner, M. J. & Green, D. J. 2009. Exercise protects the cardiovascular system: Effects beyond traditional risk factors. *J Physiol*, 587, 5551–558.

Kitas, G. D. & Erb, N. 2003. Tackling ischaemic heart disease in rheumatoid arthritis. *Rheumatology (Oxford)*, 42, 607–613.

Kitas, G. D. & Gabriel, S. E. 2011. Cardiovascular disease in rheumatoid arthritis: State of the art and future perspectives. *Ann Rheum Dis*, 70, 8–14.

Kumar, V., Abbas, A. K. & Aster, J. C. 2015. *Robbins and Cotran pathologic basis of disease*, Philadelphia: Elsevier/Saunders.

Landre-Beauvais, A. J. 2001. The first description of rheumatoid arthritis: Unabridged text of the doctoral dissertation presented in 1800. *Joint Bone Spine*, 68, 130–143.

Lemmey, A. B., Marcora, S. M., Chester, K., Wilson, S., Casanova, F. & Maddison, P. J. 2009a. Effects of high-intensity resistance training in patients with rheumatoid arthritis: A randomized controlled trial. *Arthritis Rheum*, 61, 1726–1734.

Lemmey, A. B., Marcora, S. M., Chester, K., Wilson, S., Casanova, F. & Maddison P. J. 2009b. Effects of high-intensity resistance training in patients with rheumatoid arthritis: A randomized controlled trial. *Arthritis Rheum*, 61, 1726–1734.

Liff, M. H., Hoff, M., Fremo, T., Wisløff, U., Thomas, R. & Videm, V. 2019. Cardiorespiratory fitness in patients with rheumatoid arthritis is associated with the patient global assessment but not with objective measurements of disease activity. *RMD Open*, 5, e000912.

Lopez-Vargas, P. A., Tong, A., Howell, M. & Craig, J. C. 2016. Educational interventions for patients with CKD: A systematic review. *Am J Kidney Dis*, 68, 353–370.

Louie, G. H. & Ward, M. M. 2009. Changes in the rates of joint surgery among patients with Rheumatoid Arthritis in California, 1983–2007. *Ann Rheum Dis*, 69.

Malik, A. & Lo, S. 1996. Vascular endothelial adhesion molecules and tissue inflammation. *Pharmacol Rev*, 48, 213–229.

Marcora, S. M., Chester, K. R., Mittal, G., Lemmey, A. B. & Maddison, P. J. 2006. Randomized phase 2 trial of anti-tumor necrosis factor therapy for cachexia in patients with early rheumatoid arthritis. *Am J Clin Nutr*, 84, 1463–1472.

Marcora, S. M., Lemmey, A. B. & Maddison, P. J. 2005. Can progressive resistance training reverse cachexia in patients with rheumatoid arthritis? Results of a pilot study. *J Rheumatol*, 32, 1031–1039.

Marrelli, A., Cipriani, P., Liakouli, V., Carubbi, F., Perricone, C., Perricone, R. & Giacomelli, R. 2011. Angiogenesis in rheumatoid arthritis: A disease specific process or a common response to chronic inflammation? *Autoimmunity Rev*, 10, 595–598.

Maruthur, N. M., Wang, N. Y. & Appel, L. J. 2009. Lifestyle interventions reduce coronary heart disease risk: Results from the PREMIER Trial. *Circulation*, 119, 2026–2031.

McCarthy, B., Casey, D., Devane, D., Murphy, K., Murphy, E. & Lacasse, Y. 2015. Pulmonary rehabilitation for chronic obstructive pulmonary disease. *Cochrane Database Syst Rev*, CD003793.

Mechanic, D. & Schlesinger, M. 1996. The impact of managed care on patients' trust in medical care and their physicians. *JAMA*, 275, 1693–1697.

Metsios, G. S., Koutedakis, Y., Veldhuijzen Van Zanten, J. J., Stavropoulos-Kalinoglou, A., Vitalis, P., Duda, J. L., Ntoumanis, N., Rouse, P. C. & Kitas, G. D. 2015a. Cardiorespiratory fitness levels and their association with cardiovascular profile in patients with rheumatoid arthritis: A cross-sectional study. *Rheumatol (Oxford)*, 54, 2215–2220.

Metsios, G. S. & Lahart, I. M. 2015. Exercise as medicine in rheumatoid arthritis. *Mediterr J Rheumatol*, 26, 54–61.

Metsios, G. S. & Lemmey, A. 2015. Exercise as medicine in rheumatoid arthritis: Effects on function, body composition, and cardiovascular disease risk. *J Clin Exerc Physiol*, 4, 14–22.

Metsios, G. S., Stavropoulos-Kalinoglou, A., Douglas, K. M., Koutedakis, Y., Nevill, A. M., Panoulas, V. F., Kita, M. & Kitas, G. D. 2007. Blockade of tumour necrosis factor-alpha in rheumatoid arthritis: Effects on components of rheumatoid cachexia. *Rheumatol (Oxford)*, 46, 1824–1827.

Metsios, G. S., Stavropoulos-Kalinoglou, A. & Kitas, G. D. 2015b. The role of exercise in the management of rheumatoid arthritis. *Expert Rev Clin Immunol*, 11, 1121–1130.

Metsios, G. S., Stavropoulos-Kalinoglou, A., Panoulas, V. F., Koutedakis, Y., Nevill, A. M., Douglas, K. M., Kita, M. & Kitas, G. D. 2008a. New resting energy expenditure prediction equations for patients with rheumatoid arthritis. *Rheumatol (Oxford)*, 47, 500–506.

Metsios, G. S., Stavropoulos-Kalinoglou, A., Panoulas, V. F., Sandoo, A., Toms, T. E., Nevill, A. M., Koutedakis, Y. & Kitas, G. D. 2009a. Rheumatoid cachexia and cardiovascular disease. *Clin Exp Rheumatol*, 27, 985–988.

Metsios, G. S., Stavropoulos-Kalinoglou, A., Panoulas, V. F., Wilson, M., Nevill, A. M., Koutedakis, Y. & Kitas, G. D. 2009b. Association of physical inactivity with increased cardiovascular risk in patients with rheumatoid arthritis. *Eur J Cardiovasc Prev Rehabil*, 16, 188–194.

Metsios, G. S., Stavropoulos-Kalinoglou, A., Treharne, G. J., Nevill, A. M., Sandoo, A., Panoulas, V. F., Toms, T. E., Koutedakis, Y. & Kitas, G. D. 2011. Disease activity and low physical activity associate with number of hospital admissions and length of hospitalisation in patients with rheumatoid arthritis. *Arthritis Res Ther*, 13, R108.

Metsios, G. S., Stavropoulos-Kalinoglou, A., Veldhuijzen Van Zanten, J. J., Nightingale, P., Sandoo, A., Dimitroulas, T., Kitas, G. D. & Koutedakis, Y. 2014. Individualised exercise improves endothelial function in patients with rheumatoid arthritis. *Ann Rheum Dis*, 73, 748–751.

Metsios, G. S., Stavropoulos-Kalinoglou, A., Veldhuijzen Van Zanten, J. J., Treharne, G. J., Panoulas, V. F., Douglas, K. M., Koutedakis, Y. & Kitas, G. D. 2008b. Rheumatoid arthritis, cardiovascular disease and physical exercise: A systematic review. *Rheumatol (Oxford)*, 47, 239–248.

Mojcik, C. F. & Shevach, E. M. 1997. Adhesion molecules: a rheumatologic perspective. *Arthritis Rheum*, 40, 991–1004.

Moonaz, S. H., Bingham, C. O., Wissow, L. & Bartlett, S. J. 2015. Yoga in sedentary adults with arthritis: Effects of a randomized controlled pragmatic trial. *J Rheumatol*, 42, 1194–1202.

Morgan, O. 2005. Approaches to increase physical activity: Reviewing the evidence for exercise-referral schemes. *Public Health*, 119, 361–370.

Munoz-Canoves, P., Scheele, C., Pedersen, B. K. & Serrano, A. L. 2013. Interleukin-6 myokine signaling in skeletal muscle: A double-edged sword? *FEBS J*, 280, 4131–4148.

Nassonov, E. L., Samsonov, M. Y., Chichasova, N. V., Nikiphorova, E. L., Tilz, G. P., Demel, U., Widner, B. & Fuchs, D. 2000. Soluble adhesion molecules in rheumatoid arthritis. *Rheumatol*, 39, 808–810.

NICE (National Institute of Health and Care Excellence). 2014. *Physical activity: Exercise referral schemes*. www.nice.org.uk/guidance/ph54.

Okamoto, H., Cujec, T. P., Yamanaka, H. & Kamatani, N. 2008. Molecular aspects of rheumatoid arthritis: role of transcription factors. *Febs J*, 275.

Onions, C. T., Friedrichsen, G. W. S. & Burchfield, R. W. 1996. *The Oxford Dictionary of English etymology*, Oxford: Oxford University Press.

Ospelt, C. & Gay, S. 2008. The role of resident synovial cells in destructive arthritis. *Best Pract Res Clin Rheumatol*, 22, 239–252.

Panoulas, V. F., Douglas, K. M., Milionis, H. J., Stavropoulos-Kalinglou, A., Nightingale, P., Kita, M. D., Tselios, A. L., Metsios, G. S., Elisaf, M. S. & Kitas, G. D. 2007. Prevalence and associations of hypertension and its control in patients with rheumatoid arthritis. *Rheumatol (Oxford)*, 46, 1477–1482.

Panoulas, V. F., Metsios, G. S., Pace, A. V., John, H., Treharne, G. J., Banks, M. J. & Kitas, G. D. 2008. Hypertension in rheumatoid arthritis. *Rheumatol (Oxford)*, 47, 1286–1298.

Pedersen, B. K. & Febbraio, M. A. 2008. Muscle as an endocrine organ: Focus on muscle-derived interleukin-6. *Physiol Rev*, 88, 1379–1406.

Radner, H., Neogi, T., Smolen, J. S. & Aletaha, D. 2014. Performance of the 2010 ACR/EULAR classification criteria for rheumatoid arthritis: A systematic literature review. *Ann Rheum Dis*, 73, 114–123.

Rahnama, N. & Mazloum, V. 2012. Effects of strengthening and aerobic exercises on pain severity and function in patients with knee rheumatoid arthritis. *Int J Prev Med*, 3, 493–498.

Ralston, G. W., Kilgore, L., Wyatt, F. B., Buchan, D. & Baker, J. S. 2018. Weekly training frequency effects on strength gain: A meta-analysis. *Sports Med – Open*, 4, 36.

Repping-Wuts, H., Fransen, J., Van Achterberg, T., Bleijenberg, G. & Van Riel, P. 2007. Persistent severe fatigue in patients with rheumatoid arthritis. *J Clin Nurs*, 16, 377–383.

Riebe, D., Franklin, B. A., Thompson, P. D., Garber, C. E., Whitfield, G. P., Magal, M. & Pescatello, L. S. 2015. Updating ACSM's recommendations for exercise preparticipation health screening. *Med Sci Sports Exerc*, 47, 2473–2479.

Rongen-Van Dartel, S. A., Repping-Wuts, H., Flendrie, M., Bleijenberg, G., Metsios, G. S., Van Den Hout, W. B., Van Den Ende, C. H., Neuberger, G., Reid, A., Van Riel, P. L. & Fransen, J. 2015. Effect of aerobic exercise training on fatigue in rheumatoid arthritis: A meta-analysis. *Arthritis Care Res (Hoboken)*, 67, 1054–1062.

Roubenoff, R., Roubenoff, R. A., Cannon, J. G., Kehayias, J. J., Zhuang, H., Dawson-Hughes, B., Dinarello, C. A. & Rosenberg, I. H. 1994. Rheumatoid cachexia: Cytokine-driven hypermetabolism accompanying reduced body cell mass in chronic inflammation. *J Clin Invest*, 93, 2379–2386.

Rouse, P. C., Veldhuijzen Van Zanten, J. J., Metsios, G. S., Ntoumanis, N., Yu, C. A., Koutedakis, Y., Fenton, S. A., Coast, J., Mistry, H., Kitas, G. D. & Duda, J. L. 2014. Fostering autonomous motivation, physical activity and cardiorespiratory fitness in rheumatoid arthritis: Protocol and rationale for a randomised control trial. *BMC Musculoskelet Disord*, 15, 445.

Saltiel, A. R. & Olefsky, J. M. 2017. Inflammatory mechanisms linking obesity and metabolic disease. *J Clin Invest*, 127, 1–4.

Sandstad, J., Stensvold, D., Hoff, M., Nes, B. M., Arbo, I. & Bye, A. 2015. The effects of high intensity interval training in women with rheumatic disease: A pilot study. *Eur J Appl Physiol*, 115, 2081–2089.

Scherr, J., Wolfarth, B., Christle, J. W., Pressler, A., Wagenpfeil, S. & Halle, M. 2013. Associations between Borg's rating of perceived exertion and physiological measures of exercise intensity. *Eur J Appl Physiol*, 113, 147–155.

Scott, D. L., Pugner, K., Kaarela, K., Doyle, D. V., Woolf, A., Holmes, J. & Hieke, K. 2000. The links between joint damage and disability in rheumatoid arthritis. *Rheumatol*, 39, 122–132.

Seo, D. I., Kim, E., Fahs, C. A., Rossow, L., Young, K., Ferguson, S. L., Thiebaud, R., Sherk, V. D., Loenneke, J. P., Kim, D., Lee, M. K., Choi, K. H., Bemben, D. A., Bemben, M. G. & So, W.-Y. 2012. Reliability of the one-repetition maximum test based on muscle group and gender. *J Sports Sci Med*, 11, 221–225.

Sherrer, Y. S., Bloch, D. A., Mitchell, D. M., Young, D. Y. & Fries, J. F. 1986. The development of disability in rheumatoid arthritis. *Arthritis Rheum*, 29, 494–500.

Shields, G. E., Wells, A., Doherty, P., Heagerty, A., Buck, D. & Davies, L. M. 2018 Cost-effectiveness of cardiac rehabilitation: A systematic review. *Heart*, 104.

Shin, J. H., Lee, Y., Kim, S. G., Choi, B. Y., Lee, H. S. & Bang, S. Y. 2015. The beneficial effects of Tai Chi exercise on endothelial function and arterial stiffness in elderly women with rheumatoid arthritis. *Arthritis Res Ther*, 17, 380.

Singh, V. K., Bhandari, R. B. & Rana, B. B. 2011. Effect of yogic package on rheumatoid arthritis. *Indian J Physiol Pharmacol*, 55, 329–335.

Sokka, T., Hakkinen, A., Kautiainen, H., Maillefert, J. F., Toloza, S., Mork Hansen, T., Calvo-Alen, J., Oding, R., Liveborn, M., Huisman, M., Alten, R., Pohl, C., Cutolo, M., Immonen, K., Woolf, A., Murphy, E., Sheehy, C., Quirke, E., Celik, S., Yazici, Y., Tlustochowicz, W., Kapolka, D., Skakic, V., Rojkovich, B., Muller, R., Stropuviene, S., Andersone, D., Drosos, A. A., Lazovskis, J., Pincus,

T. & Group, Q. R. 2008. Physical inactivity in patients with rheumatoid arthritis: Data from twenty-one countries in a cross-sectional, international study. *Arthritis Rheum*, 59, 42–50.

Stavropoulos-Kalinoglou, A., Metsios, G. S., Koutedakis, Y. & Kitas, G. D. 2011a. Obesity in rheumatoid arthritis. *Rheumatol*, 50, 450–462.

Stavropoulos-Kalinoglou, A., Metsios, G. S., Koutedakis, Y. & Kitas, G. D. 2011b. Obesity in rheumatoid arthritis. *Rheumatol (Oxford)*, 50, 450–462.

Stavropoulos-Kalinoglou, A., Metsios, G. S., Koutedakis, Y., Nevill, A. M., Douglas, K. M., Jamurtas, A., Van Zanten, J. J., Labib, M. & Kitas, G. D. 2007. Redefining overweight and obesity in rheumatoid arthritis patients. *Ann Rheum Dis*, 66, 1316–1321.

Stavropoulos-Kalinoglou, A., Metsios, G. S., Veldhuijzen Van Zanten, J. J., Nightingale, P., Kitas, G. D. & Koutedakis, Y. 2013. Individualised aerobic and resistance exercise training improves cardiorespiratory fitness and reduces cardiovascular risk in patients with rheumatoid arthritis. *Ann Rheum Dis*, 72, 1819–1825.

Steinbrocker, O., Traeger, C. H. & Batterman, R. C. 1949. Therapeutic criteria in rheumatoid arthritis. *J Am Med Assoc*, 140, 659–662.

Summers, G. D., Metsios, G. S., Stavropoulos-Kalinoglou, A. & Kitas, G. D. 2010. Rheumatoid cachexia and cardiovascular disease. *Nat Rev Rheumatol*, 6, 445–451.

Telles, S., Naveen, K. V., Gaur, V. & Balkrishna, A. 2011. Effect of one week of yoga on function and severity in rheumatoid arthritis. *BMC Res Note*, 4, 118.

Terpstra, S. J., De Witte, L. P. & Diederiks, J. P. 1992. Compliance of patients with an exercise program for rheumatoid arthritis. *Physiother Can* 44, 37–41.

Treharne G. J., Douglas K. M. J., Iwaszko J., Panoulas V. F., Hale E. D., Mitton D. L., Piper H., Erb N. & Kitas G. D. 2007. Polypharmacy among people with rheumatoid arthritis: The role of age, disease duration and comorbidity. *Musculoskeletal Care*, 5, 175–190.

Tugwell, P., Singh, J. A. & Wells, G. A. 2011. Biologicals for rheumatoid arthritis. *BMJ*, 343, d4027.

Uhlig, T., Fongen, C., Steen, E., Christie, A. & Ødegård, S. 2010. Exploring Tai Chi in rheumatoid arthritis: A quantitative and qualitative study. *BMC Musculoskeletal Disorders*, 11, 43.

Vane, J. R. & Botting, R. M. 1996. Mechanism of action of anti-inflammatory drugs. *Scand J Rheumatol*, 25, 9–21.

Veldhuijzen Van Zanten, J. J., Rouse, P. C., Hale, E. D., Ntoumanis, N., Metsios, G. S., Duda, J. L. & Kitas, G. D. 2015. Perceived barriers, facilitators and benefits for regular physical activity and exercise in patients with rheumatoid arthritis: A review of the literature. *Sports Med*, 45, 1401–1412.

Verheggen, R. J., Maessen, M. F., Green, D. J., Hermus, A. R., Hopman, M. T. & Thijssen, D. H. 2016. A systematic review and meta-analysis on the effects of exercise training versus hypocaloric diet: Distinct effects on body weight and visceral adipose tissue. *Obes Rev*, 17, 664–690.

Wadley, A. J., Veldhuijzen Van Zanten, J. J., Stavropoulos-Kalinoglou, A., Metsios, G. S., Smith, J. P., Kitas, G. D. & Aldred, S. 2014. Three months of moderate-intensity exercise reduced plasma 3-nitrotyrosine in rheumatoid arthritis patients. *Eur J Appl Physiol*, 114, 1483–1492.

Walsmith, J. & Roubenoff, R. 2002. Cachexia in rheumatoid arthritis. *Int J Cardiol*, 85, 89–99.

Wang, C. 2008. Tai Chi improves pain and functional status in adults with rheumatoid arthritis: results of a pilot single-blinded randomized controlled trial. *Med Sport Sci*, 52, 218–229.

Wilcox, S., Der Ananian, C., Abbott, J., Vrazel, J., Ramsey, C., Sharpe, P. A. & Brady, T. 2006. Perceived exercise barriers, enablers, and benefits among exercising and nonexercising adults with arthritis: Results from a qualitative study. *Arthritis Rheum*, 55, 616–627.

WHO (World Health Organisation). 2015. *Global recommendations of physical activity and health*. Factsheet No. 385. www.who.int/dietphysicalactivity/pa/en/.

Zangi, H. A., Ndosi, M., Adams, J., Andersen, L., Bode, C., Boström, C., Van Eijk-Hustings, Y., Gossec, L., Korandová, J., Mendes, G., Niedermann, K., Primdahl, J., Stoffer, M., Voshaar, M. & Van Tubergen, A. 2015. EULAR recommendations for patient education for people with inflammatory arthritis. *Ann Rheum Dis*, 74, 954–962.

18

OSTEOARTHRITIS AND JOINT REPLACEMENT

Liba Sheeran, Nicola Pease, Kate Button and Joseph M. Moore

Chapter aims

The aims of this chapter are to:

- Describe the pathology of osteoarthritis (OA) within a continuum of early joint changes to patients requiring joint replacement
- Explore up-to-date evidence-based management guidelines for OA
- Evaluate the effect of OA and joint replacement (including the impact of drug therapies and associated age-related co-morbidities) on a person's ability to exercise and respond to exercise
- Evaluate the effect of exercise on people with OA and joint replacement
- Overview the current methods for fitness testing and exercise programming suitable for people with OA and joint replacement

Introduction

Osteoarthritis (OA) is a degenerative disease of the musculoskeletal system inextricably linked with joint pain, swelling, stiffness, muscle weakness and subsequent loss of function and independence. Although OA is characterised as a progressive degradation of articular cartilage that is irreversible, OA can be successfully managed by exercise, which is now widely accepted as a critical pillar of OA management. Nevertheless, the significant physical, psychological, emotional, cognitive and environmental challenges associated with exercising with OA limit the uptake of and adherence to regular exercise in people living with OA. In addition, OA is a disease most prevalent in ageing populations with likely (although not invariably) lower exercise tolerance and co-morbidities bringing further obstacles impacting on motivation, capability and eventually opportunity to exercise and benefit from exercise.

To appropriately advise, prescribe and deliver exercise management for people with OA and joint replacement, this chapter aims to provide exercise practitioners with current understanding and knowledge of the OA pathology and treatment options with particular focus

DOI: 10.4324/9781315102399-18

on how it affects a person's ability to participate in and respond to exercise. The impact of exercise on OA and how to best ensure the most favourable response through appropriate exercise and fitness testing and programming are also discussed. Finally, a practical approach to exercise programming in this population is described in the form of a case study of exercise management of a person with OA in the knee.

1. Overview of pathology

OA is the most common form of arthritis and one of the leading causes of pain and disability worldwide. It most commonly affects the spine, knees, hips and hand joints in ageing populations or patients with previous joint trauma. Knee and hip OA are the 11th highest contributors to global disability (Cross et al. 2014). In the US, the age-standardised prevalence of radiographic OA is reported to range from 19% to 28% in individuals over 45 years of age (Zhang et al. 2010). In the UK, one-third of those over 45 years old (8.15 million) have sought treatment for OA, with over 20% of these seeking treatment for OA in multiple joints (Versus Arthritis 2019).

OA is characterised by a localised loss of cartilage, leading to subchondral bone changes, synovial inflammation, meniscal degeneration, remodelling of adjacent bone and associated inflammation (Poole 1999; Loeser et al. 2012). Loss of cartilage results from a failure to fully repair joint damage that can be caused by a number of mechanisms. Whilst OA is primarily a pathology of joint cartilage, the disease process can impact all structures within a joint, such as nerves, synovium, menisci and bones. These associated outcomes of OA have a direct impact on joint health and patient quality of life.

Cartilage damage can occur through acute and chronic mechanisms; however certain risk factors have been identified that appear to increase the risk of OA development. Risk factors for the development of OA are increasing age from late 40s onwards, sex (more common in females), high body mass, physical injury, biomechanical abnormalities, genetic factors, previous joint pathology, family history of knee replacement and nutritional and vitamin deficiencies (Allen and Golightly 2015; Versus Arthritis 2019; NICE 2020). Whilst many of these factors are not modifiable, some can be mitigated through interventions, including physical activity and exercise, and help inform the basis of non-operative treatment and management of OA.

OA is a long-term condition, and the rate of progression that individuals report pain and loss of function varies among patients. In some individuals, OA will demonstrate rapid progression, and in others, it can remain unchanged for many years (Deveza et al. 2017). Factors that have been suggested to be associated with a more rapid disease and symptom progression are higher body mass index (BMI), male sex, higher pain levels, greater cartilage damage and higher levels of certain biomarkers. Additional factors that are associated with a worse trajectory for pain and function are lower education, lower social class, passive coping strategies, poorer general health, presence of co-morbidities, presence of psychological issues, worse baseline symptoms, joint line space and bony tenderness (Deveza et al. 2017).

2. Management and medications

Individuals with OA will normally be managed in a primary care setting first by contact with clinicians such as general practitioners, physiotherapists, podiatrists, occupational therapists or nurses. If symptoms worsen, consultation with an orthopedic surgeon is often arranged to evaluate surgical options, including joint replacement.

Diagnosis is made after assessment of the patient's history and symptoms and manual examination of the joint and assessment of images of the joint (e.g. magnetic resonance imaging and X-rays). Individuals with OA often report pain that may or may not be localised around the joint and loss of function. Symptoms that an individual with OA may present with include tenderness around the joint line, joint crepitus, swelling, reduced motion and giving way of the joint. OA should be expected in anyone who is over the age of 45 years, has sports- or activity-related joint pain and has no morning stiffness or stiffness that lasts no longer than 30 minutes (NICE 2020; Versus Arthritis 2019). X-rays and MRI can support the diagnosis of OA; however, there can be poor correlation between baseline and changes in tissue degradation severity visible on images of the joint and the symptoms individuals experience (NICE 2020; Versus Arthritis 2019). In the knee, early OA may be present in individuals who have an X-ray Kellgren-Lawrence score (NICE 2020; Versus Arthritis 2019) of less than 2 but have had two episodes of pain for at least ten days in the past year and have arthroscopic or MRI evidence of articular cartilage damage and subchondral bone marrow lesions (Luyten et al. 2012).

While current treatments to restore cartilage and joint health are limited, the symptoms associated with OA can be successfully managed through a variety of conservative or surgical approaches. Conservative management can be further split into non-pharmacological and pharmacological. The first line of management will normally be conservative; however, where symptoms become more severe, surgical intervention is then performed, often through joint replacement. A number of clinical guidelines, consensus statements and recommendations have been published based on the research evidence for these interventions (NICE 2020; Jevsevar et al. 2013; Hochberg et al. 2012). These guidelines are often based on evidence of knee and hip OA potentially limiting their efficacy in the management of OA in other joints. This chapter focuses on the use of exercise to manage OA; however, details of general recommendations for other management tools are presented as well. Due to the complexity of factors influencing OA symptoms, patients will often be treated with a number of methods; therefore, any possible interactions between the described approaches and exercise are also described.

Conservative non-pharmacological

Advice and education: This involves providing individuals with information about OA and can cover areas such as the natural history and progression of OA, diagnosis and treatment options. Information can be tailored to individual needs, and people with OA should be signposted to websites or written information that they can access at home. This also needs to ensure that individuals have an appropriate skill set in exercise prescription, pain coping and coping strategies (Nicolson et al. 2017; Holden et al. 2020; Deveza et al. 2017).

Exercise: One of the most highly recommended management options as it is safe and low cost. There is a large body of evidence that supports the effectiveness of exercise at reducing pain and increasing function compared to no exercise. The effects of exercise on OA are discussed in detail later.

Weight management: This is seen as an essential component in the treatment of OA to reduce the load placed on the affected joints. Individuals should be directed to appropriate information or structured programmes based on their needs. A number of generic guidelines on weight management and obesity for long-term conditions are available; these are not specific to OA (NICE 2020).

Self-management programmes: These multi-modal interventions are often based on behaviour change theory. One of the most widely recognised programmes is ESCAPE for hip and knee OA (Hurley et al. 2007) and MOSAICS for hand OA (Dziedzic et al. 2018). Despite the recommendation, a recent review by Kroon et al. (2014) concluded that overall, there was a low level of evidence that these programmes benefited patients with knee OA. Future studies need to define the self-management intervention better and use different models of self-management to underpin these interventions.

Insoles: Insoles with shock-absorbing properties or shock-absorbing footwear are often recommended to individuals with hip or knee OA.

Manual therapy and electrotherapy: This can be offered as part of a multi-modal rehabilitation programme alongside other non-pharmacological interventions, such as exercise and information provision.

Walking aids and braces: These are offered on an individual basis when an individual is at risk of falling or requires assistance during gait by unloading the joint and therefore reducing pain.

Conservative pharmacological

Pharmacological options in OA can be broadly divided into oral analgesics and topical treatments. Whilst the prescription or recommendation of pharmacological treatment is the responsibility of health-care practitioners, it is important to understand the possible implications of pharmaceutical treatments and their interactions with other interventions such as exercise.

Oral analgesics

- Paracetamol
- Opioids
- Non-steroidal anti-inflammatories (NSAIDs)

Sufferers of OA often experience chronic pain, rather than acute episodes of severe pain, meaning analgesics are taken on a regular basis. Prescription is often done in accordance with the World Health Organization's three-step analgesic ladder (Reid & Davies 2004):

Step 1 – Non-opioid (e.g. paracetamol)
Step 2 – Weak opioid (e.g. cocodamol)
Step 3 – Strong opioid (e.g. morphine)

The intended outcome of analgesics is to reduce discomfort and pain. In addition to improving the patient's quality of life, a reduction in pain can also increase patient mobility and remove a possible barrier to exercise. In addition to any possible contraindications being checked with a health-care professional prior to commencing exercise, it should also be noted that opioid-based analgesics can also result in increased fatigue in a patient. This increased sleepiness may result in a reduced drive to perform exercise.

TABLE 18.1 Medication considerations for exercise for people with osteoarthritis

Class name	*Generic name*	*Brand name*	*Indication*	*Action*	*Side effects*	*Exercise considerations*
Analgesic	painkiller	Paracetamol Nurofen	Musculoskeletal pain or discomfort	Reduce pain	Possible drowsiness	Painkillers may reduce the perception of pain; therefore care should be taken in case this effect masks musculoskeletal injury

NSAIDs (e.g. ibuprofen, naproxen, celecoxib) are of benefit in managing pains associated with OA-related inflammation; however, they are associated with serious side effects limiting their long-term use. NSAIDs as a group are known to cause renal toxicity leading to renal failure, increase the risk of gastrointestinal ulcer and bleeds, worsen heart failure and increase the risk of myocardial infarction/thrombotic CVA. Whilst the impact of NSAIDs on exercise is minimal, there is evidence to suggest that their use may reduce muscular adaptations to exercise by inhibiting the natural inflammatory response to exercise (Schoenfeld 2012).

The effects of analgesics on the exercise response are indicated in Table 18.1.

Surgery

Where conservative management has been unable to control a patient's pain to within a bearable level or where the severity of the OA is having significant effects on a patient's mobility, surgical intervention may be suggested by an orthopaedic surgeon. Whilst orthopaedic lavage and debridement are no longer recommended unless the patient has a history of joint locking (NICE 2020), treatments such as osteotomy or arthroplasty are commonly performed.

Osteotomy is an operation that shortens or changes the alignment of a bone that unloads the diseased compartment and is effective for relieving pain and improving function in individuals with knee OA. The limitation of the research in this field is that no high-quality randomised controlled trial has compared surgery to non-surgical treatment options (Brouwer et al. 2014; van Outeren et al. 2017). It has not been established that this is more beneficial than arthroplasty, but the advantage of this operation is that it salvages the individual's own joint, which may be advisable for younger patients (Brouwer et al. 2014, Santoso & Wu 2017).

Joint arthroplasty or replacement surgery is only considered in individuals who have tried and received no benefit from conservative management options. This is even the case for individuals with severe osteoarthritic changes. Joint replacement should be considered in individuals who have pain and limited function that is severely impacting their everyday activities and quality of life. Not everyone has an optimal outcome after joint replacement, and it is reported that, on average, 20% of individuals are dissatisfied and have ongoing pain or loss of function following total knee arthroplasty. Therefore, careful patient selection is required based on age, health, level of activity and expectations (NICE 2020; Scott et al. 2010; Atkinson 2017).

Osteotomy and arthroplasty can both be effective at reducing a patient's pain and discomfort in a joint with OA or other disease causing joint degradation. During the acute recovery stage from surgery rehabilitation, exercises should be prescribed by a health-care professional; however, it is also important to include exercise as part of the long-term management of the affected joint or joints. This is particularly important where another joint is suffering from OA but is not yet resulting in symptoms severe enough to warrant surgical intervention. As the goals of exercise prescription in patients who have undergone surgery to manage OA are closely aligned with conservative management of the disease, recommendations presented here can be applied to a person who received arthroplasty for OA.

3. Effects of OA on exercise

This section explores how OA affects a person's ability to exercise and respond to exercise. Exercise is a core pillar of non-pharmacological management of OA and forms a critical part of recovery from joint replacement surgery (NICE 2020). The problem is that OA is a disease that can affect the locomotor system, so movement of the affected joint or a body region is associated with pain that impacts a person's motivation and ability to be physically active and exercise. An effective exercise specialist needs to have a good understanding of all the possible effects of OA on exercise to appreciate a patient's perspective when designing and developing exercise protocols for this population.

OA as a disease may impact on exercise in several ways (Figure 18.1):

- Directly through the pathophysiological process of OA with synovial inflammation mediating cartilage degradation and manifesting itself as joint stiffness, swelling, loss of movement, muscle weakness, instability and pain (NICE 2020; McNair et al. 2011; Fransen et al. 2015)
- Through treatment of OA in terms of the side effects of the pharmacological analgesic agents, such as weak and strong opioids causing fatigue, somnolence and weight gain and non-steroidal anti-inflammatory agents causing gut problems with potential impact on energy levels

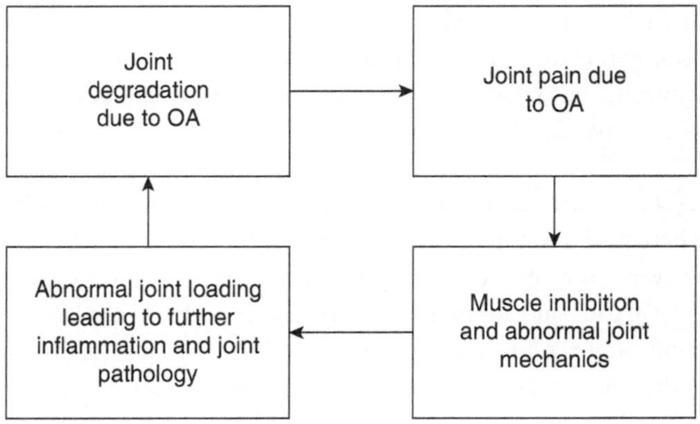

FIGURE 18.1 The cycle of osteoarthritis (OA) on pain, muscle inhibition, joint loading and joint pathology

- By association with ageing and related co-morbidities frequently seen in patients with OA (e.g. cardiovascular problems, obesity and diabetes all influencing person's exercise capacity and response)

Whether a patient living with OA is burdened with one, two or all three of these conditions, the overall impact of this multifaceted disease will be negative, resulting in physical inactivity and subsequent physical deconditioning associated with changes in aerobic fitness, muscle strength, muscular endurance, flexibility and body composition.

Physical activity and exercise in people with OA

An inextricable feature and chief complaint of OA is pain most noticeable during movement, including daily function and exercise. Subsequently, people with OA are expected to be less physically active than those without joint pain. Reduction in physical activity behaviour may be further compounded when people with OA believe that exercise is harmful, causing further damage to and deterioration of the joint or replaced joint structures (Holden et al. 2012). Current physical activity guidelines recommend 150 minutes of moderate to vigorous physical activity (MVPA) per week (Tucker et al. 2011). This equates to about 7,000 to 10,000 steps per day (Sisson et al. 2012). A systematic review of literature measuring physical activity in people with OA (knee and hip) using activity monitors revealed that 13% (knee OA) and 60% (hip OA) reached these recommended levels of physical activity (Wallis et al. 2013). Whilst this data suggests that the majority of people with OA do not reach the recommended levels, this is not far away from the physical activity of age-matched people without OA, as indicated by large epidemiological studies indicating that only 16% of the general population reach the 10,000 steps daily target (Sisson et al. 2012). However, these studies also include those with chronic disease, and comparisons between age-matched individuals with and without OA found that those with OA are, in fact, less physically active (Winter et al. 2010). Reductions in walking intensity and volume compared to their age-matched controls with knee OA were only 76.4% compared to the control group, patients with hip OA achieved only 65.3% compared to their non-OA peers, and patients with spinal stenosis only achieved 58.2%. This is in line with studies tracking the physical activity of those with and without OA, which estimated that people with knee and hip OA reach approximately 8,835 steps per a day compared to 11,859 steps for people without OA, which equates to a 25% drop in physical activity levels in OA populations (Wallis et al. 2013).

Physical activity and exercise behaviour are influenced by psychological factors related to pain experienced during daily function. Exercise-related pain is associated with a sense of causing harm and further deterioration of the joint or the surgical implant. These thoughts may have a profound effect on a person's attitudes towards exercise, causing fear, anxiety, low self-efficacy and avoidance, leading to low exercise adherence and physical inactivity. The progressive long-term nature of OA is associated with low mood, depression and anxiety, which may further affect a person's motivation to exercise. Exercise adherence is demonstrated as the key aspect of a positive exercise response in people in OA. Enhancing and maintaining exercise adherence are among the key evidence-based recommendations for exercise in managing OA (Roddy et al. 2005). Generally, there is withdrawal from society, social isolation, loneliness, loss of role, unemployment, reduced income and all the consequences of this. Spiritually, the person may ask, 'Why me?' All these factors associated with OA have a profound effect on the three key pillars required for successful, long-term change in behaviour – a person's:

1. Capability (physical and psychological abilities)
2. Opportunity (mobility, transport, family support)
3. Motivation (Michie et al. 2011)

Of course. the effect of OA on exercise and physical activity extends beyond the direct impact on the patient and affects the patient's family, employer and social circumstances as well as the effects on health economics further extended to a wider society. All these multi-factorial elements of the disease will have a further overall effect on the physical conditioning of people with OA, impacting aerobic fitness, muscle strength, flexibility, metabolism and body composition.

Aerobic fitness

Reduced physical activity associated with OA leads to subsequent deconditioning in all domains of physical fitness, including aerobic capacity. Up to 80% of people with OA report limitation in their ability to move, with 25% unable to perform functional tasks such as shopping and walking (Centers for Disease Control and Prevention 2021). It would be reasonable to assume that this drop in daily activities is likely to influence cardiorespiratory function. People with OA tend to have significantly lower walking speeds across men and women of different ages and after controlling for demographic and health factors (Dunlop et al. 2011). Whilst this reduced walking speed could be due to the OA population being older, people with OA generally only operate at approximately 80% of the intensity (measured as maximum oxygen uptake and self-reported effort measures) of their healthy age-matched and sex-matched counterparts. This reduced intensity suggests that OA-related symptoms have a direct impact on relative physical activity intensity, regardless of aerobic fitness, and may therefore contribute to the deconditioning of patients with OA (Beals et al. 1985; Ekdahl & Broman 1992; Metsios et al. 2015).

Despite the limited accuracy of the aforementioned estimates of aerobic fitness, OA and cardiovascular disease (CVD) are among the most common dyads seen in clinical practice (Hawker et al. 2014). There are some suggestions that fear of movement and injury with subsequent physical inactivity, deconditioning and obesity, combined with ageing, may accelerate declines in aerobic function, potentially mediating the disease process. Although this link has been hypothesised in literature, the evidence is not clear with research in other areas (e.g. sub-acute low back pain) demonstrating no link between aerobic capacity and level of fear avoidance (Smeets et al. 2009). Nevertheless, improving aerobic fitness in people with OA is associated with significant reductions in pain and disability and enhanced function and mood (Brosseau et al. 2004), in addition to the associated reduction in CVD risk (Aspenes et al. 2011).

Neuromuscular function

Muscle weakness and atrophy are key clinicals feature in OA and are considered the main attributors of physical deconditioning in people with OA (Petterson et al. 2008). The muscle strength deficit is partly caused by neural inhibition that prevents the central nervous system

(CNS) from fully activating the muscle, a process known as arthrogenic muscle inhibition (AMI) (Rice & McNair 2010). In OA, this process is not solely limited to the muscle of the involved limb but also affects muscles of the contralateral limb (Pietrosimone et al. 2011a). The effect of muscle inhibition is even more striking in those undergoing surgery, with a reported 80% to 90% reduction in knee extensor peak torque observed within 36 hours post joint arthroplasty (Holm et al. 2010). Although this diminishes with time, the muscle peak torque deficits are still present four years later (Becker et al. 2004). OA also appears to affect a person's ability to strengthen muscles (Hart et al. 2012; Pietrosimone et al. 2011b) through the impaired afferent signaling from the arthritic joint negatively influencing motor firing rates (Petterson et al. 2008). Ongoing muscle weakness and atrophy that is difficult to reverse are clinically important as they are associated with increased rate of joint loading (Mikesky et al. 2000), impaired joint stability (Felson et al. 2007) associated with clinical manifestations of poor physical function, poor balance and fear of falling (Nguyen et al. 2014).

The impact of pain on muscle function is also significant. In early OA, pain is a result of the synovial inflammation activating the afferent pain fibres (nociceptors) within the joint structures (except healthy cartilage) and all surrounding ligaments and muscles (Petersen et al. 2019). Exposure of nociceptors to the inflammatory mediators causes a transient increase in their excitability, resulting in hyperalgesia (increased sensitivity to pain) and allodynia (normally painless stimulus: e.g. touch causes pain) through the process of peripheral sensitisation (PS), which is pain inhibition whereby the pain signals interfere with muscle function (Kavelaars et al., 2011). In the context of OA, pain is frequently of a chronic nature where a prolonged noxious stimulation eventually leads to an amplified pain response caused by the impairment of the naturally occurring pain suppression mechanisms within the central nervous system (CNS) through a process known as central sensitisation (CS) (Bajaj et al. 2001). CS is characterised by the expansion of the receptive fields from adjacent areas contributing to the spread of pain to non-injured areas (Woolf & Salter 2000). In addition, CS engages a complex set of neural circuits in the CNS that modulate the perception of touch, temperature and pain amplified by signals from the higher CNS centres involved in emotions, reasoning and motor planning. All these processes are responsible for transition from acute to chronic pain with a person experiencing constant, widespread, unremitting pain unrelated to the joint damage and void of any mechanical behaviour (Kavelaars et al. 2011). This, in turn, may significantly influence a person's attitudes towards exercise and subsequent behaviours with growing levels of fear avoidance. This, in turn, affects exercise adherence levels, which are shown to be lower in people with OA than in healthy age-matched controls (Winter et al. 2010).

Body composition/metabolic changes

OA is most prevalent in people of older age, with 44% of the OA population being over the age of 80 years (Felson et al. 1992). Ageing is associated with a slowing down of metabolic processes with an impact on energy expenditure and subsequent changes in body composition. There is a rapid decline in skeletal muscle at a rate of 4% per decade until the age of 50 years and 10% per decade after this age (Fielding 1995). This reduced muscle mass is accompanied by declines in muscle function such as maximum muscle strength and endurance (Fisher et al. 1994), muscle fibre atrophy, loss of fibre number, motor unit remodelling and decrease in axonal sprouting (Brooks 1996). With skeletal muscle being the 'powerhouse' of energy consumption, its decline reduces energy expenditure, leading to increased adipose tissue, weight gain and likelihood of altered response to exercise. High levels of adipose tissue are associated with low-level systemic inflammation, which may predispose patients to develop OA, suggesting that OA may be a metabolic disorder (Bacardit et al. 2016; Kluzek et al. 2015). In support of this hypothesis, middle-aged people with OA (in weight-bearing and non-weight-bearing joints) were found to be five times more likely to have metabolic disorder (hypertension, dyslipidemia, insulin resistance, abdominal obesity) than individuals without OA (Puenpatom & Victor 2009). The full impact and mechanisms are not yet known, but increased body mass, which typically increases joint loads and subsequent pain, appears to negatively impact physical activity behaviours (Felson et al. 2013). Obesity is also thought to increase risk of OA progression, although this is not entirely clear since no increased risk was identified in knee OA with varus alignment, but increased risk was shown in neutral and valgus alignment OA knee (Niu et al. 2009). The effect of weight gain is more clear since the risk of subsequent joint replacement is > 40% to 100% higher in people with obesity than in those of normal weight (Leyland et al. 2016). Irrespective of the mechanisms, the impact of greater age associated with loss of skeletal muscle and co-existing metabolic disorders affects a person with OA's ability to exercise and response to exercise.

4. Effects of exercise on osteoarthritis

Evidence for overall benefits of exercise on osteoarthritis

A significant amount of research has been carried out to evaluate the potential benefits of exercise for individuals with OA in terms of symptom relief, increased function and, in some cases, improved quality of life. Whilst most of this research has been carried out on the knee joint, high-quality reviews have compiled data on the effectiveness of exercise interventions delivered for hip, knee and hand OA (Fransen et al. 2014, 2015; Bartels et al. 2016; Østerås et al. 2017). There is moderate- to high-quality evidence to support the short-term benefits of land- and water-based exercise as part of a therapeutic intervention to improve symptoms, function and quality of life in individuals with hip and knee OA. The benefits of exercise for the treatment of hand OA are small and based on low-quality evidence (Østerås et al. 2017).

The mechanisms by which exercise helps manage OA symptoms are complex; however, it is accepted that benefits can be split into localised joint improvements and systemic effects. As abnormal joint biomechanics, leading to increased joint loading, is one of the main causes of cartilage degradation and joint inflammation, a goal of exercise is to reestablish healthy joint biomechanics (Fransen et al. 2015). Muscle strength, neuromuscular control and flexibility can all contribute to joint loading; therefore, exercise prescription often focuses on developing these aspects of fitness. A secondary goal of exercise is to develop aerobic capacity to help improve quality of life by reducing the relative intensity of daily tasks, thereby improving physical function. It also can help manage metabolic syndromes and the altered metabolic state of this syndrome (type 2 diabetes, obesity and increased blood pressure) that are associated with OA that can contribute to joint damage (Yoshimura et al. 2012; Courties et al. 2017). The goals of improving joint biomechanics and increasing aerobic capacity are also the goals for patients who have undergone joint arthroscopy.

Evidence on specificity of training

Despite the evidence supporting the use of exercise to manage OA, there is limited practice-based evidence to provide firm recommendations on the most effective way to structure an exercise programme or on the specificity of training. Whilst a number of modes of exercise can help achieve the goals for OA management, factors such as the ordering of the exercises within an exercise programme, the length of time of recovery between exercises, the intensity of training, the volume of training and the types of exercise performed still lack clear evidence- based guidelines. The key is to treat each client on an individual basis and adapt and progress their exercise programme accordingly, based on their symptoms and main barriers to improved quality of life.

Exercise type

Therapeutic exercise programmes used in rehabilitation often contain a combination of exercise types, such as muscle strengthening, flexibility, balance and control, aerobic or endurance training and agility exercises (Button et al. 2012). This means there is a great deal of heterogeneity in the content of the exercise programmes that have been researched. For example, some exercise interventions have been designed to specifically target improvement in muscle strength or aerobic fitness, whilst other programmes are generalised and contain a range of different exercise types that are targeted at flexibility, balance, strength and function (Brosseau et al. 2017). This heterogeneity makes determining the most effective exercise type difficult. In an attempt to identify which exercise type was the most effective, Uthman et al. (2013) compared the quality of the evidence across different exercise types. They concluded that combining strengthening, flexibility and aerobic exercise was most effective, but these findings should be applied with caution as they were based on a limited amount of data.

Each of these different exercise types has a different training aim and underlying mechanism or molecular pathway. Aerobic exercise aims to train muscle to develop resistance to fatigue and to improve cardiopulmonary function; this is achieved through a molecular profile that results in mitochondrial biogenesis. In contrast, strengthening exercise aims to increase the power in skeletal muscle, which is achieved through hypertrophy of individual muscle fibres (Coffey & Hawley 2017). Until recently, combining different exercise types in concurrent training was thought to result in an inferior training outcome by not being specific enough to gain training benefits from either exercise type. New evidence suggests that this may not be the case and that combined training may be beneficial, especially to previously untrained or recreational athletes. It could result in its own general adaptive training profile, resulting in both mitochondrial biogenesis and muscle hypertrophy (Coffey & Hawley 2017; Murach & Bagley 2016). It may only be in the longer term that there is interference with concurrent training, with the aerobic exercise attenuating the strength/power gains (Coffey & Hawley 2017). There is still a significant amount of research that needs to be conducted in this field, and the molecular pathway for benefit in individuals with OA remains unclear.

Training intensity

The intensity of training is increasingly being seen as an important component in the design of an exercise programme for individuals with OA (Regnaux et al. 2015). In a review evaluating the training intensity of exercise interventions for knee and hip OA, high-intensity training did not result in superior clinical benefit to low-intensity training. The limitation of the research included in this review was that there was often no justification of the training intensity levels, and it was unclear if the training was sufficiently challenging to have the desired training effect (Regnaux et al. 2015). The recommendations from these reviews are that the minimum level of training needed to have a beneficial dose-response relationship is required and needs to be included in the design of future trials.

Exercise adherence

Despite the reported widespread benefits of exercise to individuals with OA, there is some evidence of poor long-term adherence. Some recommendations for improving this include taking into consideration the patient's preference for the type of exercise, including the environment; providing feedback, reinforcement and education, especially if individual holds the belief that exercise is harming the joint; supplementing face-to-face sessions with other methods or material, such as internet delivery of care or information leaflets; and ensuring that the patient has the skills they require to undertake an exercise program and in pain coping and management (Jordan et al. 2010, Dobson et al. 2016).

5. Recommendations for fitness testing and exercise programming

OA as a disease of the locomotor system means that any concerted effort to move is likely to cause pain. This very nature of OA means that simply encouraging (nudging) people towards being physically active, such as 'increase number of steps' or 'use stairs' is unlikely to produce the desired outcome for patients, other than potentially creating more pain, more fear, avoidance, further inactivity and loss of fitness. For exercise to be effective in the management of OA, the preferred option (in the early stages at least) would be to use a structured and progressive approach controlling for variables such as pain. Exercise programming also allows for individualisation addressing specific needs (function-based aims), requirements (e.g. strength, joint range, pain relief) and preferences and opportunities (gym or home based). Considering all these factors may result in better exercise adherence, with a person eventually achieving enough fitness and physical and, importantly, psychological resilience to cross over from a sedentary, fearful, inactive and self-limiting way of life to a more enduring and sustainable physically active lifestyle.

As outlined previously, in OA, a person's response to exercise is likely to be highly individual, depending on the stage of the disease, joint/joints affected, pain control, age, associated co-morbidities and medications with associated side effects. This section outlines a system of needs analysis as a useful method for exercise specialists to gain understanding and appreciation of all these parameters to be considered in planning and designing an exercise programme in line with the frequency, intensity, time and type (FITT) principles for a person with OA. Recommendations for fitness testing to obtain a baseline measure and parameters for exercise progression are outlined in this section.

Needs analysis for OA

An exercise programme for a person with OA needs to reflect the multi-faceted nature of the disease. This means that as well as standard fitness testing to establish baseline aerobic capacity, muscle strength, neuromuscular control and function, an exercise specialist needs to importantly consider:

- Disease specifics (disease progression, which joints affected, pain levels)
- General health (age, body composition, co-morbidities)
- Medications (energy levels, diet requirements)
- Exercise preferences (one to one or group based)
- Opportunities available (transport, carer/family support, local initiatives etc.)

This information can then be used to design a fit-for-purpose exercise programme that is set at the appropriate level, progressive, relevant (specific) and highly measurable and modifiable based on response. It is important to obtain quantitative measures that are both accurate and relevant to the patient (i.e. aligned to individually agreed-upon goals).

There are a number of measures included within the four domains of general fitness, disease specifics, general health and well-being used in OA populations to assess baseline levels and monitor response to exercise. It is also important to consider other psychosocial aspects characterised within the disease process, such as a person's perception of coping. A variety of psychosocial variables have been identified as impacting the severity of OA symptoms (Eberly et al. 2018) and, therefore, may impact exercise uptake and adherence. The next section presents a summary of relevant tests and fitness measures to assess fitness and function for exercise management and progression in people with OA (American College of Sports Medicine). Exercise referral guidelines using patient-reported screening tools were used:

1. Physical fitness measures
   a. Aerobic capacity
      i. **VO_2max**, in which an individual is asked to perform exercise at a maximum aerobic capacity on a treadmill or a bike, is considered a gold standard. Executing this form of testing, however, requires specialist training and laboratory equipment often unavailable in clinical and fitness settings. In addition, people with OA are typically at a lower level of function, in pain and with co-existing chronic cardiovascular and metabolic conditions, making this test prohibitive. Submaximal aerobic capacity tests are therefore more readily used, affording higher sensitivity for the given populous and greater ease of delivery.
      ii. **Six-minute walk test**, a test to assess cardiorespiratory function. Inexpensive, easy to use and sensitive to people with low levels of physical function. Basic testing parameter is a set distance walkway, which individuals are asked to walk at their own pace for six minutes, with the objective of covering as much distance as possible.
   b. Muscle strength/flexibility
      i. **Isokinetic muscle strength testing**, in which an isolated muscle group (e.g. quadriceps, hamstrings) is measured using isokinetic systems such as Biodex or Cybex, is the gold standard of muscle testing. In people with OA, isokinetic muscle strength was found highly valuable, revealing significant muscle strength deficits that were undetected with manual muscle testing and circumference measures commonly used in clinical practice (Dıraçoğlu et al. 2009). Recent systematic review also revealed isokinetic muscle training to reduce pain and

disability in people with OA (Coudeyre et al. 2016). The versatile nature of the protocols with modifiable contraction types (eccentric, concentric, isometric), joint ranges and testing velocities (range of 30–240 deg/s) brings advantages offering measures of strength (slow velocities), power (moderate velocities) and resistance (fast velocities). The disadvantage is that these systems are not readily available in clinical and fitness settings. In OA, the functionality of the system may also be limited by joint pain and subsequent neural inhibition, with velocities limited to 60 to 180 deg/s (Coudeyre et al. 2016).

ii. **One-repetition maximum (1RM)** score, in which an individual is asked to perform a single maximum-effort exercise as a measure of maximum muscle strength. In people with OA, however, pain and neural inhibition are significant factors in their ability to maximally contract, thus making this test not a truly sensitive measure of strength in this population. Submaximal measures of RM (6–12RM), in which a person performs a set number of repetitions at a lower resistance, are recommended as safer, more reliable and sensitive estimates of strength in people with OA.

iii. **Multiple repetition maximums** relate to the number of repetitions a person can complete at a certain resistance or the maximum load that can be lifted for a set number of reps (e.g. five repetition maximum). This approach to strength testing has the advantage over 1RM testing as the participant is not required to lift a maximal load that may place too much stress on the joints or muscles of the individual.

iv. **Sit-and-reach test** is a functional mobility test in which the individual sits against a wall and bends forwards to reach as far as they can. There are variations of this test to accommodate lower levels of mobility in which the individual sit in a chair with one leg extended.

c. Neuromuscular control

i. **Tests for substitution patterns (TSP)** is a quantifiable observation test of movement quality and postural orientation (alignment), in which an individual performs five movement tests: 1) body-weight altering test, 2) single-leg tiptoe squat, 3) single-leg squat, 4) forward lunge from stair and 5) double-leg squat – in the assessment. Predefined movement alterations (substitution pattern [SP]) are defined as unfavourable strategies since such compensations have been associated with negative consequences in, for example, OA (Tanamas et al. 2009). Performance of these tests is scored on scale 0 to 3 (0 = no SP, 1 = SP may be present, 2 = clearly present, 3 = very clearly present), as previously described (Trulsson et al. 2010, 2015, 2016).

ii. **Star excursion balance test (SEBT)** is a lower-limb function test in which an individual performs a series of single-leg squats, reaching with the non-stance leg as far as possible on one out of eight lines arranged in a 45° grid. The aim is to remain stable on the stance limb in the middle of the testing grid whilst reaching in one of the directions (Gribble et al. 2012). This inexpensive and easy-to-use test is considered a reliable and valid measure of dynamic balance in people with lower limb pathologies (Gribble et al. 2012), including knee OA (Al-Khlaifat et al. 2016).

2. Physical activity and OA specific function measures:

   a. **International Physical Activity Questionnaire (IPAQ)** is a self-reported measure of physical activity level expressed in units of metabolic equivalent of task (MET) by evaluating physical activities performed within one week, classifying people into 'sedentary, insufficiently active, active and very active' categories. Although IPAQ is not a strict measure of exercise behaviour, it asks how much time a person spent doing low, moderate and vigorous activity in different contexts (work, leisure, domestic), allowing for inclusion of exercise. Although in adolescents, IPAQ score overestimated physical activity when compared to accelerometry data (Ottevaere et al. 2011), in healthy adults, IPAQ was shown to have acceptable concurrent validity (Hagströmer et al. 2006) and has been used to measure levels of activity in people with OA (Mesci et al. 2015), indicating positive correlations with quality of life in OA (Figueiredo Neto et al. 2011).
   b. **Wearable sensors** are increasingly adopted to monitor physical activity and exercise in people with OA. Although this area of research is still in its infancy, there is growing evidence that such devices can feasibly capture the FITT components of physical activity in the daily life of people with end-stage OA (Holsgaard-Larsen & Roos 2012; Verlaan et al. 2015).

3. Joint function:

   a. **KOOS, HOOS** (the Knee Injury and Osteoarthritis Outcome Score and Hip Disability and Osteoarthritis Outcome Score) (Collins et al. 2011) are two self-reported questionnaires that assess a patient's perception of their knee or hip health and associated problems. These questionnaires provide a valid and reliable method of evaluating baseline joint function and monitoring progression during exercise prescription.

4. General health

   a. **QOL** (quality of life questionnaires) are common clinical practice in a number of chronic conditions; a number of disease-specific questionnaires are available. For example the OAKHQOL questionnaire was developed by Rat et al. (2005) for specific use in patients suffering from knee or hip OA.
   b. **Body composition** is an important factor for a patient's general health, and where OA is affecting a load-bearing joint (e.g. knee or hip) can also directly impact the amount of force going through the joint. Simple measures of total body mass can be used to indicate changes in body composition, although where exercise prescription involves resistance training, some form of estimation of body fat percentage may also provide insight into increases in fat free mass.
   c. **General wellness/disease to map co-morbidities**. Whilst OA is a debilitating disease, the main goal of management is to reduce the impact the disease has on quality of life and physical activity levels. As reduced physical activity is directly related to increased risk of other diseases, it is often pertinent to understand how an exercise intervention can also impact other co-morbidities in an OA patient.

The following recommendations for fitness testing can be drawn:

- Tests need to reflect the preferred mode of exercise (aerobic vs. strength testing).
- Tests need to be aligned to the functional goals set by the patient.
- Use of submaximal testing over maximal testing is preferable, given the likely deconditioning in this population.
- Consider pain levels that may change during the day based on medications, which may need to be reflected in the time of day the exercise is programmed and fitness levels are obtained.
- Consider the time of testing. With co-morbidities such as DM, an individual needs to have time for breakfast and insulin prior to attending the measurement session.

Guidelines for exercise programming

Universal guidelines for exercise programming for the management of OA are difficult to determine due to the complexity of the disease, the individual needs of each patient and the heterogeneity of exercise programmes within the research. This section aims to present some of the key considerations for programming exercises for exercise referral patients suffering from OA.

As described in Section 6, evidence supports the use of aerobic, resistance and flexibility training modalities to manage OA symptoms. Whilst evidence is limited on which of these is the most effective, due to the different mechanisms by which they may improve patient outcomes, a combination of exercise modalities is advocated here.

Frequency

The number of exercise bouts prescribed is a key consideration when providing patients with exercise plans. Patient availability and capacity may limit the selection of a suitable frequency; however, a recent review of the effects of exercise on OA concluded that regular exercise sessions had a greater effect than fewer sessions, even when total exercise volume was equivalent (Brosseau et al. 2017). It is recommended that exercise bouts are completed at least twice a week, although this can be up to six sessions a week when session time and intensity are lower, and the patient is able to tolerate such volume.

Aerobic exercise

Intensity

As the main goal of aerobic exercise is to increase a patient's aerobic capacity, the exercise needs to be conducted at a high enough intensity to elicit a physiological adaptation. Commonly in research studies, intensity is monitored as a patient's heart rate, with common intensities ranging between 50% and 70% of a theoretical peak heart rate. In practice, it may be more suitable to use more field tests, such as rate of perceived exertion (e.g. 10–14 on the Borg scale) or the talk test (e.g. the patient should be able to hold a conversation whilst exercising but with a mild level of breathlessness) to adjust exercise intensity.

Type

Walking, cycling and swimming are the most commonly prescribed aerobic exercises within the body of research. As the goal of this exercise is to improve a patient's aerobic capacity and, therefore, improve quality of life, it stands to reason that all these exercises would be effective in the management of OA. This principle is supported by the literature, with exercise programmes based on any of the exercise types shown to be effective, meaning that the selection of aerobic exercise types should be influenced by other factors. The most notable factors to consider are patient access to any required resources (e.g. gym) and patent perception of the exercise that could influence adherence rates.

Time

This variable is highly dependent on the frequency and intensity of the exercise, as well as the proportion of the exercise that is focused on this type of training. ACSM guidelines (Liguori & ACSM 2020) suggest a minimum of 150 minutes of exercise per week; however, this includes all exercise types. Recommendations are for aerobic exercise bouts to last at least 20 minutes and no longer than 60 minutes.

Resistance exercise

Intensity

The intensity of resistance exercise is more commonly discussed in terms of relative load compared to the maximum load a patient could perform the exercise for one repetition. Ranges of this relative load are then understood to target certain aspects of strength, such as 65% to 80% one-repetition maximum (1RM) being more suited to hypertrophy and 80% to 90% 1RM to maximum strength. In an inactive population, 1RM testing may be unsuitable, and therefore, intensity is more easily managed through repetition maximums. Repetition maximums relate to the number of repetitions a patient could complete at a set load and have been shown to be an estimate of someone's 1RM. To achieve the intended goal of increased strength, resistance training can increase muscle mass either through hypertrophy training or through improved neuromuscular characteristics of skeletal muscle. Due to this range in physiological adaptations that can impact OA symptoms, the recommendations are broad, ranging from 65% 1RM (i.e. 15 repetitions) to 90% (i.e. 4 repetitions).

Type

Resistance training can be achieved using different equipment and contraction types. Research has supported that no one type of resistance training appears to be more effective than another. Therefore, recommendations are to use the modality that is both most accessible to the patient and likely to have the highest adherence rates. Some examples include using resistance bands, free weights or resistance machines to elicit concentric, eccentric and isometric contractions within muscle groups surrounding the affected joint.

Time

Session length in resistance training is commonly discussed in relation to the number of sets per muscle group. It is common practice to conduct between three and five sets per muscle group to ensure that sufficient volume is completed to elicit physiological adaptations. Between-set rest is commonly between two and three minutes to allow muscles to partially recover between sets.

Flexibility exercise

Intensity

The goal of flexibility exercise is to increase the maximum range of motion of a joint by increasing the length of muscle tendon units. To achieve this goal, muscle tendon units should be stretched to near the end of their range of motion and held for a short period of time. When considering intensity of flexibility exercise, this refers to the amount of stretch that is applied and is often discussed in terms of the patient's level of comfort during the stretch. Whilst stretching of a muscle should result in a feeling of tightness to ensure that there is an adequate stimulus for lengthening to occur, the patient should never be in pain as this may suggest the stretch is causing damage to the tissues of the muscle tendon unit or joint.

Type

Flexibility training should predominantly be focused on improving the range of motion of the affected joint and the surrounding muscles. This can be achieved through targeted stretching exercises or through activities such as yoga. Whilst targeted stretching will have the most direct impact on joint range of motion, yoga or equivalent exercises have the added benefit of potentially improving muscular strength and aerobic capacity. The type of flexibility should be driven by the patient's needs and preferences.

Time

Stretches should be held for at least 15 seconds but up to 60 seconds to ensure a sufficient stimulus. Where stretching is achieved through activities such as yoga, the duration should be based on achieving the time requirements for other types of exercise described previously.

6. Case study

Age and *gender*: 52 years of age, female

Reason for referral: right knee OA

History of present complaint: Over past 18 months, had intermittent medial knee pain after physical activity but subsided after ten days so didn't seek treatment.

Symptoms developed so that her knee was aching all the time and had a small amount of swelling. Experienced sharp pain with any sudden twisting movements. Experiences stiffness in her knee after prolonged sitting and in the mornings; gets easier once taken a few steps. No locking. Concerned as her knee is now impacting her day-to-day activities, and this is coinciding with a further reduction in her physical activity levels, resulting in weight gain. Knee is still aching, but swelling has resolved, but patient reports she is concerned exercising will cause further damage to the joint. Wants guidance on exercise and other non-surgical management.

Past medical history: Ten years ago had a skiing accident and had a bucket handle tear of medial meniscus. This wasn't repairable at the time of surgery, so had a medial meniscus debridement. Made a full recovery. OA identified through MRI and X-ray imaging reviewed by an orthopedic clinician. General health good and not taking any medication other than occasionally painkillers to manage OA related pain.

Social history: Office-based job, walks 15 minutes twice a day from the train station to the office. Used to go on walks on a weekend but has ceased this since her knee symptoms have worsened due to a perceived negative impact on joint health. Her preference is to exercise on the way home from the office but not confident about what to do in a gym.

Investigations

Based on the recommendations presented in this chapter and the information provided, the following assessments were conducted to allow a needs analysis to be carried out.

TABLE 18.2 Health-fitness assessments for a person with OA

Assessment	*Outcome*	*Interpretation*
Body mass index	32 $kg \cdot m^{-2}$	The patient's BMI is categorised as being with obesity, and this excess body mass may be increasing the loading on the affected joint.
Six- minute walk	510 m	This result is below the average distance for normative data of health participants (Casanova et al. 2011), suggesting the participant's aerobic capacity is below average.
Leg extension repetition maximum (15 kg)	Four repetitions	Four repetitions suggest that 15 kg is 90% of the patient's 1RM, which is approximately 17 kg.
Tests for substitution patterns	Combined score: 9	The test identified that the patient does exhibit substitution patterns to avoid their affected limb.

(Continued)

TABLE 18.2 (Continued)

Assessment	*Outcome*	*Interpretation*
International Physical Activity Questionnaire	MVPA* per week = 700 mins Sedentary time per week = 270 mins	The IPAQ results support that the patient isn't participating in enough physical activity, possibly increasing the risk of other diseases.
KOOS	Pain 57, Function 65, Sport 0, Symptoms 60, Quality of life 68	These results clearly show the impact OA is having on the participant, and the goal of exercise should be to improve these scores.

MVPA = moderate to vigorous physical activity
Goal setting:
1. Increase KOOS pain and function by 8 points
2. Increase physical activity: attend gym 2x week 60 mins and attend 1x yoga
3. Reduce BMI to within normal weight

Management plan

Information provided on OA (pathology, symptoms, treatments, progression) and signposted to suitable website.

TABLE 18.3 Exercise programme

	Aerobic	*Resistance*	*Flexibility*
Frequency (sessions per week)	3	2	3
Intensity	Moderate intensity (40–60% VO_2R)	10 repetitions at 75% 1RM (e.g. leg extension – 17 kg × 0.75 = 13 kg)	Range-of-motion exercises at the knee joint; stretches to quadriceps, hamstrings, calf, hip flexors and gluteal muscle
Time	Initially 30 minutes Gym 2x week Pool 1x week	10 repetitions 2–5 sets 2 minute rest between sets	10 repetitions of range of motion exercises, nudge into pain; stretches hold for 20–30 seconds
Type	Static bike and cross trainer at gym; swimming	Machine weights for quadriceps, hamstrings and gluteal muscles; concurrent training with gym-based aerobic training	Dynamic stretching at the knee joint; static stretches across all major lower limb joints

Given reassurance about importance of exercise as a treatment and role of exercise in management of OA.

Provided with the following exercise programme to help reduce the impact of OA symptoms and improve quality of life.

Additional notes on the exercise programme

Program demonstrated and practiced; feedback given on exercise technique. Patient directed to YouTube exercise videos as a reminder of exercise type and technique.

Exercise progression

Progression of aerobic exercise will be based on level of exertion using Borg RPE scale.

Progression of strengthening exercise will be based on retesting the multiple repetition maximum after six weeks.

Addition of a yoga session will be based on visual analogue scale for pain levels 24 hours after an exercise session after six weeks.

7. Summary and key points

Exercise interventions are beneficial in reducing pain and increasing function and physical activity compared to no exercise in patients suffering from OA. The evidence around exercise specificity in patients with OA is still emerging, and whilst it is not possible to identify the most effective exercise type, there appear to be potential benefits in a multi-modal programme – in particular, one that contains both muscle-strengthening and aerobic exercise. It is essential that the intensity of the exercise is sufficient to have a training effect, and it needs to be individualised to the patient. A major barrier to exercise adherence within OA populations is the perception that exercise does more harm than good due to an acute exacerbation of symptoms. Therefore, education on the benefits of exercise and physical activity should form a key component of any exercise intervention.

When implementing exercise interventions, care should be taken to assess the patient's perceptions of their current joint health and quality of life. As the progression or level of osteoarthritis is predominantly characterised by the patient's perceptions of their symptoms (e.g. pain or instability), the patient's reported outcome measures provide a useful monitoring tool to assess the success of any exercise intervention.

The evidence surrounding exercise and osteoarthritis focused on managing symptoms; however, where symptoms become too severe, joint replacement surgery is often conducted. The goals of exercise for patients with joint replacements match those with OA, and therefore, the presented guidance can also be applied to patients who have undergone surgical treatment.

TABLE 18.4 At-a-glance summary guide to exercise considerations or people with osteoarthritis

Condition name	*Osteoarthritis*
Pathophysiology summary	A degradation of joint cartilage through acute or chronic abnormal loading, leading to inflammation, pain and muscle inhibition.
Aims of exercise	Reduce abnormal joint loading through increased joint stability and improve aerobic capacity with the ultimate goal of minimising the impact of symptoms and improving patient quality of life.
Exercise considerations (including contraindications)	Exercise should be conducted within patient pain limits to minimise the association of exercise with increased pain, even if this is just in the short term. There are no pharmaceutical treatments for osteoarthritis; however, many sufferers take analgesics to manage the symptoms. Whilst analgesics are not associated with major side effects, there is a chance the patient may be drowsy, particularly if they are taking opioid-based analgesics.
Frequency	Evidence supports regular exercise bouts having a greater effect than fewer sessions, even when volume is matched. Therefore, it is recommended that exercise bouts are completed at least twice a week, although this can be up to six sessions a week where session time and intensity is lower, and the patient is able to tolerate such volume.
Intensity	Intensity is primarily driven by the patient's tolerance to load on their affected joint. Where possible, intensity should be high enough to result in a physiological adaptation in the component of fitness being targeted (e.g. aerobic capacity, strength or flexibility).
Time	Due to the multimodal nature of exercise for the management of osteoarthritis, it is difficult to provide a singular guideline for exercise time. It is recommended that total exercise volume over a week should be at least 150 minutes, but how this is achieved should vary based on the patient's circumstances.
Type	As exercise has the ability to manage symptoms of osteoarthritis through different pathways, exercise type should vary to maximise the effectiveness of interventions. Specifically, it is recommended to include aerobic, strength and flexibility training when managing osteoarthritis.
Common medications associated	There are no pharmaceutical treatments for osteoarthritis; however, many sufferers take analgesics to manage the symptoms.
Key safety considerations	As osteoarthritis directly affects the musculoskeletal system, care should be taken when completing exercise involving the affected joints. Exercise of too great an intensity is associated with increase in other musculoskeletal injuries, particularly where there is muscle weakness or inhibition.
Effect of exercise on conditions	There is a large body of evidence supporting the role of exercise in managing the symptoms of osteoarthritis, with positive effects on perceived pain, quality of life and joint health. Osteoarthritis is also associated with reduced physical activity, meaning exercise interventions can also reduce the risk of further disease that is associated with physical inactivity and sedentary behaviours.

References

Al-Khlaifat, L., Herrington, L.C., Tyson, S.F., Hammond, A. and Jones, R.K. (2016) 'The effectiveness of an exercise programme on dynamic balance in patients with medial knee osteoarthritis: a pilot study', *The Knee*, 23(5), pp. 849–856.

Allen, K.D. and Golightly, Y.M. (2015) 'Epidemiology of osteoarthritis: state of the evidence', *Current Opinion in Rheumatology*, 27(3), p. 276.

Aspenes, S. T., Nilsen, T. I., Skaug, E. A., Bertheussen, G. F., Ellingsen, Ø., Vatten, L. and Wisløff, U. (2011) 'Peak oxygen uptake and cardiovascular risk factors in 4631 healthy women and men', *Medicine and Science in Sports and Exercise*, 43(8), pp. 1465–1473.

Atkinson, H.D.E. (2017) 'The negatives of knee replacement surgery: complications and the dissatisfied patient', *Orthopaedics and Trauma*, 31(1), pp. 25–33.

Bacardit, J., Mobasheri, A., Kluzek, S., Edwards, M., Spector, T., Hart, D., Cooper, C. and Arden, N. (2016) 'Metabolic profiles associated with radiographic knee osteoarthritis in a population-based cohort of middle-aged women', *Osteoarthritis and Cartilage*, 24, p. S70.

Bajaj, P., Bajaj, P., Graven-Nielsen, T. and Arendt-Nielsen, L. (2001) 'Osteoarthritis and its association with muscle hyperalgesia: an experimental controlled study', *Pain*, 93(2), pp. 107–114.

Bartels, E.M., Juhl, C.B., Christensen, R., Hagen, K.B., Danneskiold-Samsøe, B., Dagfinrud, H. and Lund, H. (2016) 'Aquatic exercise for the treatment of knee and hip osteoarthritis', *Cochrane Database of Systematic Reviews*, 3.

Beals, C.A., Lampman, R.M., Banwell, B.F., Braunstein, E.M., Albers, J.W. and Castor, C.W. (1985) 'Measurement of exercise tolerance in patients with rheumatoid arthritis and osteoarthritis', *The Journal of Rheumatology*, 12(3), pp. 458–461.

Becker, R., Berth, A., Nehring, M. and Awiszus, F. (2004) 'Neuromuscular quadriceps dysfunction prior to osteoarthritis of the knee', *Journal of Orthopaedic Research*, 22(4), pp. 768–773.

Brooks, B.R. (1996) 'Natural history of ALS: symptoms, strength, pulmonary function, and disability', *Neurology*, 47(4 Suppl 2), pp. 71S–82S.

Brosseau, L., Pelland, L., Wells, G., Macleay, L., Lamothe, C., Michaud, G., Lambert, J., Robinson, V. and Tugwell, P. (2004) 'Efficacy of aerobic exercises for osteoarthritis (part II): a meta-analysis', *Physical Therapy Reviews*, 9(3), pp. 125–145.

Brosseau, L., Taki, J., Desjardins, B., Thevenot, O., Fransen, M., Wells, G.A., Imoto, A.M., Toupin-April, K., Westby, M., Gallardo, I.C.Á. and Gifford, W. (2017) 'The Ottawa panel clinical practice guidelines for the management of knee osteoarthritis. Part one: introduction, and mind-body exercise programs', *Clinical Rehabilitation*, 31(5), pp. 582–595.

Brouwer, R.W., Huizinga, M.R., Duivenvoorden, T., van Raaij, T.M., Verhagen, A.P., Bierma-Zeinstra, S.M. and Verhaar, J.A. (2014) 'Osteotomy for treating knee osteoarthritis', *Cochrane Database of Systematic Reviews*, 12.

Button, K., Iqbal, A.S., Letchford, R.H. and van Deursen, R.W. (2012) 'Clinical effectiveness of knee rehabilitation techniques and implications for a self-care treatment model', *Physiotherapy*, 98(4), pp. 287–299.

Casanova, C., Celli, B.R., Barria, P., Casas, A., Cote, C., De Torres, J.P., Jardim, J., Lopez, M.V., Marin, J.M., De Oca, M.M. and Pinto-Plata, V. (2011) 'The 6-min walk distance in healthy subjects: reference standards from seven countries', *European Respiratory Journal*, 37(1), pp. 150–156.

Centers for Disease Control and Prevention (2021) *Arthritis* [Online]. Available at: www.cdc.gov/arthritis/ (Accessed: 28 June 2021).

Coffey, V.G. and Hawley, J.A. (2017) 'Concurrent exercise training: do opposites distract?', *The Journal of Physiology*, 595(9), pp. 2883–2896.

Collins, N.J., Misra, D., Felson, D.T., Crossley, K.M. and Roos, E.M. (2011) 'Measures of knee function: international knee documentation committee (IKDC) subjective knee evaluation form, knee injury and osteoarthritis outcome score (KOOS), knee injury and osteoarthritis outcome score physical function short form (KOOS-PS), knee outcome survey activities of daily living scale (KOS-ADL), Lysholm knee scoring scale, Oxford knee score (OKS), Western Ontario and McMaster universities osteoarthritis index (WOMAC), activity rating scale (ARS), and tegner activity score (TAS)', *Arthritis Care & Research*, 63(S11), pp. S208–S228.

Coudeyre, E., Jegu, A.G., Giustanini, M., Marrel, J.P., Edouard, P. and Pereira, B. (2016) 'Isokinetic muscle strengthening for knee osteoarthritis: a systematic review of randomized controlled trials with meta-analysis', *Annals of Physical and Rehabilitation Medicine*, 59(3), pp. 207–215.

Courties, A., Sellam, J. and Berenbaum, F. (2017) 'Metabolic syndrome-associated osteoarthritis', *Current Opinion in Rheumatology*, 29(2), pp. 214–222.

Cross, M., Smith, E., Hoy, D., Nolte, S., Ackerman, I., Fransen, M., Bridgett, L., Williams, S., Guillemin, F., Hill, C.L. and Laslett, L.L. (2014) 'The global burden of hip and knee osteoarthritis: estimates from the global burden of disease 2010 study', *Annals of the Rheumatic Diseases*, 73(7), pp. 1323–1330.

Deveza, L.A., Melo, L., Yamato, T.P., Mills, K., Ravi, V. and Hunter, D.J. (2017) 'Knee osteoarthritis phenotypes and their relevance for outcomes: a systematic review', *Osteoarthritis and Cartilage*, 25(12), pp. 1926–1941.

Dıraçoğlu, D., Başkent, A., Yağcı, İ., Oezcakar, L. and Aydın, R. (2009) 'Isokinetic strength measurements in early knee osteoarthritis', *Acta Reumatologica Portuguesa*, 34(1).

Dobson, F., Bennell, K.L., French, S.D., Nicolson, P.J., Klaasman, R.N., Holden, M.A., Atkins, L. and Hinman, R.S. (2016) 'Barriers and facilitators to exercise participation in people with hip and/or knee osteoarthritis: synthesis of the literature using behavior change theory', *American Journal of Physical Medicine & Rehabilitation*, 95(5), pp. 372–389.

Dunlop, D.D., Song, J., Semanik, P.A., Sharma, L. and Chang, R.W. (2011) 'Physical activity levels and functional performance in the osteoarthritis initiative: a graded relationship', *Arthritis & Rheumatism*, 63(1), pp. 127–136.

Dziedzic, K.S., Healey, E.L., Porcheret, M., Afolabi, E.K., Lewis, M., Morden, A., Jinks, C., McHugh, G.A., Ryan, S., Finney, A. and Main, C. (2018) 'Implementing core NICE guidelines for osteoarthritis in primary care with a model consultation (MOSAICS): a cluster randomised controlled trial', *Osteoarthritis and Cartilage*, 26(1), pp. 43–53.

Eberly, L., Richter, D., Comerci, G., Ocksrider, J., Mercer, D., Mlady, G., Wascher, D. and Schenck, R. (2018) 'Psychosocial and demographic factors influencing pain scores of patients with knee osteoarthritis', *PloS One*, 13(4), p.e0195075.

Ekdahl, C. and Broman, G. (1992) 'Muscle strength, endurance, and aerobic capacity in rheumatoid arthritis: A comparative study with healthy subjects', *Annals of the Rheumatic Diseases*, 51(1), pp. 35–40.

Felson, D.T., Niu, J., McClennan, C., Sack, B., Aliabadi, P., Hunter, D.J., Guermazi, A. and Englund, M. (2007) 'Knee buckling: prevalence, risk factors, and associated limitations in function', *Annals of Internal Medicine*, 147(8), pp. 534–540.

Felson, D.T., Niu, J., Yang, T., Torner, J., Lewis, C.E., Aliabadi, P., Sack, B., Sharma, L., Guermazi, A., Goggins, J. and Nevitt, M.C. (2013) 'Physical activity, alignment and knee osteoarthritis: data from MOST and the OAI', *Osteoarthritis and Cartilage*, 21(6), pp. 789–795.

Felson, D.T., Zhang, Y., Anthony, J.M., Naimark, A. and Anderson, J.J. (1992) 'Weight loss reduces the risk for symptomatic knee osteoarthritis in women: the Framingham study', *Annals of Internal Medicine*, 116(7), pp. 535–539.

Fielding, R.A. (1995) 'Effects of exercise training in the elderly: impact of progressive-resistance training on skeletal muscle and whole-body protein metabolism', *Proceedings of the Nutrition Society*, 54(3), pp. 665–675.

Figueiredo Neto, E.M.D., Queluz, T.T. and Freire, B.F.A. (2011) 'Physical activity and its association with quality of life in patients with osteoarthritis', *Revista Brasileira de Reumatologia*, 51, pp. 544–549.

Fisher, N.M., Kame Jr, V.D., Rouse, L. and Pendergast, D.R. (1994) 'Quantitative evaluation of a home exercise program on muscle and functional capacity of patients with osteoarthritis', *American Journal of Physical Medicine & Rehabilitation*, 73(6), pp. 413–420.

Fransen, M., McConnell, S., Harmer, A.R., Van der Esch, M., Simic, M. and Bennell, K.L. (2015) 'Exercise for osteoarthritis of the knee: a Cochrane systematic review', *British Journal of Sports Medicine*, 49(24), pp. 1554–1557.

Fransen, M., McConnell, S., Hernandez-Molina, G. and Reichenbach, S. (2014) 'Exercise for osteoarthritis of the hip', *Cochrane Database of Systematic Reviews*, 4.

Gribble, P.A., Hertel, J. and Plisky, P. (2012) 'Using the Star Excursion Balance Test to assess dynamic postural-control deficits and outcomes in lower extremity injury: a literature and systematic review', *Journal of Athletic Training*, 47(3), pp. 339–357.

Hagströmer, M., Oja, P. and Sjöström, M. (2006) 'The international physical activity questionnaire (IPAQ): a study of concurrent and construct validity', *Public Health Nutrition*, 9(6), pp. 755–762.

Hart, J.M., Kuenze, C.M., Pietrosimone, B.G. and Ingersoll, C.D. (2012) 'Quadriceps function in anterior cruciate ligament-deficient knees exercising with transcutaneous electrical nerve stimulation and cryotherapy: a randomized controlled study', *Clinical Rehabilitation*, 26(11), pp. 974–981.

Hawker, G.A., Croxford, R., Bierman, A.S., Harvey, P.J., Ravi, B., Stanaitis, I. and Lipscombe, L.L. (2014) 'All-cause mortality and serious cardiovascular events in people with hip and knee osteoarthritis: a population based cohort study', *PloS One*, 9(3), p.e91286.

Hochberg, M.C., Altman, R.D., April, K.T., Benkhalti, M., Guyatt, G., McGowan, J., Towheed, T., Welch, V., Wells, G. and Tugwell, P. (2012) 'American college of rheumatology 2012 recommendations for the use of nonpharmacologic and pharmacologic therapies in osteoarthritis of the hand, hip, and knee', *Arthritis Care & Research*, 64(4), pp. 465–474.

Holden, M.A., Button, K., Collins, N.J., Henrotin, Y., Hinman, R.S., Larsen, J.B., Metcalf, B., Master, H., Skou, S.T., Thoma, L.M. and Wellsandt, E. (2020) 'Guidance for implementing best practice therapeutic exercise for people with knee and hip osteoarthritis: what does the current evidence base tell us?', *Arthritis Care & Research*. doi:10.1002/acr.24434.

Holden, M.A., Nicholls, E.E., Young, J., Hay, E.M. and Foster, N.E. (2012) 'Role of exercise for knee pain: what do older adults in the community think?', *Arthritis Care & Research*, 64(10), pp. 1554–1564.

Holm, B., Kristensen, M.T., Bencke, J., Husted, H., Kehlet, H. and Bandholm, T. (2010) 'Loss of knee-extension strength is related to knee swelling after total knee arthroplasty', *Archives of Physical Medicine and Rehabilitation*, 91(11), pp. 1770–1776.

Holsgaard-Larsen, A. and Roos, E.M. (2012) 'Objectively measured physical activity in patients with end stage knee or hip osteoarthritis', *European Journal of Physical and Rehabilitation Medicine*, 48(4), pp. 577–585.

Hurley, M.V., Walsh, N.E., Mitchell, H.L., Pimm, T.J., Patel, A., Williamson, E., Jones, R.H., Dieppe, P.A. and Reeves, B.C. (2007) 'Clinical effectiveness of a rehabilitation program integrating exercise, self-management, and active coping strategies for chronic knee pain: a cluster randomized trial', *Arthritis Care & Research*, 57(7), pp. 1211–1219.

Jevsevar, D.S., Brown, G.A., Jones, D.L., Matzkin, E.G., Manner, P.A., Mooar, P., Schousboe, J.T., Stovitz, S., Sanders, J.O., Bozic, K.J. and Goldberg, M.J. (2013) 'The American Academy of Orthopaedic Surgeons evidence-based guideline on: treatment of osteoarthritis of the knee', *JBJS*, 95(20), pp. 1885–1886.

Jordan, J.L., Holden, M.A., Mason, E.E. and Foster, N.E. (2010) 'Interventions to improve adherence to exercise for chronic musculoskeletal pain in adults', *Cochrane Database of Systematic Reviews*, 1.

Kavelaars, A., Eijkelkamp, N., Willemen, H.L., Wang, H., Carbajal, A.G. and Heijnen, C.J. (2011) 'Microglial GRK2: a novel regulator of transition from acute to chronic pain', *Brain, Behavior, and Immunity*, 25(6), pp. 1055–1060.

Kluzek, S., Newton, J.L. and Arden, N.K. (2015) 'Is osteoarthritis a metabolic disorder?', *British Medical Bulletin*, 115(1), pp. 112–121.

Kroon, F.P., van der Burg, L.R., Buchbinder, R., Osborne, R.H., Johnston, R.V. and Pitt, V. (2014) 'Self-management education programmes for osteoarthritis', *Cochrane Database of Systematic Reviews*, 1.

Leyland, K.M., Judge, A., Javaid, M.K., Diez-Perez, A., Carr, A., Cooper, C., Arden, N.K. and Prieto-Alhambra, D. (2016) 'Obesity and the relative risk of knee replacement surgery in patients with knee osteoarthritis: a prospective cohort study', *Arthritis & Rheumatology*, 68(4), pp. 817–825.

Liguori, G. and American College of Sports Medicine. (2020) *ACSM's guidelines for exercise testing and prescription*. Lippincott Williams & Wilkins.

Loeser, R.F., Goldring, S.R., Scanzello, C.R. and Goldring, M.B. (2012) 'Osteoarthritis: a disease of the joint as an organ', *Arthritis and Rheumatism*, 64(6), pp. 1697–1707.

Luyten, F.P., Denti, M., Filardo, G., Kon, E. and Engebretsen, L. (2012) 'Definition and classification of early osteoarthritis of the knee', *Knee Surgery, Sports Traumatology, Arthroscopy*, 20(3), pp. 401–406.

McNair, P.J., Colvin, M. and Reid, D. (2011) 'Predicting maximal strength of quadriceps from submaximal performance in individuals with knee joint osteoarthritis', *Arthritis Care & Research*, 63(2), pp. 216–222.

Mesci, E., Icagasioglu, A., Mesci, N. and Turgut, S.T. (2015) 'Relation of physical activity level with quality of life, sleep and depression in patients with knee osteoarthritis', *Northern Clinics of Istanbul*, 2(3), p. 215.

Metsios, G.S., Koutedakis, Y., Veldhuijzen van Zanten, J.J., Stavropoulos-Kalinoglou, A., Vitalis, P., Duda, J.L., Ntoumanis, N., Rouse, P.C. and Kitas, G.D. (2015) 'Cardiorespiratory fitness levels and their association with cardiovascular profile in patients with rheumatoid arthritis: a cross-sectional study', *Rheumatology*, 54(12), pp. 2215–2220.

Michie, S., Van Stralen, M.M. and West, R. (2011) 'The behaviour change wheel: a new method for characterising and designing behaviour change interventions', *Implementation Science*, 6(1), pp. 1–12.

Mikesky, A.E., Meyer, A. and Thompson, K.L. (2000) 'Relationship between quadriceps strength and rate of loading during gait in women', *Journal of Orthopaedic Research*, 18(2), pp. 171–175.

Murach, K.A. and Bagley, J.R. (2016) 'Skeletal muscle hypertrophy with concurrent exercise training: contrary evidence for an interference effect', *Sports Medicine*, 46(8), pp. 1029–1039.

National Institute for Health and Care Excellence (2020) *Osteoarthritis: care and management* [Online]. Available at: www.nice.org.uk/guidance/cg177 (Accessed: 29 June 2021).

Nguyen, U.S., Felson, D.T., Niu, J., White, D.K., Segal, N.A., Lewis, C.E., Rasmussen, M. and Nevitt, M.C. (2014) 'The impact of knee instability with and without buckling on balance confidence, fear of falling and physical function: the multicenter osteoarthritis study', *Osteoarthritis and Cartilage*, 22(4), pp. 527–534.

Nicolson, P.J., Bennell, K.L., Dobson, F.L., Van Ginckel, A., Holden, M.A. and Hinman, R.S. (2017) 'Interventions to increase adherence to therapeutic exercise in older adults with low back pain and/or hip/knee osteoarthritis: a systematic review and meta-analysis', *British Journal of Sports Medicine*, 51(10), pp. 791–799.

Niu, J., Zhang, Y.Q., Torner, J., Nevitt, M., Lewis, C.E., Aliabadi, P., Sack, B., Clancy, M., Sharma, L. and Felson, D.T. (2009) 'Is obesity a risk factor for progressive radiographic knee osteoarthritis?', *Arthritis Care & Research*, 61(3), pp. 329–335.

Østerås, N., Kjeken, I., Smedslund, G., Moe, R.H., Slatkowsky-Christensen, B., Uhlig, T. and Hagen, K.B. (2017) 'Exercise for hand osteoarthritis', *Cochrane Database of Systematic Reviews*, 1.

Ottevaere, C., Huybrechts, I., De Bourdeaudhuij, I., Sjöström, M., Ruiz, J.R., Ortega, F.B., Hagströmer, M., Widhalm, K., Molnár, D., Moreno, L.A. and Beghin, L. (2011) 'Comparison of the IPAQ-A and actigraph in relation to VO_2max among European adolescents: the HELENA study', *Journal of Science and Medicine in Sport*, 14(4), pp. 317–324.

Petersen, K.K., Simonsen, O., Olesen, A.E., Mørch, C.D. and Arendt-Nielsen, L. (2019) 'Pain inhibitory mechanisms and response to weak analgesics in patients with knee osteoarthritis', *European Journal of Pain*, 23(10), pp. 1904–1912.

Petterson, S.C., Barrance, P., Buchanan, T., Binder-Macleod, S. and Snyder-Mackler, L. (2008) 'Mechanisms underlying quadriceps weakness in knee osteoarthritis', *Medicine and Science in Sports and Exercise*, 40(3), p. 422.

Pietrosimone, B.G., Hertel, J., Ingersoll, C.D., Hart, J.M. and Saliba, S.A. (2011a) 'Voluntary quadriceps activation deficits in patients with tibiofemoral osteoarthritis: a meta-analysis', *PM&R*, 3(2), pp. 153–162.

Pietrosimone, B.G., Saliba, S.A., Hart, J.M., Hertel, J., Kerrigan, D.C. and Ingersoll, C.D. (2011b) 'Effects of transcutaneous electrical nerve stimulation and therapeutic exercise on quadriceps activation in people with tibiofemoral osteoarthritis', *Journal of Orthopaedic & Sports Physical Therapy*, 41(1), pp. 4–12.

Poole, A.R. (1999) 'An introduction to the pathophysiology of osteoarthritis', *Frontiers in Bioscience*, 4(1), pp. D662–D670.

Puenpatom, R.A. and Victor, T.W. (2009) 'Increased prevalence of metabolic syndrome in individuals with osteoarthritis: an analysis of NHANES III data', *Postgraduate Medicine*, 121(6), pp. 9–20.

Rat, A.C., Coste, J., Pouchot, J., Baumann, M., Spitz, E., Retel-Rude, N., Le Quintrec, J.S., Dumont-Fischer, D. and Guillemin, F. (2005) 'OAKHQOL: a new instrument to measure quality of life in knee and hip osteoarthritis', *Journal of Clinical Epidemiology*, 58(1), pp. 47–55.

Regnaux, J.P., Lefevre-Colau, M.M., Trinquart, L., Nguyen, C., Boutron, I., Brosseau, L. and Ravaud, P. (2015) 'High-intensity versus low-intensity physical activity or exercise in people with hip or knee osteoarthritis', *Cochrane Database of Systematic Reviews*, 10.

Reid, C. and Davies, A. (2004) 'The World Health Organisation three-step analgesic ladder comes of age', *Palliative Medicine*, 18, pp. 175–176.

Rice, D.A. and McNair, P.J. (2010) 'Quadriceps arthrogenic muscle inhibition: neural mechanisms and treatment perspectives', *Seminars in Arthritis and Rheumatism*, 40(3), pp. 250–266.

Roddy, E., Zhang, W., Doherty, M., Arden, N.K., Barlow, J., Birrell, F., Carr, A., Chakravarty, K., Dickson, J., Hay, E. and Hosie, G. (2005) 'Evidence-based recommendations for the role of exercise in the management of osteoarthritis of the hip or knee – the MOVE consensus', *Rheumatology*, 44(1), pp. 67–73.

Santoso, M.B. and Wu, L. (2017) 'Unicompartmental knee arthroplasty, is it superior to high tibial osteotomy in treating unicompartmental osteoarthritis? A meta-analysis and systemic review', *Journal of Orthopaedic Surgery and Research*, 12(1), pp. 1–10.

Schoenfeld, B. J. (2012) 'The use of nonsteroidal anti-inflammatory drugs for exercise-induced muscle damage', *Sports Medicine*, 42(12), pp. 1017–1028.

Scott, C.E.H., Howie, C.R., MacDonald, D. and Biant, L.C. (2010) 'Predicting dissatisfaction following total knee replacement: a prospective study of 1217 patients', *The Journal of Bone and Joint Surgery*, 92(9), pp. 1253–1258.

Sisson, S.B., Camhi, S.M., Tudor-Locke, C., Johnson, W.D. and Katzmarzyk, P.T. (2012) 'Characteristics of step-defined physical activity categories in US adults', *American Journal of Health Promotion*, 26(3), pp. 152–159.

Smeets, R.J., van Geel, K.D. and Verbunt, J.A. (2009) 'Is the fear avoidance model associated with the reduced level of aerobic fitness in patients with chronic low back pain?', *Archives of Physical Medicine and Rehabilitation*, 90(1), pp. 109–117.

Tanamas, S., Hanna, F.S., Cicuttini, F.M., Wluka, A.E., Berry, P. and Urquhart, D.M. (2009) 'Does knee malalignment increase the risk of development and progression of knee osteoarthritis? A systematic review', *Arthritis Care & Research*, 61(4), pp. 459–467.

Trulsson, A., Garwicz, M. and Ageberg, E. (2010) 'Postural orientation in subjects with anterior cruciate ligament injury: development and first evaluation of a new observational test battery', *Knee Surgery, Sports Traumatology, Arthroscopy*, 18(6), pp. 814–823.

Trulsson, A., Miller, M., Gummesson, C. and Garwicz, M. (2016) 'Associations between altered movement patterns during single-leg squat and muscle activity at weight-transfer initiation in individuals with anterior cruciate ligament injury', *British Medical Journal Open Sport & Exercise Medicine*, 2(1).

Trulsson, A., Miller, M., Hansson, G.Å., Gummesson, C. and Garwicz, M. (2015), 'Altered movement patterns and muscular activity during single and double leg squats in individuals with anterior cruciate ligament injury', *BMC Musculoskeletal Disorders*, 16(1), pp. 1–11.

Tucker, J.M., Welk, G.J. and Beyler, N.K. (2011) 'Physical activity in US adults: compliance with the physical activity guidelines for Americans', *American Journal of Preventive Medicine*, 40(4), pp. 454–461.

Uthman, O.A., Van Der Windt, D.A., Jordan, J.L., Dziedzic, K.S., Healey, E.L., Peat, G.M. and Foster, N.E. (2013) 'Exercise for lower limb osteoarthritis: systematic review incorporating trial sequential analysis and network meta-analysis', *British Medical Journal*, 347.

Van Outeren, M.V., Waarsing, J.H., Brouwer, R.W., Verhaar, J.A.N., Reijman, M. and Bierma-Zeinstra, S.M.A. (2017) 'Is a high tibial osteotomy (HTO) superior to non-surgical treatment in patients with varus malaligned medial knee osteoarthritis (OA)? A propensity matched study using 2 randomized controlled trial (RCT) datasets', *Osteoarthritis and Cartilage*, 25(12), pp. 1988–1993.

Verlaan, L., Bolink, S.A.A.N., Van Laarhoven, S.N., Lipperts, M., Heyligers, I.C., Grimm, B. and Senden, R. (2015) 'Accelerometer-based physical activity monitoring in patients with knee osteoarthritis: objective and ambulatory assessment of actual physical activity during daily life circumstances', *The Open Biomedical Engineering Journal*, 9, p. 157.

Versus Arthritis (2019) *State of Musculoskeletal Health 2019* [Online]. Available at: www.versusarthritis.org/about-arthritis/data-and-statistics/state-of-musculoskeletal-health-2019/ (Accessed: 30 June 2021).

Wallis, J.A., Webster, K.E., Levinger, P. and Taylor, N.F. (2013) 'What proportion of people with hip and knee osteoarthritis meet physical activity guidelines? A systematic review and meta-analysis', *Osteoarthritis and Cartilage*, 21(11), pp. 1648–1659.

Winter, C.C., Brandes, M., Müller, C., Schubert, T., Ringling, M., Hillmann, A., Rosenbaum, D. and Schulte, T.L. (2010) 'Walking ability during daily life in patients with osteoarthritis of the knee or the hip and lumbar spinal stenosis: a cross sectional study', *BMC Musculoskeletal Disorders*, 11(1), pp. 1–7.

Woolf, C.J. and Salter, M.W. (2000) 'Neuronal plasticity: increasing the gain in pain', *Science*, 288(5472), pp. 1765–1768.

Yoshimura, N., Muraki, S., Oka, H., Tanaka, S., Kawaguchi, H., Nakamura, K. and Akune, T. (2012) 'Accumulation of metabolic risk factors such as overweight, hypertension, dyslipidaemia, and impaired glucose tolerance raises the risk of occurrence and progression of knee osteoarthritis: a 3-year follow-up of the ROAD study', *Osteoarthritis and Cartilage*, 20(11), pp. 1217–1226.

Zhang, W., Doherty, M., Peat, G., Bierma-Zeinstra, M.A., Arden, N.K., Bresnihan, B., Herrero-Beaumont, G., Kirschner, S., Leeb, B.F., Lohmander, L.S. and Mazières, B. (2010) 'EULAR evidence-based recommendations for the diagnosis of knee osteoarthritis', *Annals of the Rheumatic Diseases*, 69(3), pp. 483–489.

19
BONE HEALTH

Victoria Stiles and Karen Knapp

Chapter aims

The aims of this chapter are to:

- Define osteoporosis, including its incidence, financial cost and societal burden
- Describe the aetiology and clinical diagnosis of the disease
- Identify risk factors for the development of osteoporosis and fragility fractures with particular focus on modifiable (lifestyle) risk factors for the disease
- Identify characteristics of physical activity associated with better bone health
- Describe exercise recommendations to promote bone health for osteoporosis prevention
- Describe exercise recommendations to promote bone health for those living with osteoporosis but who are not at risk of falling and do not have a vertebral fracture

Overview of pathology

Definition, incidence and cost of the disease

Osteoporosis is a progressive skeletal disease that is characterised by low bone mass, deterioration of the bone's microarchitecture and an increased susceptibility to fragility (low-trauma) fracture (Kanis, 2002). One in three women and one in five men over the age of 50 years will suffer a fracture in the UK, mostly as a result of osteoporosis (van Staa et al., 2001), resulting in over 300,000 fragility fractures per year (Mitchell et al., 2010) and over 2 million per year in the US (Burge et al., 2007). Osteoporosis is also a significant public health concern in developing countries (Zhao et al., 2014). Fragility fractures, which occur as a result of a fall from a standing height or lower, cause significant pain, disability, loss of independence and increased risk of morbidity, especially in the first three to six months after fracture (Haentjens et al., 2010; Mitchell et al., 2010). As a result of an increasingly ageing population, fragility fractures, which can occur anywhere in the body but most commonly affect the wrist, hip and spine, are predicted to double over the next 50 years (NOGG, 2014). By 2025, over

DOI: 10.4324/9781315102399-19

3 million fragility fractures costing over $25 billion per year are expected in the US (Burge et al., 2007). Fragility fractures alone cost the NHS over £1.7 billion per year (NOGG, 2014), which is expected to rise to over £2.1 billion by 2020 (Gauthier et al., 2011). Currently, the combined cost to the NHS of treating fragility fractures and the consequences of them is estimated to be £4.4 billion per year (NOGG, 2017).

Hip fractures are considered to be the most severe type of fragility fracture as they almost always require hospitalisation and surgical fixation. They are associated with significant human and financial costs, with the index cost for hospitalisation estimated at $10,075 and health and social care costs at one year of $43,669 (NICE, 2011; Williamson et al., 2017). The one-year mortality rates associated with hip fractures are approximately 20%, and they are also associated with significant morbidity and reduced quality of life (Hagino et al., 2012; Menendez-Colino et al., 2018). Women who have sustained one hip fracture are four times more likely to sustain a second hip fracture, and while age-adjusted hip fracture incidence in the US had been falling in recent years as a result of earlier detection and treatment of osteoporosis, this decrease has plateaued in recent years, with the number of hip fractures exceeding predictions (Lewiecki et al., 2017).

While hip fractures are considered the most severe osteoporotic fracture type by many health-care professionals, vertebral fractures are also associated with a significant reduction in quality of life (Svedbom et al., 2017). It is estimated that one in twelve men and one in six women will suffer a symptomatic vertebral fracture during their lifetime (Gerdhem, 2013), which, again, poses a significant burden to public health. Eight percent of patients presenting with vertebral fracture require hospitalisation, and 2% require long-term nursing care (Lippuner et al., 1997). Vertebral fractures are associated with both increased morbidity and mortality (van der Jagt-Willems et al., 2013; Waterloo et al., 2013), significant pain, functional disability, gastro-intestinal symptoms, height loss, depression, breathing difficulties and an increased risk of further fractures (Gerdhem, 2013; Triantafyllopoulos et al., 2014; van Schoor et al., 2008). The risk of new (incident) vertebral fractures increases with the number of prevalent vertebral fractures, with the relative risk increasing from 3.2 to 23.3 for one to three or more prevalent vertebral fractures, respectively (Lunt et al., 2002). One in five women with an incident vertebral fracture will suffer a further vertebral fracture within a year (Lindsay et al., 2001). These risks can be mitigated through treatment with the chance of sustaining a further fracture reduced by half with bone-sparing therapies (e.g. bisphosphonates such as alendronic acid) (Kaptoge et al., 2004). However, not all vertebral fractures come to clinical attention, and therefore, methods are required to identify those with subclinical and missed vertebral fractures (Delmas et al., 2005), whilst also elevating the possibility of vertebral fracture with health-care professionals.

Aetiology

Bone remodelling continues throughout life, allowing adaptation of bone material properties to the mechanical demands placed upon it and preventing the accumulation of fatigue damage (Morgan et al., 2013). Bone remodelling involves a quantum of mineralised bone being removed by osteoclasts, followed by the synthesis and mineralisation of osteoid by osteoblasts within the cavity created (Arden & Spector, 1997). Under normal circumstances, the sequence is always resorption followed by formation, and the amounts of bone resorbed and formed are equally balanced (Arden & Spector, 1997). Bone remodelling occurs on the surface of bones, on periosteal, endosteal, Haversian canal and trabecular surfaces. The rate of remodelling in trabecular bone is proportionally higher than cortical bone throughout life and may be five to ten times higher in the adult (Morgan et al., 2013).

Attaining the genetic potential for peak bone mass in early life is a major factor for subsequent bone mass and fracture risk in later life (Arden & Spector, 1997). During childhood, bone mass accretion is relatively slow (Figure 19.1); however, after puberty, which is approximately 12.5 years in girls and 14 years in boys (Bailey et al., 1999), the highest rate of bone mass accretion occurs and accounts for approximately 22% of adult peak bone mass (Baxter-Jones et al., 2011). Peak bone mass occurs between the second and third decade of life, followed by a period of varying length during which skeletal mass is relatively stable (Morgan et al., 2013). Some studies have found little evidence of premenopausal bone loss (Baran, 1994; Chapurlat et al., 2000). However, there is strong evidence of perimenopausal bone loss (Baran, 1994; Chapurlat et al., 2000). After the menopause, women experience an accelerated loss of bone mass, and from mature to late adulthood, bone mass in men and women declines to approximately half its maximum level by the eighth or ninth decade (Buckwalter et al., 1995). In ageing, osteocytes become senescent, lose function and stop dividing and more fat cells appear in bone (Brown, 2017). Both osteoblasts and fat cells originate from the same mesenchymal stem cells, which differentiate to form one or the other of these cell types. In ageing, mesenchymal stem cells suffer DNA damage and are more likely to differentiate to become fat cells rather than osteoblasts; thus, the number of osteocytes and osteoblasts are reduced, and this impacts the ability for form new bone (Singh et al., 2016; Wang et al., 2012).

Osteoporosis is more prevalent in females than in males as there is a direct impact of hormonal influences on bone, predominantly due to the decline in 17β-oestradiol, which is the major oestrogen in premenopausal women (Wardell et al., 2013). The hormonal changes that

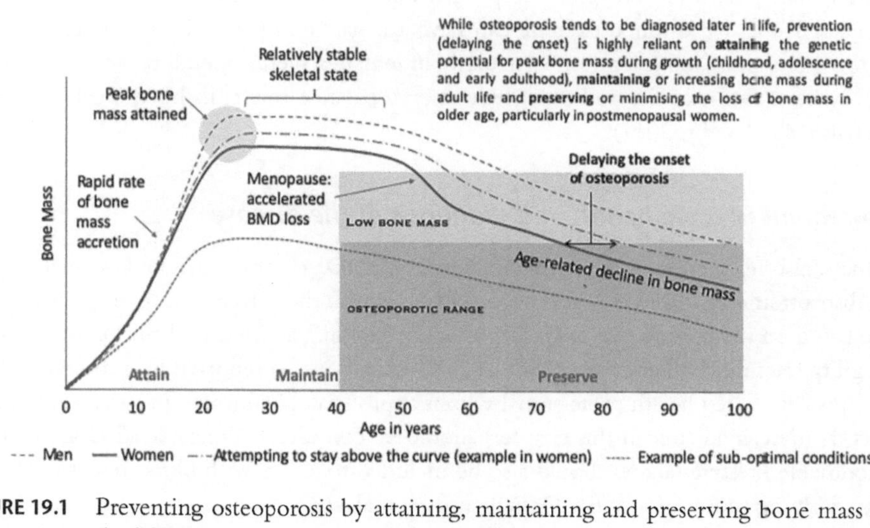

FIGURE 19.1 Preventing osteoporosis by attaining, maintaining and preserving bone mass across the lifespan

signal decreased ovarian function begin in the decade prior to the development of irregular cycles and the cessation of menstruation (Khosla & Pacifici, 2013). Although oestrogen has the greatest impact as a regulator of mineral metabolism, progesterone and ovarian androgens may also have an influence (Favus, 1999). Following menopause, indices of bone resorption are approximately twice the levels found in premenopausal women, and markers of bone formation are approximately 50% above premenopausal levels (Ebeling et al., 1996; Khosla & Pacifici, 2013). This imbalance between bone resorption and formation (relative excess of bone resorption) results in postmenopausal bone loss.

In addition to hormonal regulation of bone density, bone responds to the forces applied to it (Wolff's Law). Frost, in his mechanostat theory, proposed that a positive adaptive response (increased bone mass) to mechanical load occurs when a minimum effective strain, otherwise known as a 'mechanical set-point', is exceeded (Frost, 1987). Certain thresholds of local strain (e.g. 800–1500 or > 1500 microstrain [rodent studies]) on the surfaces of bone are proposed to maintain bone mass and architecture (homeostasis) or provide an 'overload' stimulus to trigger bone resorption and formation. The mechanostat theory continues to be refined as research takes steps to overcome the challenges of accurately measuring and modelling the effect of mechanical load and stimulation on cellular responses thought to be responsible for bone resorption and formation across the lifespan (Castillo & Leucht, 2015). It is known, however, that this threshold-driven response to loading means that magnitudes of strain below a certain threshold or the absence of any loading at all results in a reduction in bone mass (Frost, 1987; Jee, 2000). In vivo, for example, loss of bone density is reported in disuse situations, such as following a fracture, post orthopaedic surgery, a stroke and in spinal cord injury (Uebelhart et al., 1995; Poole et al., 2002, 2005; Knapp, 2010; Hopkins et al., 2016). Conversely, weight-bearing activity of a sufficient magnitude can increase bone density in adolescents (Vlachopoulos et al., 2017) and premenopausal women (Greenway et al., 2015). Although previous evidence of exercise benefiting postmenopausal women has been less compelling (Segev et al., 2017), recent methods enabling daily physical activity to be analysed more precisely have revealed a positive association between moderate-impact activity and better bone health in both pre- and postmenopausal women (Stiles et al., 2017). There is also evidence that too much exercise can have a negative impact on bone density, resulting in low bone mass and fractures, particularly in female athletes in endurance sports and in dancers, where over-exercise and a negative energy balance results in hormonally deficient individuals (MacKnight, 2017).

Measurement of bone health and diagnosis of the disease

Bone mass, also referred to as bone mineral density (BMD, g/cm^2), is assessed by dual-energy X-ray absorptiometry (DXA). Referrals for DXA scans in the UK are made via primary care and are based on the presence of clinical risk factors yielding an increased risk of osteoporosis and fragility fracture (Hillier et al., 2011). A DXA scan must be reported by a specialist clinician or specialist allied health professional who is appropriately educated in this area. Clinical risk factors (described later in this chapter) should be considered alongside all DXA reports, and modifiable lifestyle factors should also be included together with blood tests to rule out other underlying causes of low BMD, such as osteomalacia.

DXA is commonly considered to be the gold standard for the diagnosis of osteoporosis (Table 19.1), and it is supported by the widest evidence base and clinical utilisation (Blake &

TABLE 19.1 Definitions of osteoporosis and fracture risk based on measurement of bone mineral density

Definition	*BMD T-score**	*BMD measurement and fragility fracture risk*
Normal	≥ −1.0	Individuals with normal levels of BMD that are no more than 1.0 standard deviations (SD) below the mean of the reference group with no clinical risk factors for fracture are described as being at 'low risk' of fragility fracture.
Low bone mass (osteopenia)	−1.0 to −2.5	Osteopenia is defined as a BMD between 1.0 and 2.5 SD below the mean of the reference group. Individuals with BMD in this range are described as being at 'moderate risk' of fragility fracture. especially if they possess other clinical risk factors for fracture.
Osteoporosis	≤ −2.5	A diagnosis of osteoporosis is made in individuals who have a BMD of more than 2.5 SD below the mean of the reference group. Individuals with a BMD in this range are described as being at 'high risk' of fragility fracture.
Severe osteoporosis	≤ −2.5	Severe osteoporosis is defined as BMD more than 2.5 SD below the mean of the reference group and in the presence of one or more fragility fractures.

* Bone mineral density (BMD) at the hip (femoral neck) is measured using DXA and presented as a T-score to describe how far the measurement is away from a reference group average. Some centres will compare all patients, even men and other ethnicities, to the female Caucasian reference data, while others will use sex- and or ethnicity-matched data (WHO, 1994; Shepherd, et al., 2015). In premenopausal women and men under the age of 50, it is more usual to use a Z-score cut-off of more than 2.0 SD below the mean for young adults to indicate low bone mass and to explore any underlying causes of this (Baim et al., 2008).

Fogelman, 2009; Kanis et al., 2013), but it is not without its limitations (Garg & Kharb, 2013). Patients diagnosed with osteoporosis using DXA do not all go on to fracture. Instead, the majority of fractures occur in women diagnosed with osteopenia (low bone mass) or classified 'normal' by BMD criteria (Hillier et al., 2011). The potential for spurious results or uninterpretable scans leading to inappropriate management advice is also a problem in some patients, particularly the elderly (Knapp & Blake, 2014). In recognition of some of these issues, the Royal Osteoporosis Society (ROS, 2018) guards against using BMD-derived fracture risk classifications to prescribe or restrict an individual's physical activity for fear of denying them the opportunity to engage in a physically active lifestyle that reaps benefits to health and well-being which outweigh any concerns about its exacerbating the condition.

Alternative methods which measure the macro- or microarchitecture of bone to improve fracture prediction have been explored, either based on DXA measurements such as trabecular bone score (Bousson et al., 2012; Hopkins et al., 2012) or from other technologies such as peripheral quantitative computed tomography (pQCT), which provides separate measurements of cortical and trabecular bone along with accurate volumetric measurements of bone geometry, which have been demonstrated to be a better predictor of long bone fractures than DXA (Siu, et al., 2003).

Quantitative ultrasound (QUS) is a method of measuring bone, most commonly at the calcaneus, which uses the attenuation and speed of sound of ultrasound waves propagating through bone to assess its strength. QUS is reported to measure both the elasticity and microarchitectural components of bone, but it does not directly measure BMD (Knapp, 2009). While QUS is reported to predict hip fractures in the elderly population (Moayyeri et al., 2012), this measurement method has a smaller evidence base and is considered inferior to DXA. Precision errors are also higher than DXA, which precludes its use for monitoring responses to treatment (Hans & Krieg, 2009). The use of QUS in longitudinal studies where small bone changes are likely to occur or in individuals for clinical practice is also inhibited by larger measurement errors. However, QUS devices are highly portable and do not use ionising radiation, which means they can be easily utilised in many research populations and are an acceptable method for assessing cross-sectional data (Knapp, 2009).

Clinical risk factors for the development of osteoporosis and fragility fractures

Genetic factors account for 60% to 80% of an adult's BMD (Weaver et al., 2016). Low BMD is therefore a highly heritable risk factor for fragility fractures (Kanis et al., 2005), with every standard deviation decrease in BMD and diagnosis of osteoporosis being associated with an approximately 1.5- to 3-fold increase in the risk of encountering a fragility fracture (Cummings et al., 1993; Marshall et al., 1996). However, other risk factors are also taken into account when trying to predict future fracture risk. Clinical risk factors for fracture include age, sex, low body mass index, previous fragility fracture, parental history of fracture, current smoking status, alcohol exposure, glucocorticoid treatment, rheumatoid arthritis and conditions strongly associated with osteoporosis (secondary osteoporosis risk) such as type 1 (insulin-dependent) diabetes, untreated long-standing hyperthyroidism and hypogonadism or premature menopause (< 45 years). These factors predict the ten-year probability of fragility fracture risk, and when combined with BMD, they are a better predictor of fragility fracture than BMD or clinical risk factors alone. These risk factors have been incorporated into a fracture risk assessment tool developed at the University of Sheffield called FRAX (Kanis et al., 2007; www.sheffield.ac.uk/FRAX).

Screening for risk factors is an important part of decision making and can determine whether someone should be referred for further medical assessment and treatment or whether lifestyle advice and reassurance is sufficient to promote good bone health and help prevent development of the disease.

Management and medications

Pharmacological interventions

There are a number of pharmacological therapies available for the treatment of osteoporosis, and while no 'cure' is available, the current treatments are evidenced to be effective at reducing fractures in osteoporosis sufferers. The current first-line treatments are oral bisphosphonates, and these have been shown to reduce the rates of vertebral and non-vertebral fractures (Boonen et al., 2005; Jansen et al., 2011). Oral bisphosphonates include alendronic acid, risedronate and ibandronate. All must be taken on an empty stomach (usually first thing in the morning) with just a glass of water 30 to 60 minutes before any food or other drugs are taken (NICE, 2019). Ibandronate can also be administered as an injectable phamaceutical once every three months, while zolendronate can be administered via an infusion once a year. These drugs work by supressing bone resorption, and as a result, care must be taken not to oversupress bone turnover and cause adverse events such as atypical femoral fracture (Donnelly et al., 2012). Atypical femoral fractures are a rare but serious complication of bisphosphonate therapy, and it is now common to reassess BMD at five years to consider a drug treatment holiday for the patient (Brown et al., 2014). The most common side effect of oral bisphosphonates are gastrointestinal disorders, and if these occur, the patient should discuss other options with their health-care provider (NICE, 2019).

In addition to bisphosphonates, hormone replacement therapy (HRT) has a positive effect on bone and will afford protection against osteoporotic fractures for the period of use (Torgerson & Bell-Syer, 2001). However, the use of HRT primarily for osteoporosis remains a contentious matter, and it is currently used primarily to manage menopausal symptoms.

Other drugs available include raloxifene, a selective oestrogen receptor modulator (SERM), denosumab (a monoclonal antibody), strontium ranelate and parathyroid hormone (teriparatide). Parathyroid hormone (PTH) is the only one of these to exert a strong anabolic action on bone and will therefore increase BMD as well as rebuilding bone microarchitecture. PTH has to be injected daily over the period of use, and this is restricted to a maximum of 24 months (Eastell & Walsh, 2017).

Modifiable lifestyle behaviours

Lifestyle factors such as smoking, diet, alcohol use and inactivity influence 20% to 40% of an adult's peak bone mass (Weaver et al., 2016) and are considered highly modifiable behavioural and clinical risk factors for the development of osteoporosis. Whilst engaging in a healthy lifestyle does not guarantee an individual will remain disease-free, there are clear advantages for health and well-being to educate and encourage as many people as possible to modify their behaviour and adopt a balanced, healthy lifestyle.

Smoking cessation

Smoking, due to its nicotine content, has direct toxic effects on the activity of osteoblasts and osteoclasts, thus reducing BMD and increasing fracture risk. Furthermore, smoking tobacco has an indirect action on sex and adrenocortical hormones, whilst vitamin D may also be affected, thus reducing intestinal calcium absorption (Abate et al., 2013). Therefore, smoking cessation is a key recommendation for anyone at risk of osteoporosis in addition to the other health benefits yielded through stopping smoking.

Dietary requirements

Bone is metabolically active and is the major reservoir for calcium and mineral homeostasis within the body. Therefore, if there are inadequacies in blood calcium through a poor diet or due to disease, then calcium will be released from the bone through increased bone resorption to maintain blood calcium levels. It is therefore essential to have a diet replete in calcium (1,000 mg daily recommended intake), and a useful way to check this is by using a calcium calculator (e.g. www.iofbonehealth.org/calcium-calculator). It is also important to have sufficient vitamin D to support calcium absorption from the gut. In the UK, the majority of vitamin D comes from sun exposure, so it is recommended that arms, legs and the face are exposed to the sun, without skin reddening, for approximately 20 minutes three times per week between April and October. Public Health England are now recommending supplementation with 10μg per day of vitamin D to ensure the population remain vitamin D replete.

Caffeine is present in commonly consumed drinks such as coffee, tea and, Coca-Cola. Despite multiple health benefits from drinking a moderate amount (three to four cups) of caffeine-containing drinks per day, there is a negative effect on fracture risk in women, particularly those who are high caffeine consumers (relative risk 1.14, 95% confidence interval 1.05 to 1.24), but a decreased fracture risk in men (relative risk 0.76, 95% confidence interval 0.62 to 0.94) (Poole et al., 2017). Therefore, lifestyle advice can be provided to women at risk of fracture to moderate their caffeine intake. Pregnant women should also avoid caffeine or limit their intake since it's been associated with low birth weight and pregnancy loss (Poole et al., 2017).

Alcohol moderation

Alcohol affects bone metabolism by reducing bone cell proliferation and functional activity, with serum osteocalcin levels also reduced in alcoholics. Calcium metabolism is also affected by alcohol, and alcoholics frequently have low serum 25-hydroxy and 1,25-dihydroxyvitamin D and raised serum concentration of parathyroid hormone (PTH). Chronic alcohol abuse results in low bone mass, although the microarchitecture of bone is preserved (Ulhoi et al., 2017. Alcohol has a negative impact on bone in heavy drinkers but, paradoxically, a protective effect in light to moderate drinkers of one or two glasses, two or three times per week (Jang et al., 2017). Alcohol can also increase the risk of falls, and frequent fallers are at a greater risk of fracture than those who don't fall regularly (Reid & Gentius, 2017).

Physical activity

While sufficient doses of physical activity are important in helping attain the genetic potential for peak bone mass in early life, physical inactivity has long been considered a highly modifiable lifestyle risk factor at all ages for the development of osteoporosis and fragility fractures in later life (Bass et al., 1998; Kanis et al., 2007; Carter & Hinton, 2014; Weaver et al., 2016). However, the specific contribution that different doses of physical activity (frequency, intensity, duration) can make in attaining, maintaining or preserving (minimising bone loss) across the lifespan has been less well understood than environmental, behavioural or nutritional risk factors for the disease (Vainionpää et al., 2007; Jämsä et al., 2011; Weaver et al., 2016).

With regards to weight-bearing activity, the general prevailing advice for osteoporosis prevention has been to perform a large amount of vigorous high-impact jumping activity (e.g. maximal height jumping, tuck jumps, star jumps) on multiple days per week, which typically yields impact forces of over four times the individual's body weight (> 4 BW). While high-impact exercise plays an important role in positively modifying bone health (Rubin & Lanyon, 1985), research using more precise methods for analysing physical activity found that a small amount (one to two minutes per day) of moderate-impact activity (> 2 BW) (Weeks & Beck, 2008; Rowlands & Stiles, 2012; Stiles et al., 2013) equivalent to slow- or medium-paced running in post- and premenopausal women respectively, was associated with better bone health than less or lower-impact activity (Stiles et al., 2017). This is an important finding as the benefits of exercise on bone health, particularly in postmenopausal women, have not always been found in previous research (Bassey et al., 1998). Defining a dose-response relationship between volume, intensity and type of physical activity with measures of bone health in an older population is key to developing effective interventions that prevent bone loss in this population (Tobias et al., 2014).

New exercise recommendations from the ROS ('Strong, Steady and Straight') also advocate building up gradually to include moderate-impact activity (e.g. low jumps, running, hopping) to promote bone health in those who are living with osteoporosis but who are not at risk of falling and do not have vertebral fractures (ROS, 2018) (Table 19.2). The volume, intensity and frequency of these exercise recommendations is similar to the most recent exercise advice from Australia, which highlights the benefits of engaging in weight-bearing activity of at least moderate impact for osteoporosis prevention (Beck et al., 2017). For improved continuity and strength in the message for specific and achievable doses of physical activity to help attain, maintain or minimise the loss of bone strength across the lifespan, promoting engagement in small amounts of moderate-impact weight-bearing activity in everyday life or as part of an exercise programme is most appealing.

Effects of acute exercise response

Bone continually responds to meet the demands of the load encountered (mechanostat theory) (Frost, 1987), and the response is site-, mode-, dose- and intensity-specific. Evidence mainly from animal studies indicates that high external loads applied rapidly, dynamically and cyclically to bone produce high external rates of loading (large force applied over a short period of time) and, consequently, high levels of internal mechanical strain, which exceed a minimum effective strain and act as a load-induced mechanical stimulus to trigger bone formation (Frost, 1987; Burr et al., 2002; Castillo & Leucht, 2015). A proportional dose-response relationship exists whereby higher-strain magnitudes lead to a greater osteogenic response (Rubin & Lanyon, 1985). However, to maintain the responsiveness and mechanical sensitivity of bone cells, enabling external mechanical stimuli to be converted into a bone-remodelling response (mechanotransduction), it is important not to subject bone to too many loading cycles in quick succession. The greatest osteogenic response to loading has been found to occur at the beginning of a bout of activity rather than during or at the end of a lengthy continuous bout (Turner, 1998).

The frequency with which bone-specific activity is accumulated across the week has been found to be important, with nearly 2% higher BMD found in the femoral neck of the exercised limb in those who performed 50 hops (five set of ten reps performed unilaterally on exercise days) seven days of the week than in those who did not complete the intervention (control group) or completed it on two days of the week (Bailey & Brooke-Wavell, 2010). This type of evidence helps inform exercise recommendations for brief weight-bearing activity of a sufficient intensity to be performed on most days of the week, with provision for rest between repeated cycles or bouts of loading.

Experiencing odd and unfamiliar (unaccustomed) strains that act in multiple directions to create a variety of compressive, tensile and shear loading conditions is also important for maximising the osteogenic effect from exercise (Rubin & Lanyon, 1984; Nikander et al., 2008; Beck et al., 2017). Variety in movement (movement diversity) is therefore encouraged to improve, maintain or reduce rates of loss in bone and muscle strength across all sites of the body, but particularly at key fragility fracture sites such as the hip, spine and wrist (ROS, 2018).

Response to loading also differs depending on an individual's existing physical activity habits (Weaver et al., 2016), which means those who are less active and have lower bone strength experience a greater osteogenic effect from an increase in activity than healthy, more habitually active individuals. For a given level of impact, older populations with lower bone strength also experience higher levels of strain than younger populations (Tobias et al., 2014). Research findings indicate that if the activity message focused on accumulating weight-bearing activity such as running in short bursts at a comfortable speed, sufficient levels of bone health–promoting loads would likely be achieved irrespective of age.

Effects of exercise training

Weight-bearing exercise

Weight-bearing exercise refers to activity that forces you to work against the effects of gravity to maintain an upright position with different types and speeds of activity creating different levels of impact. Labels such as 'low', 'moderate' and 'high' describe the intensity of the impact experienced during different weight-bearing activities and are most useful when classifying exercise and activity in relation to bone health. However, these classifications are not always apparent or interpretable when general physical activity guidelines are presented.

General physical activity guidelines recommend either the accumulation of at least 150 minutes of moderate-intensity aerobic activity (e.g. walking) per week in bouts of ten minutes or more, 75 minutes of vigorous-intensity aerobic activity per week or a combination of the two (O'Donovan et al., 2010; Garber et al., 2011). By defintion, general guidelines are not optimised for all health outcomes and, in this instance, may cause confusion regarding the potential for certain activities to benefit bone health. For example, general physical activity guidelines use an exercise intensity classification system based on energy expenditure from steady-state activity to classify brisk walking as a moderate-intensity aerobic activity for cardiovascular health benefits. While the term 'moderate intensity' could reasonably be expected to involve activity that is sufficiently dynamic to influence bone health, there remains conflicting evidence on whether walking benefits bone health in any meaningful way (Vainionpää et al., 2007; Stiles et al., 2017; Beck et al., 2017). In contrast, applying a blanket 'vigorous intensity' term based on energy expenditure to more dynamic activities that can promote bone health does not allow activities that yield different levels of impact within this category to be differentiated. Compared to high impacts (> 4 BW) yielded by high-level jumping or drop landings, blanket use of the 'vigorous intensity' term does not accurately inform existing exercisers or those new to exercise of potentially more achievable and accessible forms of moderate-impact activity (> 2 BW) that can also benefit bone health, such as those derived from jogging/running, low jumps, skips and hops. To better inform the exerciser of the potential for certain activities to benefit a range of different health outcomes, including bone health, future activity guidelines and the terms used to describe them would need to be reconsidered. However, for a more timely solution and to supplement existing physical activity guidelines for wider benefits to overall health, a separate impact-intensity classification system based on forces experienced during weight-bearing activity (e.g. moderate-impact activity: > 2 BW) can be employed to prescribe bone-specific activity.

Low-impact activity

Walking is an important aerobic activity that helps meet general physical activity guidelines for benefits to cardiovascular and metabolic health. It is also a common daily activity that helps maintain a baseline level of bone health as it guards against disuse and the consequences of immobilisation. It is therefore an accepted low-impact activity that can help those living with osteoporosis-related vertebral fractures remain as active as possible and interrupt long periods of sitting (ROS, 2018). However, a review of exercise interventions concluded that whilst moderate gains in muscle strength can result from Nordic walking, normal walking activity confers no more than small gains in muscle strength with insufficient evidence of it benefiting bone strength or balance or reducing the risk of falling (Foster et al., 2018). A recent small study of postmenopausal women (N = 14; 64 years) has suggested that brisk walking at five kilometres per hour may provide sufficient load to either improve or preserve femoral neck BMD (Pellikaan et al., 2018), but this requires replication in a larger sample. Therefore, walking can be most helpful to promote gains in bone health for those not at risk of falling or living with vertebral fractures by acting as a warm-up activity prior to more dynamic exercise (e.g. walk-runs) and can be used as a recovery activity between repeated bouts or sets of moderate- or high-impact exercise or muscle-strength training.

Moderate-impact activity

Moderate-impact activities (see examples in Table 19.2) typically involve both feet briefly leaving the ground and yield impact forces > 2 BW upon landing (Weeks & Beck, 2008). Activities of at least moderate impact form the lower boundary of activity intensity in recent exercise prescription guidelines to prevent osteoporosis (Beck et al., 2017), and moderate-impact activity is the target intensity in new exercise guidelines to promote bone health in those living with osteoporosis who are not at risk of falling and do not have vertebral fractures (ROS, 2018).

The benefits of moderate-impact activity have also been supported by recent findings from a large cross-sectional study of habitual physical activity in free-living women (Stiles et al., 2017). This study found that the accumulation of just one to two minutes of activity per day (0.5% of the total daily activity) at an intensity equivalent to slow running (approximately 8 km/h) in healthy postmenopausal women or moderate-paced running (approximately 10 km/h) in healthy premenopausal women was associated with approximately 4% better bone health (measured using QUS of the heel) than in those who did less. Those who did over two minutes of moderate-impact weight-bearing activity had 6% better bone health than those who did less than a minute. The effect of having at least 4% higher BMD is particularly meaningful if you consider that, after menopause, the age-related rate of loss in BMD in women is approximately 1% per year. The accumulation of short bursts of running activity on most days of the week supports efforts to maintain and preserve BMD above the curve for as long as possible to help prevent osteoporosis by delaying or avoiding the point at which levels of BMD move into the osteoporotic range (see Figure 19.1). Whilst these findings indicate that accumulating more than two minutes of moderate-impact activity is associated with even better bone health, it is not necessary for everyone to become 'a runner'. As the animal studies demonstrate, there is a point at which continuing to load bone during an extended bout of activity will not provide any further osteogenic effect (diminishing returns).

Whilst the type of exercise one might engage in is down to personal choice and has cross-over benefits for a range of different health outcomes, it is important to also state that exercising to extremes and continually loading bone without adequate recovery can result in fatigue damage and possibly a stress fracture. If coupled with insufficient calorie intake to support extreme levels of activity, an individual would also become underweight, which could affect their hormonal status and put them at risk of being 'fit but fragile' (MacKnight, 2017; ROS, 2018).

High-impact activity

Before the benefits of moderate-impact activity on bone health were understood, the most-researched phsyical activity in relation to bone health was high-impact jumping activity, which typically yields > 4 BW in impact force (Weeks & Beck, 2008) or slightly lower (3–4 BW), depending on the population being tested. Jumping interventions have ranged in design but typically required participants to perform various amounts of jumping activity: for example, five sets of ten vertical jumps (approximately 8.5 cm high; ground reaction forces of 3 and 4 body weights in premenopausal and postmenopausal women, respectively) on six days of the week for a minimum of six months (Bassey et al., 1998). Other interventions have tested a higher volume on fewer days of the week (e.g. 100 impacts three days per week) (Weaver et al., 2016) or designed a 12-month progressive supervised training programme consisting of 40 minutes of moderate- to high-impact activity (running, stamping and jumping) three times per week, supplemented with a daily 10-minute home exercise programme involving similar activities (Vainionpää et al., 2005). A meta-analysis (summary of effect sizes from a selection of studies to provide greater statisical power to quantify the size of benefit, if any, from an intervention) of six studies in premenopausal women showed that the effects of jumping interventions demonstrated significant positive effects on sites at the femoral neck and troachanter (absolute increases of 0.017 ± 0.474 and 0.021 ± 0.443 g/cm^2 respectively) but were less effective on influencing BMD at the spine (Zhao et al., 2014). One suggestion for jumping to initiate less osteogenic effect at the spine is the greater attenuation of force as it travels higher up the body, which may reduce the strength of the mechancial signal to stimulate bone cells (mechanotransduction) and trigger a remodelling response. Positive effects on spine BMD, however, are suggested to be more likely in multi-modal exercise interventions that include both weight-bearing impact activity and progressive resistance training (PRT) to build muscle strength (Martyn-St James & Carroll, 2010). Further research is required to quantify any additional benefit or burden from engaging in high-impact activity versus moderate-impact activity in relation to bone health.

Exercise interventions including progressive resistance training (PRT)

Progressive resistance training (PRT) is a training protocol in which the individual repeatedly lifts or presses (e.g. 8–12 reps) an amount of weight (resistance), typically at an intensity that is 80% of the maximum amount they can lift in one repetition (80% 1RM) and, after a short break or alternative activity, repeats the exercise set again (e.g. 2–3 sets) within the same training session. Over time, as muscle strength improves, the resistance can be gradually increased, and the number of repetitions reduced (e.g. 8–10 reps) in each set as the individual continues to work towards muscle fatigue. This provides a progressive overloading training stimulus to improve muscle strength (ACSM, 2009). As an alternative to calculating 80% of

1RM, 'Strong, Steady and Straight' advises an amount that can only be lifted 8 to 12 times before tiredness in the muscle prevents any further repetitions (ROS, 2018). The theory behind PRT improving BMD is that it gradually builds muscle mass (muscle strength), which, in turn, pulls more strongly on bones during resistance exercise, creating strain that initiates bone formation to result in stronger bones. A review of evidence from studies ranging in duration, compliance and randomisation to intervention indicates that PRT alone is of limited benefit to preserving BMD at the hip (femoral neck) or lumbar spine (Hillsdon & Foster, 2018). However, multi-modal programmes that combine suitable weight-bearing exercise and PRT have the greatest chance of increasing or maintaining BMD in both hip and spine regions in either middle-aged or older women, irrespective of menopausal status (Hillsdon & Foster, 2018). The evidence from randomised controlled trials (6–12 month interventions) and meta-analyses that use either high-impact weight-bearing exercise, PRT or multi-modal interventions indicate a positive effect on the maintenance of BMD and, in some cases, a 1% to 3% increase in BMD at the end of the intervention.

A randomised controlled trial (RCT) in postmenopausal women with low or very low bone mass (LIFTMOR) assessed the effects of an eight-month, twice-weekly, bone-specific supervised high-intensity PRT training programme (> 85% 1RM; 5 sets of 5 repetitions; deadlifts, squats, overhead presses) and high-impact (jumping chin-ups with drop landings onto flat feet; 5 sets of 5 repetitions) and found significant improvements in BMD at the lumbar spine (2.9 ± 3.1%) and femoral neck (0.3 ± 3.0) (Watson et al., 2017), together with improved measures of kyphosis (Watson et al., 2019). Importantly, the intensity of this programme was not found to increase the risk of vertebral fracture, and the high levels of compliance (92%) in the supervised high-intensity exercise group also counters previous perceptions of this level of intensity not being well tolerated (Watson et al., 2019). These findings may provide reassurance to those living with osteoporosis but without vertebral fracture who might be concerned about increasing their fracture risk when engaging in moderate-impact weight-bearing activity.

Recommendations for fitness testing and exercise programming

Fitness testing

Prior to starting an exercise programme, everyone should complete a Participant Activity Readiness Questionnaire (PAR-Q+) (Warburton et al., 2011; www.eparmedx.com). It is important to clarify whether any historical fractures were due to one-off slips or falls or whether they occurred as a result of low-level, awkward movements which could indicate underlying poor levels of bone health, in which case referral for a medical consultation is required. If an individual presents with a vertbral fracture, then it is important to refer them to seek specialist supervision for a tailored exercise programme.

It would also be informative to understand someone's risk for developing an osteoporosis-related fracture in the spine, hip, shoulder or wrist in the next ten years in case referral for a medical consultation might be pertinent. The online fracture risk assessment tool (FRAX) (www.sheffield.ac.uk/FRAX/) can be used to self-assess the probability of fracture risk in an individual between the ages of 40 and 90 years, either with or without knowledge of femoral neck BMD. If an individual is < 40 years old, then the tool can be used to identify clinical risk factors present, and advice regarding modification of risk factors can be provided.

A further link on the FRAX calculation site to the National Osteoporosis Guideline Group (NOGG) helps interpret whether fracture risk is sufficiently low (their 'x' should appear in the green zone on the graph) to enable an exercise professional to provide lifestyle advice and exercise programming or whether an individual should be referred to their GP for further assessment (their 'x' may appear in the amber zone on the graph). If an adult has experienced a low-trauma fracture (fracture resulting from a fall from standing height or less), then considertation of any underlying bone disease is warranted. In this scenario, for adults over 40 years, FRAX and a DXA scan would be recommended. In younger adults, consideration of clinical risk factors for osteoporosis and any potential underlying co-morbidities should be explored. If repeated fractures are occurring, then a DXA scan and referral into a specialist bone service are recommended, along with assessment of blood to identify any underlying bone disease. A low BMI (< 22 kg/m^2) is a risk factor for osteoporosis, and this should be considered in athletic populations and alongside menstrual history in women (De Laet et al., 2005; Kmietowicz, 2008).

The NHS also provide a link on their website (www.nhs.uk/live-well/healthy-body/osteoporosis-fracture-risk-assessment-tool-frax/) to an online training video for a 'timed up and go' (TUG) test (Podsiadlo & Richardson, 1991), which is a test that anyone can do, but which is especially important for individuals who present as being unsteady on their feet or are suspected to be at risk of falling. This test measures the time taken for an individual to get up from a standard chair (46 cm in height) and walk at a comfortable pace to a marker three metres away and back to the chair. If this is completed in under 15 seconds, the individual is considered to be at low risk of falling and can continue with an appropriately tailored exercise programme. If they take longer than 15 seconds, then the exercise programme should primarily focus on improving strength and balance in the initial stages, in a supervised programme (please refer to the 'Steady' theme from 'Strong, Steady and Straight' (ROS, 2018). Consideration should also be given to whether the individual needs to be referred to their GP to help them gain access to services related to falling (health and well-being assessment, eye assessment etc).

Exercise programming

Findings from the latest research and bone-specific exercise recommendations that recognise the benefits of moderate-impact weight-bearing exercise to promote bone health (Beck et al., 2017; Stiles et al., 2017; ROS, 2018) are used to inform exercise programming for osteoporosis prevention and the preservation of bone health for those living with osteoporosis who are not at risk of falling and don't have vertebral fractures. Any additional benefit of high-impact activity over moderate-impact activity on bone health is not currently known; however, individuals who currently undertake high-impact exercise are encouraged to continue doing so as long as the activities match their levels of experience, fitness and ability. Readers are directed to 'Strong, Steady and Straight' for specific exercise and activity recommendations for those living with vertebral fracture and/or having falls, which should be delivered by specialist health or exercise practitioners (ROS, 2018).

As a supplement to existing physical activity guidelines to promote bone health, it is important to increase the volume and intensity of activity gradually, with the aim of performing approximately 50 moderate impacts in which both feet leave the floor for a brief period of time (e.g. low jumps, skipping, hopping, side steps with a small jump, dynamic dance steps) on most days of the week. If performing in quick succession, it is advisable to split these impacts into five sets of 10 impacts with at least one minute of active recovery (e.g. walking) between sets. If the accumulation of short bursts of running at a comfortable speed sounds more appealing, then once the body feels warm (for example, during a purposeful brisk walk), repeated short bouts of running at a slow-moderate pace for 10 to 20-seconds adding up to one to two minutes in total could be achieved. Others might want to be more creative, if the environment safely permits, by running at least the last 30 seconds to the corner shop and running at least 30 seconds on the way home. Taking part in sports such as those outlined in Table 19.2 for at least 30 minutes per session also counts towards accumulating daily/weekly moderate-impact activity to promote bone health.

Undertaking 20 to 30 minutes of PRT using weights (preferable) or a resistance band on two or three non-consecutive days per week whilst working with the highest amount of resistance (approximately 80% 1RM) one can lift or pulling 8 to 12 repetitions for three sets is also advised for benefits to muscle and bone strength. If performed in a standing position, PRT involving large multi-joint compound exercises (e.g. squat or deadlift or a sequence of these) that work multiple muscle groups at the same time (e.g. quadriceps, glutes and calves) can especially contribute to building bone strength by increasing BMD at the spine and hip. Participating in group exercise classes that use similar principles to progressively build muscle strength also counts towards meeting the recommended target for PRT.

Many weight-bearing and muscle strength exercises have crossover benefits for improving balance, but Public Health England advises that all adults, including older adults, should also engage specifically in balance training at least twice a week to help reduce the risk of falling (Foster et al., 2018). Balance training exercises should each be performed for at least ten seconds and present sufficient challenge to the individual by working towards reducing the base of support to a narrow or single-leg stance. As ever, it is important that the level of challenge is tailored for each individual. Balancing on uneven surfaces and/or closing the eyes can be used to increase the intensity of the challenge, although performing next to a rail or similar object is advised to provide safety and support as necessary (Beck et al., 2017). Balance training exercises such as toe/heel raises, toe/heel walking and single-leg standing can be incorporated into multi-modal exercise programmes and can also be used as a form of active recovery between exercise sets. Engaging in exercise classes such as tai chi, yoga or Pilates provides a structured, supervised environment for encountering and improving performance in balancing activities.

While this chapter focuses primarily on exercise for the prevention of osteoporosis in later life and the preservation of bone health for those living with osteoporosis brief comment is made here regarding exercise for older frail adults. As long as there is no previous history of vertebral fractures or existing conditions that prevent the individual from engaging in physical movement, older frail adults are also recommended to engage in structured exercise programmes of 60-minutes duration two or three times per week in a supervised environment with sufficiently experienced and trained practitioners either in a one-to-one or small-group setting (Foster et al., 2018). To help maintain strength and improve balance, exercise programmes for these individuals could include standing or chair-based yoga (tailored to individual needs) or tai chi, in which the level of challenge in terms of balance can be steadily increased over time. As long as the choice of exercise is appropriately tailored to the individual, alongside balance training, these programmes, even for very frail older adults, could include elements of progressive resistance training and endurance work (Foster et al., 2018).

Exercise considerations

Providing there are no medical reasons someone should not take part in exercise, anyone looking to increase their exercise should build up gradually. PRT exercises that repeatedly and forcibly load the spine while it is compressed, twisted or flexed should be avoided. Forward flexion of the back is acceptable as long as this arises from hinging at the hip and not from curving the spine forward. A 'spine-caring' approach is always advised when lifting, which involves hinging at the hip, flexing the knees, engaging the core muscles and keeping the back straight (to help avoid kyphosis). Exercises should also be performed smoothly with good control and without holding the breath at any point. Supervision from a qualified exercise professional is important, at least in the initial stages, to learn and maintain correct movement techniques, especially when introducing large multi-joint compound exercises into a programme.

Case study

Abi was 40 years old when she was diagnosed with coeliac disease following a period of weight loss and fatigue, which had lasted for over two years. During this time, Abi had noted some stomach bloating regularly but thought it was the bread in the sandwiches she was buying at work, and she put her increasing fatigue down to her new job and the pressures that had brought with it. After friends mentioned her weight loss, Abi decided to see her doctor as she was concerned that this, along with her other symptoms, meant she had something wrong.

Her blood tests demonstrated anaemia and subsequent tests proved positive for coeliac disease. Abi commenced her gluten-free diet under the supervision of a dietician and, after six months, was gaining weight well and feeling much better. However, Abi began to get concerned about her weight gain as she had become accustomed to eating significantly more food than usual prior to her diagnosis. Adjusting to more normal levels and managing her weight gain so she maintained a healthy weight was important to her. Abi was sent for a DXA scan by her consultant to check her for low bone density in light of her coeliac diagnosis, and this came back with a Z-score of −2.3 at her spine and −1.9 at her total hip. Abi was told that she had low bone mass, and this was likely as a result of her coeliac disease, which had been undiagnosed and untreated in previous years.

Abi had her vitamin D measured and was found to be vitamin D insufficient at 35 mmol/L and was prescribed calcium and vitamin D for a year until her absorption had improved and was counselled on safe sun exposure and foods rich in vitamin D. Abi was advised that weight-bearing impact and PRT exercise (multimodal exercise) would be beneficial for her bone health as well as maintaining her weight and cardiovascular health since, despite her low Z-scores, her fracture risk was still relatively low due to her age.

Abi fancied an indoor cycling exercise class, but she was advised that this would not support bone improvements, so she decided to join a gym and attend a group exercise class containing PRT and balancing exercises at least once a week and go to the gym on at least one other occasion during the week. In conversation with Abi, an exercise referral practitioner at the gym was able to put together a multi-modal programme, which, amongst PRT exercises, contained rope skipping (a favourite activity of Abi's) and a small cone drill that required Abi to perform short shuttles, side-steps and lunges towards four cones laid out in a cross-shape. Abi enjoyed performing these bursts of activity, which were interspersed with balancing exercises between sets. Abi was also encouraged to think about ways she could increase her weight-bearing impact activity on days of the week when she wouldn't be attending the gym.

After an encouraging conversation with her exercise referral practitioner, Abi decided that, whilst out walking her dog, when her body was warm, she would be happy to begin incorporating at least three 10- to 20-second bursts of running at a slow, self-selected pace, initially for two to four weeks on most days when she wasn't doing any structured exercise. She would then build up to include at least three 20-second bursts of running at a faster moderate pace in future weeks. Two years on, Abi had a further DXA scan, in which she was pleased to see a 4% increase in her hip bone density and an 5% increase in her spine BMD as a result of treating her coeliac disease, being calcium and vitamin D replete and incorporating regular weight-bearing impact and PRT exercise in her weekly routine.

Summary

Although genetics strongly influence the capacity of attaining high levels of bone mass, there are a number of highly modifiable lifestyle risk factors that also play their part (20–40%) in attaining, maintaining and preserving bone mass across the lifespan. Positively modifying these risks can help prevent osteoporosis and reduce the risk of encountering painful fragility fractures in later life. Physical activity is a highly modifiable factor that can influence bone health across the lifespan. Compared to high-impact activity, recent research using more precise methods for analysing physical activity and new exercise prescriptions for bone health advocate the osteogenic benefits of potentially more pallitable doses of moderate-impact weight-bearing activity. As a supplement to existing physical activity guidelines, multi-modal exercise programmes that combine moderate-impact weight-bearing activity (e.g. 1–2 minutes of running or 50 impacts [5 sets × 10 reps] from low jumping, hopping, rope skipping or sports participation) accumulated throughout the day on most days of the week and progressive resistance training (3 sets of 8–12 reps working at 80% 1RM on 2–3 non-consecutive days per week) are most beneficial for promoting bone health at key fracture sites (hip, wrist and spine). For greatest osteogenic effect, it important to try and vary the type, speed and direction of impact that bone experiences (movement diversity), as well as incorporating periods of rest into exercise programmes and between exercise sessions to maintain the mechanosensitivity of bone cells to stimulation. Balance-training exercises that present a sufficient challenge to the individual should also be performed two or three times per week to aid falls prevention.

Key points

- Physical inactivity is a highly modifiable risk factor for the development of osteoporosis.
- Bone continually responds to meet the demands of the load encountered, and its reponse to physical activity is site, mode, dose and intensity specific.
- With suitable levels of tailoring and supervision, new recommendations from 'Strong, Steady and Straight: An Expert Consensus Statement on Physical Activity and Exercise for Osteoporosis' (ROS, 2018) positively encourage engagement in physical activity and exercise for everyone living with osteoporosis.
- Engaging in a small amount of moderate-impact weight-bearing activity on most days can be recommended to promote bone health for prevention (Beck et al., 2017) and management (ROS, 2018) of osteoporosis for those not at risk of falling and without vertebral fracture.
- For greatest osteogenic effect, it is important to subject bone to a range of different speeds and directions of loading (movement diversity) and schedule periods of rest into the exercise programme to maintain the mechanosensitivity of bone cells to trigger bone remodelling (mechanotransduction).
- Multi-modal exercise programmes that combine moderate-impact weight-bearing activity (e.g. 1–2 minutes of running or 50 impacts [5 sets × 10 reps] from low jumping, hopping, rope skipping or sports) accumulated throughout the day on most days of the week, progressive resistance training (3 sets of 8–12 reps working at 80% 1RM, 2–3 non-consecutive days per week) and sufficiently challenging balance activities (2–3 times per week), are recommended to promote bone health at key fracture sites (hip, wrist and spine) and prevent falls.

Study tasks

1. Using lay language, define osteoporosis, the consequences of it and its prevalence in the general population.
2. List the four main modifiable lifestyle risk factors for the development of osteoporosis.
3. Describe the clinical risk factors that the online FRAX calculation tool uses to predict the ten-year probability of fracture.
4. Describe the exercise and activity impact classification system that is more relevant to bone health and include example exercises, activities, sports and exercise classes that represent activities from each category.
5. List the three themes, which can also be considered as entry points prioritising certain types of exercise, around which the 2018 Expert Consensus Statement on Exercise and Physical Activity for Osteoporosis from the Royal Osteoporosis Society (2018) is centred.
6. What sort of attitude does 'Strong, Steady and Straight': An Expert Consensus Statement on Exercise and Physical Activity for Osteoporosis (ROS, 2018) encourage exercise practitioners to adopt when promoting exercise for bone health?
7. Recent research (Stiles et al., 2017) has used information from wrist-worn activity monitors (high-resolution accelerometers) to more precisely measure bone-specific characteristics of daily physical activity in large population samples. Can you summarise the main findings from this research and how it supports the inclusion of moderate-impact activity in recent exercise prescriptions for osteoporosis prevention and management?

8. To reduce the risk of developing osteoporosis and to preserve bone health in those living with osteoporosis (but not at risk of falling and without vertebral fracture), describe characteristics of the exercise programme recommended in this chapter to promote bone health.
9. For those living with osteoporosis and vertebral fractures, what is the advice regarding the intensity of weight-bearing activity?
10) Gradual increases in exercise intensity are important for everyone undertaking an exercise programme, but what are the other key exercise considerations, including exercises to avoid when performing PRT or lifting?

TABLE 19.2 Summary of key messages for those living with osteoporosis but who are not at risk of falling and do not have vertebral fractures*

Themes and priorities	To promote bone strength, reduce the risk of falls and improve posture, this statement centres around the themes 'strong', 'steady' and 'straight', with the aim of incorporating all aspects into an exercise programme. Each theme acts as a point of entry so activities can be tailored and prioritised to meet the immediate needs of the individual. Those with osteoporosis but not at risk of falling and without vertebral fracture can prioritise muscle- and bone-strengthening exercises under 'strong'. Some exercises will have crossover benefits or can be supplemented to satisfy the aims of 'steady' and 'straight' too.
Positive attitude and reassurance	The statement encourages health-care practitioners and exercise professionals to adopt a positive, how-to attitude to help those living with osteoporosis to 'do more'. Individuals not at risk of falling and without vertebral fractures can be reassured that the risk of exercise causing a fragility fracture is low, and the benefits of exercise for health and well-being outweigh the risks of restricting activity or doing nothing.
Build up gradually	Exercise progression should be gradual, and starting points should be graded according to ability and experience. The message for beginner exercisers is that every increase in activity counts towards the aim of 'doing more'.
Moderate-impact weight-bearing activity	Moderate-impact weight-bearing activity, in which both feet leave the floor for a brief period of time, is the target intensity to promote bone health in those living with osteoporosis who are not at risk of falling and do not have vertebral fractures. Example activities include running, rope jumping, low jumps, Highland-type dancing, dynamic side steps and hops. Certain group exercise classes (e.g. Zumba) that include a mixture of these activities, together with racquet sports, track athletics, team sports/ball games and martial arts that include foot stamping are all accepted ways to experience moderate-impact activities.
Brief outline of the statement's exercise guidelines to promote bone health	**Strong**: **Weight-bearing impact** – On most days, aim for 50 moderate impacts (e.g. jumps/hops/running) split into five sets of ten, with one minute active recovery (e.g. walking) between sets. Vary movement, speed and direction. **Build muscle** – On two or three days per week, undertake progressive muscle-resistance exercise (three sets of 10–12 reps; upper and lower body including spine), using the maximum weight (or resistance band) you can lift until fatigue.

(*Continued*)

TABLE 19.2 (Continued)

	Steady: Many weight-bearing and muscle-strengthening exercises have crossover benefits for improving balance, but less steady individuals and those over 65 years should specifically perform balancing activities two or three days a week and focus on reducing the base of support to increase the level of challenge. Pilates, yoga and tai chi are also suitable.
	Straight: Many exercise programmes will cover this, but specific back-strengthening exercises should be performed two or three days a week (ten reps each, hold for three to five seconds). Pilates, yoga, swimming, hydrotherapy and aqua-aerobics are also suitable.
Learn correct technique	When lifting, a 'spine-caring' approach is advised. This involves hinging at the hip, flexing knees, engaging core muscles and keeping the back straight.
Complements other methods	Bone-specific exercise should complement rather than replace pharmacological methods for managing osteoporosis.
Supplement activity guidelines	Bone-specific exercise should supplement rather than replace general physical activity guidelines.

* For greater focus on 'steady' and 'straight' and activity recommendations for those at risk of falling and/or living with vertbral fractures, please consult 'Strong, Steady and Straight' (ROS, 2018)

Source: 'Strong, Steady and Straight': An Expert Consensus Statement on Physical Activity and Exercise for Osteoporosis from the Royal Osteoporosis Society, UK (2018)

References

Abate, M., Vanni, D., Pantalone, A. and Salini, V. (2013). Cigarette smoking and musculoskeletal disorders. *Muscles Ligaments Tendons J*, 3(2), pp. 63–69. doi:10.11138/mltj/2013.3.2.063

American College of Sports Medicine. (2009). Progression models in resistance training for healthy adults. *Medicine and Science in Sports and Exercise*, 41(3), pp. 687–708.

Arden, N. and Spector, T. (1997). *Osteoporosis illustrated*. Current Medical Literature.

Bailey, C.A. and Brooke-Wavell, K. (2010). Optimum frequency of exercise for bone health: Randomised controlled trial of a high-impact unilateral intervention. *Bone*, 46(4), pp. 1043–1049.

Bailey, D.A., McKay, H.A., Mirwald, R.L., Crocker, P.R.E., and Faulkner, R.A. (1999). A six-year longitudinal study of the relationship of physical activity to bone mineral accrual in growing children: The university of Saskatchewan bone mineral accrual study. *Journal of Bone and Mineral Research*, 14(10), pp. 1672–1679.

Baim, S., Binkley, N., Bilezikian, J.R., Kendler, D.L., Hans, D.B., Lewiecki, E.M. and Silverman, S. (2008). Official positions of the international society for clinical densitometry and executive summary of the 2007 ISCD position development conference. *Journal of Clinical Densitometry*, 11(1), pp. 75–91. doi:10.1016/j.jocd.2007.12.007

Baran, D.T. (1994). Magnitude and determinants of premenopausal bone loss. *Osteoporosis International*, 4(1), S31–S34. doi:10.1007/bf01623432

Bass, S., Pearce, G., Bradney, M., Hendrich, E., Delmas, P.D., Harding, A. and Seeman, E. (1998). Exercise before puberty may confer residual benefits in bone density in adulthood: studies in active prepubertal and retired female gymnasts. *J Bone Miner Res*, 13(3), pp. 500–507.

Bassey, E.J., Rothwell, M.C., Littlewood, J.J. and Pye, D.W. (1998). Pre- and post-menopausal women have different bone mineral responses to the same high-impact exercise. *J Bone Miner Res*, 13(12), pp. 1805–1813.

Baxter-Jones, A.D., Faulkner, R.A., Forwood, M.R., Mirwald, R.L. and Bailey, D.A. (2011). Bone mineral accrual from 8 to 30 years of age: An estimation of peak bone mass. *Journal of Bone and Mineral Research*, 26(8), pp. 1729–1739.

Beck, B.R., Daly, R.M., Fiatarone Singh, M.A. and Taaffe, D.R. (2017). Exercise and sports science Australia (ESSA) position statement on exercise prescription for the prevention and management of osteoporosis. *Journal of Science and Medicine in Sport*, 20(5), pp. 438–445.

Blake, G.M. and Fogelman, I. (2009). The clinical role of dual energy X-ray absorptiometry. *European Journal of Radiology*, 71(3), pp. 406–414. doi:10.1016/j.ejrad.2008.04.062

Boonen, S., Laan, L.A., Barton, I.P. and Watts, N.B. (2005). Effect of osteoporosis treatments on risk of non-vertebral fractures: Review and meta-analysis of intention-to-treat studies. *Osteoporosis International*, 16(10), pp. 1291–1298.

Bousson, V., Bergot, C., Sutter, B., Levitz, P., Cortet, B. and Grio. (2012). Trabecular bone score (TBS): Available knowledge, clinical relevance, and future prospects. *Osteoporosis International*, 23(5), pp. 1489–1501. doi:10.1007/s00198-011-1824-6

Brown, C. (2017). Osteoporosis: Staying strong. *Nature*, 550(7674), S15–S17. doi:10.1038/550S15a

Brown, J. P., Morin, S., Leslie, W., Papaioannou, A., Cheung, A. M., Davison, K. S. et al. (2014). Bisphosphonates for treatment of osteoporosis: Expected benefits, potential harms, and drug holidays. *Can Fam Physician*, 60(4), pp. 324–333.

Buckwalter, J., Glimcher, M., Cooper, R. and Recker, R. (1995). Bone biology. *J Bone Joint Surg Am*, 77(8), pp. 1256–1275.

Burge, R., Dawson-Hughes, B., Solomon, D.H. Wong, J.N., King, A. and Tosteson, A. (2007). Incidence and economic burden of osteoporosis-related fractures in the United States, 2005–2025. *J Bone Miner Res*, 22(3), pp. 465–475.

Burr, D.B., Robling, A.G. and Turner, C.H. (2002). Effects of biomechanical stress on bones in animals. *Bone*, 30(5), pp. 781–786.

Carter, M.I. and Hinton, P.S. (2014). Physical activity and bone health. *Missouri Med*. 111(1), pp. 59–64.

Castillo, A.B. and Leucht, P. (2015). Bone homeostasis and repair: forced into shape. *Curr Rheumatol Rep*, 17(9). doi:10.1007/s11926-015-0537-9

Chapurlat, R.D., Garnero, P., Sornay-Rendu, E., Arlot, M.E., Claustrat, B. and Delmas, P.D. (2000). Longitudinal study of bone loss in pre- and perimenopausal women: Evidence for bone loss in perimenopausal women. *Osteoporosis International*, 11(6), pp. 493–498. doi:10.1007/s001980070091

Cummings, S.R., Black, D.M., Nevitt, M.C., Browner, W., Cauley, J., Ensrud, K., Genant, H.K., Palermo, L., Scott, J. and Vogt, T.M. (1993). Bone density at various sites for prediction of hip fractures. *The Study of Osteoporotic Fractures Research Group. Lancet*, 341(8837), pp. 72–75.

De Laet, C., Kanis, J., Odén, A., Johanson, H., Johnell, O., Delmas, P. et al. (2005). Body mass index as a predictor of fracture risk: A meta-analysis. *Osteoporosis International*, 16(11), pp. 1330–1338.

Delmas, P.D., van de Langerijt, L., Watts, N.B., Eastell, R., Genant, H., Grauer, A. and Cahall, D. L. (2005). Underdiagnosis of vertebral fractures is a worldwide problem: The IMPACT study. *J Bone Miner Res*, 20(4), pp. 557–563. doi:10.1359/jbmr.041214

Donnelly, E., Saleh, A., Unnanuntana, A. and Lane, J. M. (2012). Atypical femoral fractures: Epidemiology, etiology, and patient management. *Current Opinion in Supportive and Palliative Care*, 6(3), pp. 348–354. doi:10.1097/SPC.0b013e3283552d7d

Eastell, R. and Walsh, J. S. (2017). Anabolic treatment for osteoporosis: Teriparatide. *Clinical Cases in Mineral and Bone Metabolism*, 14(2), pp. 173–178. doi:10.11138/ccmbm/2017.14.1.173

Ebeling, P.R., Atley, L.M., Guthrie, J.R., Burger, H.G., Dennerstein, L., Hopper, J L. and Wark, J.D. (1996). Bone turnover markers and bone density across the menopause transition. *J Clin Endocrinology Metab*, 81(9), pp. 3366–3371.

Favus, M.J. (1999). *Primer on the metabolic bone diseases and disorders of mineral metabolism*. 4th Edition. American Society for Bone and Mineral Research.

Foster, C., Armstrong, M., Hillsdon, M., Skelton, D., Mavroeidi, A., Cavill, N. and Milton, K. (2018). *Muscle and bone strengthening and balance activities for general health benefits in adults and older adults*. Public Health England.

Frost, H.M. (1987). Bone "mass" and the "mechanostat": A proposal. *The Anatomical Record*, 219(1), pp. 1–9. doi:10.1002/ar.1092190104

Garber, C.E., Blissmer, B., Deschenes, M.R., Franklin, B.A., Lamonte, M.J., Lee, I.M., Nieman, D.C. and Swain, D.O. (2011). American college of sports medicine position stand. Quantity and quality of exercise for developing and maintaining cardiorespiratory, musculoskeletal, and neuromotor fitness in apparently healthy adults: Guidance for prescribing exercise. *Med Sci Sports Exerc*, 43(7), pp. 1334–1359.

Garg, M.K. and Kharb, S. (2013). Dual energy X-ray absorptiometry: Pitfalls in measurement and interpretation of bone mineral density. *Indian Journal of Endocrinology and Metabolism*, 17(2), pp. 203–210. doi:10.4103/2230-8210.109659

Gauthier, A., Kanis, J.A., Jiang, Y. Martin, M., Compston, J.E., Borgström, F., Cooper, C. and McCloskey, E.V. (2011). Epidemiological burden of postmenopausal osteoporosis in the UK from 2010 to 2021: Estimations from a disease model. *Arch Osteoporosis*, 6, pp. 179–188.

Gerdhem, P. (2013). Osteoporosis and fragility fractures: Vertebral fractures. *Best Pract Res Clin Rheumatol*, 27(6), pp. 743–755. doi:10.1016/j.berh.2014.01.002

Greenway, K.G., Walkley, J.W. and Rich, P.A. (2015). Relationships between self-reported lifetime physical activity, estimates of current physical fitness, and aBMD in adult premenopausal women. *Arch Osteoporos*, 10, p. 34. doi:10.1007/s11657-015-0239-y

Haentjens, P., Magaziner, J., Colón-Emeric, C.S., Vanderschueren, D., Milisen, K., Velkeniers, B. and Boonen, S. (2010). Meta-analysis: Excess mortality after hip fracture among older women and men. *Annals of Internal Medicine*, 152(6), 380–390.

Hagino, H., Sawaguchi, T., Endo, N., Ito, Y., Nakano, T. and Watanabe, Y. (2012). The risk of a second hip fracture in patients after their first hip fracture. *Calcified Tissue International*, 90(1), pp. 14–21.

Hans, D. and Krieg, M. A. (2009). Quantitative ultrasound for the detection and management of osteoporosis. *Salud Publica Mex*, 51, Suppl 1, S25–S37.

Hillier, T.A., Cauley, J.A., Rizzo, J.H., Pedula, K.L., Ensrud, K.E., Bauer, D.C. et al. (2011). WHO absolute fracture risk models (FRAX): Do clinical risk factors improve fracture prediction in older women without osteoporosis? *Journal of Bone and Mineral Research*, 26(8), pp. 1774–1782. doi:10.1002/jbmr.372

Hillsdon, M. and Foster, C. (2018). What are the health benefits of muscle and bone strengthening and balance activities across life stages and specific health outcomes? *Journal of Frailty, Sarcopenia and Falls*, 3(2), pp. 66–73.

Hopkins, S.J., Smith, C., Toms, A., Brown, M., Appelboam, A., Welsman, J. and Knapp, K. (2012). Relationship between spine bone mineral density and trabecular bone score in postmenopausal populations following total knee replacement or leg fracture. *Osteoporosis International*, Suppl 5, p. S582.

Hopkins, S.J., Toms, A.D., Brown, M., Welsman, J.R., Ukoumunne, O.C. and Knapp, K.M. (2016). A study investigating short- and medium-term effects on function, bone mineral density and lean tissue mass post-total knee replacement in a Caucasian female post-menopausal population: Implications for hip fracture risk. *Osteoporos Int*, 27(8), pp. 2567–2576. doi:10.1007/s00198-016-3546-2

Jämsä, T., Ahola, R. and Korpelainen, R. (2011). Measurement of osteogenic exercise – how to interpret accelerometric data? *Frontiers in Physiol*, 2, p. 73.

Jang, H.D., Hong, J.Y., Han, K., Lee, J.C., Shin, B.J., Choi, S.W. et al. (2017). Relationship between bone mineral density and alcohol intake: A nationwide health survey analysis of postmenopausal women. *PLoS One*, 12(6), p. e0180132. doi:10.1371/journal.pone.0180132

Jansen, J.P., Bergman, G.J., Huels, J. and Olson, M. (2011). The efficacy of bisphosphonates in the prevention of vertebral, hip, and nonvertebral-nonhip fractures in osteoporosis: A network meta-analysis. *Semin Arthritis Rheum*, 40(4), pp. 275–284.

Jee, W.S.S. (2000). Principles in bone physiology. *J Musculoskeletal Neuron Interactions*, 1, pp. 11–13.

Kanis, J.A. (2002). Diagnosis of osteoporosis and assessment of fracture risk. *The Lancet*, 359(9321), pp. 1929–1936.

Kanis, J.A. (2007). *Assessment of osteoporosis at the primary health care level.* On behalf of the World Health Organisation Scientific Group. WHO Collaborating Centre for Metabolic Bone Diseases, University of Sheffield.

Kanis, J.A., Borgstrom, F., De Laet, C., Johansson, H., Johnell, O, Jonsson, B., Oden, A., Zethraeus, N., Pfleger, B. and Khaltaev, N. (2005). Assessment of fracture risk. *Osteoporosis International*, 16(6), pp. 581–589.

Kanis, J.A., McCloskey, E.V., Johansson, H., Cooper, C., Rizzoli, R., Reginster, J.Y. et al. (2013). European guidance for the diagnosis and management of osteoporosis in postmenopausal women. *Osteoporosis International*, 24(1), pp. 23–57. doi:10.1007/s00198-012-2074-y

Kaptoge, S., Armbrecht, G., Felsenberg, D., Lunt, M., O'Neill, T.W., Silman, A.J. and Reeve, J. (2004). When should the doctor order a spine X-ray? Identifying vertebral fractures for osteoporosis care: Results from the European prospective osteoporosis study (EPOS). *J Bone Miner Res*, 19(12), pp. 1982–1993. doi:10.1359/jbmr.040901

Khosla, S. and Pacifici, R. (2013). Estrogen deficiency, postmenopausal osteoporosis, and age-related bone loss. In R. Marcus, D. Feldman, D.W. Dempster, M. Luckey, and J. Cauley (Eds.), *Osteoporosis*. 4th edition, pp. 1113–1138. Academic Press.

Kmietowicz, Z. (2008). NICE publishes osteoporosis guidance after more than six years of consultation. *BMJ: British Medical Journal (Online)*, 337.

Knapp, K.M. (2009). Quantitative ultrasound and bone health. *Salud Publica Mex*, 51, Suppl 1, pp. S18–S24.

Knapp, K.M. and Blake, G.M. (2014). Dual Energy X-ray Absorptiometry: Quality Assurance and Governance. *Osteoporosis Review*, 22(1), pp. 1–6.

Knapp, K.M., Welsman, J.R. and MacLeod, K.M. (2010). Prolonged unilateral disuse osteopenia 14 years post external fixator removal: A case history and critical review. *Case Reports in Medicine*, p. 629020.

Lewiecki, E.M., Wright, N.C., Curtis, J.R., Siris, E., Gagel, R.F., Saag, K.G., Singer, A.J., Steven, P.M. and Adler, R.A. (2017). Hip fracture trends in the United States, 2002 to 2015. *Osteoporos Int*, 29(3), pp. 717–722. doi:10.1007/s00198-017-4345-0

Lindsay, R., Silverman, S. L., Cooper, C., Hanley, D.A., Barton, I., Broy, S.B. et al. (2001). Risk of new vertebral fracture in the year following a fracture. *JAMA*, 285(3), pp. 320–323.

Lippuner, K., von Overbeck, J., Perrelet, R., Bosshard, H. and Jaeger, P. (1997). Incidence and direct medical costs of hospitalizations due to osteoporotic fractures in Switzerland. *Osteoporos Int*, 7(5), pp. 414–425.

Lunt, M., Ismail, A.A., Felsenberg, D., Cooper, C., Kanis, J.A., Reeve, J. et al. (2002). Defining incident vertebral deformities in population studies: A comparison of morphometric criteria. *Osteoporos Int*, 13(10), pp. 809–815. doi:10.1007/s001980200112

MacKnight, J.M. (2017). Osteopenia and osteoporosis in female athletes. *Clin Sports Med*, 36(4), pp. 687–702. doi:10.1016/j.csm.2017.05.006

Marshall, D., Johnell, O. and Wedel, H. (1996) Meta-analysis of how well measures of bone mineral density predict occurrence of osteoporotic fractures. *BMJ*, 312(7041), pp. 1254–1259.

Martyn-St James, M. and Carroll, S. (2010). Effects of different impact exercise modalities on bone mineral density in premenopausal women: A meta-analysis. *J Bone Miner Metab*, 28(3), pp. 251–267.

Menendez-Colino, R., Alarcon, T., Gotor, P., Queipo, R., Ramirez-Martin, R., Otero, A. and Gonzalez-Montalvo, J.I. (2018). Baseline and pre-operative 1-year mortality risk factors in a cohort of 509 hip fracture patients consecutively admitted to a co-managed orthogeriatric unit (FONDA Cohort). *Injury*, 49(3), pp. 656–661. doi:10.1016/j.injury.2018.01.003

Mitchell, P., Dolan, L., Sahota, O., Cooper, A., Elliot, M., McQuillian, C., Stone, M., Hosking, D., Sandhu, B., Shervington, P., Moger, S. and Mullan, K. (2010). *Osteoporosis in the UK at breaking point*. Available from The British Menopause Society. https://thebms.org.uk/wp-content/uploads/2010/10/Osteo_Report2010.pdf (15 August 2019, date last accessed).

Moayyeri, A., Adams, J.E., Adler, R.A., Krieg, M.A., Hans, D., Compston, J. and Lewiecki, E. M. (2012). Quantitative ultrasound of the heel and fracture risk assessment: An updated meta-analysis. *Osteoporos Int*, 23(1), pp. 143–153. doi:10.1007/s00198-011-1817-5

Morgan, E.F., Barnes, G.L. and Einhorn, T.A. (2013). The bone organ system: Form and function. In R. Marcus, D. Feldman, D.W. Dempster, M. Luckey, and J. Cauley (Eds.), *Osteoporosis*. 4th edition, pp. 3–20. Academic Press.

National Osteoporosis Guideline Group. (2014). *Osteoporosis – clinical guideline for prevention and treatment: Executive summary*, November. www.sheffield.ac.uk/NOGG/NOGG_Executive_Summary.pdf (15th February 2018, date last accessed).

National Osteoporosis Guideline Group. (2017). *Osteoporosis – clinical guideline for prevention and treatment*, March. www.sheffield.ac.uk/NOGG/NOGG%20Guideline%202017.pdf (15 February 2018, date last accessed).

NICE. (2011/2019). CG124 hip fracture: The management of hip fracture in adults. *BNF.* https://bnf.nice.org.uk/drug/alendronic-acid.html#directionsForAdministration

Nikander, R., Sievanen, H., Heinonen, A., Karstila, T. and Kannus, P. (2008). Load-specific differences in the structure of femoral neck and tibia between world-class moguls skiers and slalom skiers. *Scand J Med Sci Sports*, 18(12), pp. 145–153.

O'Donovan, G., Blazevich, A.J., Boreham, C., Cooper, A.R., Crank, H., Ekelund, U., Fox, K.R., Gately, P., Giles-Corti, B., Gill, J.M., Hamer, M., McDermott, I., Murphy, M., Mutri, N., Reilly, J.J., Saxton, J.M. and Stamatakis, E. (2010). The ABC of physical activity for health: A consensus statement from the British association of sport and exercise sciences. *J Sports Sci*, 28(6), pp. 573–591.

Pellikaan, P., Giarmatzis, G., Vander Sloten, J., Verschueren, S. and Jonkers, I. (2018). Ranking of osteogenic potential of physical exercises in postmenopausal women based on femoral neck strains. *PLoS One,* 13(4), p. e0195463. doi:10.1371/journal.pone.0195463

Podsiadlo, D. and Richardson, S. (1991). The timed "up & go": A test of basic functional mobility for frail elderly persons. *Journal of the American Geriatrics Society*, 39(2), pp. 142–148.

Poole, K.E., Reeve, J. and Warburton, E. A. (2002). Falls, fractures, and osteoporosis after stroke: Time to think about protection? *Stroke*, 33(5), pp. 1432–1436.

Poole, K.E., Warburton, E.A. and Reeve, J. (2005). Rapid long-term bone loss following stroke in a man with osteoporosis and atherosclerosis. *Osteoporos Int*, 16(3), pp. 302–305. doi:10.1007/s00198-004-1682-6

Poole, R., Kennedy, O.J., Roderick, P., Fallowfield, J.A., Hayes, P.C. and Parkes, J. (2017). Coffee consumption and health: Umbrella review of meta-analyses of multiple health outcomes. *BMJ*, 359, j5024. doi:10.1136/bmj.j5024

Reid, S.D. and Gentius, J. (2017). Type and context of alcohol-related injury among patients presenting to emergency departments in a Caribbean Country. *Int J Environ Res Public Health*, 14(8). doi:10.3390/ijerph14080877

Rowlands, A.V. and Stiles, V.H. (2012). Accelerometer counts and raw acceleration output in relation to mechanical loading. *J Biomech*, 45(3), pp. 448–454.

Royal Osteoporosis Society. (2018). *Strong, steady and straight: An expert consensus statement on physical activity and exercise for osteoporosis.* https://theros.org.uk/forms/documents/strong-steady-and-straight/ (14 August 2019, date last accessed).

Rubin, C.T. and Lanyon, L.E. (1984). Regulation of bone formation by applied dynamic loads. *Journal of Bone and Joint Surgery*, 66A, pp. 397–402.

Rubin, C.T. and Lanyon, L.E. (1985). Regulation of bone mass by mechanical strain magnitude. *Calcif Tissue Int*, 37(4), pp. 411–417.

Segev, D., Hellerstein, D. and Dunsky, A. (2017). Physical activity – does it really increase bone density in postmenopausal women? A review of articles published between 2001–2016. *Curr Aging Sci,* 11(1), pp. 4–9. doi:10.2174/1874609810666170918170744

Shepherd, J.A., Schousboe, J.T., Broy, S.B., Engelke, K. and Leslie, W.D. (2015). Executive summary of the 2015 ISCD position development conference on advanced measures from DXA and QCT: Fracture prediction beyond BMD. *J Clin Densitom*, 18(3), pp. 274–286. doi:10.1016/j.jocd.2015.06.013

Singh, L., Brennan, T.A., Russell, E., Kim, J.H., Chen, Q., Brad Johnson, F. and Pignolo, R.J. (2016). Aging alters bone-fat reciprocity by shifting in vivo mesenchymal precursor cell fate towards an adipogenic lineage. *Bone*, 85, pp. 29–36. doi:10.1016/j.bone.2016.01.014

Siu, W.S., Qin, L. and Leung, K.S. (2003). pQCT bone strength index may serve as a better predictor than bone mineral density for long bone breaking strength. *J Bone Miner Metab*, 21(5), pp. 316–322. doi:10.1007/s00774-003-0427-5

Stiles, V.H., Griew, P.J. and Rowlands, A.V. (2013). Use of accelerometry to classify activity beneficial to bone in premenopausal women. *Med Sci Sports Exerc*, 45(12), pp. 2353–2361.

Stiles, V.H., Metcalf, B.S., Knapp, K.M. and Rowlands, A.V. (2017) A small amount of precisely measured high-intensity habitual physical activity predicts bone health in pre- and post-menopausal women in UK Biobank. *Int Journal of Epidemiology*, 46(6), pp. 1847–1856.

Svedbom, A., Borgstom, F., Hernlund, E., Strom, O., Alekna, V., Bianchi, M.L. et al. (2017). Quality of life for up to 18 months after low-energy hip, vertebral, and distal forearm fractures-results from the ICUROS. *Osteoporos Int*, 29(3), pp. 557–566. doi:10.1007/s00198-017-4317-4

Tobias, J.H., Gould, V., Brunton, L., Deere, K., Rittweger, J. and Lipperts, M. (2014). Physical activity and bone: May the force be with you. *Frontiers in Endocrinology*, 5(20).

Torgerson, D.J. and Bell-Syer, S.E. (2001). Hormone replacement therapy and prevention of nonvertebral fractures: A meta-analysis of randomized trials. *JAMA*, 285(22), pp. 2891–2897. doi:10.1001/jama.285.22.2891

Triantafyllopoulos, I.K., Lambropoulou-Adamidou, K., Nacopoulos, C.C., Papaioannou, N.A., Ceausu, I., Depypere, H. et al. (2014). EMAS position statement: The management of postmenopausal women with vertebral osteoporotic fracture. *Maturitas*, 78(2), pp. 131–137. doi:10.1016/j.maturitas.2014.03.002

Turner, C.H. (1998). Three rules for bone adaptation to mechanical stimuli. *Bone*, 23(5), pp. 399–407.

Uebelhart, D., Demiaux-Domenech, B., Roth, M. and Chantraine, A. (1995). Bone metabolism in spinal cord injured individuals and in others who have prolonged immobilisation: A review. *Paraplegia*, 33(11), pp. 669–673. doi:10.1038/sc.1995.140

Ulhoi, M.P., Meldgaard, K., Steiniche, T., Odgaard, A. and Vesterby, A. (2017). Chronic alcohol abuse leads to low bone mass with no general loss of bone structure or bone mechanical strength. *J Forensic Sci*, 62(1), pp. 131–136. doi:10.1111/1556-4029.13256

Vainionpää, A., Korpelainen, R., Leppäluoto, J. and Jämsä, T. (2005). Effects of high-impact exercise on bone mineral density: A randomized controlled trial in premenopausal women. *Osteoporosis Int*, 16(2), pp. 191–197.

Vainionpää, A., Korpelainen, R., Sievänen, H., Vihriälä, E., Leppäluoto, J. and Jämsä, T. (2007). Effect of impact exercise and its intensity on bone geometry at weight-bearing tibia and femur. *Bone*, 40(3), pp. 604–611.

van der Jagt-Willems, H.C., Vis, M., Tulner, C.R., van Campen, J.P., Woolf, A.D., van Munster, B.C. and Lems, W.F. (2013). Mortality and incident vertebral fractures after 3 years of follow-up among geriatric patients. *Osteoporos Int*, 24(5), pp. 1713–1719. doi:10.1007/s00198-012-2147-y

van Schoor, N.M., Ewing, S.K., O'Neill, T.W., Lunt, M., Smit, J.H. and Lips, P. (2008). Impact of prevalent and incident vertebral fractures on utility: Results from a patient-based and a population-based sample. *Qual Life Res*, 17(1), pp. 159–167. doi:10.1007/s11136-007-9287-0

van Staa, T.P., Dennison, E.M., Leufkens, H.G. and Cooper, C. (2001). Epidemiology of fractures in England and Wales. *Bone*, 29(6), pp. 517–522.

Vlachopoulos, D., Barker, A.R., Ubago-Guisado, E., Ortega, F.B., Krustrup, P., Metcalf, B. et al. (2017). The effect of 12-month participation in osteogenic and non-osteogenic sports on bone development in adolescent male athletes. The PRO-BONE study. *J Sci Med Sport*, 21(4), pp. 404–409. doi:10.1016/j.jsams.2017.08.018

Wang, H., Chen, Q., Lee, S.H., Choi, Y., Johnson, F.B. and Pignolo, R.J. (2012). Impairment of osteoblast differentiation due to proliferation-independent telomere dysfunction in mouse models of accelerated aging. *Aging Cell*, 11(4), pp. 704–713. doi:10.1111/j.1474-9726.2012.00838.x

Warburton, D.E.R., Jamnik, V.K., Bredin, S.S.D. and Gledhill, N. on behalf of the PAR-Q+ Collaboration (2011). The physical activity readiness questionnaire for everyone (PAR-Q+) and electronic physical activity readiness medical examination (ePARmed-X+). *Health and Fitness Journal of Canada*, 4(2), pp. 3–23.

Wardell, S.E., McDonnell, D.P. and Nelson, E.R. (2013). Regulation of bone cell function by estrogens. In R. Marcus, D. Feldman, D.W. Dempster, M. Luckey, and J. Cauley (Eds.), *Osteoporosis*. 4th edition, pp. 329–344. Academic Press.

Waterloo, S., Sogaard, A.J., Ahmed, L.A., Damsgard, E., Morseth, B. and Emaus, N. (2013). Vertebral fractures and self-perceived health in elderly women and men in a population-based cross-sectional study: The Tromso Study 2007–08. *BMC Geriatr*, 13, p. 102. doi:10.1186/1471-2318-13-102

Watson, S., Weeks, B., Weis, L., Harding, A., Horan, S. and Beck, B. (2017). High-intensity resistance and impact training improves bone mineral density and physical function in postmenopausal women with osteopenia and osteoporosis: The LIFTMOR randomised controlled trial. *Journal of Bone and Mineral Research*, 33(2), pp. 211–220.

Watson, S., Weeks, B., Weis, L., Harding, A., Horan, S. and Beck, B. (2019). High-intensity exercise did not cause vertebral fractures and improves thoracic kyphosis in postmenopausal women with low to very low bone mass: The LIFTMOR trial. *Osteoporosis International*, 30(5), pp. 957–964.

Weaver, C.M., Gordon, C.M., Janz, K.F., Kalkwarf, H.J., Lappe, J.M., Lewis, R., O'Karma, M., Wallace, T.C. and Zemel, B.S. (2016). The national osteoporosis foundation's position statement on peak bone mass development and lifestyle factors: A systematic review and implementation recommendations. *Osteoporosis Int*, 27(4), pp. 1281–1386.

Weeks, B.K. and Beck, B.R. (2008). The BPAQ: X a bone-specific physical activity assessment instrument. *Osteoporos Int*, 19(11), pp. 1567–1577.

Williamson, S., Landeiro, F., McConnell, T., Fulford-Smith, L., Javaid, M.K., Judge, A. and Leal, J. (2017). Costs of fragility hip fractures globally: A systematic review and meta-regression analysis. *Osteoporos Int*, 28(10), pp. 2791–2800. doi:10.1007/s00198-017-4153-6

World Health Organisation. (1994). Assessment of fracture risk and its application to screening for postmenopausal osteoporosis: A report of a WHO study group. *WHO Tech Report Series*, 843, pp. 1–129.

Zhao, R., Zhao, M. and Zhang, L. (2014). Efficiency of jumping exercise in improving bone mineral density among premenopausal women: A meta-analysis. *Sports Medicine*, 44(10), pp. 1393–1402.

20

MENTAL HEALTH AND ILLNESS

Kemi Wright, Simon Rosenbaum and Bonnie Furzer

Chapter Aims

The aims of this chapter are to:

- Explain the mental-health, mental-illness continuum
- Illustrate the basic mechanisms by which exercise can help improve mental health
- Understand the collective prevalence and burden of both common and severe mental disorders
- Describe the key characteristics associated with various categories of mental disorders
- Outline common medical management of mental disorders
- Review the evidence for exercise as both a treatment for and preventative strategy against mental disorders
- Apply basic principles of exercise screening and assessment
- Identify contraindications and/or considerations for exercise for people living with mental illness

Introduction – Including Prevalence

In the early 1990s, Britain's Health of the Nation initiative outlined a number of aims including 'adding years to life', commonly referred to as reducing premature mortality and/or improving life expectancy (Department of Health, 1999). Additionally, an equally important aim adding 'life to years' was noted or said differently: to improve the quality of life throughout the years lived (HM Government, 2011). This focus on quality, not just quantity, of life was and continues to be mirrored internationally and across varied medical, allied health and societal contexts.

With an estimated 30% of the population experiencing a common mental disorder (depression or anxiety) in their lifetime (Steel et al., 2014), mental and substance use disorders are a global health priority and collectively responsible for the leading cause of years lived with disability worldwide (Whiteford et al., 2013). In addition to the personal and social costs of

DOI: 10.4324/9781315102399-20

mental illness, the direct treatment costs are estimated upwards of £22 billion per year in the UK alone (McCrone et al., 2008). This figure is likely to be significantly higher if also considering indirect costs and the costs associated with disability and loss of productivity (Centre for Mental Health, 2010).

There is a bi-directional relationship between poor physical and mental health, with people who experience poor physical health more likely to develop co-morbid mental health conditions (Stubbs et al., 2016b; Luppino et al., 2010). Furthermore, individuals who experience mental illness exhibit significantly poorer physical health than the general population, with an estimated 10 to 15 year reduction in life expectancy due to multiple factors such as cardiovascular and metabolic diseases (De Hert et al., 2009; Olfson et al., 2015; Vancampfort et al., 2016a; Walker et al., 2015).

The benefits of physical activity on quantity and quality of life for both physical and mental health concerns are well acknowledged and the 'exercise as medicine' concept has progressed rapidly, most notably in the domains of physical medicine (Lobelo et al., 2014). With the emergence of mental and substance use disorders as a global health priority, research into novel strategies such as physical activity and structured exercise programmes for the prevention and treatment of mental illness is urgently required.

Mental-Health, Mental-Illness Continuum

The World Health Organization (WHO, 2018) defined mental health as 'a state of well-being in which the individual realises his or her own abilities, can cope with the normal stresses of life, can work productively and is able to make a contribution to his or her community'. The three core components of this definition are 1) well-being, 2) effective functioning of an individual and 3) effective functioning of a community (WHO, 2018). As a result, mental health is more than just the absence of mental illness (e.g. depression and anxiety) but encompasses a positive phenomenon related to emotional, psychological and social well-being, or the presence of mental health (Westerhof and Keyes, 2010). Therefore, an individual can experience 'languishing' mental health without the presence or diagnosis of mental illness. Regardless, anything less than complete mental health results in worse outcomes in terms of physical disease, health-care utilisation, work productivity and psychosocial functioning (Keyes, 2002).

Mental Disorders

Mental disorders encompass a wide variety of signs, symptoms, experiences and disorders which are diagnosed by a medical professional and significantly interfere with an individual's cognitive, emotional or social abilities (American Psychiatric Association, 2013). Much like cardiovascular disease being a group of diseases that affect the heart, mental disorders are a group of disorders that affect the mind. Individuals can experience symptoms of poor mental health (e.g. low mood, sadness) for a short period of time; however, in order to be considered a mental disorder, it needs to be long lasting and impair the individual's psychosocial functioning. Depressive or mood (affective) disorders and anxiety disorders are often referred to as common mental disorders, with a worldwide prevalence at 4.4% and 3.6%, respectively (WHO, 2017). Both broad disorders are more prevalent in women than men and have seen an 18.4% and 14.9% increase, respectively, between 2005 and 2015 (GBD Disease And Injury Incidence And Prevalence Collaborators, 2016).

Mental disorders are typically classified according to the *Diagnostic and Statistical Manual of Mental Disorders* (see Table 20.1) (American Psychiatric Association, 2013), *International Classification of Disease* (ICD) (WHO, 1992) or other structured diagnostic classification. Whilst each mental disorder may be viewed in isolation with distinct characteristics, co-morbidity with other mental health disorders (and physical disorders) is common (Amerio et al., 2015; Fornaro et al., 2016).

TABLE 20.1 Summary of Mental Disorders

Diagnostic Classifications	*Examples*	*Key Features and Prevalence*
Neurodevelopmental Disorders	Attention-deficit/hyperactivity disorder Autism spectrum disorder Intellectual disabilities Motor disorders	Onset in developmental period, with resultant impairments of personal, social, academic or occupational functioning
Schizophrenia Spectrum and Other Psychotic Disorders	Schizophrenia Schizoaffective disorder	Defined by abnormalities in one or more of the following five domains: delusions, hallucinations, disorganised thinking, grossly disorganised or abnormal motor behaviour and negative symptoms (e.g. diminished emotional expression, decreased participation in work or social activities)
Bipolar and related disorders	Bipolar I disorder Bipolar II disorder Cyclothymic disorder	Category forming a bridge between two diagnostic classes: schizophrenia spectrum and other psychotic disorders and depressive disorders, based on symptomatology (e.g. mood fluctuations), family history and genetics
Depressive Disorders	Major depressive disorder Persistent depressive disorder (dysthymia)	Presences of sad, empty or irritable mood, accompanied by somatic and cognitive changes that significantly affect the individual's capacity to function.
Anxiety Disorders	Separation anxiety disorder Specific phobia Panic disorder	Excessive fear (emotional response to real or perceived imminent threat) and anxiety (anticipation of future threat) and related behavioural disturbances
Obsessive-Compulsive and Related Disorders	Obsessive-compulsive disorder (OCD) Body dysmorphic disorder Hoarding disorder Trichotillomania (hair-pulling disorder)	Presences of obsessions and/or compulsions and/or preoccupations and repetitive behaviours. Related disorders are characterised primarily by recurrent body-focused repetitive behaviours (e.g. hair pulling, skin picking) and repeated attempts to decrease or stop the behaviours
Trauma- and Stressor-Related Disorders	Reactive attachment disorder Post-traumatic stress disorder (PTSD) Acute stress disorder Adjustment disorders	Exposure to a traumatic or stressful event is listed explicitly as a diagnostic criterion, with a close relationship between these diagnoses and anxiety disorders, obsessive-compulsive and related disorders and dissociative disorders

(*Continued*)

TABLE 20.1 (Continued)

Diagnostic Classifications	*Examples*	*Key Features and Prevalence*
Feeding and Eating Disorders	Anorexia nervosa Bulimia nervosa Binge-eating disorder	Persistent disturbance of eating or eating-related behaviour, resulting in the altered consumption or absorption of food, significantly impairing health
Disruptive, Impulse-Control and Conduct Disorders	Oppositional defiant disorder Intermittent explosive disorder Conduct disorder Antisocial personality disorder	Problems in the self-control of emotions and behaviours, unique in that these problems are manifested in behaviours that violate the rights of others (e.g. aggression, destruction of property) and/or bring the individual into significant conflict with societal norms or authority figures
Substance-Related and Addictive Disorders	Substance-related disorders: Substance use disorder Substance-induced disorders (separated based on substance): Gambling disorder	The substance-related disorders encompass ten separate classes of drugs, all of which, when taken in excess, result in direct activation of the brain reward system, resulting in the reinforcement of behaviours; also includes gambling disorder, based on similar activation of reward systems and similar behavioural symptoms
Additional classifications listed in *DSM-5* but not summarised here:		
Dissociative Disorders		Neurocognitive Disorders (NCD)
Sleep-Wake Disorders		Personality Disorders
Somatic Symptom and Related Disorders		Paraphilic Disorders
Elimination Disorders		Other Mental Disorders
Sexual Dysfunctions		Medication-Induced Movement Disorders and Other Adverse Effects of Medication
Gender Dysphoria		

Source: *Diagnostic and Statistical Manual of Mental Disorders: DSM-5*. (2013). (Fifth edition). Arlington, VA: American Psychiatric Publishing

Common Medical Management for Mental Disorders

Various treatment types and supports are available to aid individuals with mental disorders to improve function and aid in their recovery. Whilst there is no one-size-fits-all approach in the treatment of mental disorders, a combination of medication and psychological therapy (i.e. talking-based therapy) form the basis of treatment. Despite effective treatments being available, evidence suggests that only 1 in 5 people in high-income and 1 in 27 in low-/lower-middle-income countries received minimally adequate treatment (Thornicroft et al., 2017).

Medical Interventions

- *Antipsychotics*: Used primarily to treat psychotic disorders, these are the primary drugs used to control positive symptoms (e.g. delusions, hallucinations). Common adverse metabolic effects include weight gain, hyperglycaemia, hypertension and hyperlipidaemia, with a two- to three-fold increased likelihood of developing cardiovascular disease in those with schizophrenia (Olfson et al., 2015). This is a significant concern with cardiovascular disease the single biggest cause of early preventable death in those experiencing psychosis and is responsible for an estimated 15- to 20-year shortened lifespan (Walker et al., 2015). Early detection and monitoring for cardiometabolic risks (see screening and assessment later in this chapter), lifestyle and medical interventions and tailoring of antipsychotic medications can help improve long-term outcomes.

- *Antidepressants*: A variety of drugs including selective serotonin re-uptake inhibitors (SSRIs), serotonin and noradrenaline reuptake inhibitors (SNRIs) and monoamine oxidase inhibitors (MAOIs) are prescribed to treat depression. Whilst they all have different mechanisms of action, the underlying premise is that they act on chemicals in the brain related to emotion and motivation. There is strong evidence, particularly in depression of moderate to severe intensity, that antidepressants are an effective treatment. In mild depression, antidepressants have demonstrated no greater benefit than placebo, with psychological and/or adjuvant therapies recommended (Moncrieff et al., 2004). Additionally, antidepressants can be used to treat anxiety and have shown effectiveness in most types of anxiety disorders, PTSD and OCD (Kendall et al., 2011). There are a variety of generally mild, common side effects depending on the type of antidepressant prescribed, including nausea, headaches and drowsiness. However, some antidepressants have been associated with increased suicidal thoughts, notably in those under the age of 25, and everyone prescribed antidepressants should be carefully monitored.
- *Antianxiety drugs*: Pharmacological therapies for anxiety disorders, such as benzodiazepines and antipsychotics, are associated with tolerance, dependence and adverse side effects (see antipsychotics) and are not advocated for routine use unless there are specific clinical reasons for short-term benefit.
- *Electroconvulsive therapy (ECT)*: ECT is a medical treatment whereby across a course of treatment, electrical currents are passed through the brain while the individual is under a general anaesthetic with the aim of inducing a seizure and stimulating regions of the brain. In severely depressed adults, ECT has been shown to effectively reduce symptoms immediately pos -treatment, with limited high-quality studies exploring its effectiveness in other mental disorders (The U. K. Ect Review Group, 2003).

Psychological Interventions

- *Cognitive Behavioural Therapy (CBT)*: In CBT, individuals work alongside a therapist to explore their cognitive (thinking) and behavioural (actions) patterns, which may be contributing to their mental disorder or preventing/impacting recovery. Recognition of these patterns of thinking and action allows a person to work on adjusting potentially detrimental patterns. Extensive evidence has explored the efficacy of CBT across a variety of mental disorders including a range of anxiety disorders, depressive disorders, PTSD, and OCD, and across a range of different populations (Butler et al., 2006).

Table 20.2 illustrates the effects of commonly prescribed medications for mental ill health on the exercise response.

TABLE 20.2 Medication Considerations for Exercise for People with Mental Illness and Disease

Class Name	*Generic Name*	*Brand Name*	*Indication*	*Side Effects*	*Exercise Considerations*
Antipsychotic, 1st generation (typical)	haloperidol chlorpromazine	Haldol Thorazine	Used in treatment of psychotic disorders (e.g. schizophrenia)	Metabolic effects include weight gain, hyperglycaemia, hypertension, and hyperlipidaemia; increased prolactin levels; nausea, drowsiness, dizziness, dry mouth; extra pyramidal symptoms such as tremor, restlessness, rigidity	Conduct appropriate cardiometabolic screening to ensure participant is safe to exercise; modify exercise prescription (frequency, intensity, time) based on side effects experienced
Antipsychotics, 2nd generation (atypical)	aripiprazole clozapine risperidone quetiapine olanzapine paliperidone	Abilify Clozaril Risperdal Seroquel Zyprexa Invega	Used in treatment of psychotic disorders (e.g. schizophrenia)	Metabolic effects include weight gain, hyperglycaemia, hypertension, and hyperlipidaemia; nausea, drowsiness, constipation, tachycardia, excess salivation/ drooling (night); extra pyramidal symptoms such as tremor, restlessness, rigidity	Conduct appropriate cardiometabolic screening to ensure participant is safe to exercise; modify exercise prescription (frequency, intensity, time) based on side effects experienced
Antidepressants (SSRI)	fluoxetine citalopram sertraline escitalopram fluvoxamine	Prozac Celexa/ Lexapro Zoloft Lexapro Luvox	Used in treatment of mood disorders (e.g. depression), some anxiety disorders and PTSD	Headache, GI distress, insomnia, fatigue, anxiety, sexual dysfunction, weight gain	Conduct appropriate cardiometabolic screening to ensure participant is safe to exercise; modify exercise prescription (frequency, intensity, time) based on side effects experienced
Antidepressants (SNRI)	venlafaxine duloxetine desvenlafaxine atomoxetine	Effexor Cymbalta Pristiq Strattera	Used in treatment of mood disorders (e.g. depression) some anxiety disorders and ADHD	Nausea, insomnia, dry mouth, headache, increased blood pressure sexual dysfunction, weight gain	Conduct appropriate cardiometabolic screening to ensure participant is safe to exercise; modify exercise prescription (frequency, intensity, time) based on side effects experienced
Benzodiazepines	diazepam lorazepam alprazolam clonazepam	Valium Ativan Xanax Klonopin	Used in treatment of anxiety disorders (e.g. generalised anxiety disorder)	Nausea, drowsiness, dizziness, confusion, constipation, memory problems, slurred speech, muscle weakness	Conduct appropriate cardiometabolic screening to ensure participant is safe to exercise; modify exercise prescription (frequency, intensity, time) based on side effects experienced

Flourishing Mental Health and Exercise

'Flourishing' or complete mental health is to be filled with positive emotion and to be functioning well psychologically, emotionally and socially and is the opposite of those 'languishing' in life with low well-being (Keyes, 2002). Numerous population studies incorporating young people, adults, varied genders, clinical and non-clinical populations, conducted in Western countries including Britain and North America, have shown clear associations between physical activity and psychological well-being (Biddle, 2006). A growing body of experimental research demonstrating the effects of exercise on affect and mood supports this; however, it should be noted that exercise responses may vary based on individuals and exercise variables (e.g. exercise type and intensity). Other factors that warrant consideration for exercise to promote 'flourishing' mental health include enjoyment (Ekkekakis, 2003) and motivation (Kwan et al., 2018), along with exercise context and experience (Boutcher et al., 1997). However, participation in and motivation for physical activity is likely a reciprocal relationship in which 'enhancing mental health through increasing physical activity may have the added benefit of enhancing people's motivation to maintain regular physical activity'(Rebar et al., 2015).

In addition to psychological mechanisms, it is widely accepted that exercise enhances well-being due to the interaction between the psychological and the biological, with a growing body of research linking exercise to improvements in brain function and cognition (Mandolesi et al., 2018). Research has progressed from animal studies looking at the impacts of exercise-enriched environments on growth and structure of the nervous system through to advances in neuroimaging that have enabled researchers to explore exercise-induced changes in human brain structure and function (Firth et al., 2018c). A large body of research in this domain is related to older adults and findings that lifestyle factors, such as physical activity, intellectual engagement, social interaction and diet are associated with the maintenance of cognitive function and reduction in risk of neurodegenerative disorders (Mandolesi et al., 2018). Whilst there is a greater volume of research in older adults, data suggests that physical activity can have significant beneficial effects throughout the lifespan (Hillman et al., 2008, Suetani et al., 2018, Suetani et al., 2017). There is a consensus that any level of physical activity is likely to be beneficial; however, it is worth noting that a number of unanswered questions remain, including exercise prescription specifics (e.g. frequency, intensity, time, type) and the interaction and implications of other important lifestyle factors, such as diet and social interaction.

Mechanisms by which exercise promotes flourishing mental health and/or changes in brain structure and function are multifactorial and likely due to the contribution of several mechanisms across psychological (e.g. mood, self-efficacy) (Biddle, 2006), social (McAuley et al., 2000) and neurophysiological domains (e.g. dopamine, serotonin) (Mandolesi et al., 2018). A number of neurophysiological hypotheses have been posited, and there is a likely contribution from some or interactions between all these mechanisms, including:

- Dopaminergic responses (Stubbs and Rosenbaum, 2018): Research has demonstrated that chronic exercise induces changes in dopaminergic functioning, which has been linked to behavioural characteristics (e.g. reward and motivation) (Beeler et al., 2016). However, acute effects remain unclear.
- Serotonin responses (Chaouloff, 1997): Refers to changes in serotonin in several brain regions following acute and chronic exercise; however, responses vary depending on exercise intensity and duration.

- Endocannabinoid responses (Raichlen et al., 2012): Exercise has been shown to activate the endocannabinoid responses, with activation of this system linked to positive mood effects such as anxiolysis and a sense of well-being, along with a role in neurogenesis. As with other neurophysiological responses, this appears to vary with exercise variables, including duration and intensity (Raichlen et al., 2012).
- Neuroplasticity and brain-derived neurotrophic factor (BDNF) (Szuhany et al., 2015): Acute and chronic exercise has been shown to induce changes in BDNF levels and BDNF-induced neurogenesis with links to cognitive benefits, stress resiliency and neuroprotective effects.

Whilst the mechanisms related to exercise, physical activity and mental health are multifactorial and are still being explored, there is consistency in the research and consensus within the medical community that exercise is a key aspect for flourishing mental health, and throughout the lifespan, individuals should be encouraged to meet the minimum recommended participation guidelines (Kim et al., 2012). Further exploration of the neurophysiological mechanisms and impact of exercise variables (e.g. type, intensity, duration) may offer further insight to guide participation guidelines and clinical decision making.

Exercise for Prevention of Mental Disorders

The growing costs and burden of disease associated with mental disorders, along with limitations in availability and cost effectiveness of optimal treatment, has turned a spotlight on the primary prevention of common mental illnesses. Whilst a number of known risk factors for depression and anxiety are non-modifiable (e.g. life events, familial risk), lifestyle factors such as physical activity participation and diet have emerged as potential strategies for prevention (Schuch et al., 2018).

Across a number of large-scale population studies and meta-analyses, protective effects for emergent or future depression have been shown with low volumes of exercise, regardless of intensity (Harvey et al., 2018), age or geographical region (Schuch et al., 2018). Even after adjustment for cofounders, Harvey and colleagues found 12% of all cases of depression could have been prevented with at least one hour of physical activity each week (Harvey et al., 2018). Conversely, and not surprisingly given the symptoms associated with depression (i.e. lack of motivation), depressive symptoms can predict whether someone will drop out of an exercise programme (Swardfager et al., 2016), and baseline depression can predict decreased future physical activity (Gunnell et al., 2016). This is an important consideration for exercise practitioners looking to engage and maintain exercise participation.

In addition to the widespread understanding and acceptance of the antidepressant effects of exercise, there is a growing body of evidence supporting the protective effects of physical activity against symptoms of anxiety and/or anxiety disorders (Aylett et al., 2018; Stubbs et al., 2017b). McDowell and colleagues (2018) demonstrated that meeting the World Health Organization's physical activity guidelines is associated with lower odds of incident generalised anxiety disorder among older adults, along with a number of meta-analytic reviews that support the effect of exercise of varied durations, intensities and time on both state and trait anxiety symptoms (McDowell et al., 2018).

Given that mental disorders are associated with increased co-morbidity, health-care costs and premature mortality, the role of exercise as an effective preventive and protective modality is crucial, and population-based strategies to encourage and maintain participation to meet the minimum recommended levels are vital.

Exercise and Mental Disorders

Despite the preventative and protective effects of exercise, and in addition to the well-known benefits for health and well-being in the general population, people with mental illness are significantly less likely to meet physical activity guidelines (Vancampfort et al., 2017). High levels of physical inactivity behaviour are often coupled with additional negative health behaviours (e.g. poor nutritional intake, high smoking rates), all of which contribute to the significantly higher morbidity and premature mortality seen in those with mental health disorders when compared to the general population (Vancampfort et al., 2017; Stubbs et al., 2016a, 2017a). Increased physical activity and/or tailored exercise interventions can not only improve cardiometabolic health in order to help address the deficits in quality and quantity of life, but have also been shown to have positive effects on symptoms across a variety of mental health disorders (Rosenbaum et al., 2014). Whilst there is variation in specific outcomes, exercise interventions demonstrate consistently positive effects across a variety of mental health disorders, with specific improvements evident in cognitive function, mood, depression and anxiety (Schuch et al., 2016b; Rosenbaum et al., 2014; Firth et al., 2017; Melo et al., 2016; Stubbs et al., 2018).

Aerobic Training

Aylett and colleagues (2018) completed a meta-analysis (15 studies with 675 patients) incorporating 9 studies of individuals with diagnosed anxiety disorders and an additional 6 studies of individuals with elevated levels of anxiety (Aylett et al., 2018). There was high variability in aerobic exercise variables, with programmes ranging from four weeks to six months in duration; two to five sessions per week; high to low intensity; and various exercise types, including walking, running, treadmill training and/or supervised aerobic training sessions. Despite the variability in exercise variables and the relatively small number of studies, results demonstrated that aerobic exercise was effective in treating elevated anxiety when compared to non-exercise controls. Whilst there was no significant difference in positive effects seen between those with a diagnosed anxiety disorder and those experiencing elevated symptoms, a dose-response relationship was evident for exercise intensity, with greater efficacy for higher-intensity exercise. Varied responses based on exercise variables are not uncommon in the literature and highlight the need for further research and consideration of key exercise variables (e.g. volume, duration, intensity and type) in order to tailor exercise prescription for individuals with mental health disorders.

When examining other types of mental health disorders and populations including young people, adults and those with complex mood disorders, similar beneficial effects of aerobic exercise have been demonstrated (Bailey et al., 2018; Rebar et al., 2015; Schuch et al., 2016a). A 2016 meta-analysis of exercise for depression pooled data from 25 separate studies and found a clinically significant reduction of depressive symptoms on average of 4.5 and 6.5

points on the Beck depression inventory and Hamilton depression scale, respectively. Over 1,000 additional negative studies would be needed to nullify the significance of the findings (fail safe N = 1,057), with larger effects found for moderate-intensity aerobic exercise, and interventions supervised by exercise professionals (Schuch et al., 2016b).The largest trial to date of exercise and depression compared the effects of exercise versus internet-based cognitive behavioural therapy (iCBT) versus treatment as usual (TAU). The trial recruited 946 patients with mild to moderate depression through primary health-care centres in Sweden and found that both exercise and iCBT were more effective than TAU over a three-month period (Hallgren et al., 2015).

Similar findings were replicated by Keating and colleagues, who explored the impact of a group running programme on adults (n = 19) and young people (16–25 years; n = 29) with bipolar disorder, major depressive disorder or anxiety disorder, in addition to co-morbid diagnoses and cognitive and social impairment (Keating et al., 2018). Whilst some variation in results were shown based on clinical factors (e.g. age at onset and duration of illness), a significant decrease in depression, anxiety and stress scores was seen following the 12-week group running program. Additionally, higher attendance and perceived levels of friendship within the group were associated with positive mental health outcomes. Along with providing further evidence for aerobic exercise – in this case, specifically running – this study also emphasises the importance of exercise environment. In this case, aerobic exercise in combination with a supportive group setting improved mood symptoms in young people and adults with complex mood disorders (Keating et al., 2018).

The impact of the exercise environment may have a relationship to the social elements of mental health and well-being; however, given the links between aerobic exercise and neurophysiological effects (e.g. BDNF release; see earlier in this chapter), it is not surprising that aerobic training has also been consistently linked to changes in brain structure and cognitive function in a variety of populations (Hillman et al., 2008; Smith et al., 2010). Importantly, improvements in cognitive function have also been demonstrated in those experiencing mental health disorders such as schizophrenia and depression (Nuechterlein et al., 2016; Su et al., 2016; Khatri et al., 2001; Greer et al., 2017). A meta-analysis combining ten studies and 385 participants demonstrated improvements in cognitive outcomes in people with schizophrenia, and notably greater improvements were seen from interventions using higher dosages of aerobic exercise and supervised by an exercise professional (Firth et al., 2017).

In addition to the overall benefits of aerobic exercise on physical and mental health outcomes, attention has also been directed to the potential use of exercise to augment or supplement other treatment modalities. On that basis, single bouts of aerobic exercise have demonstrated acute anxiolytic effects in people with specific phobias or panic disorder (Ströhle et al., 2009; Lindenberger et al., 2017). Bischoff and colleagues (2018) investigated the effect of aerobic exercise to augment an exposure-based CBT. Seventy-seven patients with panic disorder and agoraphobia completed low- or moderate-intensity treadmill exercise alongside exposure- based CBT, with results pointing to a potential accelerating effect of moderate-intensity aerobic exercise within the standard psychotherapeutic approach (Bischoff et al., 2018). A similar supplementary effect of aerobic exercise was demonstrated in a small pilot study incorporating nine participants undergoing prolonged exposure therapy for PTSD who completed 30 minutes of treadmill walking prior to therapy sessions (Powers et al., 2015).

Resistance Training

Whilst the majority of exercise-based research has focused on aerobic types of training, there is increasing interest in and evidence around the relationship between resistance training, mental health and mental illness. Gordon and colleagues completed two meta-analyses exploring symptoms of depression (combining 33 randomised control trials and 1,877 participants) and symptoms of anxiety (combining 16 studies and 922 participants), finding resistance training improved symptoms of depression and anxiety, respectively, regardless of age, sex or exercise intervention specifics (Gordon et al., 2017, 2018).

When investigating symptoms of anxiety, greater effects were seen in healthy participants than in those with a mental or physical illness, but regardless, resistance training significantly reduced anxiety symptoms in both groups (Gordon et al., 2017). Notably, the impact on depressive symptoms was independent of improvements in participants' strength, reiterating findings from other studies that whilst responses may vary, any level of exercise can be helpful for those experiencing mental illness (Gordon et al., 2018). This is also interesting, given that research has demonstrated weak handgrip strength, when used as a measure of global strength, is associated with an increased prevalence of depression (Ashdown-Franks et al., 2019), and handgrip strength is significantly associated with cognitive functioning in the general population and individuals with schizophrenia and depressive and bipolar disorders (Firth et al., 2018a, 2018b). Consequently, resistance training appears to have both protective and preventive mental health impacts, in addition to a role in the treatment of mental illness, further highlighting the multi-faceted mechanisms underpinning exercise-induced changes.

Mixed Modalities

Whilst large portions of the available research have focused on either resistance or aerobic training modalities in isolation, it is not uncommon in practice to see a mixed-modality approach as supported by physical activity recommendations, which call for both 'aerobic activity' and 'muscle-strengthening activities' (WHO, 2011). In a cohort of 40 inpatients with anxiety, bipolar or depressive disorder, Stanton and colleagues (2015) explored the acute effects of 20 minutes of aerobic exercise and 30 minutes of body weight or resistance band activities, with all exercise performed at preferred and self-selected intensities (Stanton et al., 2016). In agreement with previous studies that have demonstrated a positive acute effect of exercise on mood (Bartholomew et al., 2005, Hays et al., 2008, Stark et al., 2012), significant acute improvements for bipolar and depressive disorder were seen following exercise.

Additionally, Martin and colleagues completed a meta-analysis including seven eligible studies with 389 individuals with schizophrenia (Martin et al., 2017). Whilst programme variables were poorly reported, and there were limited studies (which also demonstrated a high risk of bias), combined exercise was found to improve strength, symptoms of schizophrenia and overall mental health. Additionally, clinically meaningful improvements in cardiovascular fitness were seen, despite not reaching statistical significance.

Whilst consistently positive responses have been demonstrated for exercise and mental illness, responses are dependent on exercise prescription variables including type, duration and intensity, as well as diagnostic or clinical characteristics. Despite the growing evidence demonstrating the efficacy of exercise interventions for individuals with mental health disorders, this is still a vulnerable and complex cohort, and sufficiently trained exercise professionals with links to interdisciplinary mental health treatment teams should be engaged to decrease dropout, optimise outcomes and ensure the safety of individuals (Vancampfort et al., 2016b; Stubbs et al., 2016c).

For exercise professionals working with mental health disorders, key fundamentals include:

- Comprehensive knowledge of mental health disorders and treatment pathways, including pharmacology and interdisciplinary management (Stanton et al., 2018)
- Awareness of unique barriers and facilitators to physical activity participation and strategies to maximise engagement (Lederman et al., 2017)
- Understanding and current knowledge of evidence-based practice around exercise, mental health and mental illness (Lederman et al., 2016)
- Ability to perform pre-screening and assessment practices and appropriate knowledge and skills to address special considerations, contraindications and signs of crisis (see the next section)

Screening and Assessment

Whilst exercise is considered a safe and beneficial adjunct treatment in the majority of mental health disorders, it is important for all exercise practitioners working in community/outpatient or inpatient mental health to conduct a pre-exercise screening, in addition to regular monitoring and assessment in order to:

1. Ensure safety of the participant to exercise
2. Monitor for emerging signs of crisis
3. Provide appropriate exercise prescription and delivery

In accordance with best-practice guidelines for all exercise practitioners, pre-exercise screening and assessment should take place for all participants prior to undertaking exercise. In addition to the standard protocols around medical screening (e.g. signs of cardiovascular risk via physical activity readiness questionnaire [PAR-Q]), a number of mental health–specific screening and assessment considerations are recommended by various mental health agencies and collaborative groups due to the increased risk and/or potential co-morbidities (Shiers et al., 2014).

Antipsychotics/Psychotropic Medication

In order to support and ensure positive cardiometabolic for people taking antipsychotics or psychotropic medication, an early-intervention framework (Lester UK Adaptation, HETI Positive Cardiometabolic Health Algorithm) has been developed and advocated worldwide (Shiers et al., 2014; Curtis et al., 2012).Given the high rate of co-morbidities and significant reduction in lifespan due to cardiovascular disease, a number of items have been identified for screening and ongoing health monitoring, including:

- Smoking habits

- Lifestyle and life skills – diet and physical activity. Assessment options employed in various mental health settings include, but are not limited to:
  - The Simple Physical Activity Questionnaire (SIMPAQ), a five-item clinical tool designed to assess physical activity among populations at high risk of sedentary behaviour (www.simpaq.org/about-us/)
  - Physical Activity as a Vital Sign (PAVS), a quick, single-item method of determining if a patient is compliant with international physical activity guidelines of 150 minutes of moderate-vigorous physical activity per week (www.exerciseismedicine.org/support_page.php/resources/)
- Body composition – weight (gain of > 5 kg over a three-month period), BMI (≥ 25 kg/m^3 or ≥ 23 if South Asian or Chinese) and waist circumference (Male ≥ 94 cm; female ≥ 80 cm or waist ↑ > 5 cm)
- Blood pressure – > 140 mmHg systolic and/or > 90 mmHg diastolic)
- Blood glucose regulation – HbA_{1c} ≥ 42 mmol/mol (≥ 6%) and/or fasting blood glucose ≥ 5.5 mmol/L or random blood glucose ≥ 11.1 mmol/L
- Blood lipids – total cholesterol–to–high-density lipoprotein ratio to detect high (> 10%) risk of CVD based on QRISK-2 Tool (http://qrisk.org)

Caution When Delivering Exercise

Exercise should not be commenced or ceased immediately if:

- A participant is under the influence of any substances
- A participant is not in compliance with prescribed medication
- During self-imposed detoxification in the absence of medical management
- A participant demonstrates signs of mania
- A participant shows signs of nutritional or cardiovascular decompensation (see section on eating and feeding disorders)
- Any physical or mental distress emerges or is exacerbated during exercise (e.g. cardiac distress, acute psychotic distress, mental health crisis)

Mental Health Crisis

Any exercise practitioner working in a setting likely to come across individuals experiencing mental distress or mental disorders should be familiar with the signs and an appropriately robust action plan in the event of an emerging mental health crisis. A mental health crisis may be considered as a situation in which an individual is experiencing significant distress, and/or is at risk of injuring themselves or others (Kitchener et al., 2017). Examples may include suicidal ideation, non-suicidal self-injury, panic attack, manic episode and/or psychotic episode.

In the event of a mental health crisis, the aim is to reduce the level of distress and ensure the safety of the individual and others. In order to achieve this, mental health first aid training (https://mhfaengland.org/), Applied Suicide Intervention Skills Training (ASIST) or similar can provide exercise professionals with the skill set to help manage crisis situations and liaise with appropriate follow-on services (www.nhs.uk/NHSEngland/AboutNHSservices/mental-health-services-explained/Pages/mental-health-emergencies.aspx). Additionally, clear processes and referral pathways should be developed and articulated in the given exercise setting due to the variations in community, national and international settings.

Case Study – Schizophrenia

Steven is as a 41-year-old male, living alone, with a history of schizophrenia diagnosed 13 years prior. Steven reports a history of depression, anxiety and gastro-esophageal reflux disease (GORD). Steven reports a recent exacerbation in psychological symptoms and was subsequently prescribed an increased dose of sertraline hydrochloride (Zoloft, antidepressant SSRI) from 50 mg daily to 100 mg three times daily. Other medications include clozapine 50 mg (antipsychotic) and pantoprazole 40 mg (Somac).

Referral Information: Steven has a body weight of 129 kg, waist circumference of 117 cm, and a body mass index (BMI) of 38.0 kg/m^2, classified as class II obesity. Steven reported being unsuccessful in losing weight, despite exercising regularly (3–5 times per week for the past six months) at a local gymnasium. Steven reported minor pain in his left knee when exercising (3/10 on a visual analogue scale), with no other conditions or limitations noted. Steven is referred to you (three sessions) and a dietitian (two sessions) working in the same practice under a general practitioner–initiated chronic disease management plan.

Key Questions to Consider (Before Reading the Additional Information Provided)

- What factors must be considered when developing Steven's exercise programme?
- Describe the assessments that you would use with Steven to guide the exercise programming.
- What contact, if any, will the exercise practitioner have with the dietitian?
- How does Steven's medication impact your management?
- What strategies would you use to motivate Steven and help manage his programme?

Results and Client Progression

As a starting point, you contact the GP to determine clearance for exercise and any screening completed in line with recommendations for positive cardiometabolic health (e.g. Lester UK Adaptation). Given that Steven is taking an antipsychotic and based on risks already identified, you determine it is crucial to screen and assess for risk of CVD and guide future monitoring. The GP advises that screening has taken place, with additional information provided:

- Smoking habits – previous smoker, but not currently
- Blood pressure – no indication of elevated risk
- Blood glucose regulation – no indication of elevated risk
- Blood lipids – no indication of elevated risk

The GP has highlighted body composition as the key physical health risk factor to be addressed by the EP and dietician, in addition to management of psychological symptoms.

Additionally, you contact the dietician to ensure a person-centred, team-management approach is taken to optimise Steven's outcomes. You determine an appointment schedule across seven weeks in order to maximise contact between Steven and the relevant health professional at the appropriate times. Furthermore, in the assessments completed by the EP and dietician, you determine key outcome measures and additional lifestyle-related risk information relevant to Steven's treatment, including:

- Poor diet with limited knowledge of what/how to improve it = prioritise dietician consult in the early phases on management, with communication between dietician and EP to ensure principles and diet management are reinforced by all health professionals.
- Low physical activity despite previously stating three to five times per week = when further discussing with Steven his physical activity, it became clear that for the last one or two months, it was closer to less than twice per week at the gym, and Steven often spent a lot of his time at the gym not exercising ('wandering around') as he was unsure what to do and did not want to ask staff for fear of embarrassment.

Key Questions to Consider

- What are some concerns for Steven's long-term adherence to an exercise programme, and what strategies could be used to maximise this?
- How may Steven's social isolation impact the prescribed program?
- What other outcomes could be used to evaluate the effectiveness of the intervention?

Implementation and Results

Following implementation of a coordinated exercise and diet programme alongside medical management, Steven has seen improvements in key outcome measures (waist circumference, weight, body mass index).

The coordinated approach has been effective for maximising Steven's engagement and support over a seven-week programme, and strategies have been implemented to assist Steven in self-management moving forward, including:

Education:

- Both you and the dietician tailored education strategies with Steven to improve his knowledge of diet and exercise and his confidence to apply the principles in order to lose weight.

TABLE 20.3 Summary of Consultation and Measurements Obtained

Weeks Since Commencement	*Consult**	*Waist Circumference (cm)*	*Weight (kg)*	*Body Mass Index (m²/kg)*
0	GP	N/A	129	37.69
0	EP	117	129	37.69
0	Diet	117	129	37.69
1	Diet	N/A	126	36.82
4	EP	114.5	124	36.23
7	EP	112	120	35.06
Change (%)		5 cm (4%)	9 kg (7%)	2.63 m²/kg

* GP = general practitioner; EP = exercise physiologist; Diet = dietician

Person-centred approach:

- Focusing on the specific barriers to Steven's participation in exercise (i.e. fear of embarrassment at the gym, minor knee pain) has facilitated an increased confidence, effort and attendance at gym sessions (two to three times per week over the seven-week period).
- Looking at long-term strategies, given the likelihood that Steven will be under medical and pharmacological management of schizophrenia throughout his lifetime, a key outcome for you was finding what is enjoyable and efficacious for Steven.
- You established that Steven loved football and would be interested in joining a local club. From the perspective of adherence and optimal outcomes for Steven, this would be ideal, as it would address not only the physical aspects of health management but also socialisation. You developed a program for Simon in the gym around this goal (e.g. improving aerobic fitness, strength and skills) to keep him engaged and moving toward his goal of joining a local team. Before the end of the 7-week period, you contacted some local teams to find a suitable club to transition Steven into. You have told Steven you will be following him up in week ten to see how he is going, and he has a review with the GP scheduled at 12-week mark.

Exercise and Mental Disorders – Special Considerations

Feeding and Eating Disorders

Eating and feeding disorders have a lifetime prevalence of 5%, with the highest incidence occurring between 10 and 19 years of age and are associated with profound and long-term physical and psychosocial morbidity (Treasure et al., 2010). Whilst there are a variety of different diagnostic classifications (see Table 20.1), a common feature is the significant impairment to health and function as a result of feeding/eating behaviours (American Psychiatric Association, 2013).

Broadly, causal factors or contributors can include biological, cultural, social, environmental and interpersonal elements which can trigger the onset, with subsequent changes to brain structure and function contributing to the extended duration and recovery from illness (Treasure et al., 2010). The impact of nutritional deficits or starvation on the brain are noteworthy given that most eating disorders emerge during adolescence, a crucial and vulnerable period of brain reorganisation (Dishman et al., 2009). 'Comorbidity is the rule rather than the exception for patients with eating disorders', including anxiety disorders, neurodevelopmental disorders and SUDs, along with long-term medical complications such as growth disturbances, dental problems, osteoporosis and reproductive changes (Treasure et al., 2010; Bhadoria et al., 2010).

When working with feeding and eating disorders, there are a number of acute complications that signal the need for increased or urgent care. These outcomes should be monitored by a medical team based on recommended markers of nutritional and cardiovascular decompensation, including:

- Systolic blood pressure < 90 mmHg
- Diastolic blood pressure < 60 mmHg
- BMI < 15 kg/m^2
- Pulse rate < 50 bpm
- Oxygen saturation < 90%
- Core temperature < 35°C

See Treasure et al., 2010 and Bhadoria et al., 2010 for a comprehensive list of markers signalling the need for urgent care.

In many feeding and eating disorders (notably anorexia nervosa), compulsive exercise or exercise dependence may present as a prominent characteristic to control weight, is often associated with worse prognosis and greater chances of relapse and is often one of the last symptoms to subside (Meyer and Taranis, 2011).

> Compulsive exercise describes a condition characterised by an association with weight and shape concerns, and persistent continuation in order to: (a) mitigate the experience of extreme guilt and/or negative affect when unable to exercise; and (b) avoid the perceived negative consequences of stopping.
>
> *(Meyer et al., 2011)*

Compulsive exercise may be considered a primary behaviour of concern, where exercise itself is an addiction, or secondary to another mental health disorder or behaviour: for example, exercising as a strategy to manage weight in feeding and eating disorder (Muller et al., 2015). A key feature of compulsive exercise is individuals continuing to exercise despite exhaustion or serious physical impairment, and individuals with primary or secondary exercise dependence should be monitored closely for adverse responses when exercising.

In addition to the general benefits of exercise – specifically in those with eating and feeding disorders – research has demonstrated the safety and efficacy of supervised exercise with specific benefits including improvements in strength, cardiovascular fitness, and bone density (Stubbs and Rosenbaum, 2018; Chapter 9). However, a balance between physical activity (energy expenditure) and nutritional strategies (energy intake) to ensure weight restoration is essential, along with monitoring for signs of exercise compulsion (Danielsen et al., 2018).

Whilst defining what level of exercise is appropriate or detrimental for any given individual with feeding or eating disorders is challenging, individualised assessment, including activity levels, physical fitness and health risks, should be conducted in consultation with the medical team. In the event signs and symptoms of compulsive exercise become apparent, consultation with an expert in obsessive-compulsive disorders is required.

Substance-Related Disorders

Substance use disorders (SUD) are recognised as mental health disorders and occur when substance use becomes habitual, resulting in a cluster of cognitive, behavioural and physiological symptoms, with the diagnosis of SUD based on evidence of impaired control, social impairment, risky use and pharmacological criteria (American Psychiatric Association, 2013). Co-morbidity of SUD and other mental health disorders is common, with researchers reporting that 93% of youth with SUD experience co-occurring mental health disorders (Lichtenstein et al., 2010). All drugs that are taken in excess have commonality in the direct activation of the brain reward system, which is involved in the reinforcement of behaviours and the production of memories. They produce such an intense activation of the reward system that normal activities may be neglected, and they reinforce the drug-taking behaviour (Koob and Volkow, 2016).

In both adult and youth SUD populations, exercise interventions can provide effective, low-cost adjunct therapies with numerous secondary physical and mental health benefits during treatment (Abrantes et al., 2011; Giesen et al., 2015; More et al., 2018, 2017; Wang et al., 2014). Whilst the mechanisms behind these benefits are likely multi-faceted and require further investigation, some of the proposed pathways through which exercise-induced benefits may occur include:

- Behavioural factors (e.g. substituting exercise for unhealthy behaviours such as substance use) (Weinstock et al., 2017; Zubala et al., 2017; More et al., 2018)
- Psychological factors (e.g. improved well-being) (Penedo and Dahn, 2005)
- Neurobiological factors (e.g. activation of reward pathways in the brain) (Linke and Ussher, 2015)

When working with a SUD population, caution should be taken to ensure appropriate screening and management of any drug-induced (e.g. cardiac failure) or physical and mental co-morbidities, with medical clearance to participate in exercise likely required. Additionally, exercise should not be commenced or be ceased immediately if a participant is under the influence of any substance, and any detoxification should be medically managed and carefully monitored.

Post-Traumatic Stress Disorder (PTSD)

PTSD can develop following exposure to a potentially life-threatening or traumatic event and is highly prevalent among those exposed to occupational trauma, including emergency service workers (e.g. police, fire, ambulance) and veterans. PTSD is characterised by symptoms including hyperarousal, hypervigilance, avoidance and reexperiencing. People with PTSD are also at high risk of experiencing poor cardiometabolic health, including metabolic syndrome and cardiovascular disease (Vancampfort et al., 2015a; Wolf et al., 2016). Increases in PTSD severity are associated with greater reductions in physical activity (Winning et al., 2017), while physical activity and structured exercise have been shown to play a role in reducing symptoms and improving physical health outcomes (Rosenbaum et al., 2015). Comparable to the evidence and recommendations in other mental disorders, no optimal exercise prescription for PTSD exists. Both aerobic and resistance-based exercise appear to be effective, with emerging evidence demonstrating a positive impact of yoga and other mind-body types of physical activity (Cramer et al., 2018). Ensuring engagement and rapport and addressing motivational deficits common in people with PTSD are critical to maximising adherence to and engagement with exercise interventions in this population.

Psychosis

Psychosis refers to a distortion in the perception of reality and is a component of some severe forms of mental illness, including schizophrenia. Psychosis has a substantial impact on overall psychosocial functioning and can be a costly and debilitating condition. Available treatments, including anti-psychotic medication, while effective in treating symptoms, often have a devastating impact on cardiovascular health, including rapid and pronounced weight gain of up to seven to eight kilograms within 12 weeks (Álvarez-Jiménez et al., 2008). There is strong evidence that appropriately supervised exercise (Vancampfort et al., 2015b, 2015a), ideally conducted at a moderately vigorous intensity, can be effective in reducing both positive and negative symptoms of schizophrenia (Firth et al., 2015), improve cognition (Firth et al., 2017) and improve cardiorespiratory fitness (Vancampfort et al., 2015b, 2015a).

Summary/Key Points

There is an overwhelming body of evidence demonstrating the mental health benefits of exercise, not only in promoting positive mental well-being, but also in reducing the incidence and severity of mental disorders. Ensuring adequate referral pathways for people experiencing poor mental health, by which they can see exercise practitioners as part of routine mental healthcare, is clearly justified. For exercise practitioners, designing and delivering engaging, tailored and individualised exercise programs that incorporate evidence-based motivational strategies can reduce the burden of mental disorders and simultaneously improve both physical and mental health outcomes.

- Mental health and mental illness exist on separate continuums, whereby at any point in time, people experiencing poor mental health (e.g. feeling down) may not necessarily be experiencing a mental illness. Regardless of where along the two continuums someone is, exercise has an important role to play in improving mental health.
- Exercise is an evidence-based, fundamental component of treatment for a range of mental illnesses.
- It's not about what type of exercise is the best kind; it's about what works for the individual and that doing something is better than doing nothing at all.

- 'Exercise should be seen as a "tool in the tool belt" for people living with mental illness and as a strategy for helping to manage symptoms, improve physical health, improve sleep quality, and improve overall quality of life' (Exercise & Sport Science Australia, 2018).

Study Tasks

1. What are some of the broad mechanisms by which exercise promotes mental health?
2. Provide an example of a 'common mental illness' and its key features.
3. List and describe briefly or provide examples of common medical management strategies for mental disorders.
4. What are the purposes of a pre-exercise screening and assessments?
5. In addition to mental health outcomes, what key outcomes should be assessed and monitored to support positive cardiometabolic health in individuals taking psychotropic medication?
6. When delivering exercise to an individual with high risk of cardiovascular disease and/or evidence of metabolic disease due to psychotropic medication, what should you monitor pre-, during and/or post-exercise to ensure client safety?
7. When working in feeding and/or eating disorders, what are key signs of diminished health indicating need for immediate or emergency medical care?
8. What are the aims of structured exercise interventions within mental health services?
9. What are some of the proposed mechanisms (and examples) behind the benefits seen from exercise in SUDs?

   Consider whether you agree or disagree with the following statements and provide your justification or evidence for why.

10. Resistance training is contraindicated for people experiencing mental illness.
11. Exercise is beneficial for optimising mental health but is not effective for those with diagnosed mental disorders.

TABLE 20.4 At-a-Glance Summary Guide to Exercise Considerations for People with Major Depressive Disorder

Condition Name	*Major depressive disorder*
Symptomology	Presence of sad, empty or irritable mood, accompanied by somatic and cognitive changes that significantly affect the individual's capacity to function.
Aims of Exercise	To encourage the participant to reach the international physical activity guidelines of 150 minutes of moderately vigorous physical activity per week. This will assist in reducing mental health symptomology and improving overall physical health.
Exercise Considerations (Including Contraindications)	In accordance with best-practice guidelines for all exercise professionals, pre-exercise screening and assessment should take place for all participants prior to undertaking exercise. Exercise should not be commenced or be ceased immediately if any indication of physical or mental distress emerges or is exacerbated during exercise (e.g. cardiac distress, acute psychotic distress, mental health crisis).

Condition Name	*Major depressive disorder*
Frequency	Most days of the week, with resistance training on two. non-consecutive days each week.
Intensity	Low to moderate intensity or within the participant's current physical capacity.
Time	30 to 60 minutes per session. Starting with short sessions of 5 to 10 minutes may also be effective.
Type	Any exercise that the participant finds enjoyable: for example, aerobic activity (e.g. walking, cycling or swimming). Most resistance training (e.g. machines, free weights, body weight exercise).
Common Medications Associated	Antidepressants (SSRI, SNRI).
Key Safety Considerations	Consider impact of medication and any potential side effects on exercise prescription and delivery.
Effect of Exercise on Conditions	Improvement in depressive symptomology and overall physical health.

TABLE 20.5 At-a-Glance Summary Guide to Exercise Considerations for People with Schizophrenia

Condition Name	*Schizophrenia*
Symptomology	Defined by abnormalities in one or more of the following five domains: delusions, hallucinations, disorganised thinking, grossly disorganised or abnormal motor behaviour and negative symptoms (e.g. diminished emotional expression, decreased participation in work or social activities).
Aims of Exercise	To encourage the participant to reach the international physical activity guidelines of 150 minutes of moderately vigorous physical activity per week. This will assist in reducing mental health symptomology and improving overall physical health.
Exercise Considerations	In accordance with best-practice guidelines for all exercise professionals, pre-exercise screening and assessment should take place for all participants prior to undertaking exercise. Exercise should not be commenced or be ceased immediately if: • A participant is under the influence of any substances • A participant is not in compliance with prescribed medication • During self-imposed detoxification in the absence of medical management • A participant demonstrates signs of mania • Any physical or mental distress emerges or is exacerbated during exercise (e.g. cardiac distress, acute psychotic distress, mental health crisis)
Frequency	Most days of the week, with resistance training on two non-consecutive days each week.
Intensity	Low to moderate intensity or within the participant's current physical capacity.
Time	30 to 60 minutes per session. Starting with short sessions of 5 to 10 minutes may also be effective

(*Continued*)

TABLE 20.5 (Continued)

Condition Name	*Schizophrenia*
Type	Any exercise that the participant finds enjoyable: for example: aerobic activity (e.g. walking, cycling or swimming). Most resistance training (e.g. machines, free weights, body weight exercise)
Common Medications Associated	Antipsychotics (typical, atypical)
Key Safety Considerations	Consider impact of medication and any potential side effects on exercise prescription and delivery
Effect of Exercise on Conditions	Improvement in mental health symptomology and overall physical health. Management of secondary physical health co-morbidities.

TABLE 20.6 At-a-Glance Summary Guide to Exercise Considerations for People with Generalised Anxiety Disorder

Condition Name	*Generalised anxiety disorder*
Symptomology	Excessive fear (emotional response to real or perceived imminent threat) and anxiety (anticipation of future threat) and related behavioural disturbances.
Aims of Exercise	To encourage the participant to reach the international physical activity guidelines of 150 minutes of moderately vigorous physical activity per week. This will assist in reducing mental health symptomology and improving overall physical health.
Exercise Considerations (Include Contraindications)	In accordance with best-practice guidelines for all exercise professionals, pre-exercise screening and assessment should take place for all participants prior to undertaking exercise. Exercise should not be commenced or be ceased immediately if any indication of physical or mental distress emerges or is exacerbated during exercise (e.g. cardiac distress, acute psychotic distress, mental health crisis)
Frequency	Most days of the week with resistance training on two non-consecutive days each week.
Intensity	Moderate intensity or within the participant's current physical capacity.
Time	30 to 60 minutes per session. Starting with short sessions of 5 to 10 minutes may also be effective
Type	Any exercise that the participant finds enjoyable: for example, aerobic activity (e.g. walking, cycling or swimming). Most resistance training (e.g. machines, free weights, body weight exercise).
Common Medications associated	Antidepressants; benzodiazepines.
Key Safety Considerations	Consider impact of medication and any potential side effects on exercise prescription and delivery.
Effect of Exercise on Conditions	Improvement in mental health symptomology and overall physical health.

References

Abrantes, A. M., Battle, C. L., Strong, D. R., Ing, E., Dubreuil, M. E., Gordon, A. & Brown, R. A. 2011. Exercise preferences of patients in substance abuse treatment. *Mental Health and Physical Activity*, 4, 79–87.

Álvarez-Jiménez, M., González-Blanch, C., Crespo-Facorro, B., Hetrick, S., Rodriguez-Sánchez, J., Pérez-Iglesias, R. & Luis, J. 2008. Antipsychotic-induced weight gain in chronic and first-episode psychotic disorders. *CNS Drugs*, 22, 547–562.

American Psychiatric Association. 2013. *Diagnostic and statistical manual of mental disorders: DSM-5*, Arlington, VA, American Psychiatric Publishing.

Amerio, A., Stubbs, B., Odone, A., Tonna, M., Marchesi, C. & Ghaemi, S. N. 2015. The prevalence and predictors of comorbid bipolar disorder and obsessive – compulsive disorder: A systematic review and meta-analysis. *Journal of Affective Disorders*, 186, 99–109.

Ashdown-Franks, G., Stubbs, B., Koyanagi, A., Schuch, F., Firth, J., Veronese, N. & Vancampfort, D. 2019. Handgrip strength and depression among 34,129 adults aged 50 years and older in six low- and middle-income countries. *Journal of Affective Disorders*, 243, 448–454.

Aylett, E., Small, N. & Bower, P. 2018. Exercise in the treatment of clinical anxiety in general practice – a systematic review and meta-analysis. *BMC Health Services Research*, 18.

Bailey, A. P., Hetrick, S. E., Rosenbaum, S., Purcell, R. & Parker, A. G. 2018. Treating depression with physical activity in adolescents and young adults: A systematic review and meta-analysis of randomised controlled trials. *Psychological Medicine*, 48, 1068–1083.

Bartholomew, B. J., Morrison, T. D. & Ciccolo, T. J. 2005. Effects of acute exercise on mood and well-being in patients with major depressive disorder. *Medicine & Science in Sports & Exercise*, 37, 2032–2037.

Beeler, J. A., Faust, R. P., Turkson, S., Ye, H. & Zhuang, X. 2016. Low dopamine D2 receptor increases vulnerability to obesity via reduced physical activity, not increased appetitive motivation. *Biological Psychiatry*, 79, 887–897.

Bhadoria, R., Webb, K. & Morgan, J. F. 2010. Treating eating disorders: A review of the evidence. *Evidence Based Mental Health*, 13, 1.

Biddle, S. J. H. 2006. *Psychology of physical activity determinants, well-being and interventions*, London, Taylor and Francis.

Bischoff, S., Wieder, G., Einsle, F., Petzold, M. B., Jansse, C., Mumm, J. L. M., Wittchen, H.-U., Fydrich, T., Plag, J. & Ströhle, A. 2018. Running for extinction? Aerobic exercise as an augmentation of exposure therapy in panic disorder with agoraphobia. *Journal of Psychiatric Research*, 101, 34–41.

Boutcher, S. H., Mcauley, E. & Courneya, K. S. 1997. Positive and negative affective response of trained and untrained subjects during and after aerobic exercise. *Australian Journal of Psychology*, 28–32.

Butler, A. C., Chapman, J. E., Forman, E. M. & Beck, A. T. 2006. The empirical status of cognitive-behavioral therapy: A review of meta-analyses. *Clinical Psychology Review*, 26, 17–31.

Centre For Mental Health. 2010. *Economic and social costs of mental health problems in 2009/10*, London, Centre for Mental Health.

Chaouloff, F. 1997. Effects of acute physical exercise on central serotonergic systems. *Medicine & Science in Sports & Exercise*, 29, 58–62.

Cramer, H., Anheyer, D., Saha, F. J. & Dobos, G. 2018. Yoga for posttraumatic stress disorder – a systematic review and meta-analysis. *BMC Psychiatry*, 18.

Curtis, J., Newall, H. D. & Samaras, K. 2012. The heart of the matter: Cardiometabolic care in youth with psychosis. *Early Intervention in Psychiatry*, 6, 347–353.

Danielsen, M., Rø, Ø. & Bjørnelv, S. 2018. How to integrate physical activity and exercise approaches into inpatient treatment for eating disorders: fifteen years of clinical experience and research. *J Eat Disord*, 6, 34. https://doi.org/10.1186/s40337-018-0203-5

De Hert, M., Dekker, J. M., Wood, D., Kahl, K. G., Holt, R. I. G. & Möller, H. J. 2009. Cardiovascular disease and diabetes in people with severe mental illness position statement from the

European psychiatric association (EPA), supported by the European association for the study of diabetes (EASD) and the European society of cardiology (ESC). *European Psychiatry*, 24, 412–424.

Department of Health. 1999. *Saving lives: Our healthier nation*, London, Stationary Office.

Dishman, R. K., Amp, A. & Connor, P. J. 2009. Lessons in exercise neurobiology: The case of endorphins. *Mental Health and Physical Activity*, 2, 4–9.

Ekkekakis, P. 2003. Pleasure and displeasure from the body: Perspectives from exercise. *Cognition and Emotion*, 17, 213–239.

Exercise & Sport Science Australia. 2018. *Exercise & mental health*, Rosenbaum, S. & Hobson-Powell, A. (eds.), Queensland, Camilla Brightman.

Firth, J., Cotter, J., Elliott, R., French, P. & Yung, A. R. 2015. A systematic review and meta-analysis of exercise interventions in schizophrenia patients. *Psychological Medicine*. 45, 1343–1361.

Firth, J., Firth, J. A., Stubbs, B., Vancampfort, D., Schuch, F. B., Hallgren, M., Veronese, N., Yung, A. R. & Sarris, J. 2018a. Association between muscular strength and cognition in people with major depression or bipolar disorder and healthy controls. *JAMA Psychiatry*, 75, 740.

Firth, J., Stubbs, B., Rosenbaum, S., Vancampfort, D., Malchow, B., Schuch, F., Elliott, R., Nuechterlein, K. H. & Yung, A. R. 2017. Aerobic exercise improves cognitive functioning in people with schizophrenia: A systematic review and meta-analysis. *Schizophrenia Bulletin*, 43, 546–556.

Firth, J., Stubbs, B., Vancampfort, D., Firth, J. A., Large, M., Rosenbaum, S., Hallgren, M., Ward, P. B., Sarris, J. & Yung, A. R. 2018b. Grip strength is associated with cognitive performance in schizophrenia and the general population: A UK biobank study of 476559 participants. *Schizophrenia Bulletin*, 44, 728.

Firth, J., Stubbs, B., Vancampfort, D., Schuch, F., Lagopoulos, J., Rosenbaum, S. & Ward, P. B. 2018c. Effect of aerobic exercise on hippocampal volume in humans: A systematic review and meta-analysis. *NeuroImage*, 166, 230–238.

Fornaro, M., Orsolini, L., Marini, S., De Berardis, D., Perna, G., Valchera, A., Ganança, L., Solmi, M., Veronese, N. & Stubbs, B. 2016. The Prevalence and predictors of bipolar and borderline personality disorders comorbidity: Systematic review and meta-analysis. *Journal of Affective Disorders*, 195, 105–118.

Gbd Disease and Injury Incidence and Prevalence Collaborators. 2016. Global, regional, and national incidence, prevalence, and years lived with disability for 310 diseases and injuries, 1990–2015: A systematic analysis for the global burden of disease study 2015. *Lancet*, 388.

Giesen, E. S., Deimel, H. & Bloch, W. 2015. Clinical exercise interventions in alcohol use disorders: A systematic review. *Journal of Substance Abuse Treatment*, 52, 1–9.

Gordon, B., Mcdowell, C., Hallgren, M., Meyer, J., Lyons, M. & Herring, M. 2018. Association of efficacy of resistance exercise training with depressive symptoms meta-analysis and meta-regression analysis of randomized clinical trials. *JAMA Psychiatry*, 75, 566.

Gordon, B., Mcdowell, C., Lyons, M. & Herring, M. 2017. The effects of resistance exercise training on anxiety: A meta-analysis and meta-regression analysis of randomized controlled trials. *Sports Medicine*, 47, 2521–2532.

Greer, T. L., Furman, J. L. & Trivedi, M. H. 2017. Evaluation of the benefits of exercise on cognition in major depressive disorder. *General Hospital Psychiatry*, 49, 19–25.

Gunnell, K. E., Flament, M. F., Buchholz, A., Henderson, K. A., Obeid, N., Schubert, N. & Goldfield, G. S. 2016. Examining the bidirectional relationship between physical activity, screen time, and symptoms of anxiety and depression over time during adolescence. *Preventive Medicine*, 88, 147–152.

Hallgren, M., Kraepelien, M., Öjehagen, A., Lindefors, N., Zeebari, Z., Kaldo, V. & Forsell, Y. 2015. Physical exercise and internet-based cognitive-behavioural therapy in the treatment of depression: Randomised controlled trial. *British Journal of Psychiatry*, 207, 227.

Harvey, S. B., Øverland, S., Hatch, S. L., Wessely, S., Mykletun, A. & Hotopf, M. 2018. Exercise and the prevention of depression: Results of the HUNT cohort study. *American Journal of Psychiatry*, 175, 28–36.

Hays, A. E., Goss, F., Aaron, D., Abt, K., Friedman, E., Gallagher, M. & Nagle, E. 2008. Hormonal and perceptual changes in bipolar subjects after acute aerobic exercise: 584. *Medicine & Science in Sports & Exercise*, 40, S17.

Hillman, C. H., Erickson, K. I. & Kramer, A. F. 2008. Be smart, exercise your heart: Exercise effects on brain and cognition. *Nature Reviews Neuroscience*, 9, 58.

HM Government. 2011. *No health without mental health*, London, Department of Health.

Keating, L. E., Becker, S., Mccabe, K., Whattam, J., Garrick, L., Sassi, R. B., Frey, B. N. & Mckinnon, M. C. 2018. Effects of a 12-week running programme in youth and adults with complex mood disorders. *BMJ Open Sport & Exercise Medicine*, 4.

Kendall, T., Cape, J., Chan, M. & Taylor, C. 2011. Management of generalised anxiety disorder in adults: Summary of NICE guidance. *BMJ*, 342.

Keyes, C. L. M. 2002. The mental health continuum: From languishing to flourishing in life. *Journal of health and social behavior*, 43, 207.

Khatri, P., Blumenthal, J., Babyak, M. A., Craighead, W., Herman, S., Baldewicz, T., Madden, D., Doraiswamy, M., Waugh, R. & Krishnan, K. 2001. Effects of exercise training an cognitive functioning among depressed older men and women. *Journal of Aging and Physical Activity*, 9, 43–57.

Kim, Y. S., Park, Y. S., Allegrante, J. P., Marks, R., Ok, H., Ok Cho, K. & Garber, C. E. 2012. Relationship between physical activity and general mental health. *Preventive Medicine*, 55, 458–463.

Kitchener, B. A., Jorm, A. F., Kelly, C. & Australia, M. H. F. A. 2017. *Mental health first aid manual*, Parkville, VIC, Mental Health First Aid Australia.

Koob, G. F. & Volkow, N. D. 2016. Neurobiology of addiction: a neurocircuitry analysis. *The Lancet Psychiatry*, 3, 760–773.

Kwan, B. M., Bryan, A. D. & Sheeran, P. 2018. The dynamics of success and failure: How post-behaviour evaluations relate to subsequent exercise intentions and behaviour. *Psychology & Health*, 33, 1–18.

Lederman, O., Grainger, K., Stanton, R., Douglas, A., Gould, K., Perram, A., Baldeo, R., Fokas, T., Nauman, F., Semaan, A., Hewavasam, J., Pontin, L. & Rosenbaum, S. 2016. Consensus statement on the role of accredited exercise physiologists within the treatment of mental disorders: A guide for mental health professionals. *Australasian Psychiatry*, 24, 347–351.

Lederman, O., Suetani, S., Stanton, R., Chapman, J., Korman, N., Rosenbaum, S., Ward, P. B. & Siskind, D. 2017. Embedding exercise interventions as routine mental health care: Implementation strategies in residential, inpatient and community settings. *Australasian Psychiatry*, 25, 451–455.

Lichtenstein, D., Spirito, A. & Zimmermann, R. 2010. Assessing and treating co-occurring disorders in adolescents: Examining typical practice of community-based mental health and substance use treatment providers. *Community Mental Health Journal*, 46, 252–257.

Lindenberger, B. L., Plag, J., Schumacher, S., Gaudlitz, K., Bischoff, S., Bobbert, T., Dimeo, F., Petzold, M. B., Kirschbaum, C., Dudás, Z. & Ströhle, A. 2017. Clinical and neurobiological effects of aerobic exercise in dental phobia: A randomized controlled trial. *Depression and Anxiety*, 34, 1040–1048.

Linke, S. E. & Ussher, M. 2015. Exercise-based treatments for substance use disorders: evidence, theory, and practicality. *Am J Drug Alcohol Abuse*, 41(1), 7–15, January. doi:10.3109/00952990.2014.976708.

Lobelo, F., Stoutenberg, M. & Hutber, A. 2014. The exercise is medicine global health initiative: A 2014 update. *British Journal of Sports Medicine*, 48, 1627.

Luppino, F. S., De Wit, L. M., Bouvy, P. F., Stijen, T., Cuijpers, P., Penninx, B. W. J. H. & Zitman, F. G. 2010. Overweight, obesity, and depression: A systematic review and meta-analysis of longitudinal studies. *Arch Gen Psychiatry*, 67, 220–229.

Mandolesi, L., Polverino, A., Montuori, S., Foti, F., Ferraioli, G., Sorrentino, P. & Sorrentino, G. 2018. Effects of physical exercise on cognitive functioning and wellbeing: Biological and psychological benefits. *Frontiers in Psychology*, 9.

Martin, H., Beard, S., Clissold, N., Andraos, K. & Currey, L. 2017. Combined aerobic and resistance exercise interventions for individuals with schizophrenia: A systematic review. *Mental Health and Physical Activity*, 12, 147–155.

McAuley, E., Blissmer, B., Marquez, D. X., Jerome, G. J., Kramer, A. F. & Katula, J. 2000. Social relations, physical activity, and well-being in older adults. *Preventive Medicine*, 31, 608–617.

McCrone, P., Dhanasiri, S., Patel, A., Knapp, M. & Lawton-Smith, S. 2008. *Paying the price: The cost of mental health care in England to 2026*, London, The King's Fund.

McDowell, C. P., Dishman, R. K., Vancampfort, D., Hallgren, M., Stubbs, B., Macdonncha, C. & Herring, M. P. 2018. Physical activity and generalized anxiety disorder: Results from The Irish longitudinal study on ageing (TILDA). *International Journal of Epidemiology*, 47(5), 1443–1453. doi: 10.1093/ije/dyy141.

Melo, M. C. A., Daher, E. D. F., Albuquerque, S. G. C. & De Bruin, V. M. S. 2016. Exercise in bipolar patients: A systematic review. *Journal of Affective Disorders*, 198, 32–38.

Meyer, C. & Taranis, L. 2011. Exercise in the eating disorders: terms and definitions. *European Eating Disorders Review*, 19 (3), 169–73.

Meyer, C., Taranis, L., Goodwin, H. & Haycraft, E. 2011. Compulsive exercise and eating disorders. *European Eating Disorders Review*, 19(3), 174–189.

Moncrieff, J., Wessely, S. & Hardy, R. 2004. Active placebos versus antidepressants for depression. *The Cochrane Database of Systematic Reviews*, CD003012.

More, A., Jackson, B., Dimmock, J., Thornton, A. L., Colthart, A. & Furzer, B. 2017. Exercise in the treatment of youth substance use disorders: Review and recommendations. *Frontiers in Psychology*, 8.

More, A., Jackson, B., Dimmock, J. A., Thornton, A. L., Colthart, A. & Furzer, B. J. 2018. "It's like a counselling session . . . but you don't need to say anything": Exercise program outcomes for youth within a drug and alcohol treatment service. *Psychology of Sport and Exercise*, 39, 1–9.

Muller, A., Loeber, S., Sochtig, J., Te Wildt, B. & De Zwaan, M. 2015. Risk for exercise dependence, eating disorder pathology, alcohol use disorder and addictive behaviors among clients of fitness centers. *Journal of Behavioral Addictions*, 4, 273–280.

Nuechterlein, K. H., Ventura, J., Mcewen, S. C., Gretchen-Doorly, D., Vinogradov, S. & Subotnik, K. L. 2016. Enhancing cognitive training through aerobic exercise after a first schizophrenia episode: Theoretical conception and pilot study. *Schizophrenia Bulletin*, 42, S44–S52.

Olfson, M., Gerhard, T., Huang, C., Crystal, S. & Stroup, T. S. 2015. Premature mortality among adults with schizophrenia in the United States. *JAMA Psychiatry*, 72, 1172–1181.

Penedo, J. F. & Dahn, R. J. 2005. Exercise and well-being: A review of mental and physical health benefits associated with physical activity. *Current Opinion in Psychiatry*, 18, 189–193.

Powers, M. B., Medina, J. L., Burns, S., Kauffman, B. Y., Monfils, M., Asmundson, G. J. G., Diamond, A., Mcintyre, C. & Smits, J. A. J. 2015. Exercise augmentation of exposure therapy for PTSD: Rationale and pilot efficacy data. *Cognitive Behaviour Therapy*, 44, 1–14.

Raichlen, D. A., Foster, A. D., Gerdeman, G. L., Seillier, A. & Giuffrida, A. 2012. Wired to run: Exercise-induced endocannabinoid signaling in humans and cursorial mammals with implications for the 'runner's high'. *The Journal of Experimental Biology*, 215, 1331.

Rebar, A. L., Stanton, R., Geard, D., Short, C., Duncan, M. J. & Vandelanotte, C. 2015. A meta-meta-analysis of the effect of physical activity on depression and anxiety in non-clinical adult populations. *Health Psychology Review*, 9, 366–378.

Rosenbaum, S., Sherrington, C. & Tiedemann, A. 2015. Exercise augmentation compared with usual care for post-traumatic stress disorder: A randomized controlled trial. *Acta Psychiatrica Scandinavica*, 131, 350–359.

Rosenbaum, S., Tiedemann, A., Sherrington, C., Curtis, J. & Ward, P. 2014. Physical activity interventions for people with mental illness: A systematic review and meta-analysis. *Journal of Clinical Psychiatry*, 75, 964–U171.

Schuch, F., Vancampfort, D., Rosenbaum, S., Richards, J., Ward, P., Veronese, N., Solmi, M., Cadore, E. & Stubbs, B. 2016a. Exercise for depression in older adults: A meta-analysis of randomized controlled trials adjusting for publication bias. *Revista Brasileira De Psiquiatria*, 38, 247–254.

Schuch, F. B., Vancampfort, D., Firth, J., Rosenbaum, S., Ward, P. B., Silva, E. S., Hallgren, M., Ponce De Leon, A., Dunn, A. L., Deslandes, A. C., Fleck, M. P., Carvalho, A. F. & Stubbs, B. 2018. Physical activity and incident depression: A meta-analysis of prospective cohort studies. *American Journal of Psychiatry*, 175, 631–648.

Schuch, F. B., Vancampfort, D., Richards, J., Rosenbaum, S., Ward, P. B. & Stubbs, B. 2016b. Exercise as a treatment for depression: A meta-analysis adjusting for publication bias. *Journal of Psychiatric Research*, 77, 42–51.

Shiers, D., Rafi, I., Cooper, S. & Holt, R. I. G. 2014. *Positive cardiometabolic health resource: An intervention framework for patients with psychosis and schizophrenia*, London, Royal College of Psychiatrists.

Smith, P., Blumenthal, J., Hoffman, B. M., Cooper, H., Strauman, T. A., Welsh-Bohmer, K., Browndyke, J. & Sherwood, A. 2010. *Aerobic exercise and neurocognitive performance: A meta-analytic review of randomized controlled trials*, Psychosom, Lippincott Williams & Wilkins.

Stanton, R., Reaburn, P. & Happell, B. 2016. The effect of acute exercise on affect and arousal in inpatient mental health consumers. *The Journal of Nervous and Mental Disease*, 204, 658–664.

Stanton, R., Rosenbaum, S., Lederman, O. & Happell, B. 2018. Implementation in action: How Australian exercise physiologists approach exercise prescription for people with mental illness. *Journal of Mental Health*, 27, 150–156.

Stark, R., Schöny, W. & Kopp, M. 2012. Acute effects of a single bout of moderate exercise on psychological well-being in patients with affective disorder during hospital treatment. Neuropsychiatrie: Klinik, Diagnostik. *Therapie und Rehabilitation: Organ der Gesellschaft Osterreichischer Nervenarzte und Psychiater*, 26, 166.

Steel, Z., Marnane, C., Iranpour, C., Chey, T., Jackson, J. W., Patel, V. & Silove, D. 2014. The global prevalence of common mental disorders: A systematic review and meta-analysis 1980–2013. *International Journal of Epidemiology*, 43, 476–493.

Ströhle, A., Graetz, B., Scheel, M., Wittmann, A., Feller, C., Heinz, A. & Dimeo, F. 2009. The acute antipanic and anxiolytic activity of aerobic exercise in patients with panic disorder and healthy control subjects. *Journal of Psychiatric Research*, 43, 1013–1017.

Stubbs, B., Koyanagi, A., Hallgren, M., Firth, J., Richards, J., Schuch, F., Rosenbaum, S., Mugisha, J., Veronese, N., Lahti, J. & Vancampfort, D. 2017a. Physical activity and anxiety: A perspective from the world health survey. *Journal of Affective Disorders*, 208, 545–552.

Stubbs, B., Koyanagi, A., Schuch, F. B., Firth, J., Rosenbaum, S., Veronese, N., Solmi, M., Mugisha, J. & Vancampfort, D. 2016a. Physical activity and depression: a large cross-sectional, population-based study across 36 low- and middle-income countries. *Acta Psychiatrica Scandinavica*, 134, 546–556.

Stubbs, B., Koyanagi, A., Thompson, T., Veronese, N., Carvalho, A. F., Solomi, M., Mugisha, J., Schofield, P., Cosco, T., Wilson, N. & Vancampfort, D. 2016b. The epidemiology of back pain and its relationship with depression, psychosis, anxiety, sleep disturbances, and stress sensitivity: Data from 43 low- and middle-income countries. *General Hospital Psychiatry*, 43, 63–70.

Stubbs, B. & Rosenbaum, S. 2018. *Exercise-based interventions for mental illness: physical activity as part of clinical treatment*, London, Academic Press, an imprint of Elsevier.

Stubbs, B., Vancampfort, D., Hallgren, M., Firth, J., Veronese, N., Solmi, M., Brand, S., Cordes, J., Malchow, B., Gerber, M., Schmitt, A., Correll, C. U., De Hert, M., Gaughran, F., Schneider, F., Kinnafick, F., Falkai, P., Möller, H.-J. & Kahl, K. G. 2018. EPA guidance on physical activity as a treatment for severe mental illness: a meta-review of the evidence and Position Statement from the European Psychiatric Association (EPA), supported by the International Organization of Physical Therapists in Mental Health (IOPTMH). *European Psychiatry*, 54, 124–144.

Stubbs, B., Vancampfort, D., Rosenbaum, S., Firth, J., Cosco, T., Veronese, N., Salum, G. A. & Schuch, F. B. 2017b. An examination of the anxiolytic effects of exercise for people with anxiety and stress-related disorders: A meta-analysis. *Psychiatry Research*, 249, 102–108.

Stubbs, B., Vancampfort, D., Rosenbaum, S., Ward, P. B., Richards, J., Soundy, A., Veronese, N., Solmi, M. & Schuch, F. B. 2016c. Dropout from exercise randomized controlled trials among people with depression: A meta-analysis and meta regression. *Journal of Affective Disorders*, 190, 457–466.

Su, C.-Y., Wang, P.-W., Lin, Y.-J., Tang, T.-C., Liu, M.-F. & Chen, M.-D. 2016. The effects of aerobic exercise on cognition in schizophrenia: A 3-month follow-up study. *Psychiatry Research*, 244, 394–402.

Suetani, S., Mamun, A., Williams, G. M., Najman, J. M., Mcgrath, J. J. & Scott, J. G. 2017. Longitudinal association between physical activity engagement during adolescence and mental health outcomes in young adults: A 21-year birth cohort study. *Journal of Psychiatric Research*, 94, 116–123.

Suetani, S., Mamun, A., Williams, G. M., Najman, J. M., Mcgrath, J. J. & Scott, J. G. 2018. The association between adolescent psychopathology and subsequent physical activity in young adulthood: a 21-year birth cohort study. *Psychol Med*, 48, 269–278.

Swardfager, W., Yang, P., Herrmann, N., Lanctôt, K. L., Shah, B. R., Kiss, A. & Oh, P. I. 2016. Depressive symptoms predict non-completion of a structured exercise intervention for people with Type 2 diabetes. *Diabetic Medicine*, 33, 529–536.

Szuhany, K. L., Bugatti, M. & Otto, M. W. 2015. A meta-analytic review of the effects of exercise on brain-derived neurotrophic factor. *Journal of Psychiatric Research*, 60, 56–64.

The U. K. ECT Review Group 2003. Efficacy and safety of electroconvulsive therapy in depressive disorders: a systematic review and meta-analysis. *The Lancet*, 361, 799–808.

Thornicroft, G., Chatterji, S., Evans-Lacko, S., Gruber, M., Sampson, N., Aguilar-Gaxiola, S., Al-Hamzawi, A., Alonso, J., Andrade, L., Borges, G., Bruffaerts, R., Bunting, B., De Almeida, J. M. C., Florescu, S., De Girolamo, G., Gureje, O., Haro, J. M., He, Y., Hinkov, H., Karam, E., Kawakami, N., Lee, S., Navarro-Mateu, F., Piazza, M., Posada-Villa, J., De Galvis, Y. T. & Kessler, R. C. 2017. Undertreatment of people with major depressive disorder in 21 countries. *The British journal of psychiatry*, 210, 119.

Treasure, J., Claudino, A. M. & Zucker, N. 2010. Eating disorders. *The Lancet*, 375, 583–593.

Vancampfort, D., Correll, C. U., Galling, B., Probst, M., De Hert, M., Ward, P. B., Rosenbaum, S., Gaughran, F., Lally, J. & Stubbs, B. 2016a. Diabetes mellitus in people with schizophrenia, bipolar disorder and major depressive disorder: a systematic review and large scale meta-analysis. *World Psychiatry*, 15, 166–174.

Vancampfort, D., Firth, J., Schuch, F. B., Rosenbaum, S., Mugisha, J., Hallgren, M., Probst, M., Ward, P. B., Gaughran, F., De Hert, M., Carvalho, A. F. & Stubbs, B. 2017. Sedentary behavior and physical activity levels in people with schizophrenia, bipolar disorder and major depressive disorder: a global systematic review and meta-analysis. *World Psychiatry*, 16, 308–315.

Vancampfort, D., Rosenbaum, S., Probst, M., Soundy, A., Mitchell, A. J., De Hert, M. & Stubbs, B. 2015a. Promotion of cardiorespiratory fitness in schizophrenia: a clinical overview and meta-analysis. *Acta Psychiatrica Scandinavica*, 132, 131–143.

Vancampfort, D., Rosenbaum, S., Schuch, F. B., Ward, P. B., Probst, M. & Stubbs, B. 2016b. Prevalence and predictors of treatment dropout from physical activity interventions in schizophrenia: a meta-analysis. *General Hospital Psychiatry*, 39, 15–23.

Vancampfort, D., Rosenbaum, S., Ward, P. B. & Stubbs, B. 2015b. Exercise improves cardiorespiratory fitness in people with schizophrenia: A systematic review and meta-analysis. *Schizophrenia Research*, 169, 453–457.

Walker, E. R., Mcgee, R. E. & Druss, B. G. 2015. Mortality in mental disorders and global disease burden implications: A systematic review and meta-analysis. *JAMA Psychiatry*, 72, 334–341.

Wang, D., Wang, Y., Wang, Y., Li, R. & Zhou, C. 2014. Impact of physical exercise on substance use disorders: A meta-analysis. *PLoS One*, 9(10):e110728. doi:10.1371/journal.pone.0110728.

Weinstock, J., Farney, M. R., Elrod, N. M., Henderson, C. E. & Weiss, E. P. 2017. Exercise as an adjunctive treatment for substance use disorders: Rationale and intervention description. *Journal of Substance Abuse Treatment*, 72, 40–47.

Westerhof, G. J. & Keyes, C. L. M. 2010. Mental illness and mental health: The two continua model across the lifespan. *Journal of Adult Development*, 17, 110.

Whiteford, H. A., Degenhardt, L., Rehm, J., Baxter, A. J., Ferrari, A. J., Erskine, H. E., Charlson, F. J., Norman, R. E., Flaxman, A. D., Johns, N., Burstein, R., Murray, C. J. & Vos, T. 2013. Global burden of disease attributable to mental and substance use disorders: Findings from the global burden of disease study 2010. *The Lancet*, 382, 1575–1586.

WHO. 1992. *The ICD-10 classification of mental and behavioural disorders clinical descriptions and diagnostic guidelines*, Geneva, World Health Organization.

WHO. 2011. *Recommended levels of physical activity for adults aged 18–64 years* [Online]. World Health Organization. Available: www.who.int/dietphysicalactivity/factsheet_adults/en/.

WHO. 2017. *Depression and Other Common Mental Disorders: Global Health Estimates*, Geneva, World Health Organisation.

WHO. 2018. *Mental health: Strengthening our response*. Geneva, World Health Organization.

Winning, A., Gilsanz, P., Koenen, K. C., Roberts, A. L., Chen, Q., Sumner, J. A., Rimm, E. B., Maria Glymour, M. & Kubzansky, L. D. 2017. Post-traumatic stress disorder and 20-year physical activity trends among women. *American Journal of Preventive Medicine*, 52, 753–760.

Wolf, E. J., Bovin, M. J., Green, J. D., Mitchell, K. S., Stoop, T. B., Barretto, K. M., Jackson, C. E., Lee, L. O., Fang, S. C., Trachtenberg, F., Rosen, R. C., Keane, T. M. & Marx, B. P. 2016. Longitudinal associations between post-traumatic stress disorder and metabolic syndrome severity. *Psychol Med*, 46, 2215–2226.

Zubala, A., Macgillivray, S., Frost, H., Kroll, T., Skelton, D., Gavine, A., Gray, N., Toma, M. & Morris, J. 2017. Promotion of physical activity interventions for community dwelling older adults: A systematic review of reviews. *PLoS One*, 12, e0180902.

INDEX

Taylor & Francis Group
an informa business

Taylor & Francis eBooks

www.taylorfrancis.com

A single destination for eBooks from Taylor & Francis with increased functionality and an improved user experience to meet the needs of our customers.

90,000+ eBooks of award-winning academic content in Humanities, Social Science, Science, Technology, Engineering, and Medical written by a global network of editors and authors.

TAYLOR & FRANCIS EBOOKS OFFERS:

A streamlined experience for our library customers

A single point of discovery for all of our eBook content

Improved search and discovery of content at both book and chapter level

REQUEST A FREE TRIAL

support@taylorfrancis.com

Routledge Taylor & Francis Group

CRC Press Taylor & Francis Group